DEDICATION

To the contributors to this and future editions, who took time to share their knowledge, insight, and humor for the benefit of residents and clinicians.

and

To our families, friends, and loved ones, who supported us in the task of assembling this guide.

CONTENTS

NICHOLAS DANIEL ANDERSEN

Harvard Medical School
Class of 2008

ALEXANDER ARRIAGA

Weill Medical College of Cornell University
Class of 2007

ANNA AWDANKIEWICZ, MD

Resident
Department of Internal Medicine
Vanderbilt Medical Center

ALI BEHBAHANI, BSE

University of Pennsylvania School of Medicine

DAVID T. BRAUN, MBA

Temple University School of Medicine
Class of 2007

DAVID M. BROWN, MD

Resident
Department of Otolaryngology
University of Chicago

WHITNEY K. BRYANT

Columbia University College of Physicians and Surgeons
Class of 2007

DANIEL BURDICK

Johns Hopkins School of Medicine

VICKI KAI CHAN, MD

Resident
UCLA Jules Stein Eye Institute

POOJA P. CHANDRA

Weil Medical College of Cornell University
Class of 2007

STEPHEN CHANG, MD

Transitional Year Intern
York Hospital

KEVIN CHEUNG, MD

Intern
Department of Internal Medicine
Brigham and Women's Hospital

FELICIA CHE-SHUEN CHOW

Johns Hopkins School of Medicine
Class of 2007

JULIA TING CHU

Harvard Medical School
Class of 2007

CHRISTINA E. CLARK

Drexel University College of Medicine
Class of 2007

SARAH K. COLLINS

Weill Medical College of Cornell University
Class of 2007

LARA DEVGAN, MD

Johns Hopkins University School of Medicine

PRABHJOT SINGH DHADIALLA

Tri-Institutional MD/PhD Program of Weill Medical College of Cornell University, Rockefeller University, and Memorial Sloan-Kettering Cancer Center
Class of 2010

DEREK J. DONEGAN, MD

Resident
Department of Orthopedic Surgery
University of Pennsylvania

JOHN EIFLER

Weill Medical College of Cornell University
Class of 2007

DAWN M. EMICK, MD

Resident
Department of Surgery
Duke University Medical Center

VICTOR ESENWA, MD

Transitional Year Intern
New York Hospital Queens

ROBERT FLAVELL

Tri-Institutional MD/PhD Program of Weill Medical College of Cornell University, Rockefeller University, and Memorial Sloan-Kettering Cancer Center
Class of 2010

AARON M. FLETCHER, MD

Surgical Intern
University of Iowa Hospitals and Clinics

KATHLEEN FORCIER

Weill Medical College of Cornell University
Class of 2007

JORGE GALVEZ

Resident
Department of Anesthesiology
Yale Primary Care Program
Yale University School of Medicine

GEOFFREY GEIGER

University of Pennsylvania School of Medicine

POURYA M. GHAZI, MD

Senior Fellow
Department of Laboratory Medicine
University of Washington, Seattle

RANI K. HASAN, MD

Intern
Department of Medicine
Hospital of the University of Pennsylvania

EMILY PARKER HYLE, MD

Resident
Department of Internal Medicine
Massachusetts General Hospital

DANIEL JAMIESON, MD

Resident
Department of Internal Medicine
University of Colorado

BLUMA LESCH

Tri-Institutional MD/PhD Program of Weill Medical College of Cornell
   University, Rockefeller University, and Memorial Sloan-Kettering
   Cancer Center

ILYA LEYNGOLD, MD

Resident
Wilmer Ophthalmological Institute
Johns Hopkins University School of Medicine

MARK LEYNGOLD, MD

Resident
Integrated Program in Plastic and Reconstructive Surgery
University of Nevada

DAVID M. LIEBERMAN, MD

Resident
Department of Otolaryngology
Stanford University

NICHOLAS MAHONEY, MD

Resident
Scheie Eye Institute

MATTHEW McCARTHY

Harvard Medical School
Class of 2008

MARCUS A. McFERREN, PhD, MD

Resident
Department of Dermatology
Yale School of Medicine

ANUJ BHARAT MEHTA

Weill Medical College of Cornell University
Class of 2007

AMANDA MULLINS

Drexel University College of Medicine
Class of 2007

ANOMA NELLORE, MD

Resident
Department of Internal Medicine
University of Pennsylvania

FRANK OCASIO, MD

Weill Medical College of Cornell University

ANTON ORLIN

University of Pennsylvania School of Medicine
Class of 2007

BEN EUGENE PAXTON

Johns Hopkins University School of Medicine
Class of 2007

TONGUC PINAR

Harvard Medical School
Class of 2008

JASON E. PORTNOF, DMD, MD

Resident
Department of Oral and Maxillofacial Surgery
New York Presbyterian Hospital

ARIKE PRICE, MD

Resident
Department of Neurology
Albert Einstein College of Medicine

PABLO RECINOS, MD

Resident
Department of Neurosurgery
Johns Hopkins University School of Medicine

GABRIELLE RIZZUTO

Tri-Institutional MD/PhD Program of Weill Medical College of Cornell
   University, Rockefeller University, and Memorial Sloan-Kettering
   Cancer Center

JAMES S. ROSOFF, MD

Resident
Department of Urology
Weill Medical College of Cornell University

CORY JOSHUA RUBIN, MD

Resident
Department of Otolaryngology-Head and Neck Surgery
Case Western Reserve University

JONATHAN SCHOENFELD

Harvard Medical School
Class of 2008

PRITHA SEN

Harvard Medical School
Class of 2008

MOHUMMAD MINHAJ SIDDIQUI, MD

Resident
Department of Urology
Harvard Medical School

AMANDEEP SINGH

Tri-Institutional MD/PhD Program of Weill Medical College of Cornell
    University, Rockefeller University, and Memorial Sloan-Kettering
    Cancer Center
Class of 2007

JOANNA LOUISE SPENCER

Tri-Institutional MD/PhD Program of Weill Medical College of Cornell
    University, Rockefeller University, and Memorial Sloan-Kettering
    Cancer Center

TESSA A. SUNDARAM

University of Pennsylvania School of Medicine
Class of 2007

VENEE N. TUBMAN, MD

Boston Combined Residency in Pediatrics
Children's Hospital Boston
Boston Medical Center

APRIL TROY

Johns Hopkins School of Medicine
Class of 2007

JENICA UPSHAW

Weill Medical College of Cornell University
Class of 2008

KONSTANTINA M. VANEVSKI, MD

F. Edward Hébert School of Medicine
PhD Neuroscience Graduate Program
Uniformed Services University of the Health Sciences
Adjunct Scientist
NIH/National Institute of Child Health and Human Development

MARISSA A. WAGNER

Harvard Medical School
Class of 2010

ADAM M. WEITZMAN

Weill Medical College of Cornell University
Class of 2007

ELIZABETH WINTER, MD

Intern
Department of Medicine
Mount Sinai Hospital

FACULTY REVIEWERS

KHALED I. ATTIA, MD, MPH

Clincal Research Fellow
TIMI Study Group, Department of Cardiology
Brigham & Women's Hospital
Harvard Medical School

BRAD P. BARNETT

Johns Hopkins University School of Medicine

CAROL L. BECK, PharmD, PhD

Assistant Professor
Department of Pharmacology and Experimental Therapeutics
Jefferson Medical College
Thomas Jefferson University

JONATHAN W. BRESS, MD

Nephrology Fellow
Hospital of the University of Pennsylvania

JIM W. CHEUNG, MD

Attending Cardiac Electrophysiologist
Long Island Jewish Medical Center

BARBARA J. CRAIN, MD

Associate Professor
Department of Pathology
Johns Hopkins University School of Medicine

MONICA E. DE BACA, MD

Physicians Laboratory
Sioux Falls, SD

ABDEL BASSET EL ESSAWY, MD, PhD

Division of Medicine/Immunology
The Transplant Center
Beth Israel Deaconess Medical Center
Harvard Medical School

TAMIA ALISHA HARRIS

MD/PhD candidate
Johns Hopkins University School of Medicine

AMY S. KELLEY, MD

Fellow
Division of Geriatrics
New York Presbyterian Hospital

DIANA MOLAVI, MD, PhD

Department of Pathology
Johns Hopkins School of Medicine

SUHAIL K. MITHANI, MD

Resident
Division of Plastic Surgery
Johns Hopkins Hospital

DARA L. NEUMAN

Johns Hopkins University School of Medicine

AFSHAN A. NANJI

Medical Student
Johns Hopkins University School of Medicine

MICHAEL S. RAFII, MD, PhD

Chief Resident
Department of Neurology
Johns Hopkins Hospital

VÉRONIQUE TACHÉ, MD

Department of Obstetrics and Gynecology
University of California, Davis

MEREDITH L. TURETZ, MD

Clinical Fellow Pulmonary and Critical Care Medicine
New York Presbyterian Hospital

GIL WEITZMAN

Attending Physician, Division of Gastroenterology
Department of Medicine
New York Presbyterian Hospital

APRIL ZHU, MD

Payne Whitney Manhattan
New York Presbyterian Hospital

With *First Aid Q&A for the USMLE Step 1*, we continue our commitment to providing students with the most useful and up-to-date preparation guides for the USMLE Step 1. This new addition to the *First Aid* series represents an outstanding effort by a talented group of authors and includes the following:

- 1000 high-yield USMLE-style questions based on the top-rated *USMLERx Qmax Step 1 Test Bank* (www.usmlerx.com).
- Concise yet complete explanations to correct and incorrect questions
- Questions organized by general principles and organ systems
- Seven full-length test blocks simulate the actual exam experience
- High-yield images, diagrams, and tables complement the questions and answers
- Organized as a perfect complement to *First Aid for the USMLE Step 1*

We invite you to share your thoughts and ideas to help us improve *First Aid Q&A for the USMLE Step 1*. See How to Contribute, p. xv.

Louisville	Tao Le
Boston	Joshua Klein
Boston	Anil Shivaram

ACKNOWLEDGMENTS

This has been a collaborative project from the start. We gratefully acknowledge the thoughtful comments and advice of the medical students, international medical graduates, and faculty who have supported the authors in the development of *First Aid Q&A for the USMLE Step 1*.

We want to especially thank Dr. Pourya Ghazi, who spent many hours selecting and organizing quality questions from the top-rated *USMLERx Qmax Step 1 Test Bank* for this publication.

Additional thanks to the following for reviewing manuscript: Lawrence Siegel, MD; Scott Weisenberg, MD; Brian Bosworth, MD; Michael Brucculeri, MD; Elizabeth Dzeng; Ashwin K. Mani, MD; Allyson Mirabella, MD; Majd Mouded, MD; Gal Omry, MD; Assil Shaker Saleh, MPH; and Eunice Wang, MD.

For support and encouragement throughout the process, we are grateful to Thao Pham, Selina Franklin, Louise Petersen, Jonathan Kirsch, and Vikas Bhushan. Thanks to our publisher, McGraw-Hill, for the valuable assistance of their staff. For enthusiasm, support, and commitment to this challenging project, thanks to our editor, Catherine Johnson. For outstanding editorial work, we thank Emma D. Underdown. A special thanks to Rainbow Graphics for remarkable production work.

Louisville	Tao Le
Boston	Joshua Klein
Boston	Anil Shivaram

HOW TO CONTRIBUTE

To continue to produce a high-yield review source for the USMLE Step 1 exam, you are invited to submit any suggestions or corrections. We also offer paid internships in medical education and publishing ranging from three months to one year (see next page for details). Please send us your suggestions for

- Corrections or enhancements to existing questions and explanations
- New high-yield questions
- Low-yield questions to remove

For each entry incorporated into the next edition, you will receive a $10 gift certificate, as well as personal acknowledgment in the next edition. Diagrams, tables, partial entries, updates, corrections, and study hints are also appreciated, and significant contributions will be compensated at the discretion of the authors.

The preferred way to submit entries, suggestions, or corrections is via electronic mail. Please include name, address, institutional affiliation, phone number, and e-mail address (if different from the address of origin). If there are multiple entries, please consolidate into a single e-mail or file attachment. Please send submissions to:

firstaidteam@yahoo.com

Otherwise, please send entries, neatly written or typed or on disk (Microsoft Word), to:

First Aid Q&A for the USMLE Step 1
914 North Dixie Avenue, Suite 100
Elizabethtown, KY 42701
Attention: Contributions

All entries become property of the authors and are subject to editing and reviewing. Please verify all data and spellings carefully. In the event that similar or duplicate entries are received, only the first entry received will be used. Include a reference to a standard textbook to facilitate verification of the fact. Please follow the style, punctuation, and format of this edition if possible.

The First Aid Team is pleased to offer part-time and full-time paid internships in medical education and publishing to motivated medical students and physicians. Internships may range from three months (e.g., a summer) up to a full year. Participants will have an opportunity to author, edit, and earn academic credit on a wide variety of projects, including the popular *First Aid* and *USMLERx* series. Writing/editing experience, familiarity with Microsoft Word, and Internet access are desired. For more information, e-mail a résumé or a short description of your experience along with a cover letter to **firstaidteam@yahoo.com**.

General Principles

- Behavioral Science
- Biochemistry
- Embryology
- Microbiology and Immunology
- Pharmacology

CHAPTER 1

Behavioral Science

1. A group of researchers conducted a large double-blind, randomized trial comparing the efficacy of a new antibiotic with penicillin in treating streptococcal pneumonia. The results showed that 95% of the patients taking the new antibiotic cleared their pneumonia, while 90% of those taking penicillin cleared their pneumonia. A large sample size was chosen in order to generate a statistical power of 80% with a p-value of 0.21. Which of the following represents the probability that there is a difference between the two treatment groups despite the study's failure to show this difference (p-value < 0.05)?

   (A) 0.05
   (B) 0.20
   (C) 0.21
   (D) 0.80
   (E) 0.90
   (F) 0.95

2. A 70-year-old man comes into his doctor's office for a routine checkup. His past medical history is significant for a heart attack, for which he takes a daily baby aspirin and a β-blocker. He practices safe habits and always wears his seat belt while driving. His health has been "great" for the past few years, although he is concerned about his wife because she recently suffered a mild stroke. He denies any visual loss or motor or sensory weakness. The patient's physical examination is unremarkable. Which of the following is the leading cause of death among people age 65 years or older?

   (A) Congenital anomalies
   (B) Heart disease
   (C) Motor vehicle crashes
   (D) Stroke
   (E) Suicide

3. A 16-year-old boy is brought to the pediatrician by his mother, who states that the patient has been sleeping at random times during the day and that he sometimes has difficulty moving immediately after waking up. The patient also reports feeling "generally weak" when he laughs out loud. Which of the following medications can be used to treat this patient?

   (A) Chloral hydrate
   (B) Hydroxyzine
   (C) Methylphenidate
   (D) Prochlorperazine maleate
   (E) Zolpidem

4. A 52-year-old woman is being treated by a male psychiatrist for depression stemming from her recent divorce. Recently, the patient has been coming to her appointments dressed up and wearing expensive perfumes. She has also started to flirt with the doctor. The patient's demeanor and appearance had initially reminded the psychiatrist of his aunt. He is uncomfortable with the patient's new behavior patterns and tells her so. She becomes very angry and storms out of the office, canceling all remaining appointments on her way out. Which of the following behaviors is an example of negative transference?

   (A) The doctor seeing the patient as his aunt
   (B) The doctor telling the patient he is uncomfortable
   (C) The patient being angry with the doctor
   (D) The patient dressing up for appointments
   (E) The patient flirting with the doctor

5. A 24-year-old woman presents to her primary care physician because of depression and insomnia for the past 6 months. The patient states that she feels bad about herself almost all of the time. A review of the patient's history shows that she has had frequent physician visits with complaints of stomachaches, headaches, and fatigue for the past 2 years. Which of the following characteristics would differentiate between a diagnosis of dysthymic disorder and a diagnosis of major depressive disorder in this patient?

(A) Changes in appetite
(B) Changes in sleep patterns
(C) Depressed mood
(D) Fatigue/lack of energy
(E) Persistence of symptoms

6. An 8-month-old infant presents to the pediatrician for a routine checkup. His mother reports that he plays peek-a-boo at home, waves bye-bye, and will say "dada." He cannot yet drink from a cup. He seemed somewhat apprehensive when the physician entered the room. He can lift his head when lying on his stomach but cannot sit unassisted. He has a positive Babinski's reflex. Which of the following developmental milestone is lagging behind the others in this patient?

(A) Cognitive
(B) Motor
(C) Reflexes
(D) Social
(E) Verbal

7. A 20-year-old man is brought to the emergency department by friends after he became very agitated at a fraternity party. The patient is belligerent and uncooperative. Physical examination shows that he has a fever, tachycardia, horizontal nystagmus, and hyperacusis. Which of the following substances may cause the behavioral changes and physical findings exhibited by this patient?

(A) Alcohol
(B) Amphetamines
(C) Cocaine
(D) Lysergic acid diethylamide
(E) Nicotine
(F) Phencyclidine

8. The figure below is a common representation used in studying the characteristics of a test's results. Using the letters in the figure, which of the following accurately describes the prevalence of the disease?

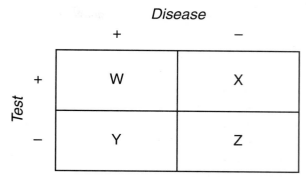

Reproduced, with permission, from USMLERx.com.

(A) W / (W+X+Y+Z)
(B) (W+X) / (W+X+Y+Z)
(C) W / (X+Y+Z)
(D) W / (X+Z)
(E) (W+Y) / (W+X+Y+Z)

9. A third-year medical resident is driving home after being on call and witnesses a car accident. He sees one person leave the car and collapse at the side of the road. He pulls over to help. The person appears to be a female in her 30s with a large laceration across her forehead. She is barely conscious. Which of the following is required and/or implied under the Good Samaritan Law?

(A) Compensation for actions
(B) Continued care until emergency service is activated
(C) Freedom from legal action
(D) Implied consent of patient
(E) Use of standard procedure

10. A battery of tests is used to evaluate a 13-year-old child's readiness to skip from seventh to ninth grade. As part of the battery, she is given an IQ test. Which of the following is an appropriate IQ test to use?

(A) Iowa Test of Educational Development
(B) Vineland Social Maturity Scale
(C) Wechsler Adult Intelligence Scale–Revised
(D) Wechsler Intelligence Scale for Children–Revised
(E) Wide-Range Achievement Test

11. A 43-year-old woman comes to her physician's office extremely nervous because she just tested positive for HIV according to a newly designed serum test. Of the 1000 patients tested, 200 patients had HIV; the test came back positive for 180 of them, while the remaining 20 tested negative. Eight hundred of the patients did not have HIV; however, the test was positive for 40 of them. The remaining 760 patients tested negative for HIV. Given this patient's positive test, which of the following is the probability that she does have HIV?

(A) 0.20
(B) 0.24
(C) 0.82
(D) 0.90
(E) 0.97

12. A 56-year-old man presents to his family doctor for a regular checkup. His past medical history is significant for long-standing hypertension and coronary artery disease. He had a myocardial infarction and percutaneous angioplasty 1 year ago. The patient initially reports no complaints, but as his physician is heading toward the door, the patient states with some embarrassment that he has had problems achieving erections since he was released from the hospital last year. He says that he has morning erections. His current medications include simvastatin and lisinopril. Which of the following is a likely cause for this man's acquired erectile dysfunction?

(A) Decreased interest in sexual activity
(B) Fear of another heart attack
(C) Increasing age of the patient
(D) Medication side effects
(E) Physical inability after the heart attack

13. A 17-year-old girl presents to her primary care physician with a complaint of missed menses. She is well known to the staff, having survived a tumultuous family life with her irresponsible parents. Tests reveal she is pregnant. She returns to the office 2 weeks later asking for recommendations on obtaining an abortion. She explains that although she has finished high school, she works full-time to support herself and her husband and is not ready for a child.

She decides that she does not want to notify anyone, and says she has chosen not to talk with her parents for many months. Her doctor understands that he must abide by her wishes because she is emancipated. Which of the following makes this patient emancipated?

(A) Age 17 years is considered an adult
(B) Full-time work
(C) High school diploma
(D) Living separately from her parents
(E) Marriage

14. A group of oncologists is interested in determining whether a relationship exists between alcohol use and pancreatic cancer. The researchers enroll 1000 patients, and subjects are placed into different groups depending on their level of alcohol consumption. The subjects are followed for 10 years; the data show no statistical difference in the number of pancreatic cancers among the groups. The above research is an example of which of the following kinds of study?

(A) Case-control study
(B) Clinical treatment trial
(C) Cohort study
(D) Cross-sectional study
(E) Historical cohort study

15. An 11-year-old girl is brought to the pediatrician because she has been complaining of back pain. On physical examination, a right thoracic scoliotic curve is seen. An x-ray film indicates that the curve is 25°. Girls with scoliosis need to be especially carefully watched during peak height velocity, during which the curvature can dramatically worsen. Given that peak height velocity occurs during Tanner stage III, what other physical attributes would one expect to occur in the girl at the same time?

(A) Elevation of the breast papilla only and no pubic hair
(B) Enlargement of the breast and areola with a single contour and darker, coarse curled pubic hair
(C) Mature breast adult quantity and pattern of pubic hair that extends to the thighs
(D) Projection of the areola and papilla with separate contours and adult-type pubic hair limited to the genital area

(E) Small breast buds with elevation of breast and papilla and sparse, straight, downy hair on the labial base

16. A 10-year-old Hispanic boy is admitted for bone marrow transplantation as treatment for chronic myelogenous leukemia. The doctor wants to enroll the patient in a clinical trial for a new pain medication. When the doctor arrives to discuss the study, she finds that both of the patient's parents speak only Spanish, and the consent form is in English. What is the best option for obtaining consent for this patient?

(A) Exclude non-English-speaking patients from the study
(B) Explain the study to the whole family
(C) Have the consent form translated into Spanish
(D) Have the patient translate the form for his parents

17. The statistical distribution of two studies is shown below. The mean is equal to the median and the mode in the first curve (labeled A). Which of the following correctly describes the mean, median, and mode in the second curve (labeled B)?

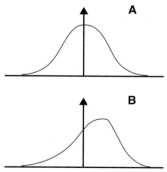

Reproduced, with permission, from USMLERx.com.

(A) Mean < median < mode
(B) Mean < mode < median
(C) Median < mean < mode
(D) Median < mode < mean
(E) Mode < mean < median
(F) Mode < median < mean

18. A 44-year-old schizophrenic patient on a psychiatric ward is interviewed daily as part of her treatment. She has been persistently reporting that she is married to Paul McCartney. This psychotic symptom is a disorder of which of the following?

(A) Cognition
(B) Form of thought
(C) Perception
(D) Thought content
(E) Thought process

19. An 18-year-old college freshman is brought to the college health clinic after her roommate confronted her about vomiting after every meal. The patient reports that she began binging and purging in high school after making the cheerleading squad. She seems to want help. Laboratory studies show a K^+ level of 3.3 mEq/L, a Cl^- level of 94 mEq/L, and a blood urea nitrogen level of 22 mg/dL. Which of the following drugs is contraindicated in this patient?

(A) Bupropion
(B) Chlorpromazine
(C) Clomipramine
(D) Fluoxetine
(E) Trazodone

20. A new antihypertensive medication is being investigated in a clinical trial. Investigators have noted a decrease in blood pressure in the group treated with the drug compared to the placebo group. While examining the study's participants, investigators notice that the experimental group has a lower mean age. What is this an example of?

(A) Confounding error
(B) Random error
(C) Recall bias
(D) Selection bias
(E) Systematic error

21. A 45-year-old patient with borderline personality disorder on a psychiatry ward is told by a staff psychiatrist to spend 2 hours in a quiet room after violently disrupting a meeting. The next morning the psychiatrist interviews her. She complains bitterly about how the nursing staff is so mean to her even though she is always nice to them. She says she has no idea why they locked her in the quiet room yesterday. This patient is using which of the following defense mechanisms?

    (A) Dissociation
    (B) Isolation
    (C) Projection
    (D) Splitting
    (E) Suppression

22. A new serum test was recently developed to detect antibodies to a certain virus in order to diagnose the infection. One thousand patients received the test, and while 100 people had the infection, only 80 of them tested positive. Of the 900 people who did not have the infection, 800 tested negative and 100 tested positive. Which of the following percentages indicates the specificity of this new test?

    (A) 10%
    (B) 44%
    (C) 80%
    (D) 89%
    (E) 98%

23. A 36-year-old man is brought to the psychiatrist by his wife. She reports that the patient has always been somewhat reclusive and introverted, but lately he has been refusing to go to friends' houses for dinner. The patient also reports that he has been reluctant to leave the house for any reason for the past few months because he is afraid people will think him bizarre or peculiar. The patient is referred for behavioral therapy. What is the best choice for pharmacologic therapy for this patient?

    (A) Amitriptyline
    (B) Buspirone
    (C) Fluoxetine
    (D) Propranolol
    (E) Valproate

24. A prospective cohort study is examining birth complications in women with diabetes. The study determines that babies are more likely to be born large for gestational age (LGA) if the mother has diabetes. The relative risk for the study is calculated to be 4. Which of the following accurately describes this relative risk?

    (A) The incidence rate of diabetes among LGA mothers is 4 times that of non-LGA mothers
    (B) The incidence rate of LGA among women with diabetes is 4 times that of women without diabetes
    (C) The incidence rate of LGA among women without diabetes is 4 times that of women with diabetes
    (D) The odds of diabetes among LGA mothers is 4 times that of non-LGA mothers
    (E) The odds of LGA among women with diabetes is 4 times that of women without diabetes

25. A 45-year-old man presents to a marriage counselor at his wife's prompting. He has been married for 10 years and believes that his wife has been unfaithful for the entire marriage, despite her protests to the contrary. He says that everyone is always betraying him, and he has a litany of slights, insults, and injuries that have been perpetrated against him. He is very defensive with the counselor and reads an attack in almost every statement. This patient most likely has which of the following personality disorders?

    (A) Antisocial
    (B) Avoidant
    (C) Borderline
    (D) Obsessive-compulsive
    (E) Paranoid
    (F) Schizoid

ANSWERS

1. **The correct answer is B.** This question is asking for the β or type II error. The p-value in the trial is 0.21, which is greater than 0.05 (p < 0.05 is commonly accepted as statistically significant), and therefore we cannot reject the null hypothesis. Because we do not reject the null hypothesis, there is a possibility for a type II error. A type II error occurs when we state that no difference exists when in fact one does exist. β is the probability of making a type II error—i.e., the probability that we fail to reject the null hypothesis when in fact it is false. β is related to power, calculated as $1 - β$, or $1 - 0.2 = 0.80$.

   Answer A is incorrect. The p-value represents the probability of making a type I error. If p < 0.05, there is less than a 5% chance that the null hypothesis was incorrectly rejected.

   Answer C is incorrect. The figure 0.21 simply represents the p-value, which is greater than 0.05. We therefore fail to reject the null hypothesis (no difference between treatment groups).

   Answer D is incorrect. The figure 0.80 represents the power of the study. Power = $1 - β$. The power increases when the sample size does.

   Answer E is incorrect. The figure 0.90 is a distracter and represents the percentage of patients taking penicillin who were able to clear the pneumonia.

   Answer F is incorrect. The figure 0.95 is a distracter and represents the percentage of patients taking the new antibiotic who were able to clear the pneumonia.

2. **The correct answer is B.** Heart disease is the leading cause of death among the elderly (65 years and older). Heart disease is also the leading cause of death if all ages are combined. This patient has already suffered a heart attack.

   Answer A is incorrect. Congenital anomalies are the leading cause of death among infants (less than 1 year of age), and not among the elderly.

   Answer C is incorrect. Motor vehicle crashes, and accidents in general, are leading causes of death. However, they are the most common cause of death among children (1–14 years of age) and adolescents (15–24 years of age) and not among the elderly.

   Answer D is incorrect. Stroke is a common cause of death among the elderly; however, it is not as common as heart disease or cancer.

   Answer E is incorrect. Suicide is not the leading cause of death in the elderly. It is a common cause of death among adolescents.

3. **The correct answer is C.** This patient exhibits some classic symptoms of narcolepsy, including cataplexy and sleep paralysis. Methylphenidate is an amphetamine derivative that is used to treat attention-deficit/hyperactivity disorder and narcolepsy.

   Answer A is incorrect. Chloral hydrate is a nonbenzodiazepine hypnotic that is used for sedation and insomnia. This patient does not need help sleeping.

   Answer B is incorrect. Hydroxyzine is a nonselective antihistamine that is used in the treatment of anxiety, pruritus, nausea/vomiting, sedation, and insomnia.

   Answer D is incorrect. Prochlorperazine maleate is a typical antipsychotic used in the treatment of nausea, vomiting, anxiety, and psychosis.

   Answer E is incorrect. Zolpidem is a nonbenzodiazepine hypnotic that is used in the treatment of insomnia.

4. **The correct answer is C.** Transference occurs when a patient projects feelings from his or her personal life onto a doctor; countertransference takes place when the doctor projects feelings onto the patient. These feelings can be either positive or negative. The patient's anger at the doctor when her sexual advances are rebuffed is an example of negative transference.

Answer A is incorrect. The doctor being reminded of his aunt by this patient is an example of countertransference.

Answer B is incorrect. The doctor telling the patient that he is uncomfortable is not an example of countertransference or transference.

Answer D is incorrect. The patient dressing up for appointments is positive transference.

Answer E is incorrect. The patient flirting with the doctor is positive transference. In its most extreme form, positive transference can take the form of sexual desire.

5. **The correct answer is E.** Mood disorders are extremely common in primary care offices. Distinguishing between dysthymia and a major depressive episode has clinical implications for this patient. This patient displays somatic symptoms in addition to a depressed mood. Dysthymic disorder requires the presence of two of six symptoms for at least 2 years, including change in appetite, change in sleep patterns, decreased energy, decreased self-esteem, decreased concentration, and increased hopelessness. Major depressive disorder is diagnosed in patients when they have five of nine symptoms for at least 2 weeks, including **S**leep changes, loss of **I**nterest (anhedonia), **G**uilt, **E**nergy loss, **C**oncentration changes, **A**ppetite changes, **P**sychomotor abnormalities, and **S**uicidal thoughts (**SIG E CAPS**).

Answer A is incorrect. Changes in appetite and/or weight are characteristics shared by major depression and dysthymia. Patients can exhibit an increased or decreased appetite or weight.

Answer B is incorrect. Changes in sleep patterns are also characteristics shared by major depression and dysthymia. Patients can have insomnia or hypersomnia.

Answer C is incorrect. Depressed mood is another characteristic shared by the two disorders. The depressed mood tends to last longer in patients with dysthymia, although there can be variation in their moods. Diagnostic criteria for dysthymia require that the depressed mood be present for more days than not.

Answer D is incorrect. Fatigue/lack of energy is a characteristic shared by the two disorders.

6. **The correct answer is B.** This baby is displaying motor skills expected for a 2- to 3-month-old infant but exhibits social, verbal, and cognitive skills appropriate for a 7- to 11-month-old baby. A 7- to 11-month-old baby should be able to sit alone, crawl, and use a pincer grasp.

Answer A is incorrect. This infant is displaying age-appropriate verbal and cognitive skills (being able to say "dada" even in a nonsensical manner).

Answer C is incorrect. While reflexes are not usually a developmental milestone, this infant is still age-appropriate. Babinski's reflex usually disappears around 12 months.

Answer D is incorrect. This infant is displaying age-appropriate social skills, including playing peek-a-boo and displaying stranger anxiety.

Answer E is incorrect. This infant is displaying age-appropriate verbal and cognitive skills (being able to say "dada" even in a nonsensical manner).

7. **The correct answer is F.** This patient has taken phencyclidine, or PCP. Patients with PCP intoxication show signs of belligerence, impulsiveness, fever, psychomotor agitation, vertical and horizontal nystagmus, tachycardia, ataxia, homicidality, psychosis, and delirium. On withdrawal, patients may demonstrate a recurrence of intoxication when the PCP, which was trapped in an ionized form in the acidic gastric lumen, is reabsorbed in the alkaline duodenum. They may also experience a sudden onset of severe, random homicidal violence. PCP users will have normal or small pupils. Death can result from a variety of causes, including respiratory depression and violent behavior.

Answer A is incorrect. Patients presenting with acute alcohol intoxication will show symptoms of disinhibition, emotional lability, slurred speech, ataxia, coma, and blackouts.

On withdrawal, they will demonstrate a tremor, tachycardia, hypertension, malaise, nausea, seizures, delirium tremens, tremulousness, agitation, and hallucinations.

Answer B is incorrect. Patients presenting with amphetamine intoxication will display psychomotor agitation, impaired judgment, pupillary dilation, hypertension, tachycardia, euphoria, prolonged wakefulness and attention, cardiac arrhythmias, delusions, hallucinations, and fever. On withdrawal, they will show a post-use "crash" that includes depression, lethargy, headache, stomach cramps, hunger, and hypersomnolence.

Answer C is incorrect. Patients presenting with acute cocaine intoxication will show symptoms of euphoria, psychomotor agitation, impaired judgment, tachycardia, pupillary dilation, hypertension, hallucinations, paranoid ideations, angina, and sudden cardiac death. On withdrawal, they will show a post-use "crash" that includes severe depression, hypersomnolence, fatigue, malaise, and severe psychological craving.

Answer D is incorrect. Patients presenting with acute lysergic acid diethylamide intoxication will display marked anxiety or depression, delusions, visual hallucinations, flashbacks, and pupillary dilation.

Answer E is incorrect. Patients presenting with acute nicotine intoxication will show symptoms of restlessness, insomnia, anxiety, and arrhythmias. On withdrawal, they will have symptoms of irritability, headache, anxiety, weight gain, craving, and tachycardia.

8. **The correct answer is E.** The prevalence is the number of individuals with a disease in a given population at a given time. Prevalence is estimated by test results but is not a measure of a test's validity. In the chart shown, the prevalence can also be determined by calculating the number of true-positive plus false-negative results divided by the total number of patients.

Answer A is incorrect. This represents true-positive results divided by the total number of patients.

Answer B is incorrect. This term represents the incidence of positive test results.

Answer C is incorrect. This represents true-positive results divided by the total number of patients tested less those with true-positive results, and would not be a meaningful calculation.

Answer D is incorrect. This represents the number of true-positive results over the total number of patients without disease. This would not be a meaningful calculation.

9. **The correct answer is E.** The Good Samaritan Law is meant to protect people (including off-duty medical professionals) who help others in emergency situations such as this. The law differs in each state, but the general concepts are the same: care providers must use standard procedures. Note that the law does not protect volunteers from gross negligence. Volunteers should limit their actions to their field of training.

Answer A is incorrect. The Good Samaritan Law stipulates that the care provider cannot request or receive any compensation for their actions.

Answer B is incorrect. The provider should call for help as soon as possible. The law requires that once a provider assumes the role, he or she must stay with the victim until further help arrives, not simply until help is called.

Answer C is incorrect. The Good Samaritan Law does not protect the volunteer from legal action. The patient is free to pursue legal recourse if the care provided is negligent and results in injury.

Answer D is incorrect. As with any other medical intervention, the patient has the right to refuse care from the provider.

10. **The correct answer is D.** Many different intelligence quotient scales have been devised. One of the first was the Stanford-Binet. The Wechsler Intelligence Scale for Children–Revised is used to evaluate children between the ages of 6 and 16½ years.

Answer A is incorrect. The Iowa Test of Educational Development is an achievement test, not an intelligence test. It is used to evaluate older children through the end of high school.

Answer B is incorrect. The Vineland Social Maturity Scale is a test used to evaluate adaptive behavior. It is typically used to evaluate children with mental retardation, but its use has been expanded to include children with other learning disabilities.

Answer C is incorrect. The Wechsler Adult Intelligence Scale–Revised is used to evaluate those patients who are older than 16½ years.

Answer E is incorrect. The Wide-Range Achievement Test is another achievement test. Unlike the Iowa tests, which are given in a group setting to almost every child in the United States, the Wide-Range Achievement Test is used for individual testing.

11. **The correct answer is C.** The probability of having a condition, given a positive test, represents the positive predictive value. This is calculated by TP/(TP + FP), where TP means true positive and FP means false positive. Therefore, the positive predictive value is 180/(180 + 40), or 0.82 (82%). As the prevalence of the disease increases in a population, so does the positive predictive value.

Answer A is incorrect. The figure 0.20 is the prevalence of the disease among tested patients (200/1000).

Answer B is incorrect. The figure 0.24 is a distracter and is the number of positive tests divided by the total number of patients.

Answer D is incorrect. The figure 0.90 is the sensitivity of the new HIV test. It is given by TP/(TP + FN), where TP means true positive and FN means false negative, or those with the disease who test negative.

Answer E is incorrect. The figure 0.97 is the negative predictive value, or the probability of not having a condition given a negative test. It is calculated by TN/(TN + FN), where TN means true negative and FN means false negative.

12. **The correct answer is B.** There is a temporal association between this man's myocardial infarction and his subsequent erectile dysfunction (ED). The presence of morning erections indicates that the cause of this patient's ED is psychological rather than physical. The patient should be reassured that if he can tolerate climbing two flights of stairs, he can tolerate sexual activity.

Answer A is incorrect. It is unlikely that a patient would complain of erectile dysfunction if he had a decreased interest in sexual activity. A problem with decreased interest is more likely to be brought up by a partner or spouse.

Answer C is incorrect. Sexual desire/interest does not decrease with age. Men can have a longer refractory period and can take longer to achieve an erection as they age.

Answer D is incorrect. This patient's medications are low on the sexual side effect scale. While antihypertensives in general can cause impotence, angiotensin-converting enzyme inhibitors are the least likely to do so. Statins are not known to cause sexual problems.

Answer E is incorrect. If patients can climb two flights of stairs without becoming short of breath or experiencing chest pain, limits on sexual activity are unnecessary.

13. **The correct answer is E.** Emancipation is a legal definition through which minors become independent of their parents and are free to make medical decisions for themselves. A minor, which is a legal condition defined by age, can generally acquire emancipation through court order or marriage. These situations usually suggest that the minor will be financially independent of his or her parents. This patient is married and is therefore emancipated.

Answer A is incorrect. While this patient has many adult responsibilities, 18 years is the legal age of consent and adulthood.

Answer B is incorrect. Full-time work suggests that the patient is financially independent, but taken alone it is not proof of emancipation.

Answer C is incorrect. A high school diploma does not provide emancipation. Even though a minor becomes the primary decision maker after high school graduation, he or she is not necessarily financially independent of the parents.

Answer D is incorrect. A teenager may state he or she has separated from the parents, but unless the courts have approved a legal separation, merely saying she is "separated" from her parents is not enough; legally, the parents are still financially responsible for the child until he or she turns 18.

14. **The correct answer is C.** This vignette illustrates a cohort study. This is an observational study in which a specific population is identified that is free of the illness at the beginning of the study. Samples are chosen based on the presence or absence of risk factors (alcohol in this case), and the incidence rate of a certain disease is compared between exposed and unexposed members.

Answer A is incorrect. Case-control studies are also observational studies, but the sample is chosen based on the presence (case) or absence (control) of a disease (pancreatic cancer). Information is then gathered regarding prior exposures of cases and controls to certain risk factors.

Answer B is incorrect. Clinical treatment trials are examples of cohort studies; however, members with a specific illness are given a treatment, while others with the same illness are given a different therapy or placebo. Information is collected regarding the treatment compared with other therapies or placebo.

Answer D is incorrect. This vignette does not exemplify a cross-sectional study. These studies involve the collection of information on a disease and risk factors in a population at one point in time.

Answer E is incorrect. This vignette is an example of a cohort study, which is prospective (taking place in the present time) as opposed to historical.

15. **The correct answer is B.** Tanner stage III is the stage when most girls experience peak height velocity (PHV). PHV occurs approximately 1 year after the initiation of breast development.

Answer A is incorrect. This description corresponds to Tanner stage I.

Answer C is incorrect. This description corresponds to Tanner stage V.

Answer D is incorrect. This description corresponds to Tanner stage IV.

Answer E is incorrect. This description corresponds to Tanner stage II.

16. **The correct answer is C.** Obtaining informed consent requires that the consenting party agree to the plan of care, that they are free from coercion, and that they have been able to engage in discussion of pertinent information. The consenting party must understand the risks, benefits, and alternative to participation. In this setting, the best option for achieving these goals is to wait for the consent to be translated into Spanish and then return with an interpreter. This allows the parents freedom to read and process the consent and to discuss it later. While this option may not be possible for every language or reasonable for every study, it is the best choice of the examples given.

Answer A is incorrect. Patients cannot be excluded from a research study solely because of language barriers. Services do exist to facilitate this.

Answer B is incorrect. With minimal Spanish, it is unlikely that the physician would be able to engage in a thorough discussion with the family or that she would be able to appropriately address their concerns.

Answer D is incorrect. Having the patient translate the form to his parents places undue pressure on the patient and removes autonomy from the parents, plus the physician cannot be certain of an accurate translation.

17. **The correct answer is A.** The first curve, with mean = median = mode, represents a normal Gaussian distribution. The second curve represents a negative skew. The mean is equal to the center of the graph. The mode is equal to the most common result. This is represented at the top of the curve. The median is the middle value if the value were ordered sequentially. It turns out that during either a positive skew or a negative skew, the median is in between the mean and the mode. Therefore, mean < median < mode.

    Answer B is incorrect. In Gaussian distributions, the median is always between the mode and the mean.

    Answer C is incorrect. In Gaussian distributions, the median is always between the mode and the mean.

    Answer D is incorrect. In Gaussian distributions, the median is always between the mode and the mean.

    Answer E is incorrect. In Gaussian distributions, the median is always between the mode and the mean.

    Answer F is incorrect. This would be the case in a positively skewed data distribution, rather than a negative skew.

18. **The correct answer is D.** This patient is suffering from delusions, which are disorders of thought content. Delusions are commonly referred to as fixed false beliefs, although they can be transitory and distressing to the patient. Delusions are not shared by others. The other disorder of thought content is ideas of reference.

    Answer A is incorrect. Disorders of cognition affect a patient's level of alertness and orientation. Cognitive disorders can manifest with problems in memory, calculation, and language. Alzheimer's disease is a classic cognitive disorder.

    Answer B is incorrect. Disorders of form of thought include loose associations and tangentiality. Both of these disorders are evident in a patient's manner of speech.

Answer C is incorrect. Disorders of perception include illusions and hallucinations. Hallucinations are false and illusions are misinterpretations.

Answer E is incorrect. Disorders of thought processes include impaired abstraction ability and neologisms. These are essentially problems with words—either with the meaning of words or with the creation of new words.

19. **The correct answer is A.** Bupropion is an atypical antidepressant that is thought to inhibit reuptake of norepinephrine and dopamine. A known complication of bupropion is that it can lower the seizure threshold in normal patients. This is an even more significant issue in bulimic patients, who may have abnormalities of electrolyte balance.

    Answer B is incorrect. Chlorpromazine is a typical antipsychotic that selectively antagonizes dopamine D_2 receptors. It can be useful in the early refeeding of anorexic patients by helping to reduce their anxiety surrounding eating.

    Answer C is incorrect. Clomipramine is a tricyclic antidepressant that is useful in maintaining the recovery phase of anorexic patients.

    Answer D is incorrect. Fluoxetine is the most widely studied of the antidepressants in the treatment of eating disorders. It also helps prevent relapse in anorexic patients. It is the only drug approved by the Food and Drug Administration for the treatment of bulimia.

    Answer E is incorrect. Trazodone is another antidepressant that can be useful in the treatment of bulimia, although it is considered a second-line treatment.

20. **The correct answer is A.** A confounding error is committed when a variable other than the one being studied is influencing the results. In this study, the treatment group's lower blood pressure may be secondary to their younger mean age rather than to the antihypertensive medication. A sampling bias could be involved, although it would refer to a systematic error in which the participants chosen for the

study where not representative of the population from which they are drawn. This would pose a problem when attempting to generalize the study's results to other situations.

Answer B is incorrect. Random error results in decreased precision of results.

Answer C is incorrect. Recall bias results in an increased likelihood that one outcome will occur.

Answer D is incorrect. Selection bias results in an increase in the likelihood of one outcome occurring.

Answer E is incorrect. Systematic errors result in decreased accuracy of results.

21. **The correct answer is D.** Splitting is a belief that people are either all good or all bad. Although the doctor had to approve the time in the quiet room, the patient blames only the nurses. She is also displaying a tendency toward acting out through tantrums. Splitting and acting out are two examples of immature defense mechanisms.

Answer A is incorrect. Dissociation is a temporary, drastic change in personality, memory, consciousness, or motor behavior that is used to avoid emotional stress. This is an immature defense mechanism.

Answer B is incorrect. Isolation is a separation of feelings from ideas and events. This is an immature defense mechanism.

Answer C is incorrect. Projection is when an unacceptable internal impulse is attributed to an external source. This is an immature defense mechanism.

Answer E is incorrect. Suppression is a voluntary withholding of an idea or feeling from conscious awareness. This is a mature defense mechanism.

22. **The correct answer is D.** The specificity of the test is 89%. It is calculated by dividing the true negatives by the sum of the true negatives and false positives. In the above case, the specificity is 800/(800 + 100). The specificity measures how well a test identifies people who are truly well. High specificity is most important

when it means that a healthy patient might undergo unnecessary and harmful treatment because of testing positive.

Answer A is incorrect. The figure 10% simply represents the prevalence of the disease in this select population (100/1000).

Answer B is incorrect. The figure 44% is the positive predictive value of the test. It is calculated by dividing true positives by the sum of true positives and false positives (80/[80 + 100]). The positive predictive value is the probability that someone with a positive test actually does have the infection.

Answer C is incorrect. The figure 80% is the sensitivity of the test. It is calculated by dividing true positives by the sum of true positives and false negatives (80/[80 + 20]). It measures how well a test identifies truly ill people.

Answer E is incorrect. The figure 98% is the negative predictive value of the test. It is calculated by dividing true negatives by the sum of true negatives and false negatives (800/[800 + 20]). The negative predictive value is the probability that a person with a negative test actually does not have the disease.

23. **The correct answer is C.** Selective serotonin reuptake inhibitors such as fluoxetine are the treatment of choice for social phobia disorders. They lack abuse potential and the side effects are generally well tolerated. Social phobia is an irrational fear of social or performance situations that the patient recognizes as irrational. Patients can begin to avoid all social situations in order to avert the unpleasant feelings that are aroused. Social phobia tends to have an insidious onset and remains a chronic problem. Relapse is common after pharmacologic therapy is stopped.

Answer A is incorrect. Tricyclic antidepressants such as amitriptyline are not first-line treatment for social phobia. They are considered to be less effective than the selective serotonin reuptake inhibitors.

Answer B is incorrect. Buspirone is not an effective treatment for social phobia. Buspirone is prescribed for patients with generalized anxiety disorder.

Answer D is incorrect. Propranolol is useful in treating patients with performance anxiety but is not as useful in patients with a nonspecific social phobia.

Answer E is incorrect. Valproate is being investigated for the treatment of social phobia, but no recommendations for its use in social phobia exist.

24. **The correct answer is B.** Relative risk is used in cohort studies. Cohort studies are based on presence or absence of risk factors. Relative risk is defined as the incidence rate in those exposed to a risk factor divided by the incidence rate of those not exposed. In this study, the risk factor is diabetes in the mothers and the incident would be LGA babies. The incidence rate of LGA births in women with diabetes is 4 times that in women without diabetes.

Answer A is incorrect. This choice describes the correct type of risk analysis but describes the relationship in reverse.

Answer C is incorrect. This choice reverses the findings of the study, which shows that the incidence of LGA is 4 times more in women with diabetes.

Answer D is incorrect. This choice incorrectly uses odds rather than incidence rates and also describes the relationship of the findings of the study in reverse.

Answer E is incorrect. This choice would be the description of an odds ratio for a case-control study. A case-control study evaluates the presence of risk factors in people with and without a disease. Although this is the opposite of a cohort study, the results are still reported in terms of disease presence with respect to risk factors; that is, the presence or absence of disease is categorized in the group with risk factors and compared to the group without. The difference, however, is that odds are used rather than incidence. The incidence rate is a percentage (e.g., 50 out of 100). Odds are calculated by dividing those with disease by those without (50 to 50).

25. **The correct answer is E.** Cluster A personality disorders include paranoid, schizoid, and schizotypal, and patients with these disorders are often characterized as eccentric and/or weird. They employ abnormal cognition (suspiciousness), abnormal self-expression (odd speech), and abnormal relation to others (seclusiveness). There is a genetic association with schizophrenia. Patients with paranoid personality disorder are not psychotic. They are distrustful and suspicious and use projection as their main defense mechanism.

Answer A is incorrect. Patients with antisocial personality disorder show a disregard for and violation of the rights of others, including a proclivity for criminal behavior. This is the only personality disorder with an age limit—patients must be above the age of 18. Minors with similar behavior are considered to have conduct disorder. This is the only conduct disorder in which males outnumber females.

Answer B is incorrect. Patients with avoidant personality disorder are sensitive to rejection, socially inhibited, and timid with overwhelming feelings of inadequacy.

Answer C is incorrect. Patients with borderline personality disorder show unstable mood and behavior and impulsiveness and have a pervasive sense of emptiness. Females outnumber males.

Answer D is incorrect. Patients with obsessive-compulsive personality disorder have a preoccupation with order and perfectionism

Answer F is incorrect. Patients with schizoid personality disorder exhibit voluntary social withdrawal and have limited emotional expressions.

CHAPTER 2

Biochemistry

1. A 16-year-old boy comes to the clinic for a routine visit. On physical examination, the patient is found to have symptoms that are consistent with Fabry's disease, including angiokeratomas, hypohidrosis, and acroparesthesias. Examination of this patient's vascular endothelium would most likely show a pathologic accumulation of which of the following substances?

   (A) Ceramide trihexoside
   (B) Galactocerebroside
   (C) Glucocerebroside
   (D) Lactosyl cerebroside
   (E) Sphingomyelin

2. A metabolic process is pictured below. Which intermediate in this process inhibits the rate-limiting enzyme of glycolysis and activates the rate-limiting enzyme of fatty acid synthesis?

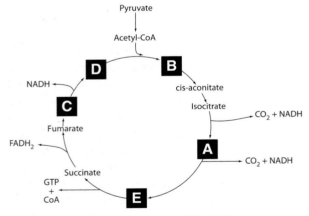

Reproduced, with permission, from USMLERx.com.

   (A) A
   (B) B
   (C) C
   (D) D
   (E) E

3. A 32-year-old woman develops polyuria. Her nephrologist monitors her closely on a water deprivation test, and she continues to have increased urine output. A diagnosis of diabetes insipidus is made. The nephrologist orders an antidiuretic hormone level and determines that it is inappropriately elevated. Which of the following is the site of pathology in this patient?

   (A) Adenohypophysis
   (B) D_1
   (C) Pituitary function
   (D) V_1
   (E) V_2

4. A 35-year-old man presents to the physician with arthritic pain in both knees along with back pain. He states that the pain has been present for months. In an effort to obtain relief, he has taken only aspirin, but this has been of little benefit. The patient is afebrile, and his slightly swollen knee joints are neither hot nor tender to palpation; however, the pain does restrict his motion. The cartilage of his ears appears slightly darker than normal. No tophi are present. A urine specimen is taken for analysis of uric acid content and turns black in the laboratory while standing. What is the most likely diagnosis at this point?

   (A) Alkaptonuria
   (B) Ankylosing spondylitis
   (C) Maple syrup urine disease
   (D) Phenylketonuria
   (E) Rheumatoid arthritis

5. The single base-pair mutation for sickle cell anemia destroys the MstII restriction enzyme recognition site represented by an asterisk in the image. The restriction enzyme-binding

sites are shown as arrows on the map. DNA from a carrier of the sickle cell trait is treated with MstII and run on an electrophoresis gel. The DNA is then hybridized with a labeled probe that binds to the normal gene in the position shown on the map. In the Southern blot shown in the image, which lane represents the patient?

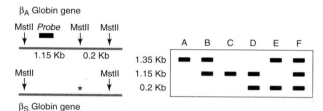

Reproduced, with permission, from USMLERx.com.

(A) A
(B) B
(C) C
(D) D
(E) E
(F) F

6. Phosphatidylcholine is a major component of red blood cell membranes, myelin, surfactant, and cholesterol. Phosphatidylcholine is synthesized through phosphorylation of choline obtained from the diet or with reused choline derived from phospholipid turnover. De novo synthesis requires an addition of three methyl groups, transferred from an amino acid. Without the turnover component, deficiency in which essential amino acid would make dietary choline essential for phosphatidylcholine synthesis?

(A) Asparagine
(B) Histidine
(C) Methionine
(D) Threonine
(E) Valine

7. The muscles that control the diameter of the pupil are triggered by a cascade of molecular events within a muscle cell. What is the function of the enzyme activated by the calcium-calmodulin complex?

(A) Binding to troponin
(B) Dephosphorylation of actin
(C) Dephosphorylation of myosin
(D) Phosphorylation of actin
(E) Phosphorylation of myosin

8. A DNA segment is treated with restriction enzymes, pipetted into a well of polyacrylamide gel, and subjected to an electric field. Next, the gel is stained with ethidium bromide and visualized under ultraviolet lights. What laboratory technique does this describe?

(A) Enzyme-linked immunosorbent assay
(B) Gel electrophoresis
(C) Northern blot
(D) Polymerase chain reaction
(E) Sequencing
(F) Southern blot
(G) Western blot

9. Ion flux across the cell membrane is tightly regulated by ion channels and ion carriers in order to maintain specific intracellular and plasma ion concentrations. Because increases in intracellular calcium can be especially detrimental to the cell, calcium homeostasis is very tightly regulated through the additional work of sequestration in endoplasmic reticulum and mitochondria. In which of the following ways does increased intracellular calcium concentration cause the most cell damage?

(A) Enzyme activation
(B) Free radical generation
(C) Increased membrane permeability
(D) Inhibition of glycolysis
(E) Inhibition of oxidative phosphorylation

10. A scientist working in a research laboratory has been examining different compounds that antagonize the microbial surface components recognizing adhesive matrix molecules (MSCRAMM) receptor, a new G-coupled receptor that has been implicated in rheumatoid arthritis. Compound A has a much higher affinity for the MSCRAMM receptor than compound B. Both compounds have a higher affinity for the receptor than the endogenous ligand. Which of the following describes the relationship between compound A and compound B?

(A) The maximum reaction rate of compound A is greater than that of compound B

(B) The maximum reaction rate of compound B is greater than that of compound A

(C) The Michaelis-Menten constant of compound A is higher than that of compound B

(D) The Michaelis-Menten constant of compound A is lower than that of compound B

(E) The Michaelis-Menten constant values of compounds A and B are the same

11. An 18-year-old woman presents to the emergency department with acute onset of severe abdominal pain. She says she had a similar attack 1 year earlier after taking some barbiturates. At that time she underwent an exploratory laparotomy, which revealed nothing. The patient no longer takes barbiturates but recently started a low-carbohydrate diet. She has a temperature of 37° C (98.6° F), a respiratory rate of 16/min, and a blood pressure of 128/83 mm Hg. Her WBC count is normal. The SMA-7 reveals a sodium level of 127 mEq/L, and a urinalysis demonstrates increased porphobilinogen levels. The physician tells the patient that she has a genetic condition involving her RBCs. What congenital disorder did the physician most likely tell the patient she has?

(A) Acute intermittent porphyria
(B) Factor V Leiden deficiency
(C) Fanconi's anemia
(D) Hereditary spherocytosis
(E) Sickle cell disease

12. A 48-year-old woman presents to a new physician because of the recent onset of fatigue, arthralgias, discomfort in her right upper quadrant, and polyuria. On physical examination, her skin seems somewhat browner than would be expected. Laboratory tests are remarkable for an elevated glucose level, indications of hemolysis, and increased transferrin saturation. Cardiac testing shows moderate restrictive cardiomyopathy. She mentions that she regularly requires blood transfusions. Which of the following is the cause of this patient's condition?

(A) Absence of the hemoglobin α chain
(B) Absence of the hemoglobin β chain
(C) Mutation resulting in increased absorption of dietary iron
(D) Mutations in the gene encoding ankyrin
(E) Mutations resulting in copper accumulation

13. A 2-month-old boy is brought to the emergency department with respiratory insufficiency and failure to thrive after an uneventful pregnancy and perinatal course. Generalized hypotonia and weakness are noted. The patient's hospital stay is remarkable for the development of tracheobronchomalacia and respiratory insufficiency that requires mechanical ventilation before the patient dies of respiratory complications. Muscle biopsy shows denervation and panfascicular atrophy. The patient's family history demonstrates other occurrences of similar disease. A genetics consult obtained prior to the patient's death yields the pedigree shown in the image. Which of the following diseases is most consistent with this patient's presentation and the pedigree shown in the image?

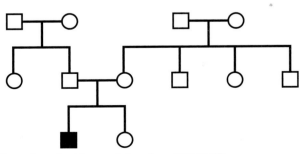

Reproduced, with permission, from USMLERx.com.

(A) Becker's muscular dystrophy
(B) Duchenne's muscular dystrophy
(C) Kugelberg-Welander disease
(D) Spinal muscular atrophy, type II
(E) Werdnig-Hoffmann disease

14. Glucose transport into cells occurs via one member of a family of glucose transporters or via cotransport with sodium. If this patient has a defect in a glucose transporter, which cell line uses an alternate method of acquiring glucose?

(A) Adipocytes
(B) Enterocytes
(C) Erythrocytes
(D) Hepatocytes
(E) Myocytes
(F) Pancreatic beta cells

15. A 31-year-old woman is trying to get pregnant. She has a niece with cystic fibrosis and would like to assess her chances of having a child with this disease. Which of the following laboratory techniques could be used to determine if this woman and/or her husband is a carrier of the cystic fibrosis gene?

(A) Enzyme-linked immunosorbent assay
(B) Gel electrophoresis
(C) Northern blot
(D) Polymerase chain reaction and sequencing
(E) Western blot

16. Consider the electron transport chain. If an agent is applied such that there is no membrane potential or pH gradient across the mitochondria, which of the following will increase?

(A) ATP consumption
(B) Free energy of the reaction adenosine diphosphate + phosphorus, yielding ATP at standard conditions
(C) Redox potential of oxygen at standard conditions
(D) Redox potential of reduced nicotinamide adenine dinucleotide at standard conditions
(E) The number of cristae

17. A 65-year-old woman develops a urinary tract infection. Urine cultures are positive for *Ente-*

rococcus faecalis. Treatment with vancomycin is attempted but is unsuccessful. Which of the following molecular changes is responsible for this patient's vancomycin resistance?

(A) D-ala D-ala to D-ala D-lac
(B) D-ala D-ala to D-ala D-leu
(C) D-ala D-lac to D-ala D-ala
(D) D-ala D-leu to D-ala D-ala
(E) D-leu D-ala to D-ala D-ala

18. A 2-year-old boy presents to the pediatrician with fever, facial tenderness, and a green, foul-smelling nasal discharge. The patient is diagnosed with sinusitis, and the physician notes that he has a history of recurrent episodes of sinusitis. An x-ray film of the chest is ordered because of the fever. It reveals some dilated bronchi and shows the heart situated on the right side of his body. A diagnosis of a congenital disorder is made. Which of the other following findings would this patient be most likely to have?

(A) Defective chloride transport
(B) Elevated blood sugar
(C) Ineffective phagocytosis
(D) Reactive airway disease
(E) Tetralogy of Fallot

19. A 9-month-old boy is brought to the emergency department after his mother is unable to rouse him. His past medical history is significant for the onset of seizures at the age of 4 months and for a delay in reaching developmental milestones. On examination, the patient is found to have poor muscle tone and an enlarged liver. Laboratory studies show a blood urea nitrogen level of 3.2 mg/dL, a creatinine level of 0.4 mg/dL, and a serum ammonia level of 300 mg/dL. A plasma amino acid analysis fails to detect citrulline, while his urinary orotic acid level is increased. This patient suffers from a deficiency of which of the following enzymes?

(A) Arginase
(B) Argininosuccinate lyase
(C) Carbamoyl phosphate synthetase II
(D) Glutamate dehydrogenase
(E) Ornithine transcarbamoylase

20. A restriction fragment length polymorphism analysis and pedigree of a family plagued with an autosomal recessive disease is shown. The grandmother, represented by the darkened circle at the top of the pedigree, is known to be affected by the disease, while the grandfather, represented by the square at the top of the pedigree, is not affected by the disease. Which of the grandchildren is a carrier of the disease?

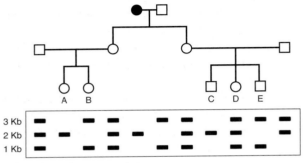

Reproduced, with permission, from USMLERx.com.

(A) A
(B) B
(C) C
(D) D
(E) E

21. A 29-year-old woman with a long-standing history of asthma and eczema presents with watery, itchy eyes and a stuffy nose of 3 days' duration. The woman states that her symptoms are similar to those she experiences during the spring. Her heart rate is 82/min, blood pressure is 117/80 mm Hg, respiratory rate is 14/min, and oxygen saturation is 96%. This patient's symptoms are due to the activation of which of the following receptors?

(A) α_1
(B) β_1
(C) β_2
(D) Histamine$_1$
(E) Histamine$_2$

22. An 8-month-old boy is brought to the pediatrician by his parents because he has recently lost the ability to crawl or hold his toys. His mother says she took him to the emergency department last week because he was wheezing. He was diagnosed with a cold and given an antihistamine, which did not relieve his symptoms. On examination, the patient is tachypneic and breathing with considerable effort; the liver is palpable five fingerwidths below the right costal margin. X-ray film of the chest reveals cardiomegaly. He has a difficult time sitting upright and cannot squeeze the physician's fingers or the ring of his pacifier with any noticeable force. Despite a number of interventions, the child's symptoms continue to worsen until his death 2 weeks later. On autopsy, it is likely that this patient's cells will contain an accumulation of which of the following substances?

(A) Glucose
(B) Glycogen
(C) Oxaloacetate
(D) Pyruvate
(E) Urea

23. After consumption of a carbohydrate-rich meal, the liver continues to convert glucose to glucose-6-phosphate. The liver's ability to continue this processing of high levels of glucose is important in minimizing increases in blood glucose after eating. What is the best explanation for the liver's ability to continue this conversion after eating a carbohydrate-rich meal?

(A) The hepatocyte cell membrane's permeability for glucose-6-phosphate
(B) The high maximum reaction rate of glucokinase
(C) The inhibition of glucokinase by high glucose-6-phosphate
(D) The lack of glucokinase level regulation by insulin
(E) The low Michaelis-Menten constant of glucokinase

24. A 30-year-old man is diagnosed with type I familial dyslipidemia. He has had recent laboratory studies showing elevated triglycerides and normal cholesterol levels. Which of the following explains the pathophysiology of this disease?

(A) Apolipoprotein E deficiency
(B) LDL receptor deficiency
(C) Lipoprotein lipase deficiency

(D) VLDL clearance deficiency
(E) VLDL overproduction

25. A 36-year-old woman returned from a trip to Japan 2 days ago. Yesterday she started experiencing left calf pain. The woman is afebrile with a heart rate of 82/min, a blood pressure of 129/86 mm Hg, and a respiratory rate of 14/min. On examination, the patient's calf pain is found to intensify on dorsiflexion of the left foot. Suspecting a deep venous thrombosis (DVT), the physician performs a duplex ultrasound, which confirms the diagnosis. Which of the following factors is most abundant locally at the site of the DVT?

(A) Leukotriene C_4
(B) Prostaglandin I_2
(C) Renin
(D) Thromboxane A_2
(E) Vascular endothelial growth factor

26. A 42-year-old woman comes to her physician because she noticed blood in her urine and has been having some low back pain. She had a hysterectomy 3 years earlier. Physical examination reveals palpable flank masses felt bilaterally as well as mild hypertension. Based on the clinical findings, the physician orders a CT scan to aid in the diagnosis (as shown in the image). Which of the following conditions is also associated with this disorder?

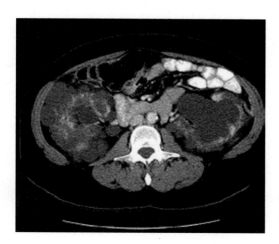

Image courtesy of PEIR Digital Library (http://peir.net).

(A) Astrocytomas
(B) Berry aneurysm
(C) Dark urine
(D) Optic nerve degeneration
(E) Squamous cell carcinoma

27. Which of the following is true of the 50S ribosomal subunit in bacterial protein synthesis?

(A) Proteins in the 50S subunit are responsible for creation of a peptide bond
(B) Streptomycin binds to the 50S subunit, disrupting the translocation step
(C) The 23S rRNA molecule within the 50S subunit is responsible for creation of a peptide bond
(D) The 50S subunit holds the binding site for both the aminoacyl-tRNA (A site) and the binding site for the elongating peptide chain (P site)
(E) The 50S subunit is a part of the initiation complex

28. A researcher investigating mechanisms of intracellular signaling develops a mouse model using recombinant DNA technology to generate a gene knockout. The F2 progeny exhibit dwarfism, hypogonadism, and hypothyroidism with low levels of follicle-stimulating hormone (FSH), luteinizing hormone (LH), and thyroid-stimulating hormone (TSH) but normal level. Which of the following is the second-messenger molecule for the intracellular signaling system that is most likely impaired in this mouse model?

(A) Cyclic adenosine monophosphate
(B) Cyclic guanosine monophosphate
(C) Inositol trisphosphate
(D) Steroid nuclear hormone receptor
(E) Tyrosine kinase

29. Hemoglobin consists of 2 α subunits and 2 β subunits. Each α unit is bound to a β unit by strong hydrophobic bonds. The β units and α units are each bound to one another by weaker polar bonds that are somewhat mobile. This change in quaternary structure changes the affinity for oxygen that hemoglobin exhibits as it shifts between its taut (T) form and relaxed form. At a given partial pressure of oxygen, which of the following will increase the amount of T hemoglobin?

    (A) Binding of CO_2 to hemoglobin
    (B) Decreasing the amount of 2,3-bisphospho-glycerate in RBCs
    (C) Increasing the number of oxygen molecules bound to a hemoglobin from one to three
    (D) Increasing the pH by moving from peripheral tissue to lung
    (E) The presence of excess CO from carbon monoxide poisoning

30. A group of scientists have recently discovered a new drug for treating hypercholesterolemia. In vitro studies with a hepatocyte cell line have revealed that the drug acts in a manner similar to that of steroids and results in increased synthesis of LDL cholesterol receptors. What is the mechanism by which this drug is acting on hepatocytes?

    (A) Allosteric regulation
    (B) Cell surface receptor antagonism
    (C) G-protein-cell receptor–mediated phosphorylation
    (D) Increased transcription
    (E) Proteolytic modification

31. A 30-year-old patient previously diagnosed with pheochromocytoma comes to the physician to explore the possibility of other endocrine disorders. On physical examination, the patient is found to have a solitary thyroid nodule. Laboratory studies show an increased serum calcitonin level and a pentagastrin-induced rise in the secretion of calcitonin. A biopsy confirms the presence of a medullary thyroid carcinoma. The patient is scheduled for a total thyroidectomy. Which of the following is a potential complication of this treatment?

    (A) Acromegaly
    (B) Cretinism
    (C) Hypertension
    (D) Hypoparathyroidism
    (E) Renal osteodystrophy

32. Consider the reaction sequence given below. E1, E2, and E3 are enzymes, while A, B, B2, C, and D are substrates. D feedback inhibits A. B2 is a partial agonist of E2 with a greater affinity for E2 than for B. Two separate experiments are performed. In the first, adequate amounts of A, E1, E2, and E3 are added. In the second, adequate amounts of A, E1, E2, and E3 are added as well as an excess of B2. The reactions are stopped after a set period of time. Which of the following most accurately describes the results of the experiments?

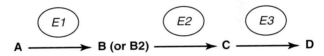

Reproduced, with permission, from USMLERx.com.

    (A) The amount of C in the second experiment is greater than the amount of C in the first experiment
    (B) The amount of D in the second experiment is greater than that in the first experiment
    (C) The amount of E1 in the first experiment is less than that in the second experiment
    (D) The amount of E2 in the first experiment exceeds that in the second experiment
    (E) There will be less feedback inhibition by D on A in the second experiment than in the first experiment

33. Scientists have discovered a new drug that appears to arrest the growth of cancer cells. In an in vitro experiment, cancer cells were arrested in metaphase. The mechanism of action of this new drug is similar to which of the following drugs?

    (A) Bleomycin
    (B) Cyclophosphamide
    (C) 5-Fluorouracil

(D) Methotrexate
(E) Paclitaxel

34. Essential amino acids are those that the body cannot synthesize de novo and must be present in an individual's diet for optimal health. These amino acids include the ketogenic amino acids leucine and lysine. Which of the following is also an essential amino acid?

(A) Alanine
(B) Cysteine
(C) Glutamine
(D) Proline
(E) Serine
(F) Threonine
(G) Tyrosine

35. A 78-year-old man with asthma went to his primary care physician for an annual checkup. The physician performed a physical examination and ordered routine blood work, which revealed a macrocytic anemia. Subsequent laboratory testing revealed an elevated level of methylmalonic acid, and results of a peripheral blood smear are shown. The physician diagnoses a vitamin deficiency. If this patient's vitamin deficiency is not corrected, what neurological symptoms may he experience?

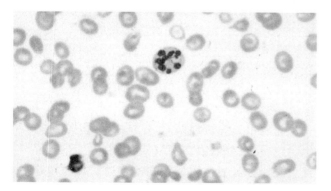

Image courtesy of PEIR Digital Library (http://peir.net).

(A) Deficiency in this vitamin does not cause neurological symptoms
(B) Dementia

(C) Paresthesias and ataxia
(D) Polyneuritis
(E) Wernicke-Korsakoff syndrome

36. A group of scientists is interested in studying how vesicles synthesized in the cell bodies of neurons are transported down the axon to the terminal boutons. Which of the following make up the cellular structures involved in axonal transport of vesicles?

(A) Actin
(B) Desmin
(C) Keratin
(D) Tubulin
(E) Vimentin

37. A term child is delivered by spontaneous vaginal delivery without complications. Upon physical examination the child has bilateral hip dislocations, restricted movement in shoulder and elbow joints, and coarse facial features. Laboratory studies show that the activities of β-hexosaminidase, iduronate sulfatase, and aryl-sulfatase A are deficient in cultured fibroblasts, but are 20 times normal in serum. This disease is associated with which of the following abnormal cellular components?

(A) Apolipoprotein B-48
(B) Collagen
(C) Mannose-6-phosphate
(D) Rough endoplasmic reticulum
(E) Sphingomyelinase

38. Patients who possess melanocytes but lack melanin in their skin, appear white-pink, and have white hair and nonpigmented irises are said to be albino. Which of the following is the most likely cause of congenital albinism?

(A) Acetaldehyde dehydrogenase deficiency
(B) Congenital abnormality in amino acid absorption
(C) Decreased consumption of phenylalanine
(D) Tryptophan hydroxylase deficiency
(E) Tyrosinase deficiency

39. Obstructive liver disease is usually characterized by which of the following qualities?

Choice	Type of Hyperbilirubinemia	Urine Bilirubin	Urine Urobilinogen
A	Conjugated	↑	Normal
B	Conjugated	↑	↓
C	Unconjugated	↑	↓
D	Unconjugated	↓	↑
E	Unconjugated	↓	↓

(A) A
(B) B
(C) C
(D) D
(E) E

40. A DNA fragment is added to four different tubes along with DNA polymerase, a radiolabeled primer, and the adenine, thymine, cytosine, and guanine deoxynucleotides. Each tube also contains one of the four bases as dideoxynucleotides. The four tubes are then run on electrophoresis gel and visualized by autoradiography. Which of the following laboratory techniques does this describe?

(A) Allele-specific oligonucleotide probe
(B) Enzyme-linked immunosorbent assay
(C) Northern blot
(D) Polymerase chain reaction
(E) Sequencing
(F) Southern blot
(G) Western blot

41. A 56-year-old man who is an alcoholic presents to the emergency department with severe epigastric pain radiating to his back. The pain was preceded by nausea and vomiting. His past medical history is notable for gallstones. Laboratory testing reveals a lipase level of 800 U/L (normal 10–140 U/L), a serum amylase level of 1020 U/L, and a WBC count of 13,200/mm³.

Which of the following pathophysiologic mechanisms is most likely responsible for this patient's presentation?

(A) Exhaustion of enzyme reserve
(B) Hyperactive renin-angiotensin system
(C) Inappropriate enzyme activation
(D) Inappropriate enzyme deactivation
(E) pH alteration of the surrounding milieu

42. A 3-year-old girl who was born at home in a rural area is brought to the local clinic because of seizures. She is pale skinned, shows marked mental retardation, and has a musty body odor. The doctor diagnoses her with a defect in tetrahydrobiopterin metabolism. Which of the following is a correct therapeutic measure for this child?

(A) Branched-chain amino acid–free diet
(B) Fructose-free diet
(C) Ketogenic diet
(D) Low-phenylalanine diet
(E) Low-tyrosine diet

43. A 3-month-old infant is rushed to the emergency department in respiratory distress. Her mother notes that she is "always sick." She has had multiple hospitalizations over the past months, including one for a severe bout of pneumonia with *Pneumocystis carinii* and another for respiratory syncytial virus. On admission, she is noted to be at the 50th percentile for weight and length and appears pale and lethargic. Her vital signs include a pulse of 150/min, respirations of 20/min, and a temperature of 38.9° C (102° F). Her mouth is coated with whitish bumps that scrape off easily. This patient is most likely to have a deficiency of which of the following enzymes?

(A) Adenosine deaminase
(B) Hexokinase
(C) Phenylalanine hydroxylase
(D) Pyruvate dehydrogenase
(E) Ribonucleotide reductase

44. A mass is felt in the groin of an infant girl during a physical examination. Surgical resection shows that it is a testicle. The baby is diagnosed with testicular feminization syndrome. In this syndrome, androgens are produced but cells fail to respond to the steroid hormones because they lack appropriate intracellular receptors. After binding intracellular receptors, steroids regulate the rate of which of the following?

(A) Initiation of protein synthesis
(B) mRNA degradation
(C) mRNA processing
(D) Protein translation
(E) Transcription of genes

45. A 27-year-old male develops a deep venous thrombosis in his left lower leg after a 4-hour car ride. His 59-year-old father had a thrombosis in a mesenteric vein last year, and his 52-year-old mother has had repeated superficial venous thromboses. Which of the following disorders does this patent most likely have?

(A) Factor V Leiden thrombophilia
(B) Familial hypercholesterolemia
(C) Fanconi's anemia
(D) Von Hippel–Lindau syndrome
(E) Von Willebrand's deficiency

46. A pediatrician examines two babies with two separate deficiencies in fructose metabolism. The first child has a deficiency of fructokinase, and the second has a deficiency of aldolase B. Although the physician states with confidence that the first child has a benign prognosis, he is concerned about the second child. What best explains the clinical severity of aldolase B deficiency?

(A) Increased ATP
(B) Increased circulating free phosphate
(C) Increased circulating fructose
(D) Sequestration of phosphate
(E) Upregulated fructokinase

47. A cyanotic patient is found to have circulating hemoglobin with high levels of oxidized iron (Fe^{3+}) instead of Fe^{2+}. Which of the following is the most appropriate treatment for this condition?

(A) Atropine
(B) Methylene blue

(C) N-acetylcysteine
(D) Naloxone
(E) Protamine

48. A neonate born 4 hours ago is having difficulty breathing. The baby was born prematurely at 28 weeks' gestation. He is tachypneic and is using his accessory muscles to breathe with nasal flaring and grunting. The baby's heart rate is 120/min, blood pressure is 100/60 mm Hg, and respiratory rate is 55/min. Analysis of amniotic fluid reveals a lecithin:sphingomyelin ratio of 0.9. What is this baby's lung lacking?

(A) Angiotensin-converting enzyme
(B) Collagen
(C) Dipalmitoyl phosphatidylcholine
(D) Elastase
(E) Myelin

49. A 69-year-old woman diagnosed with rheumatoid arthritis is being given antimetabolite therapy with methotrexate. Her physician explains to her that she can expect the greatest toxicity of the drug to cells with the shortest G_1 phase. Which cell has the shortest G_1 phase?

(A) Hepatocyte
(B) Intestinal mucosal cell
(C) Neuron
(D) Oocyte in the adult female
(E) RBC

50. A group of investigators is studying the effect that a protein has on DNA. They isolate the protein by running it on electrophoresis gel. They remove the portion of gel with the protein and purify the protein. They transfer the protein to nitrocellulose paper and expose it to a labeled DNA probe. Which of the following laboratory techniques does this describe?

(A) Enzyme-linked immunosorbent assay
(B) Northern blot
(C) Polymerase chain reaction
(D) Sequencing
(E) Southern blot
(F) Southwestern blot
(G) Western blot

1. **The correct answer is A.** Fabry's disease is an X-linked recessive disease caused by a deficiency in the enzyme α-galactosidase A, which results in the accumulation of ceramide trihexoside. This accumulation leads to pain and angiokeratomas, and the deposition of ceramide trihexoside in the vascular endothelium leads to cardiac, cerebral, and vascular involvement.

   Answer B is incorrect. Galactocerebroside accumulation occurs in Krabbe's disease as a result of galactosylceramide α-galactosidase deficiency. It causes optic atrophy, spasticity, and early death via deposition of the intermediary in the brains of affected patients.

   Answer C is incorrect. Glucocerebroside accumulation occurs in Gaucher's disease as a result of a deficiency in β-glucocerebrosidase, which leads to glucocerebroside accumulation in the brain, liver, spleen, and bone marrow.

   Answer D is incorrect. Lactosyl cerebroside is the end product of conversion of ceramide trihexoside via α-galactosidase A and is deficient in patients with Fabry's disease.

   Answer E is incorrect. Sphingomyelin and cholesterol buildup in reticuloendothelial and parenchymal cells and tissues occurs in Niemann-Pick disease and is the result of a deficiency in sphingomyelinase. Patients typically die by age 3 years.

2. **The correct answer is B.** Citrate, formed from oxaloacetate and acetyl CoA by the enzyme citrate synthase, inhibits phosphofructokinase and allosterically activates acetyl CoA carboxylase. Citrate synthase regenerates a molecule of CoA and is an important regulator of the tricarboxylic acid cycle. It is inhibited by adenosine triphosphate.

   Answer A is incorrect. α-Ketoglutarate is not an important regulator of the tricarboxylic acid cycle, but it is an important intermediate in protein metabolism.

   Answer C is incorrect. Malate is not an important regulator of the tricarboxylic acid cycle, but it is important in the malate shuttle.

   Answer D is incorrect. Oxaloacetate is not an important regulator of the tricarboxylic acid cycle, but it is important in glyconeogenesis.

   Answer E is incorrect. Succinyl-CoA downregulates its own synthesis by inhibiting the enzyme responsible for dehydrogenation of α-ketoglutarate.

3. **The correct answer is E.** This scenario describes nephrogenic diabetes insipidus, which is pathology at the antidiuretic hormone receptor in the kidney. This receptor is the V_2 receptor.

   Answer A is incorrect. The adenohypophysis is not related to the pathology of diabetes insipidus.

   Answer B is incorrect. D_1 receptors are not involved in nephrogenic diabetes insipidus.

   Answer C is incorrect. This is nephrogenic, not central, diabetes insipidus.

   Answer D is incorrect. The V_1 receptor is involved in vascular smooth muscle contraction.

4. **The correct answer is A.** Alkaptonuria is a condition corresponding to the one described in the stem. Due to a lack of the enzyme homogentisic acid oxidase, it leads to deposition of homogentisic acid in the joints and cartilage, giving them a dark color (ochronosis) and resulting in degenerative changes. Classically, the urine of these patients turns black on contact with air or when the urine is made alkaline. The associated defect is on chromosome 3.

   Answer B is incorrect. Ankylosing spondylitis is a condition associated with sacroiliac arthritis and eventual loss of mobility in the spine (bamboo spine). It is not associated with black urine or darkened cartilage.

Answer C is incorrect. Maple syrup urine disease is a metabolic disorder of autosomal recessive inheritance that affects the metabolism of branched-chain amino acids (leucine, isoleucine, and valine) and causes the urine of affected patients to smell like maple syrup. The urine does not, however, turn black upon standing. The disease is not classically associated with arthritis in middle-aged individuals.

Answer D is incorrect. Phenylketonuria is a congenital deficiency of phenylalanine hydroxylase. It is associated with mental retardation and with the presence of phenylketones in the urine (which do not classically turn black upon standing).

Answer E is incorrect. Rheumatoid arthritis (RA) is a condition characterized by symmetrical polyarticular synovitis. It causes destructive arthritis as a result of pannus formation on joint cartilage and typically presents with fatigue, lack of appetite, low-grade fever, muscle and joint aches, and stiffness. Muscle and joint stiffness are usually most notable in the morning and after periods of inactivity, and arthritis is common during disease flares. During flares, joints frequently become red, swollen, painful, and tender. The vignette does not rule out the possibility of this being RA. However, the dark urine and dark ear cartilage make alkaptonuria, while a rarer condition, the more likely diagnosis.

5. **The correct answer is B.** Lane B represents the Southern blot of a heterozygous carrier of sickle cell anemia. The β-A-globin gene results in a 1.15-kb fragment of DNA cut by the MstII restriction enzyme. The β-S-globin gene results in a 1.35-kb band because the single basepair mutation responsible for sickle cell anemia eliminates an MstII restriction site.

Answer A is incorrect. The band in lane A is from a sickle cell anemia patient with two copies of the β-S-globin gene. This gene results in a 1.35-kb band because the single basepair mutation responsible for sickle cell anemia eliminates an MstII restriction site.

Answer C is incorrect. The band in lane C is from an unaffected patient with two copies of the β-A-globin gene. The gene results in a 1.15-kb fragment of DNA cut by the MstII restriction enzyme.

Answer D is incorrect. The bands in lane D could not result from any patient. The labeled DNA probe does not bind to the 0.2-kb DNA fragment and therefore would not be visualized on the Southern blot.

Answer E is incorrect. The bands in lane E could not result from any patient. The labeled DNA probe does not bind to the 0.2-kb DNA fragment and therefore would not be visualized on the Southern blot.

Answer F is incorrect. The bands in lane F could not result from any patient. The labeled DNA probe does not bind to the 0.2-kb DNA fragment and therefore would not be visualized on the Southern blot.

6. **The correct answer is C.** The key to answering this question correctly is an understanding that phosphatidylcholine is formed by donation of methyl groups. Methionine is the only amino acid listed that can donate methyl groups. Its activated form, S-adenosyl-L-methionine is a very common methyl group donor.

Answer A is incorrect. Asparagine is an essential amino acid with a negative charge. It can serve as a hydrogen ion recipient.

Answer B is incorrect. Histidine is an essential amino acid with a positive charge. It can serve as a hydrogen ion donor.

Answer D is incorrect. Threonine is an essential amino acid with an uncharged polar side chain. It contains a hydroxy group that can serve as a hydrogen ion donor or recipient.

Answer E is incorrect. Valine is an essential amino acid with a hydrocarbon side chain; however, it is not a methyl group donor.

7. **The correct answer is E.** The calcium-calmodulin complex activates myosin light chain kinase, which phosphorylates myosin and allows it to bind to actin, leading to contraction and shortening of the muscle fiber.

Answer A is incorrect. In smooth muscle, unlike skeletal muscle, there is no troponin. Instead, calcium is the regulator of myosin on the thick filament.

Answer B is incorrect. Actin is not phosphorylated or dephosphorylated in the contraction and relaxation cycle of smooth muscle.

Answer C is incorrect. The calcium-calmodulin complex activates myosin light chain kinase, which phosphorylates myosin. Myosin light chain phosphatase removes the phosphate group from myosin.

Answer D is incorrect. Actin is not phosphorylated or dephosphorylated in the contraction and relaxation cycle of smooth muscle.

8. **The correct answer is B.** This question describes gel electrophoresis. Gel electrophoresis uses an electric field to separate molecules based on their sizes. The negatively charged DNA migrates in the electric field toward the positive end. Smaller fragments move more rapidly through the gel. Bands of DNA can be visualized by staining the gel with dyes such as ethidium bromide.

Answer A is incorrect. Enzyme-linked immunosorbent assay (ELISA) is an immunologic technique used in laboratories to determine whether a particular antibody is present in a patient's blood. Labeled antibodies are used to detect whether the serum contains antibodies against a specific antigen precoated on an ELISA plate. This is not the technique described above.

Answer C is incorrect. Northern blots are similar to Southern blots except that in Northern blotting, mRNA is separated by electrophoresis instead of DNA. This is not the technique described above.

Answer D is incorrect. Polymerase chain reaction is a laboratory technique used to produce many copies of a segment of DNA. In this procedure, DNA is mixed with two specific primers, deoxynucleotides and a heat-stable polymerase. The solution is heated to denature the DNA and is then cooled to allow synthesis. Twenty cycles of heating and cooling

amplify the DNA over a million times. This is not the procedure described above.

Answer E is incorrect. Sequencing is a laboratory technique that utilizes dideoxynucleotides to randomly terminate growing strands of DNA. Gel electrophoresis is used to separate the varying lengths of DNA. The DNA sequence can then be read based on the position of the bands on the gel. This is not the technique described above.

Answer F is incorrect. In a Southern blot procedure, DNA is separated with electrophoresis, denatured, transferred to a filter, and hybridized with a labeled DNA probe. Regions on the filter that base-pair with the labeled DNA probes can be identified when the filter is exposed to film that is sensitive to the radio-labeled probe. This is not the technique described above.

Answer G is incorrect. In a Western blot procedure, protein is separated by electrophoresis and labeled antibodies are used as a probe. This technique can be used to detect the existence of an antibody to a particular protein.

9. **The correct answer is A.** Calcium is maintained in high concentrations outside the cell and within discrete compartments within the cell (i.e., mitochondria). Free intracellular calcium can activate several enzymes whose cumulative effect is to induce significant cell injury. A few important enzyme classes include ATPases, which decrease ATP supply; phospholipases, which decrease membrane stability; endonucleases, which induce DNA damage; and several proteases.

Answer B is incorrect. Free radical generation is a common mechanism of cell injury, but calcium excess does not induce free radical generation.

Answer C is incorrect. Activation of proteases and phospholipases induces the breakdown of necessary components of cell membranes.

Answer D is incorrect. ATP depletion, resulting from the activation of ATPases, can also contribute to the inhibition of glycolysis.

Answer E is incorrect. Inhibition of oxidative phosphorylation is an effect of ATP depletion caused by enzyme activation. Although this may contribute to cell damage, it is not the best answer.

10. **The correct answer is D.** Compounds A and B are both microbial surface components recognizing adhesive matrix molecules (MSCRAMM) receptor antagonists and competitive inhibitors to the endogenous ligand. Because they are competitive inhibitors of the receptor, the two compounds will have an equal or lower Michaelis-Menten constant (K_m) for the receptor than the endogenous compound. In addition, the K_m of compound A will be lower than that of compound B because compound A has a higher affinity for the receptor than compound B.

    Answer A is incorrect. Acetaminophen overdose can cause hepatic toxicity.

    Answer B is incorrect. Competitive inhibitors do not change the maximum reaction rate of the enzyme.

    Answer C is incorrect. Competitive inhibitors do not change the maximum reaction rate of the enzyme.

    Answer E is incorrect. Given that compounds A and B have different affinities for the receptor, their Michaelis-Menten constant values cannot be the same.

11. **The correct answer is A.** Acute intermittent porphyria (AIP) is a blood disorder caused by a deficiency of uroporphyrinogen I synthetase. ∂-Aminolevulinic acid and porphobilinogen are found in the urine. Patients often present with hyponatremia and recurrent episodes of abdominal pain and can even develop neuropsychiatric problems. Barbiturates (among other drugs) and starvation diets can precipitate attacks. Patients with AIP do not have the cutaneous photosensitivity seen in other porphyrias.

    Answer B is incorrect. Factor V Leiden deficiency is a relatively common coagulopathy associated with hypercoagulability. People with

factor V Leiden deficiency have a fivefold increased risk of thrombosis. This condition could cause painful episodes, but such episodes would be the result of thrombophlebitis and would present with swollen, painful, and red extremities.

Answer C is incorrect. Fanconi's anemia is an autosomal recessive disorder in which DNA repair is defective. This results in aplastic anemia and defective DNA. Patients are at increased risk of malignancy. Abdominal pain and hyponatremia are not hallmarks of this illness.

Answer D is incorrect. Hereditary spherocytosis is an autosomal dominant disorder of the erythrocyte structural protein spectrin. The defective membrane causes erythrocytes to be culled in the spleen. While some patients may develop an anemia, abdominal pain, hyponatremia, and porphobilinogen in the urine are not observed.

Answer E is incorrect. Sickle cell disease is an autosomal recessive disease characterized by a point mutation in the β-globin chain. While painful episodes (crises) are frequent in sickle cell disease, it is not classically associated with hyponatremia or barbiturates. Additionally, urine porphobilinogen levels are normal in sickle cell disease.

12. **The correct answer is A.** This woman suffers from β-thalassemia major, a condition caused by absence of both β chains. Clinically, β-thalassemia major manifests as severe hemolysis and ineffective erythropoiesis. These individuals are transfusion-dependent and frequently develop iron overload. The consequences of iron overload due to transfusion dependency or secondary hemochromatosis are described in the question stem. These manifestations are due to iron deposition in various tissues, including the pancreas, heart, and skin.

Answer B is incorrect. Absence of α chains describes the most severe form of α-thalassemia. In this form, no functional α chains are made, and the fetus is unable to make any functional hemoglobin aside from the γ_4 tetramer, also called Hb Barts. Hb

Barts's high oxygen affinity results in poor oxygen delivery to peripheral tissues and ultimately congestive heart failure, anasarca, and intrauterine fetal death.

Answer C is incorrect. This answer describes hereditary hemochromatosis, a condition caused by iron overload due to an intrinsic defect in the body's ability to control the absorption of iron. Iron overload in hemochromatosis is not due to transfusions, and the laboratory picture is not characterized by hemolysis. Otherwise, the clinical manifestations are the same for both genetic and secondary hemochromatosis.

Answer D is incorrect. Hereditary spherocytosis (HS) is caused by mutations in either the ankyrin or the spectrin gene, both of which contribute to the erythrocyte cytoskeleton. HS is caused by erythrocytes with abnormal membranes passing through the spleen; the reticuloendothelial cells remove pieces of the membrane causing spherocyte formation. This condition is characterized by extravascular hemolysis. Clinical manifestations include gallstones, anemia, jaundice, and splenomegaly.

Answer E is incorrect. Failure of copper to enter the circulation in the form of ceruloplasmin, resulting in copper accumulation in the liver, brain, and cornea, is also known as Wilson's disease. Clinically, Wilson's disease is characterized by parkinsonian symptoms, Kayser-Fleischer rings, asterixis, and dementia. Laboratory studies demonstrate low ceruloplasmin. Heart failure, diabetes, and skin changes, as well as the hematologic manifestations of β-thalassemia, are not associated with Wilson's disease.

13. **The correct answer is E.** Spinal muscular atrophy (SMA) is one of the most common autosomal recessive diseases, affecting approximately 1 in 10,000 live births. It has a carrier frequency of approximately 1 in 50 and is characterized by symmetric proximal muscle weakness due to the degeneration of the anterior horn cells of the spinal cord. SMA is classically divided into three subtypes based on age of onset and clinical severity. Type I SMA (Werdnig-Hoffmann disease) is characterized by the onset of severe muscle weakness and hypotonia in the first few months of life and the inability to sit or walk. Fatal respiratory failure usually occurs before the age of 2 years. Muscle biopsy demonstrates large numbers of atrophic fibers that involve entire fascicles (panfascicular atrophy). Unlike SMA types II and III, this patient's disease developed at an early age, so early milestones were not achieved. This is not the case in the less severe forms of SMA.

Answer A is incorrect. Becker's muscular dystrophy involves the same genetic locus that is affected in Duchenne's muscular dystrophy (DMD), but its occurrence is less common than DMD. It follows a more indolent course, with onset often occurring in late childhood; many patients have nearly normal life spans.

Answer B is incorrect. Duchenne's muscular dystrophy (DMD) and Becker's muscular dystrophy (BMD) are both characterized by defects in the 427-kDa protein dystrophin, encoded on the Xp21 region. DMD is the most common form of muscular dystrophy, with an incidence of about 1 in 3500 live births. Onset typically occurs after infancy and before age 5 years. The clinical course is characterized by progressive muscle weakness and wasting that lead to wheelchair dependence by 10–12 years of age. Early motor milestones are met in patients with BMD and DMD.

Answer C is incorrect. Type III spinal muscular dystrophy, or Kugelberg-Welander disease, is characterized by the onset of proximal muscle weakness after the age of 2 years, the ability to walk independently until the disease progresses, and survival into adulthood.

Answer D is incorrect. Type II spinal muscular dystrophy is characterized by the onset of proximal muscle weakness before 18 months of age, the ability to sit but not to walk unaided, and survival beyond 4 years of age.

14. **The correct answer is B.** This patient likely has a defect of glucose transporter 1, which transports glucose across the blood-brain barrier. A family of glucose transporters (GLUT 1–5) is responsible for cellular uptake in many cell types. However, enterocytes and nephrons

acquire glucose through cotransport with sodium ion.

Answer A is incorrect. Adipocytes primarily use GLUT4 for glucose transport. GLUT4 is the transporter most affected by insulin.

Answer C is incorrect. Erythrocytes largely contain GLUT1.

Answer D is incorrect. Hepatocytes primarily contain GLUT2, the same transporter found in pancreatic beta cells. This transporter is especially important for equilibrating calcium inside and outside of the cell.

Answer E is incorrect. Myocytes also use GLUT4 for glucose transport.

Answer F is incorrect. Pancreatic beta cells contain GLUT2 transporters. This transporter is especially important for equilibrating calcium inside and outside of the cell.

15. **The correct answer is D.** Polymerase chain reaction (PCR) and sequencing can be used to determine if this woman and/or her husband is a carrier of the cystic fibrosis gene. PCR is used to amplify the region of interest, and sequencing is used to see if the CF mutation is present.

Answer A is incorrect. Enzyme-linked immunosorbent assay is an immunologic technique used in laboratories to determine whether a particular antibody is present in a patient's blood. This test cannot be used to determine whether the woman and her husband are carriers for the cystic fibrosis gene.

Answer B is incorrect. Gel electrophoresis uses an electric field to separate molecules based on their sizes. Gel electrophoresis cannot be used alone to determine whether the woman and her husband are carriers for the cystic fibrosis gene.

Answer C is incorrect. Northern blots test RNA levels. It cannot be used to determine whether the woman and her husband are carriers for the cystic fibrosis gene.

Answer E is incorrect. A Western blot is a test for the presence or absence of a protein. This test cannot be used to determine whether the

woman and her husband are carriers for the cystic fibrosis gene.

16. **The correct answer is A.** The equilibrium constant, or K_{eq}, of the reaction is: adenosine diphosphate + phosphorus → ATP. The reaction, which is catalyzed by the enzyme Fi/Fo ATPase in mitochondria, tends to go to the left; thus the forward reaction requires the energy of the proton gradient to produce ATP. Lacking this gradient, the reaction will proceed in the direction of K_{eq}, or negative free energy—that is, ATP consumption.

Answer B is incorrect. The free energy of any reaction at standard conditions is a constant.

Answer C is incorrect. The redox potential of oxygen at standard conditions is a constant.

Answer D is incorrect. The redox potential of reduced nicotinamide adenine dinucleotide at standard conditions is a constant.

Answer E is incorrect. Cristae are infoldings within mitochondria. The number of infoldings is not altered by changes in the proton gradient.

17. **The correct answer is A.** Vancomycin is an antibiotic that is effective only in fighting gram-positive cocci. It binds tightly to a cell wall precursor that contains the amino acid sequence D-ala D-ala and prevents cell wall synthesis. Resistance to vancomycin is transferred via plasmids and encodes enzymes that convert D-ala D-ala to D-ala D-lac, preventing vancomycin from binding. This type of resistance is seen in *Enterococcus faecium* but not in the more common *Enterococcus faecalis*.

Answer B is incorrect. D-ala D-leu is not seen in the bacterial wall precursor.

Answer C is incorrect. Wild-type *Enterococcus* species have a cell wall precursor containing D-ala D-ala, which is the binding site for vancomycin. After acquiring resistance, D-ala D-lac is substituted for D-ala D-ala, rendering the bacterium resistant.

Answer D is incorrect. D-ala D-leu is not seen in the bacterial wall precursor.

Answer E is incorrect. D-ala D-leu is not seen in the bacterial wall precursor.

18. **The correct answer is C.** Kartagener's syndrome, or immotile cilia, is caused by a defect in dynein that prevents effective movement of cilia. The full syndrome is characterized by sinusitis, bronchiectasis, situs inversus, and male infertility. Cilia play an important role in moving mucus along the airway and clearing debris; the absence of this function contributes to the pulmonary findings of the syndrome. Cilia are also very important for leukocyte movement and phagocytosis. Without functioning cilia, one would expect this patient to have ineffective phagocytosis, which contributes to these patients' frequent infections.

    Answer A is incorrect. Defective chloride transport is the cause of cystic fibrosis. Cystic fibrosis frequently causes bronchiectasis, but it is not associated with situs inversus.

    Answer B is incorrect. Patients with diabetes are predisposed to developing chronic fungal sinusitis. However, the bronchiectasis and situs inversus are not consistent with diabetes.

    Answer D is incorrect. Mucus plugging in reactive airway disease can cause atelectasis at the lung bases. On an x-ray film of the chest of a patient with reactive airway disease, one would expect hyperinflated lungs with areas of atelectasis, not bronchiectasis.

    Answer E is incorrect. Tetralogy of Fallot is a congenital heart defect, but is not associated with infections or cardiac inversion. Patients with this condition develop early cyanosis because of the malformed right-to-left shunt. The four components of the teratology are (1) ventricular septal defect, (2) overriding aorta, (3) infundibular pulmonary stenosis, and (4) right ventricular hypertrophy.

19. **The correct answer is E.** This child is suffering from an inherited form of hyperammonemia as a result of a defect in ornithine transcarbamoylase. This enzyme is a component of the urea cycle that is responsible for combining carbamoyl phosphate and ornithine to make citrulline. As a result, the patient has an excess of ammonia in circulation, which leads to mental retardation, seizures, and ultimately death. Some patients with ornithine transcarbamoylase deficiency also exhibit a very low blood urea nitrogen, but this is not enough to make a conclusive diagnosis.

    Answer A is incorrect. Arginase is the enzyme (found predominantly in the liver) that converts arginine into urea and ornithine. A defect in this enzyme would affect later steps of the urea cycle and would result in an accumulation of citrulline.

    Answer B is incorrect. A defect in argininosuccinate lyase would result in elevated citrulline levels.

    Answer C is incorrect. Carbamoyl phosphate synthetase (CPS) I is a component of the urea cycle, and combines carbon dioxide and ammonia to form carbamoyl phosphate. CPS II, however, is an enzyme in the pyrimidine synthesis pathway and would not result in hyperammonemia if deficient.

    Answer D is incorrect. Glutamate dehydrogenase is the enzyme responsible for the conversion of glutamate to α-ketoglutarate in the liver. A defect in this enzyme would result in low levels of ammonia.

20. **The correct answer is D.** Grandchild D is a carrier for the disease. She has inherited the mutant gene from her father and a copy of the normal gene from her mother.

    Answer A is incorrect. Grandchild A has inherited two copies of the mutant gene from her parents, who are both carriers. She is affected by the disease.

    Answer B is incorrect. Grandchild B has inherited two copies of the normal gene from her parents. She is unaffected by the disease.

    Answer C is incorrect. Grandchild C has inherited two copies of the mutant gene from her parents. She is affected by the disease.

    Answer E is incorrect. Grandchild E has inherited two copies of the normal gene from her parents. She is unaffected by the disease.

21. **The correct answer is D.** The patient's symptoms are consistent with those of seasonal allergies. The patient has experienced asthma, eczema, and allergies and most likely suffers from atopy. Seasonal allergies are a result of histamine$_1$-receptor activation, which results in pruritus, bronchoconstriction, and increased nasal and bronchial mucus production. Seasonal allergy symptoms can be treated with antihistamines such as loratadine, which are histamine$_1$-antagonists.

Answer A is incorrect. Activation of α_1 receptors results in vasoconstriction and increased blood pressure. α_1 Receptors are primarily found in blood vessel walls and are not associated with allergies.

Answer B is incorrect. Activation of β_1 receptors leads to inotropy and chronotropy. β_1 Receptors are typically located in the heart, and stimulation of the receptors results in increased contractility (inotropy) and heart rate (chronotropy).

Answer C is incorrect. Activation of β_2 receptors leads to vasodilation and bronchodilation. β_2 Receptors are primarily located in blood vessel walls and in the respiratory tract. Drugs that antagonize β_2 receptors are used in the treatment of asthma.

Answer E is incorrect. Activation of histamine$_2$ receptors leads to increased gastric acid production. Histamine$_2$ receptors are located in the stomach, and drugs that antagonize histamine$_2$ receptors are used to treat gastroesophageal reflux disease and peptic ulcer disease.

22. **The correct answer is B.** This patient has Pompe's disease, a glycogen storage disorder. Pompe's disease is an autosomal recessive disease that is characterized by a deficiency or defect in lysosomal α-1,4-glucosidase. This enzyme is necessary for the dissolution of the polymer linkages in glycogen. In its absence, glycogen accumulates to toxic levels in both the cytoplasm and lysosomes.

Answer A is incorrect. Glucose is stored as glycogen in the cells and is also present in blood. However, hyperglycemia is not responsible for the symptoms observed in this patient.

Answer C is incorrect. Oxaloacetate is the first intermediate in the Krebs cycle. It is regenerated with each turn of the cycle but is not present in excessive amounts in the cell.

Answer D is incorrect. Pyruvate is a component of the cellular respiration pathway and an intermediate in gluconeogenesis. It is not stored in cells in any significant quantity.

Answer E is incorrect. Disorders of the urea cycle leading to nitrogen accumulation in the body can result in progressive lethargy and coma but generally do not cause the myopathy observed in this patient.

23. **The correct answer is B.** Glucokinase is found in liver and pancreatic β cells. It catalyzes the initial step of glycolysis, phosphorylation of glucose to glucose-6-phosphate, which is catalyzed by hexokinase in other tissues. Both enzymes are found in the liver. Glucokinase has a higher Michaelis-Menten constant and a higher maximum reaction rate (V_{max}) than hexokinase, which means it has a lower affinity for substrate but processes it faster. At low glucose levels, hexokinase, with its higher affinity for glucose, processes it to glucose-6-phosphate. At higher glucose levels, hexokinase is overwhelmed—operating at its low V_{max}—and sufficient substrate is available for glucokinase to process the excess glucose even with its low affinity. Glucokinase thus helps to handle large increases in glucose from the gut.

Answer A is incorrect. The hepatocyte cell membrane is permeable to glucose, which is trapped in the cell after phosphorylation.

Answer C is incorrect. Glucokinase is not inhibited by glucose-6-phosphate.

Answer D is incorrect. Insulin- and glucose-rich diets increase glucokinase levels.

Answer E is incorrect. Glucokinase has a relatively high Michaelis-Menten constant.

24. **The correct answer is C.** Type I dyslipidemia is caused by a deficiency of lipoprotein lipase.

This enzyme exists in capillary walls of adipose and muscle tissue and cleaves triglycerides into free fatty acids and glycerol. The enzyme is activated by apolipoprotein C-II, which is found on VLDL and chylomicrons. Type I dyslipidemia is characterized by an accumulation of triglyceride-rich lipoproteins in the plasma. It can also occur with an alteration in apolipoprotein C-II.

Answer A is incorrect. VLDL remnants are removed from the circulation by apolipoprotein E receptors. Thus, apolipoprotein E deficiency results in a decreased efficiency of that clearance and elevated VLDL, triglyceride, and cholesterol levels. Dysbetalipoproteinemia often only manifests with additional factors that cause hyperlipidemia such as diabetes. Xanthomas are often present.

Answer B is incorrect. LDL receptor dysfunction is characteristic of familial hyperbetalipoproteinemia, also known as type II hyperlipidemia. In these cases, plasma LDL levels rise, which causes an increase in plasma cholesterol; triglyceride levels remain normal.

Answer D is incorrect. Mixed hypertriglyceridemia (type V) is a dyslipidemia characterized by extremely high triglyceride levels and visibly foamy plasma. Unlike type I, type V is characterized by elevated VLDL levels and is thought to be related to a VLDL clearance problem.

Answer E is incorrect. VLDL overproduction is another characteristic of type V dyslipidemias, as well as type IIb combined hyperlipidemia.

25. **The correct answer is D.** This patient's long airplane flight placed her at an increased risk of developing deep venous thrombosis (DVT). In addition, the patient has a positive Homans' sign (calf pain on dorsiflexion), which is seen in some patients with a DVT. Virchow's triad refers to three factors that predispose a patient to developing a venous thrombosis: (1) local trauma to the vessel wall, (2) stasis, and (3) hypercoagulability. Thromboxane A_2 stimulates platelet aggregation and vasoconstriction and will be elevated at the site of a clot.

Answer A is incorrect. Leukotrienes (LT)C_4, LTD_4, and LTE_4 are bronchoconstrictors that are believed to contribute to symptoms of asthma. 5-Lipoxygensase is the enzyme that converts arachidonic acid to 5-hydroperoxy-eicosatetraenoic acid, which is then used to produce leukotrienes.

Answer B is incorrect. Prostaglandin I_2 (PGI_2) is synthesized by vascular endothelium and smooth muscle. Its effects include inhibition of platelet aggregation, relaxation of smooth muscle, reduction of systemic and pulmonary vascular resistance by direct vasodilation, and natriuresis in kidney. Thus, PGI_2 is not abundant locally at the site of a deep venous thrombosis because it does not promote platelet aggregation.

Answer C is incorrect. Renin is a circulating enzyme released mainly by the kidneys in response to low blood volume or low body NaCl content. Renin activates the renin-angiotensin system by cleaving angiotensinogen in the liver to produce angiotensin I. Angiotensin I is then further converted into angiotensin II in specialized lung capillaries, ultimately leading to constriction of blood vessels, an increase in ADH and aldosterone production, and stimulation of the hypothalamus to activate the thirst reflex, leading in turn to increased blood pressure.

Answer E is incorrect. Vascular endothelial growth factor (VEGF) is a substance made by cells that stimulates new blood vessel formation. The binding of VEGF turns on the receptors, which then generate signals inside the cell, ultimately leading to the growth of new blood vessels. Although this growth factor may be elevated at the site of the clot, it is not as abundant as thromboxane A_2.

26. **The correct answer is B.** This patient has adult polycystic kidney disease, an autosomal dominant condition characterized by massive bilateral cysts in the kidneys as well as the liver. The renal cysts can eventually lead to end-stage renal disease. In addition to the cysts, patients are more prone to berry aneurysms, which can rupture and lead to strokes.

Answer A is incorrect. Astrocytomas are seen in patients with tuberous sclerosis, an autosomal dominant disorder affecting tuberin and hamartin proteins that regulate cellular growth and differentiation.

Answer C is incorrect. Dark urine can be seen in patients with alkaptonuria, a congenital deficiency of homogentisic acid oxidase, which is needed in the degradative pathway of tyrosine.

Answer D is incorrect. Optic nerve degeneration can be seen in Leber's hereditary optic neuropathy, a condition in which patients develop a rapid loss of central vision.

Answer E is incorrect. Squamous cell carcinoma is seen in increased incidence in patients with xeroderma pigmentosum, an autosomal recessive disease caused by a deficiency in DNA repair of thymine dimers.

27. **The correct answer is C.** The 50S ribosomal subunit is the larger of the two ribosomal macromolecules. Its main function in translation is the creation of a new peptide bond between the incoming aminoacyl-tRNA and the growing peptide chain. Essential for this purpose is the 23S rRNA molecule, which holds the peptidyl transferase enzyme activity.

Answer A is incorrect. The 50S subunit is responsible for the creation of the peptide bond, but the molecule that accomplishes this activity is the 23S rRNA strand, not proteins. If all proteins are removed, the peptidyl transferase activity remains intact.

Answer B is incorrect. Streptomycin is an aminoglycoside antibiotic that binds to the 30S subunit and disrupts formation of the initiation complex. Aminoglycosides are bactericidal and used to treat gram-negative rod infections. Major adverse effects include nephrotoxicity and ototoxicity, especially when combined with cephalosporins and loop diuretics, respectively.

Answer D is incorrect. The A site of the ribosome is the binding site for the incoming aminoacyl-tRNA complexes, whereas the P site refers to the binding site for the elongating peptide chain (which is still bound to the aminoacyl-tRNA of the 30′ amino acid). While the 50S subunit has moieties that interact with

each site, the 30S subunit contains the major binding sites for each.

Answer E is incorrect. The *initiation complex* is the term used to describe the complex of macromolecules necessary for the onset of translation. The complex is composed of the 30S subunit, an aminoacyl-tRNA bound to N-formylmethionine, and initiation factors. The 50S subunit is not part of the initiation complex.

28. **The correct answer is C.** The knockout mouse model described exhibits a phenotype consistent with impaired function of all of the hypothalamic hormones with the exception of corticotropin-releasing hormone (CRH). The hypothalamus produces a number of important hormones, including trophic hormone–releasing hormone, that act on the anterior pituitary; these include thyrotropin-releasing hormone and gonadotropin-releasing hormone as well as hormones to be stored and released in the posterior pituitary, such as ADH and oxytocin. All of the hypothalamic hormones exert their actions on target cells via a phospholipase C (PLC) intracellular signaling cascade with inositol trisphosphate (IP_3) as the second messenger, with the exception of CRH, which acts via adenylate cyclase–cAMP. Thus, the PLC-IP_3 signaling system is the most likely target of the gene knockout described in the vignette. Important nonhypothalamic hormones that also act via this signaling system include angiotensin II and α_1-adrenergic agonists.

Answer A is incorrect. cAMP is the second-messenger molecule for the signaling systems that mediate the mechanisms of corticotropin-releasing hormone, luteinizing hormone, follicle-stimulating hormone, thyroid-stimulating hormone, human chorionic gonadotropin, ADH (V2 receptor), parathyroid hormone, calcitonin, glucagon, and β_2-, α_1-, and α_2-adrenergic agonists.

Answer B is incorrect. cGMP is the second-messenger molecule for the signaling systems that mediate the mechanisms of atrial natriuretic peptide, endothelium-derived relaxing factor, and nitrous oxide.

Answer D is incorrect. Steroid nuclear hormone receptors are the second-messenger molecules that mediate the mechanisms of aldosterone, glucocorticoids, testosterone, estrogen, progesterone, thyroid hormones, and 1,25-dihydroxycholecalciferol (vitamin D).

Answer E is incorrect. Tyrosine kinases are the second-messenger molecules that mediate the mechanisms of insulin, insulin-like growth factor-1, prolactin, and growth hormone.

29. **The correct answer is A.** Hemoglobin carries oxygen better when it is in the relaxed form, in which it has a higher affinity for oxygen. As a result, the oxygen dissociation curve shifts to the left and decreased unloading of oxygen results. Conversely, tightening hemoglobin decreases its affinity for oxygen. Hemoglobin in the taut form is stabilized by all the processes that result in increased oxygen unloading. Binding of CO_2 stabilizes the taut form, which decreases oxygen affinity.

Answer B is incorrect. 2,3-Bisphosphoglycerate (2,3-BPG) binds to a pocket formed by the two β subunits. It can only bind when they are close together, such as in the taut form. Its binding holds the hemoglobin in this fashion and prevents oxygen binding and promotes unloading. It is essential to add inosine to stored blood for transfusions to prevent the loss of 2,3-BPG, which would make transfused blood an oxygen "trap" in peripheral tissues.

Answer C is incorrect. Binding of oxygen molecules is the major cause of the shift of hemoglobin from its T structure to R. The oxygen molecule disrupts the weak polar bonds and "opens up" the molecule for more oxygen to bind.

Answer D is incorrect. The Bohr effect comes from an increase in protons, which subsequently stabilize the T form of hemoglobin preferentially. In addition, an increase in protons means an increase in CO_2 because of the bicarbonate buffer present in blood. Remember, though, that increasing the pH means a decrease in protons.

Answer E is incorrect. CO stabilizes the R form of hemoglobin so that the dissociation curve shifts dramatically to the left.

30. **The correct answer is D.** Like steroid hormones, this drug is binding to a cytosolic receptor. The complex then travels to the nucleus, where it acts on DNA to increase the transcription of LDL cholesterol receptor mRNA, which can be translated to LDL cholesterol receptors.

Answer A is incorrect. Allosteric regulation involves the binding of a drug to a protein and either increasing or decreasing the activity of that protein.

Answer B is incorrect. Antagonism of a cell surface receptor would not result in increased transcription of LDL cholesterol receptors.

Answer C is incorrect. Many drugs bind to G-protein–coupled receptors (GPCRs) located at the cell surface. This binding would then set in motion a secondary messenger system that could result in increased transcription of LDL cholesterol receptors. However, steroids and the drug described above do not work by a GPCR-mediated mechanism.

Answer E is incorrect. Proteolytic modification involves the cleavage of a zymogen into an active enzyme. This would not explain the increased synthesis of LDL cholesterol receptor.

31. **The correct answer is D.** Hypoparathyroidism can occur if all of the parathyroid glands are accidentally removed during total thyroidectomy. Hypoparathyroidism can lead to hypocalcemia and hyperphosphatemia. Symptoms of hypocalcemia include tingling of the lips and digits and muscle spasms.

Answer A is incorrect. Acromegaly is caused by an excess of growth hormone in adults. It is not a side effect of thyroidectomy.

Answer B is incorrect. *Cretinism* is the term used for fetal hypothyroidism. Cretinism can be caused by either a defect in thyroxine formation or failure of thyroid development.

Answer C is incorrect. Hypertension can occur from a variety of mechanisms; however, thyroidectomy is not a cause.

Answer E is incorrect. Renal osteodystrophy occurs in patients with renal failure. The failing kidney retains phosphate, leading to hyper-phosphatemia and subsequent hypocalcemia; hypocalcemia causes a secondary hyperparathyroidism, which is the basis for the bone pathology.

32. **The correct answer is E.** In the second experiment, B2 is in excess and will avidly bind E2; less C and less D will be made in the second experiment. With less D produced, there will be less feedback inhibition of A.

    Answer A is incorrect. The amount of C produced in a set time interval will be decreased in the second experiment as compared to the first, since B2 is a partial agonist, will bind E2 better than B, and functions at a decreased V_{max}.

    Answer B is incorrect. The amount of D produced in a set time interval will be decreased in the second experiment as compared to the first, since B2 is a partial agonist of E2, will bind E2 better than B, and functions at a decreased V_{max}.

    Answer C is incorrect. Enzymes are neither consumed nor produced by reactions they catalyze.

    Answer D is incorrect. Enzymes are neither consumed nor produced by reactions they catalyze.

33. **The correct answer is E.** The new drug works by stabilizing the mitotic spindle and preventing the microtubules from depolymerizing. This mechanism of action is similar to that of paclitaxel, which also prevents microtubule depolymerization. The overly stable microtubules that are formed are dysfunctional, thereby causing the death of the cell. Paclitaxel is primarily used to treat advanced ovarian cancer and metastatic breast cancer.

    Answer A is incorrect. Bleomycin works by intercalating DNA. It is a mixture of different copper-chelating glycopeptides that cause scission of DNA by an oxidative process. Bleomycin is used in the treatment of testicular tumors, lymphomas, and squamous cell carcinomas. Its characteristic toxicity is pul-

monary, which progresses from rales, cough, and infiltrate, to fibrosis.

Answer B is incorrect. Cyclophosphamide is a DNA alkylator that is activated by cytochrome P-450. The most characteristic toxicity of this drug is hemorrhagic cystitis, which can be prevented through adequate hydration and intravenous injection of mesna before the administration of cyclophosphamide.

Answer C is incorrect. 5-Fluorouracil (5-FU) is an antimetabolite that does not affect metaphase. It is a pyrimidine analog with a stable fluorine atom in place of a hydrogen atom at position 5 of the uracil ring. The fluorine interferes with the conversion of deoxyuridylic acid to thymidylic acid. 5-FU is used to treat slow-growing solid tumors such as breast, ovarian, pancreatic, colorectal, and gastric carcinomas.

Answer D is incorrect. Methotrexate is an inhibitor of dihydrofolate reductase, the enzyme that converts folic acid to tetrahydrofolic acid, its active coenzyme form. Methotrexate is effective against acute lymphocytic leukemia, choriocarcinoma, Burkitt's lymphoma, breast cancer, and head and neck carcinomas.

34. **The correct answer is F.** Threonine is one of the essential amino acids, along with leucine, lysine, isoleucine, phenylalanine, tryptophan, methionine, valine, arginine, and histidine. Note that arginine and histidine are essential only during periods of growth, such as during infancy or pregnancy.

Answer A is incorrect. Alanine is not an essential amino acid.

Answer B is incorrect. Cysteine is not an essential amino acid.

Answer C is incorrect. Glutamine is not an essential amino acid.

Answer D is incorrect. Proline is not an essential amino acid.

Answer E is incorrect. Serine is not an essential amino acid.

Answer G is incorrect. Tyrosine is not an essential amino acid.

35. **The correct answer is C.** Vitamin B_{12} deficiency is frequently seen in the elderly and can be caused by pernicious anemia, bacterial overgrowth, chronic alcoholism, or decreased dietary intake. Vitamin B_{12}, like folate deficiency, causes megaloblastic anemia and a low reticulocyte count. The WBCs are affected as well and neutrophils show hypersegmented nuclei often with six or more lobes, as shown on the blood smear above. Two features distinguish folate deficiency from vitamin B_{12} deficiency: the presence of neurologic symptoms and elevated methymalonic acid levels are seen in the latter, but not in the former. Vitamin B_{12} deficiency causes a defect in myelin formation by an unknown mechanism. The patient experiences subacute combined degeneration of the posterior and lateral spinal columns that presents as paresthesias and ataxia because of loss of position and vibration sense. If untreated, neurological symptoms can progress to weakness, spasticity, clonus, and paraplegia. Because treatment with vitamin B_{12} is needed to prevent the development of neurological symptoms, vitamin B_{12} deficiency must not be confused with folate deficiency. Elevated methylmalonic acid levels in the serum are a sign of vitamin B_{12} deficiency, not folate deficiency.

Answer A is incorrect. Folic acid deficiency also causes macrocytic anemia but does not increase methylmalonic acid levels and does not cause neurological symptoms. If this patient's lab work had shown macrocytic anemia, hypersegmented neutrophils, but normal methymalonic acid levels, folic acid deficiency would have been suspected and no neurological symptoms would be anticipated.

Answer B is incorrect. Niacin (vitamin B_3) deficiency causes pellagra. Pellagra is the triad of diarrhea, dermatitis, and dementia. The patient described above does not have any of those symptoms.

Answer D is incorrect. Thiamine deficiency can cause beriberi and Wernicke-Korsakoff syndrome. The symptoms of beriberi include dilated cardiomyopathy, edema, and polyneuritis. The polyneuritis of beriberi is a peripheral neuropathy that causes foot drop or wrist drop.

Answer E is incorrect. Thiamine (vitamin B_1) deficiency causes both beriberi and Wernicke-Korsakoff syndrome. Frequently seen in alcoholics, Wernicke-Korsakoff syndrome is characterized by confusion, confabulation, and ataxia. All alcoholics brought into the hospital are treated with glucose and thiamine to prevent the development of this syndrome.

36. **The correct answer is D.** Microtubules are involved in the transport of vesicles down the axons of neurons. Microtubules are made of polymerized tubulin. The microtubule is made up of two subunits, α and β, that polymerize to form a hollow tubule. Two attachment proteins, dynein and kinesin, attach to membranous organelles and move along the tubules toward and away from the cell center.

Answer A is incorrect. Actin is polymerized to form actin filaments, which are found in the contractile apparatus of skeletal muscle. Two strings of beadlike actin subunits are twisted together like a rope to form an actin filament. The globular actin subunits are stabilized by calcium ions.

Answer B is incorrect. Intermediate filaments of muscle cells are made up primarily of desmin.

Answer C is incorrect. Intermediate filaments are cytoskeletal elements that are prominent in cells that withstand stress. Intermediate filaments of epithelial cells are composed primarily of keratin.

Answer E is incorrect. Vimentin is polymerized to form intermediate filaments that are found in cells of mesodermal origin, such as fibroblasts.

37. **The correct answer is C.** I-cell disease is caused by a failure of addition of mannose-6-phosphate, an intracellular signal sequence, to lysosomal proteins, leading to an inappropriate

release of those proteins into the extracellular space. Thus, lysosomal enzymes, including hexosaminidase, iduronate sulfatase, and aryl-sulfatase A, will be found in the extracellular space, but not intracellularly. I-cell disease is characterized by skeletal abnormalities, restricted joint movement, coarse facial features, and severe psychomotor impairment. Death usually occurs by the age of 8 years.

Answer A is incorrect. Apolipoprotein B-48 mediates the extracellular secretion of chylomicrons.

Answer B is incorrect. Collagen is an extracellular molecule. Procollagen has a specific extracellular signal sequence at its N-terminal end. Faulty collagen synthesis can lead to many diseases including scurvy, osteogenesis imperfecta, and Ehlers-Danlos syndrome.

Answer D is incorrect. Rough endoplasmic reticulum (RER) typically translates proteins meant for extracellular use. The RER in I-cell disease is not abnormal.

Answer E is incorrect. Sphingomyelinase is a lysosomal enzyme that is deficient in Niemann-Pick disease. This is an autosomal recessive disease characterized by progressive neurodegeneration, hepatosplenomegaly, and cherry red spot on the macula.

38. **The correct answer is E.** Congenital albinism is often due to a deficiency in tyrosinase, the enzyme needed for converting tyrosine to melanin. Hereditary forms can be autosomal dominant or autosomal recessive. Albinism can also result from altered neural crest migration, but this is not an option included among the answer choices. Albinos are at increased risk for skin cancer because the melanin pigment that normally absorbs ultraviolet radiation is lacking.

Answer A is incorrect. Acetaldehyde dehydrogenase converts acetaldehyde to acetate. A person lacking this enzyme will get very sick from buildup of acetaldehyde following ethanol consumption. This plays no role in pigmentation.

Answer B is incorrect. A dietary deficiency is not an established cause of congenital albinism.

Answer C is incorrect. Although phenylalanine can be converted to tyrosine, decreased dietary phenylalanine does not have a substantial effect on melanin levels, as tyrosine itself can be obtained by dietary means. This is also not a congenital cause of albinism.

Answer D is incorrect. Tryptophan hydroxylase converts tryptophan to serotonin and is not related to pigmentation.

39. **The correct answer is B.** Obstructive liver disease refers to the obstruction of intrahepatic and/or extrahepatic bile ducts with subsequent cholestasis and liver injury. This entity commonly presents with jaundice, conjugated hyperbilirubinemia, increased urine bilirubin, and decreased urine urobilinogen. The majority of bilirubin results from the breakdown of heme groups in senescent erythrocytes. After cellular release, bilirubin binds to albumin, which delivers the molecule to the liver. Hepatocellular uptake and glucuronidation in the endoplasmic reticulum generate conjugated bilirubin, which is water-soluble and readily excreted in bile. Gut bacteria deconjugate the bilirubin and degrade it to urobilinogens. The urobilinogens are excreted in the feces, with some reabsorption and excretion into urine. Based on this metabolic schema, the laboratory values in obstructive liver disease become evident. Thus, compromised excretion of conjugated bilirubin results in conjugated hyperbilirubinemia, an increase in urine bilirubin, and a decrease in urine urobilinogen.

Answer A is incorrect. Conjugated hyperbilirubinemia, increased urine bilirubin, and normal urine urobilinogen can be seen in patients with hepatocellular jaundice and not usually with obstructive jaundice. Since little conjugated bilirubin is excreted in obstructive jaundice, urine urobilinogen concentration should be low.

Answer C is incorrect. Unconjugated hyperbilirubinemia, increased urine bilirubin, and decreased urine urobilinogen can occur with hepatocellular disease if there is also concurrent conjugated hyperbilirubinemia. However, a purely obstructive condition is not characterized by unconjugated hyperbilirubinemia.

Answer D is incorrect. Unconjugated hyperbilirubinemia, decreased urine bilirubin, and increased urine urobilinogen is a classic pattern seen in hemolytic jaundice. However, none of these changes is consistent with obstructive liver disease.

Answer E is incorrect. Conjugated hyperbilirubinemia, decreased urine bilirubin, and decreased urine urobilinogen are very unlikely to occur simultaneously in any given condition.

40. **The correct answer is E.** This question describes sequencing. Sequencing is a laboratory technique that utilizes dideoxynucleotides to randomly terminate growing strands of DNA. Gel electrophoresis is used to separate the varying lengths of DNA. The DNA sequence can then be read based on the position of the bands on the gel.

Answer A is incorrect. Allele-specific oligonucleotide probes are short, labeled DNA sequences complementary to an allele of interest. These probes can be used to detect the presence of disease-causing mutations.

Answer B is incorrect. Enzyme-linked immunosorbent assay (ELISA) is an immunologic technique used to determine whether a particular antibody is present in a patient's blood. Labeled antibodies are used to detect whether the serum contains antibodies against a specific antigen precoated on an ELISA plate. This is not the technique described above.

Answer C is incorrect. Northern blots are similar to Southern blots except that in Northern blotting, mRNA is separated by electrophoresis instead of DNA. This is not the technique described above.

Answer D is incorrect. Polymerase chain reaction is a laboratory technique used to produce many copies of a segment of DNA. In the pro-

cedure, DNA is mixed with two specific primers, deoxynucleotides and a heat-stable polymerase. The solution is heated to denature the DNA and then cooled to allow synthesis. Twenty cycles of heating and cooling amplify the DNA over a million times. This is not the procedure described above.

Answer F is incorrect. In a Southern blot procedure, DNA is separated with electrophoresis, denatured, transferred to a filter, and hybridized with a labeled DNA probe. Regions on the filter that base-pair with the labeled DNA probes can be identified when the filter is exposed to film that is sensitive to the radio-labeled probe. This is not the technique described above.

Answer G is incorrect. In a Western blot procedure, protein is separated by electrophoresis and labeled antibodies are used as a probe. This technique can be used to detect the existence of an antibody to a particular protein.

41. **The correct answer is C.** Symptoms of severe epigastric pain radiating to the back, nausea, and vomiting, combined with risk factors such as chronic alcohol use and gallstones, are suggestive of acute pancreatitis. Increases in serum lipase and amylase confirm the diagnosis. Pathologically, acute pancreatitis is marked by necrosis and inflammation of the pancreatic tissue. Based on anatomic evidence of pancreatic injury, the most likely mechanism leading to acute pancreatitis is thought to be an inappropriate activation of pancreatic enzymes. There is evidence for three possible pathways by which activation of pancreatic enzymes is initiated. One possibility is pancreatic duct obstruction resulting from cholelithiasis, ampullary obstruction, or chronic alcoholism. Acinar cell injury caused by alcohol, drugs, trauma, ischemia, or viruses can also result in enzymatic activation. Finally, defective intracellular transport secondary to alcohol, duct obstruction, or metabolic injury is another possible cause of inappropriate enzyme activation.

Answer A is incorrect. Exhaustion of enzyme reserve may be a consequence of multiple injuries to the pancreas, sometimes seen in patients with chronic pancreatitis. However, it is not a mechanism responsible for acute pancreatitis.

Answer B is incorrect. A hyperactive renin-angiotensin system commonly occurs in congestive heart failure or prerenal failure; however, it is not a mechanism responsible for acute pancreatitis.

Answer D is incorrect. Inappropriate pancreatic enzyme deactivation is not a mechanism responsible for acute pancreatitis.

Answer E is incorrect. pH alteration of the surrounding milieu is not a mechanism responsible for acute pancreatitis.

42. **The correct answer is D.** This child has phenylketonuria (PKU) due to a defect of tetrahydrobiopterin metabolism, due to a deficiency of either phenylalanine hydroxylase or (less frequently) tetrahydrobiopterin cofactor. Patients therefore cannot convert phenylalanine to tyrosine. If the defect is a tetrahydrobiopterin deficiency, the patient needs supplementation with tetrahydrobiopterin in addition to a low-phenylalanine, high-tyrosine diet. Excess phenylalanine leads to a buildup of phenylketones. Children with untreated PKU display mental and growth retardation, fair skin, eczema, and a musty body odor.

Answer A is incorrect. A diet free of branched-chain amino acids is used to treat maple syrup urine disease (MSUD). MSUD is caused by a deficiency of α-ketoacid dehydrogenase. Untreated patients present with lethargy, seizures, failure to thrive, mental retardation, and urine that smells like maple syrup.

Answer B is incorrect. Low-fructose diets are used to treat hereditary fructose intolerance, an autosomal recessive inherited disease due to a deficiency of aldolase B, causing an accumulation of fructose-1-phosphate. This accumulation decreases the available phosphate, leading to inhibition of gluconeogenesis and glycogenolysis. Patients present with jaundice, cirrhosis, and hypoglycemia after ingestion of fructose.

Answer C is incorrect. A ketogenic diet will not help this patient with PKU. Diets high in ketogenic nutrients (high in fats) are used as treatment for pyruvate dehydrogenase deficiency.

Answer E is incorrect. Low-tyrosine diets are used for the treatment of type II tyrosinemia, a disorder in which patients are unable to completely metabolize tyrosine. Patients present with mental retardation and eye and skin lesions.

43. **The correct answer is A.** This child suffers from severe combined immunodeficiency (SCID). In 3 months, she has been diagnosed with a number of severe infections with unusual pathogens common in immunocompromised individuals (*Pneumocystis carinii* and *Candida albicans*). She also demonstrates failure to thrive, as evidenced by her growth charts. There are a variety of genetic causes of SCID; however, approximately 20% of cases (1 in 200,000 live births) are attributed to a deficiency of adenosine deaminase. The enzyme is a component of the purine salvage system, and its absence ultimately leads to an inability to complete DNA synthesis in B and T cells.

Answer B is incorrect. Hexokinase is the first enzyme in the glycolytic pathway. It converts glucose to glucose-6-phosphate but is not affected in severe combined immunodeficiency.

Answer C is incorrect. Phenylalanine hydroxylase is the enzyme that converts phenylalanine to tyrosine. It is deficient in patients with phenylketonuria but is not implicated in severe combined immunodeficiency.

Answer D is incorrect. Pyruvate dehydrogenase is a component of cellular respiration. It converts pyruvate into acetyl CoA in preparation for entry into the Krebs cycle. However, it is not affected in severe combined immunodeficiency.

Answer E is incorrect. Ribonucleotide reductase is the enzyme that converts ribonucleosides to deoxyribonucleosides. It is also a component of the purine salvage pathway but is not affected in severe combined immunodeficiency.

44. **The correct answer is E.** Steroid hormones enter cells and bind to receptor proteins. The receptor-hormone complex binds to specific response elements, or the regulatory region of DNA, and activates gene transcription.

   Answer A is incorrect. Steroid hormones do not regulate the initiation of protein synthesis.

   Answer B is incorrect. Steroid hormones do not regulate mRNA degradation.

   Answer C is incorrect. Steroid hormones do not regulate mRNA processing.

   Answer D is incorrect. Steroid hormones regulate gene transcription, not translation.

45. **The correct answer is A.** This patient has factor V Leiden thrombophilia, an inherited condition that predisposes patients to thromboses, especially those in unusual locations (e.g., the mesenteric veins), those suffered at an early age (before age 50), and repeated thrombotic events (superficial and/or deep). Heterozygous patients have a slightly increased risk of thrombotic events, while homozygous individuals are at a significantly increased risk.

   Answer B is incorrect. Familial hypercholesterolemia leads to increased levels of LDL cholesterol, thereby increasing the risk of atherosclerosis, myocardial infarction, and stroke.

   Answer C is incorrect. People with Fanconi's anemia have a pancytopenia that causes increased incidence of infections, anemia, fatigue, and bleeding.

   Answer D is incorrect. Von Hippel–Lindau syndrome is characterized by abnormal blood vessel growth leading to angiomas and hemangioblastomas in the retina, brain, and spinal cord as well as in other regions of the body.

   Answer E is incorrect. Von Willebrand's deficiency causes prolonged bleeding time, which manifests as increased bleeding after trauma or surgery, nosebleeds, and hematomas.

46. **The correct answer is D.** Fructose-1-phosphate → dihydroxyacetone-phosphate + glyceraldehyde. This reaction is catalyzed by aldolase B. If there is a deficiency in aldolase B,

the reactant fructose-1-phosphate accumulates in the liver. This depletes the liver's stores of free phosphate, which is necessary for the creation of ATP. Thus, aldolase B deficiency causes a fall in ATP production. Fructokinase deficiency produces an elevation of fructose in the body and does not affect essential processes such as ATP production.

   Answer A is incorrect. ATP will not be increased, because much of the free phosphate needed to combine with adenosine diphosphate to form ATP is already bound to fructose.

   Answer B is incorrect. Phosphate will be sequestered as fructose-1-phosphate, and the amount of free circulating phosphate will fall.

   Answer C is incorrect. This occurs with fructokinase deficiency.

   Answer E is incorrect. If aldolase B is deficient, the end product of the fructokinase pathway will be great, and this will feedback-inhibit the activity of fructokinase.

47. **The correct answer is B.** This patient suffers from methemoglobinemia, which may be due to a variety of causes, including a hereditary deficiency of the reduced form of nicotinamide adenine dinucleotide or a structurally abnormal hemoglobin. The oxidized form of hemoglobin (Fe^{3+}) does not bind oxygen effectively. Methylene blue has been shown to increase the conversion of Fe^{3+} back to Fe^{2+}.

   Answer A is incorrect. Atropine, an antimuscarinic, has several clinical applications, including the treatment of anticholinesterase and organophosphate toxicity.

   Answer C is incorrect. N-Acetylcysteine is used to treat acetaminophen toxicity, most likely by reducing the effects of toxic metabolites.

   Answer D is incorrect. Naloxone is an opioid antagonist that is used to reverse the effects of any opioid or to treat an opioid overdose.

   Answer E is incorrect. Protamine is used to reverse the effects of heparin. Protamine is a positively charged molecule that works by binding to negatively charged heparin.

48. **The correct answer is C.** This baby was born prematurely, and therefore his lungs have not fully developed. Type II pneumocytes in the lungs are responsible for secreting surfactant (dipalmitoyl phosphatidylcholine). Additionally, a lecithin:sphingomyelin ratio of less than 2.0 is associated with a greater risk of neonatal respiratory distress syndrome. This baby is showing signs of neonatal respiratory distress syndrome due to the lack of surfactant.

Answer A is incorrect. Collagen is an important part of the connective tissues in lungs. However, it is not associated with neonatal respiratory distress syndrome.

Answer B is incorrect. Cisplatin (as well as other platinum-based chemotherapeutics) is used in the treatment of testicular, ovarian, and lung cancers.

Answer D is incorrect. Elastase is an endogenous proteolytic enzyme in the lung that is normally broken down by α_1-antitrypsin. In patients with α_1-antitrypsin deficiency, however, there is an increased level of elastase, which leads to lung tissue destruction and emphysema.

Answer E is incorrect. Myelin is synthesized by Schwann cells. It is layered onto nerves and helps speed up the transmission of electrical impulses down a nerve. Destruction of myelin has been implicated in neurodegenerative diseases such as multiple sclerosis.

49. **The correct answer is B.** A cell with the shortest G_1 phase is a cell that is rapidly dividing, as is the case with a mucosal cell of the intestine. Neurons and myocytes replicate relatively slowly as compared to mucosal cells. The oocyte in the adult female does not undergo mitosis at all, nor does the RBC.

Answer A is incorrect. Hepatocytes do not ordinarily replicate rapidly unless part of the liver is removed, prompting hepatic regeneration.

Answer C is incorrect. Neurons replicate extremely slowly and would not have a long G_1 phase.

Answer D is incorrect. Oocytes of the adult female do not undergo mitosis. Spermatocytes of the adult male do.

Answer E is incorrect. RBCs do not divide.

50. **The correct answer is F.** This question describes a Southwestern blot. In a Southwestern blot procedure, protein is separated by electrophoresis and labeled DNA is used as a probe. This technique can be used to detect protein-DNA interactions such as those with transcription factors.

Answer A is incorrect. Enzyme-linked immunosorbent assay (ELISA) is an immunologic technique used in laboratories to determine whether a particular antibody is present in a patient's blood. Labeled antibodies are used to detect whether serum contains antibodies against a specific antigen precoated on an ELISA plate. This is not the technique described above.

Answer B is incorrect. Northern blots are similar to Southern blots except that in Northern blotting, mRNA is separated by electrophoresis instead of DNA. This is not the technique described above.

Answer C is incorrect. Polymerase chain reaction is a laboratory technique used to produce many copies of a segment of DNA. In this procedure, DNA is mixed with two specific primers, deoxynucleotides and a heat-stable polymerase. The solution is heated to denature the DNA and is then cooled to allow synthesis. Twenty cycles of heating and cooling amplify the DNA over a million times. This is not the procedure described above.

Answer D is incorrect. Sequencing is a laboratory technique that utilizes dideoxynucleotides to randomly terminate growing strands of DNA. Gel electrophoresis is used to separate the varying lengths of DNA. The DNA sequence can then be read based on the position of the bands on the gel. This is not the technique described above.

Answer E is incorrect. In a Southern blot procedure, DNA is separated with electrophoresis, denatured, transferred to a filter, and hybridized with a labeled DNA probe. Regions on the filter that base-pair with the labeled DNA probes can be identified when the filter is exposed to film that is sensitive to the radiolabeled probe. This is not the procedure described above.

Answer G is incorrect. In a Western blot procedure, protein is separated by electrophoresis and labeled antibodies are used as a probe. This technique can be used to detect the existence of an antibody to a particular protein.

CHAPTER 3

Embryology

QUESTIONS

1. A baby boy dies 2 days after birth. He was born with wrinkled skin, deformed limbs, and abnormal facies. The mother's pregnancy was complicated by oligohydramnios. Which of the following embryologic processes most likely failed in this child?

   (A) Development of dermis
   (B) Development of the kidneys
   (C) Fusion of maxillary and medial nasal prominences
   (D) Migration of neural crest cells to the distal colon
   (E) Outgrowth of limb buds

2. Immediately following delivery, a newborn is observed to have multiple abnormalities, including a small lower jaw, abnormal feet, and hands that are clenched into fists. Despite supportive therapy for a congenital heart condition, the baby dies before 1 year of age. What is the likely etiology of the patient's condition?

   (A) CAG tandem repeats
   (B) Deletion of chromosome 21
   (C) Translocation 15;17
   (D) Trisomy of chromosome 18
   (E) X chromosome fragility

3. A newborn infant is found to have a congenital urethral abnormality in which the urethral meatus opens on the ventral side of the penis, resulting in difficulty directing the urine stream and ventral curvature of the penis. Which of the following is the cause of this malformation?

   (A) Failure of urethral fold fusion
   (B) Failure of urethrorectal septum formation
   (C) Maldevelopment of the urinary sphincters
   (D) Short urethra
   (E) Urethral stricture

4. A neonate is found to have strong, bounding pulses in both upper extremities and carotids, but her femoral pulses are very weak. She is diagnosed with coarctation of the aorta and is taken to surgery to correct the defect. Subsequent follow-up examinations show no further heart abnormalities. Sixteen years later, the patient is noted to have poorly developed secondary sexual characteristics, including persistent, nonprogressive Tanner stage 2 breast and pubic hair development. She has not experienced menarche. Which of the following would most likely be found in this patient?

   (A) Decreased estrogen levels
   (B) Normal ovaries
   (C) Patent ductus arteriosus
   (D) Simian crease
   (E) 46,XY karyotype

5. A newborn boy is brought to the pediatrician for further evaluation of an extensive skin rash. Physical examination shows that this child has microcephaly, hearing loss, and a petechial skin rash. The abdominal examination reveals hepatosplenomegaly. Further questioning of the infant's mother reveals that she had "the flu" early in her pregnancy. A tissue sample from the infant is sent for culture, which confirms the diagnosis. Which of the following is the correct diagnosis?

   (A) Congenitally acquired cytomegalovirus
   (B) Congenitally acquired Epstein-Barr virus
   (C) Congenitally acquired herpes simplex virus
   (D) Congenitally acquired HIV
   (E) Congenitally acquired syphilis

6. A 13-month-old child is brought to the emergency department after his parents found blood in his stool. They state that he did not appear distressed at the time, although he now displays some tenderness to abdominal pressure. Other than this tenderness, there are no significant findings on physical examination. After performing radionuclide imaging using ^{99m}Tc pertechnetate, the doctor makes a diagnosis and recommends surgery to correct the problem. What is the probable source of this child's condition?

   (A) Blockage of the intestine due to folding of the distal ileum into the proximal colon

(B) Breakdown of the stomach mucosal barrier with erosion of the underlying mucosa

(C) Damage to the intestinal epithelium due to ingestion of coins

(D) Ectopic gastric epithelium in a persistent omphalomesenteric duct

(E) Incomplete bowel rotation resulting in obstruction of the superior mesenteric artery

7. The accompanying image shows the gross pathology of a congenital condition. Which of the following is the most common cause of death in infants with this condition?

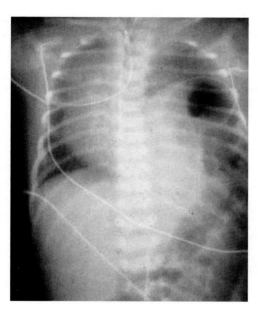

Image courtesy of PEIR Digital Library (http://peir.net).

(A) Cardiac tamponade

(B) Mediastinal shift

(C) Pulmonary hypoplasia

(D) Renal agenesis

(E) Small bowel obstruction

8. An infant girl presents with cyanosis 4 hours after birth. A physician diagnoses her with a condition that develops due to a failure of neural crest cell migration that results in a nonspiraling aorticopulmonary septum. A careful interview of the mother reveals that she has a disease that predisposed her child to this congenital condition. Which of the following

collections of symptoms is this infant's mother most likely experiencing?

(A) Arachnodactyly, hyperextensible joints, and aortic aneurysm

(B) Cold intolerance, delayed reflexes, constipation

(C) Megaloblastic anemia without neurologic symptoms

(D) Mild fever with a descending maculopapular rash and clear buccal mucosa

(E) Polydipsia, polyuria, and blurred vision

9. Spermatogenesis, the process of forming spermatozoa, occurs in the seminiferous tubules. As the cells proceed through the different stages of spermatogenesis, they contain varying numbers of chromosomes and varying amounts of DNA. Spermiogenesis describes a particular stage of spermatogenesis. When the cells are going through spermiogenesis, which of the following is the amount of DNA and the number of chromosomes that exist in those cells?

(A) 23, 1n

(B) 23, 2n

(C) 46, 1n

(D) 46, 2n

(E) 46, 4n

10. In an experimental model designed to study the process of limb development, a researcher removes the distal end of one upper limb and one lower limb just after limb bud formation. This manipulation is performed such that the apical ectodermal ridge on each of these limbs is completely obliterated. Which of the following is the expected effect of the removal of the apical ectodermal ridge on these limbs relative to the unaffected limbs?

(A) Extended length with aberrant anterior-posterior patterning

(B) Normal length with aberrant anterior-posterior patterning

(C) Normal length with aberrant digit development

(D) Normal length with aberrant dorsal-ventral patterning

(E) Shortened length with aberrant dorsal-ventral patterning

11. A 1-week-old infant presents with a urachal fistula, which occurs when the allantois fails to regress. Normally, the allantois and urachus regress to form a specific structure in the fully matured neonate. Which of the following is the mature structure derived from the fetal allantois and urachus?

    (A) Ligamentum arteriosum
    (B) Ligamentum teres hepatis
    (C) Ligamentum venosum
    (D) Medial umbilical ligament
    (E) Median umbilical ligament
    (F) Nucleus pulposus

12. The pancreas is derived from two elements of the foregut: the ventral pancreatic bud and the dorsal pancreatic bud. The ventral bud is responsible for part of the head, the uncinate process, and one other structure. Which of the following is the additional structure formed from the ventral pancreatic bud?

    (A) Body of the pancreas
    (B) Isthmus of the pancreas
    (C) Main pancreatic duct
    (D) Pancreatic acinar cells
    (E) Pancreatic islet cells
    (F) Tail of the pancreas

13. A baby is born to a 42-year-old mother. The baby has wide-spaced eyes, epicanthal folds, and simian creases. Eye examination reveals small white spots on the peripheral iris, and cytogenetic testing shows an extra autosomal chromosome. Which of the following is associated with the patient's most likely condition?

    (A) Acquired cardiac valvular disease
    (B) Chronic lymphocytic leukemia
    (C) Duodenal atresia
    (D) High IQ
    (E) Pick's disease

14. A full-term neonate presents to the pediatrician with failure to pass meconium. Digital examination of the rectum results in a gush of retained fecal material. Which of the following is the most likely diagnosis in this infant?

    (A) Carcinoma of the colon
    (B) Chagas' disease

    (C) Hirschsprung's disease
    (D) Imperforate anus
    (E) Necrotizing enterocolitis

15. A 5-year-old girl is brought to her pediatrician because her mother says she is frequently running into stationary objects when playing. Blood work reveals low levels of thyroid hormone and cortisol. A visual field examination shows bilateral peripheral vision defects. A CT scan of the head revealed calcifications in the pituitary fossa. The pediatrician tells the mother that the cause of her child's symptoms is a brain tumor of embryological origins. Which of the following is most likely this child's diagnosis?

    (A) Craniopharyngioma
    (B) Ependymoma
    (C) Hemangioblastoma
    (D) Medulloblastoma
    (E) Pituitary adenoma

16. Ensuring adequate maternal intake of a specific nutrient is especially important in reducing the incidence of the congenital anomaly shown in the image. A deficiency of this nutrient in the adult is associated with which of the following conditions?

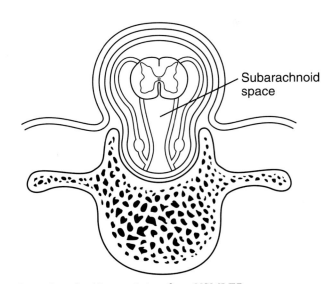

Subarachnoid space

Reproduced, with permission, from USMLERx.com.

    (A) Confabulation and anterograde amnesia
    (B) Diarrhea, dermatitis, and dementia

(C) Megaloblastic anemia with neurologic symptoms

(D) Megaloblastic anemia without neurologic symptoms

(E) Microcytic anemia

(F) Polyneuritis and cardiac pathology

(G) Swollen and bleeding gums, easy bruising, and poor wound healing

17. A 5-year-old boy presents to his pediatrician with dyspnea on exertion. His mother says that when he exercises, he becomes slightly blue and breathes unusually heavily. Physical examination reveals central cyanosis and a systolic murmur over the left upper sternal border. A subsequent echocardiogram shows a ventricular septal defect, hypertrophy of the right ventricle, and an overriding aorta. Which of the following embryologic defects underlies this condition?

(A) Anterosuperior displacement of the aorticopulmonary septum

(B) Incomplete expansion and division of the bronchial tree

(C) Incomplete formation of the tracheoesophageal septum

(D) Incomplete fusion of the right bulbar ridge, the left bulbar ridge, and the AV cushions

(E) Nonspiral development of the aorticopulmonary septum

18. The eye is a complex organ and, as such, has complex embryologic origins. Which of the following is the only structure in the eye that is derived exclusively from surface ectoderm?

(A) Choroid

(B) Cornea

(C) Extraocular muscles

(D) Iris epithelium

(E) Lens

(F) Retina

(G) Sclera

19. A physician is asked to evaluate a 5-year-old girl who has developed a mass in her neck. During the interview, he learns that the mass has appeared within the last few months and has been enlarging; however, it causes no pain or discomfort. The mass is in the midline of the neck just below the hyoid bone. Laboratory tests reveal a triiodothyronine level of 150 ng/dL, a thyroxine level of 8.0 g/dL, and a thyroid-stimulating hormone level of 10 U/mL. A CT scan of the neck is performed and the doctor recommends surgery. What is the most likely diagnosis?

(A) Branchial cleft cyst

(B) Dermoid cyst

(C) Ectopic thyroid gland

(D) Enlarged pyramidal lobe of the thyroid

(E) Lipoma

(F) Thyroglossal duct cyst

20. As part of the routine physical examination, physicians typically evaluate palatal elevation by asking the patient to "say ah." The muscles used to perform palatal elevation are derived from which of the following embryologic structures?

(A) Branchial arches 1 and 2

(B) Branchial arches 3 and 4

(C) Branchial arches 4 and 6

(D) Branchial clefts 1 and 2

(E) Branchial pouches 3 and 4

21. A 26-year-old woman learns she is pregnant shortly after discontinuing isotretinoin (13-cis-retoinic acid). During which period of development should this woman be most concerned about fetal teratogen exposure?

(A) Conception

(B) Weeks 1 and 2 of gestation

(C) Weeks 3–8 of gestation

(D) Weeks 8–10 of gestation

(E) After the 10th week of gestation

22. A 3-week-old boy presents to his pediatrician because his mother has noticed that he "looks yellow." On questioning, she elaborates that the jaundice began several days after birth and has been associated with dark urine and acholic stools. Laboratory studies show a direct bilirubin level of 5.0 mg/dL and a total bilirubin level of 5.5 mg/dL. Which of the following is the most likely diagnosis?

    (A) Congenital extrahepatic biliary atresia
    (B) Crigler-Najjar syndrome type I
    (C) Gilbert syndrome
    (D) Hereditary spherocytosis
    (E) Physiological jaundice

23. Over the course of embryologic development, the predominant location of hematopoiesis changes several times. Where does this process take place during the 11th week of fetal life?

    (A) Bone marrow
    (B) Gastric fundus
    (C) Pancreas
    (D) Liver
    (E) Yolk sac

24. A 6-year-old boy who was born prematurely presents to his pediatrician because his mother says that he tires easily. She also notes that he has had several respiratory infections. On examination, the boy is noted to be below the fifth percentile in height; jugular venous pressure is elevated; and a continuous "machine-like" murmur is heard over the left upper sternal border. The congenital anomaly responsible for these signs and symptoms produces which of the following patterns of blood flow in fetal life?

    (A) It shunts blood from the inferior vena cava to the aorta
    (B) It shunts blood from the left pulmonary artery to the aorta
    (C) It shunts blood from the left ventricle to the right ventricle
    (D) It shunts blood from the portal vein to the inferior vena cava
    (E) It shunts blood from the right atrium to the left atrium

25. A 6-month-old boy presents to the pediatrician with congenital hearing loss that the physician determines is the result of the mother's contracting a rubella infection in the eighth week of her pregnancy. Which of the following is the embryologic origin of the hearing structure that is damaged by congenital rubella infection?

    (A) Auricular hillocks
    (B) First pharyngeal (branchial) arch
    (C) Optic cup
    (D) Saccular portion of the otic vesicle
    (E) Second pharyngeal (branchial) arch

1. **The correct answer is B.** The presentation described here is consistent with Potter's syndrome, or bilateral renal agenesis. The failure of both kidneys to develop leads to oligohydramnios because the fetus cannot excrete urine into the amniotic sac. This in turn allows compression of the fetus by the uterine wall, leading to limb deformities, abnormal facies, and wrinkly skin. Death occurs shortly after birth unless an appropriate donor is found.

Answer A is incorrect. A failure of development of the dermis would not present with oligohydramnios or deformed limbs, but rather with skin abnormalities.

Answer C is incorrect. This describes the etiology of cleft lip, which does not cause oligohydramnios or wrinkly skin and is compatible with life.

Answer D is incorrect. This describes the defect in Hirschsprung's disease, which results in failure to pass meconium and in constipation, but does not share any of the symptoms in this scenario.

Answer E is incorrect. A problem with limb bud growth would not produce abnormal facies or oligohydramnios.

2. **The correct answer is D.** This newborn has Edwards' syndrome, or trisomy 18. Affected children are born with clenched fists, rocker-bottom feet, micrognathia (a small lower jaw), congenital heart disease, and mental retardation. The survival rate of less than 1 year is similar to that of trisomy 13 (Patau's syndrome), from which it should be distinguished.

Answer A is incorrect. CAG tandem repeats are found in Huntington's disease, among others. Huntington's disease is characterized by degeneration of the caudate and putamen, leading to choreiform (dancelike) movements, but not the birth defects found in this patient.

Answer B is incorrect. A deletion of chromosome 21 may cause physical deformity, but clenched fists and rocker-bottom feet are classic for trisomy 18.

Answer C is incorrect. This translocation is often found in acute promyelocytic leukemia but is not classically associated with the findings in this child.

Answer E is incorrect. This is fragile X syndrome. Associated with CGG tandem repeats, this syndrome is characterized by mental retardation, a large jaw, and large testes. Children with fragile X syndrome typically survive beyond 1 year of age.

3. **The correct answer is A.** The malformation described is hypospadias, resulting from incomplete union of the urethral folds. In the male, the urethral folds form the ventral aspect of the penis. In the female, the urethral folds develop into the labia minora.

Answer B is incorrect. Congenital failure of urethrorectal septum formation results in an abnormal communication between the urethra and the rectum. Clinical signs include feces in the urine. This is not a cause of hypospadias.

Answer C is incorrect. In males, the proximal portion of the urethra forms from the urogenital sinus. The distal urethra is formed by ectoderm that is canalized to form the navicular fossa. If the sphincters do not form properly, urethral incompetence and incontinence result.

Answer D is incorrect. A short urethra causes chordee, or poorly developed penis with ventral curvature, without hypospadias.

Answer E is incorrect. Urethral stricture causes urethral obstruction and is the second most common cause of incontinence in older men. It is not a cause of hypospadias.

4. **The correct answer is A.** The patient has Turner's syndrome, which is associated with coarctation of the aorta. Turner's patients often present in adolescence with amenorrhea, and a diagnostic workup shows a 45,XO karyotype. Turner's syndrome patients have poor development of secondary sexual characteristics and are infertile.

Answer B is incorrect. Turner's syndrome patients have rudimentary ovaries; sexual ducts and external genital structures appear normal but are very immature. When examined histologically at or after birth, the ovaries are found to be long, pale streaks of tissue devoid of primordial follicles. Early in gestation the ovaries appear normal and contain primordial germ cells, but after the third month, numbers become severely reduced, and in most patients oocytes are not present after birth. These patients are therefore infertile and do not naturally progress through puberty.

Answer C is incorrect. Turner's syndrome is not associated with a patent ductus arteriosus (PDA). Furthermore, in the vignette the patient's cardiac examination is normal. With a PDA, the patient would have a continuous machinelike murmur.

Answer D is incorrect. A simian crease is commonly seen in Down's syndrome (trisomy 21). It is not seen in Turner's syndrome.

Answer E is incorrect. Patients with Turner's syndrome have a 45,XO karyotype. In androgen insensitivity syndrome (testicular feminization), a genetically male patient can be phenotypically female; however, this is not the case with Turner's syndrome.

5. **The correct answer is A.** This is a case of congenitally acquired cytomegalovirus (CMV) infection. Fetuses exposed to CMV during the first trimester may experience intrauterine growth retardation and be afflicted with central nervous system damage, with hearing and sight impairments. Mental retardation will occur along with microcephaly. A characteristic "blueberry muffin rash" is usually present.

Answer B is incorrect. Epstein-Barr virus, the cause of infectious mononucleosis, is a rare cause of congenital defects. These defects include cataracts, hypotonia, cryptorchidism, and micrognathia.

Answer C is incorrect. Herpes simplex virus can result in a variety of congenital defects, abortions, and neonatal encephalitis.

Answer D is incorrect. Congenital HIV results in neonatal AIDS.

Answer E is incorrect. Congenital syphilis can result in cranial nerve VIII deafness, mulberry molars, saber shins, saddle nose, and Hutchinson's teeth.

6. **The correct answer is D.** The child was diagnosed with a Meckel's diverticulum, which describes the persistence after birth of part of the omphalomesenteric duct (vitelline duct or yolk stalk). Meckel's diverticulum is usually found in the mid to distal ileum and may end blindly or connect to the umbilicus. It is described by the **"rule of 2's"**: it is about **2 inches** long, **2 feet** from the ileocecal valve, occurs in about **2%** of the population, often presents before age **2 years** (60% of cases), and may contain **2 types** of epithelium (intestinal and gastric or duodenal). Ectopic gastric epithelium can cause ulcers and bleeding, but does not generally cause severe pain unless inflammation occurs. ^{99m}Tc pertechnetate is absorbed preferentially by gastric mucosa and thus may be used to detect ectopic gastric mucosa in the diverticulum.

Answer A is incorrect. Intussusception is the folding of the distal ileum into the proximal colon. It usually presents in the first 2 years of life and a Meckel diverticulum may predispose to this condition. However, it typically has an abrupt and severe presentation, with paroxysmal bouts of screaming, vomiting, diarrhea, and bloody bowel movements occurring within 24 hours of onset.

Answer B is incorrect. Breakdown of the mucosal barrier of the stomach and erosion of the underlying mucosal epithelium describes the pathology of a peptic ulcer. Peptic ulcers may present at any age, but are more common in patients 12–18 years old than in very young children. Additionally, it is not diagnosed by ^{99m}Tc pertechnetate scanning and is not treated surgically unless it perforates.

Answer C is incorrect. Ingestion of foreign objects occurs frequently in young children and may cause mechanical damage to the intestinal lining. However, they are not detected with ^{99m}Tc pertechnetate scanning and rarely require surgery.

Answer E is incorrect. Abnormal or incomplete rotation of the intestine as it returns to the abdomen after physiological herniation can trap and twist loops of bowel; twisting of these loops (volvulus) can result in obstruction of circulation and potentially lead to gangrene of the affected segment of intestine. Most affected infants present within the first 3 weeks of life with bile-containing vomit or bowel obstruction. Bloody stool is not a principal sign of malrotation or volvulus.

7. **The correct answer is C.** Pulmonary hypoplasia is the most common cause of death in infants born with congenital diaphragmatic hernia. When the pleuroperitoneal folds fail to fuse with the other components of the diaphragm during development, a hole is created that allows bowel into the thorax. The physical compression of the bowels on the lung buds then prevents full development of the respiratory system (pulmonary hypoplasia). This leads to a common presentation of dyspnea and cyanosis and, unless it can be repaired surgically, eventually leads to death.

Answer A is incorrect. Cardiac tamponade is most frequently associated with a pericardial effusion. This is not a common complication of congenital diaphragmatic hernia.

Answer B is incorrect. Mediastinal shift does occur in congenital diaphragmatic hernia, as the bowel invades the thorax and pushes the mediastinum to the right. However, this in itself is not a cause of death.

Answer D is incorrect. Renal maldevelopment is not associated with congenital diaphragmatic hernia.

Answer E is incorrect. Although it is theoretically possible for a volvulus to develop as the bowel herniates into the thorax, small bowel obstruction is not a common complication of congenital diaphragmatic hernia.

8. **The correct answer is E.** This question requires three steps to answer. First, the clinical scenario should be recognized as transposition of the great vessels. Early cyanosis is typically one of three conditions: Transposition, Tetralogy of Fallot, or Truncus arteriosus (the "3 T's"). Of these, only transposition is due to nonspiral development of the aorticopulmonary septum. Second, it must be known that maternal diabetes increases the risk of having a child with transposition. Finally, the common symptoms of diabetes must be known: polydipsia, polyuria, and blurred vision.

Answer A is incorrect. These are the symptoms seen in patients with Marfan's syndrome, a condition caused by a defect of connective tissue. This condition is not associated with transposition in the offspring of people with Marfan's syndrome.

Answer B is incorrect. These symptoms describe hypothyroidism, which does not increase the risk of congenital defects.

Answer C is incorrect. This describes the result of folate deficiency. This is associated with neural tube defects in the offspring but not with transposition of the great vessels.

Answer D is incorrect. These symptoms describe rubella, the result of infection by *Rubivirus*, a togavirus. Maternal rubella leads to many congenital defects, including patent ductus arteriosus, ventral septal defect, cataracts, and deafness, but it is not associated with transposition.

9. **The correct answer is A.** Spermiogenesis is the series of postmeiotic morphologic changes that mark the final maturation of the sperm. Spermatids are the 23, 1n cells that result from secondary spermatocyte meiosis II completion. They undergo morphologic changes to become mature sperm that include acrosome, head, neck, and tail formation.

Answer B is incorrect. Secondary spermatocytes are 23, 2n cells that result from primary spermatocytes completing meiosis I. Each primary spermatocyte forms two secondary spermatocytes.

Answer C is incorrect. At no point during male gametogenesis is there a haploid cell with 46 chromosomes.

Answer D is incorrect. Both primordial germ cells in the testes, which are dormant until puberty, and type A spermatogonia, which develop at puberty, are 46, 2n cell types. A type A spermatogonium perpetuates itself to provide a constant supply of sperm cells; it also differentiates into type B spermatogonia.

Answer E is incorrect. Primary spermatocytes are 46, 4n cells that result from type B spermatogonia DNA replication.

10. **The correct answer is E.** The apical ectodermal ridge (AER) is a region of thickened ectoderm at the distal end (or apex) of each limb. It produces two substances crucial to limb development: fibroblast growth factor, which is necessary to stimulate mitosis of the underlying mesoderm and thus produce lengthening of the limb; and the Wnt7 gene, which is necessary for proper organization along the dorsal-ventral axis. Thus, removing the AER will lead to a shortened limb and aberrant dorsal-ventral patterning.

Answer A is incorrect. Removing the apical ectodermal ridge will lead to a shortened length due to the lack of fibroblast growth factor, not extended length. Anterior-posterior patterning will likely be normal. Patterning along the anterior-posterior axis is controlled by, among other proteins, sonic hedgehog, a protein produced in the zone of polarizing activity, which is located at the base (rather than the apex) of the limb.

Answer B is incorrect. The limb will neither be of normal length nor have aberrant anterior-posterior patterning. Limb length is dependent on fibroblast growth factor produced at the apical ectodermal ridge (AER), so removing the AER will lead to a shortened limb. Anterior-posterior patterning is determined by sonic hedgehog produced in the zone of polarizing activity at the base of the limb. This will

be unaffected by removal of the apex (or distal end) of the limb.

Answer C is incorrect. Removal of the apical ectodermal ridge (AER) will have an effect on limb length due to lack of fibroblast growth factor. The digits form as a result of selected apoptosis within the AER, so it is likely that digit development will be aberrant.

Answer D is incorrect. Although removal of the apical ectodermal ridge (AER) will disrupt dorsal-ventral patterning due to the lack of expression of Wnt7, the limb will not be of normal length. Outgrowth of the limb is dependent on fibroblast growth factor produced in the AER, so the limb will be shortened.

11. **The correct answer is D.** The allantois and urachus form the median umbilical ligament. Do not confuse this with the medial umbilical ligaments, which are remnants of the umbilical arteries. Even if one did not know the answer to this question immediately, it could be deduced from the fact that, of the answer choices, only the median umbilical ligament is related to the umbilical cord, through which the allantoic duct passes.

Answer A is incorrect. The ligamentum arteriosum is the derivative of the ductus arteriosus, which serves to shunt blood from the pulmonary artery to the aorta in fetal circulation.

Answer B is incorrect. The ligamentum teres hepatis is the derivative of the umbilical vein, which brings oxygenated blood from the maternal circulation to the fetus.

Answer C is incorrect. The ligamentum venosum is the derivative of the ductus venosus, which shunts blood from the portal vein to the inferior vena cava.

Answer E is incorrect. The medial umbilical ligaments are remnants of the umbilical arteries. This should not be confused with the median umbilical ligament, which is involved in the formation of a urachal fistula.

Answer F is incorrect. The nucleus pulposus is a remnant of the notochord.

12. The correct answer is C. The ventral pancreatic bud also forms the main pancreatic duct in addition to the uncinate process and a part of the head. The dorsal pancreatic duct is responsible for the rest of the structural components of the pancreas, including the portion of the head not formed by the ventral bud.

Answer A is incorrect. The pancreatic body is formed by the dorsal pancreatic bud.

Answer B is incorrect. The pancreatic isthmus is formed by the dorsal pancreatic bud.

Answer D is incorrect. Pancreatic acinar cells, as well as duct epithelium, are formed from endoderm. In general, epithelium and glands of the gastrointestinal mucosa are formed from endoderm.

Answer E is incorrect. Pancreatic islet cells, like pancreatic acinar cells, are derived from endoderm.

Answer F is incorrect. The pancreatic tail is formed by the dorsal pancreatic bud.

13. The correct answer is C. The patient in the question has Down's syndrome, or trisomy 21. Duodenal atresia is associated with Down's syndrome.

Answer A is incorrect. Congenital cardiac disease is commonly associated with trisomy 21; especially common are endocardial cushion defects.

Answer B is incorrect. Down's syndrome is associated with acute lymphocytic leukemia, not chronic lymphocytic leukemia.

Answer D is incorrect. Trisomy 21 is the most common cause of congenital mental retardation.

Answer E is incorrect. The brains of patients with Down's syndrome have changes similar to those of Alzheimer's disease, not Pick's disease, after the age of 35.

14. The correct answer is C. This patient's inability to pass meconium, as well as the subsequent digital disimpaction, is consistent with Hirschsprung's disease, or congenital megacolon. This disorder is characterized by the ab-sence of ganglion cells in the large bowel, leading to functional obstruction and colonic dilatation proximal to the affected segment. Signs and symptoms of the disease result from failure of neural crest cell migration into the bowel wall during development.

Answer A is incorrect. Carcinoma of the colon can result in mechanical obstruction of the colon and present like acquired megacolon. However, colonic malignancies develop over time because the cells need to undergo multiple mutations before undergoing transformation. Thus, colon carcinoma would be unlikely in this infant.

Answer B is incorrect. Chronic Chagas' disease, a result of *Trypanosoma cruzi* infection, can result in acquired megacolon, an unlikely possibility in a neonate.

Answer D is incorrect. A neonate with imperforate anus will present with inability to pass meconium. However, digital examination of the rectum and subsequent disimpaction rule out this diagnosis.

Answer E is incorrect. Necrotizing enterocolitis occurs in a preterm infant and not in a full-term one. This condition usually occurs secondary to bowel ischemia.

15. The correct answer is A. The visual field defect being described is bilateral temporal hemianopia usually caused by lesions in the sella turcica that impinge on the optic chiasm, causing loss of visual input from the temporal field bilaterally. In children a tumor in this location of embryological origin is a craniopharyngioma. Craniopharyngiomas are derived from remnants of Rathke's pouch, which budded from the roof of the mouth to form the anterior pituitary. Patients usually have pituitary hypofunction, visual difficulties, and severe headaches. Diagnosis is confirmed by CT of the head, which shows calcification in the suprasellar region. Treatment includes surgery, radiotherapy, or both.

Answer B is incorrect. Ependymomas form from the cells lining the ventricles and most often occur in the fourth ventricle. Like medulloblastomas, ependymomas can block the flow of cerebrospinal fluid and cause hydrocephalus. These patients, however, do not have the hormonal or visual disturbances of the patient in this question.

Answer C is incorrect. Hemangioblastomas are vascular tumors of the central nervous system that usually occur in the cerebellum and spinal cord and thus would be unlikely to cause the visual field defects described in this case. The symptoms they do cause include cerebellar ataxia, motor weakness, and sensory dysfunction. Hemangioblastomas can occur sporadically or in patients with von Hippel–Lindau disease, which is an autosomal dominant disease in which patients develop cerebellar and retinal hemangioblastomas, pancreatic cysts, and pheochromocytomas.

Answer D is incorrect. Medulloblastoma is also an embryonic tumor that arises from primitive neuroectoderm in the fourth ventricle. It does not cause the visual symptoms seen in this patient, but the tumor may compress the fourth ventricle to cause hydrocephalus and symptoms consistent with increased intracranial pressure such as morning headache and vomiting. Treatment consists of surgery and chemoradiation.

Answer E is incorrect. Pituitary adenomas would cause bitemporal hemianopia as in this patient; however, pituitary tumors are age-linked, becoming increasingly more common in older patients, and would be unlikely in a child. Also pituitary adenomas tend to secrete one of the pituitary hormones and thus would cause an elevation of serum hormone levels rather than a decrease, as seen in this patient. The three most common forms of pituitary adenoma are prolactinomas (which secrete prolactin and cause galactorrhea and amenorrhea), growth hormone–secreting tumors (which cause acromegaly), and ACTH-producing tumors (which cause Cushing's disease). While the location of the tumor and the visual symptoms with pituitary adenomas are similar to those seen with craniopharyngioma, the patient's age and serum hormone levels as well as the tumor's "embryological origin" make the latter a more likely choice.

16. **The correct answer is D.** This question requires three steps to answer. First, it must be recognized that the image shows a meningomyelocele, a neural tube defect in which the meninges and spinal cord herniate through a defect in the spinal canal. Second, it has to be known that folate is the nutrient that, if given to a mother early in pregnancy, will lower the risk of developing neural tube defects (spina bifida occulta, meningocele, or meningomyelocele). Finally, selecting the right answer requires knowing that in the adult, folate deficiency produces a megaloblastic anemia without neurologic symptoms. Note that a deficiency of vitamin B_{12} also causes a megaloblastic anemia but produces neurologic symptoms as well.

Answer A is incorrect. This describes Wernicke-Korsakoff syndrome, which is a result of a deficiency of thiamine (vitamin B_1) and is commonly seen in alcoholism.

Answer B is incorrect. Pellagra, a deficiency of niacin (vitamin B_3), produces these symptoms.

Answer C is incorrect. Megaloblastic anemia with neurologic symptoms is produced by vitamin B_{12} deficiency. This is not associated with neural tube defects.

Answer E is incorrect. Microcytic anemia is caused by iron deficiency as well as lead poisoning and the thalassemias.

Answer F is incorrect. These are the signs of beriberi, which results from thiamine (vitamin B_1) deficiency.

Answer G is incorrect. This describes scurvy, which results from vitamin C deficiency.

17. **The correct answer is A.** **P**ulmonary valve stenosis (as evidenced here by the left upper sternal border systolic murmur), **R**ight ventricular hypertrophy, an **O**verriding aorta, and a **V**entricular septal defect are the four components of the tetralogy of Fallot (remember the

mnemonic **PROVe**). This condition results from abnormal migration of neural crest cells and results in the aorticopulmonary septum being displaced anterosuperiorly. Life-threatening hypoxia may develop. The child will often squat in an effort to relieve hypoxia; squatting increases the systemic pressure, thereby reducing the right-to-left shunt and improving oxygenation. Treatment is corrective surgery.

Answer B is incorrect. Incomplete development of the bronchial tree leads to pulmonary hypoplasia. This may produce dyspnea but is otherwise inconsistent with this presentation.

Answer C is incorrect. A tracheoesophageal fistula is the result of incomplete formation of the tracheoesophageal septum. This produces gagging and possibly cyanosis on feeding but is not associated with any of the other findings in this vignette.

Answer D is incorrect. This describes the etiology of a pure ventricular septal defect (VSD). A VSD does not produce cyanosis unless it leads to Eisenmenger's syndrome, in which pulmonary hypertension transforms a left-to-right shunt into a right-to-left shunt. Moreover, a simple VSD does not cause any of the other findings of tetralogy of Fallot.

Answer E is incorrect. Nonspiral development of the aorticopulmonary septum results in transposition of the great vessels. This does cause dyspnea and cyanosis but it is evident much earlier in life and would not result in an echocardiogram showing tetralogy of Fallot.

18. **The correct answer is E.** The lens is the only structure in the eye that is derived exclusively from surface ectoderm. The ectoderm forms the lens placode, which then invaginates to create the lens vesicle. Surface ectoderm also gives rise to the epidermis, hair, nails, and sweat and sebaceous glands as well as the epithelial lining of the lower anal canal and distal male urethra, the utricle and saccule, the olfactory placodes, and the adenohypophysis, among other structures.

Answer A is incorrect. The choroid is derived from the mesoderm around the optic cup.

Answer B is incorrect. The anterior epithelium of the cornea is derived from surface ectoderm, but the stroma and endothelium of the cornea are derived from mesoderm. Thus, the cornea is not derived exclusively from the surface ectoderm and does not satisfactorily answer the question.

Answer C is incorrect. The extraocular muscles derive from mesoderm.

Answer D is incorrect. The iris epithelium, like the retina, derives from the double-layered optic cup. It is a derivative of neuroectoderm.

Answer F is incorrect. The retina is formed by the optic cup, a derivative of the diencephalon. This is created by neuroectoderm, not surface ectoderm. The optic sulcus in the diencephalon evaginates to form the optic cup, a double-layered structure consisting of an inner neural layer and an outer pigment layer. The outer layer gives rise to the retinal pigment epithelium (RPE), while the inner layer develops into the photoreceptors (rods and cones), the bipolar cells, and the ganglion cells.

Answer G is incorrect. The sclera is derived from the mesoderm around the optic cup.

19. **The correct answer is F.** The thyroid gland originates as the thyroid diverticulum on the floor of the pharynx. It descends into the neck during development, but remains connected to the tongue by the thyroglossal duct. The thyroglossal duct eventually disappears, leaving a small cavity (the foramen cecum) at the base of the tongue. The pyramidal lobe of the thyroid can be thought of as the caudal part of the duct. Occasionally, part of the duct epithelium persists in the neck and may form cysts. Thyroglossal duct cysts are usually painless or slightly tender and appear in the midline of the neck. They often appear over or just below the hyoid, but may appear anywhere between the base of the tongue and the thyroid. If a normal thyroid gland is present, surgery is recommended to prevent infection. In this case, the presence of a normal thyroid is demonstrated by normal triiodothyronine, thyroxine, and thyroid-stimulating hormone levels and is confirmed by CT scan.

Answer A is incorrect. Branchial cleft cysts can also occur in the neck but are not always in the midline. Unlike thyroglossal duct cysts, they are often associated with fistulas or sinus tracts.

Answer B is incorrect. Dermoid cysts are the second most common cause of midline neck masses, after thyroglossal duct cysts. They tend to be more superficial than thyroglossal duct cysts and more mobile relative to underlying structures.

Answer C is incorrect. Ectopic thyroid glands are often seen in the presence of a thyroglossal duct cyst. An ectopic thyroid gland occurs when the thyroid fails to descend during development; in contrast, ectopic thyroid tissue may occur along the path of the thyroglossal duct in the presence of a normal thyroid gland. Unlike this patient, who has normal thyroid levels, about one third of patients with an ectopic gland are hypothyroid. A CT scan is usually performed to confirm the presence of a normal thyroid gland before surgery is performed on a thyroglossal duct cyst.

Answer D is incorrect. Hypertrophy of the pyramidal lobe of the thyroid is not the most likely cause of midline neck swelling in a young child. Furthermore, hypertrophic thyroid tissue would most likely alter thyroid hormone and thyroid-stimulating hormone levels.

Answer E is incorrect. Lipomas may cause neck swelling, but the location of this mass and the age of the patient make a thyroglossal duct cyst much more likely. Lipomas tend to be very superficial, with poorly defined edges.

20. **The correct answer is B.** The muscles that elevate the palate are derived from branchial arch 3 (the stylopharyngeus) and branchial arch 4 (the levator veli palatini). These are innervated by cranial nerves IX and X, respectively.

Answer A is incorrect. The first branchial arch generates "M" muscles: muscles of Mastication (teMporalis, Masseter, Medial and lateral pterygoids) and the Mylohyoid. The second arch gives rise to "S" muscles: Stapedius,

Stylohyoid, and facial expression muscles. None of these muscles is involved in palatal elevation.

Answer C is incorrect. Although branchial arch 4 does give rise to the levator veli palatini, branchial arch 6 gives rise to the intrinsic muscles of the larynx (except the cricothyroid, which is a fourth arch derivative). These muscles are not involved in elevating the palate.

Answer D is incorrect. The first branchial cleft gives rise to the external auditory meatus, while the second, third, and fourth clefts are obliterated during development. The clefts are formed from ectoderm and could not give rise to muscles, which are derived from mesoderm.

Answer E is incorrect. Branchial pouch 3 gives rise to the thymus (ventral wings) and inferior parathyroid glands (dorsal glands), while the fourth branchial pouch gives rise to the superior parathyroids. These are obviously not involved in palatal elevation. Remember that pouches give rise to endoderm-derived tissue, while the arches give rise to mesoderm-derived tissue such as muscle.

21. **The correct answer is C.** Isotretinoin is commonly prescribed for severe acne vulgaris and is a dangerous teratogen that causes defects in fetal development. As a result, women at risk of pregnancy should undergo monthly pregnancy testing and be counseled to use two forms of contraception during treatment with isotretinoin. Like most other teratogens, exposure to isotretinoin during weeks 3–8 of fetal development is especially damaging since this is the period during which organogenesis occurs and developing fetal tissues are most susceptible to the effects of teratogens.

Answer A is incorrect. Teratogen exposure at the time of conception is less damaging and typically exerts an "all-or-nothing" effect resulting in either embryo-lethality, or no malformation at all as undifferentiated cells are simply replaced.

Answer B is incorrect. Teratogen exposure in early embryogenesis (weeks 1–2 of fetal development) normally produces an "all-or-nothing" effect on malformation and is less risky than exposure during organogenesis.

Answer D is incorrect. Teratogen exposure during weeks 8–10 of fetal development is generally less risky than exposure during weeks 3–8. However, severe birth defects are still possible as organogenesis sometimes lasts until the tenth week of fetal development.

Answer E is incorrect. Risk for malformation is less severe after the 10th week of fetal development as organogenesis is complete and most fetal structures have formed. However, teratogen exposure during this interval can lead to restrictions in fetal growth, low birth weight, and disorders of the central nervous system.

22. **The correct answer is A.** The patient is presenting with congenital extrahepatic biliary atresia, which is caused by congenital occlusion of the bile ducts. During embryonic development, the hepatic diverticulum buds off from the foregut and develops into the liver. The bile ducts are formed by narrowing of the embryologic connection between the hepatic diverticulum and the foregut; congenital extrahepatic biliary atresia develops when the bile ducts close completely and fail to recanalize. While many of the other causes of neonatal jaundice result in an unconjugated (indirect) hyperbilirubinemia, biliary atresia leads to a conjugated (direct) hyperbilirubinemia, as well as dark urine and acholic stools from the complete lack of urobilinogens in the stool and the increased conjugated bilirubin excreted in the urine. Appropriate therapy of congenital biliary atresia is surgery to connect an intrahepatic bile duct directly to the small intestine, thus bypassing the area of occlusion.

Answer B is incorrect. Crigler-Najjar syndrome type I is caused by a complete deficiency in UDP-glucuronosyltransferase, the hepatic enzyme necessary to conjugate bilirubin. This disorder produces a severe unconjugated (indirect) hyperbilirubinemia that causes death within the first few years of life. The patient in this case, however, has a conjugated hyperbilirubinemia, suggesting an obstructive cause and ruling out Crigler-Najjar syndrome.

Answer C is incorrect. Gilbert's syndrome is due to a mutation in the promoter region of the same gene that causes Crigler-Najjar syndrome, however the defect leads to a mild decrease in gene expression instead of a complete deficiency. Like Crigler-Najjar syndrome, patients with Gilbert's syndrome have an unconjugated hyperbilirubinemia. However, unlike Crigler-Najjar, the patients are usually asymptomatic and have a normal life expectancy.

Answer D is incorrect. Hereditary spherocytosis can cause jaundice and hyperbilirubinemia secondary to hemolytic anemia. This autosomal dominant condition is due to mutations in spectrin or ankyrin causing RBC membrane defects that make the cells more fragile to hemolysis. Peripheral blood smears show small RBCs without central pallor and diagnosis can be confirmed with the osmotic fragility test. Unlike in this patient, hereditary spherocytosis usually presents later in life with a mixed conjugated and unconjugated hyperbilirubinemia and no acholic stools.

Answer E is incorrect. Physiologic jaundice refers to the mild unconjugated (indirect) hyperbilirubinemia that affects nearly all newborns due to the greater turnover of neonatal RBCs and the decreased bilirubin clearance in the first few weeks of life. The peak total serum bilirubin level in physiologic jaundice is typically 5–6 mg/dL, occurring between 72 and 96 hours of age, not exceeding 17–18 mg/dL, and resolving within the first few weeks of life. This patient has a severe conjugated hyperbilirubinemia that is due to complete biliary obstruction and cannot be explained by normal neonatal physiological jaundice.

23. **The correct answer is D.** Until week 5, the yolk sac is solely responsible for hematopoiesis. By week 8, the liver has taken over as the predominant location. It remains so until the bone marrow takes over around week 28. The thymus and spleen also begin producing blood cells around week 12 but are never the predominant sites of hematopoiesis.

Answer A is incorrect. The bone marrow is the predominant site of hematopoiesis beginning around week 28 and remains so throughout adult life.

Answer B is incorrect. The gastric fundus is the site of parietal cells, which produce intrinsic factor and gastric acid. The stomach plays no role in hematopoiesis.

Answer C is incorrect. The pancreas produces insulin, glucagon, and digestive enzymes. It plays no role in hematopoiesis.

Answer E is incorrect. The yolk sac is the predominant site of hematopoiesis between fetal weeks 3 and 8.

24. **The correct answer is B.** The child is presenting with common signs and symptoms of a patent ductus arteriosus (PDA). In the fetus, the ductus arteriosus serves to shunt blood from the left pulmonary artery to the aorta, allowing the blood to avoid the high-resistance lungs and delivering more oxygenated blood to the rest of the body. Failure of the ductus arteriosus to close is common in premature babies, as in this case as well as in cases of maternal rubella during pregnancy. Indomethacin, a nonsteroidal anti-inflammatory drug, blocks the production of PGE_1 and can be used to close a PDA.

Answer A is incorrect. There is no fetal structure or congenital anomaly that shunts blood from the inferior vena cava to the aorta.

Answer C is incorrect. This pattern of blood flow is seen with a ventricular septal defect. This is not a normal feature of fetal circulation. After birth, this will also present with exercise intolerance but will produce a holosystolic murmur, not a continuous murmur. Also note that the question is asking about the blood flow in the fetus; because the pressure on the right side of the fetal heart is higher than the pressure on the left, blood will always be shunted from right to left, not left to right as this answer choice describes.

Answer D is incorrect. This is the pattern of blood flow of the ductus venosus. This does not lead to cardiac pathology.

Answer E is incorrect. The foramen ovale shunts blood from the right atrium to the left atrium, also bypassing the lungs. This typically closes at birth in response to the dramatic decrease in right atrial pressure and increase in left atrial pressure as the infant takes its first breath and opens the lungs. However, should it fail to close, a patent foramen ovale results. This condition ranges in severity and may not become clinically apparent until the age of 30 or later. Signs and symptoms of a patent foramen ovale include a systolic ejection murmur (not a continuous murmur) and a widely split fixed S_2.

25. **The correct answer is D.** As one of the ToRCHeS infections that cross the placenta, rubella infection during pregnancy damages the cochlear duct (organ of Corti), resulting in congenital deafness. The cochlear duct is derived from the saccular portion of the otic vesicle. During week 4, a portion of the surface ectoderm thickens to form the otic placode, which then invaginates to create the otic vesicle. The otic vesicle divides into the saccular portion, which forms the saccule, cochlear duct, and spiral ganglion of cranial nerve VIII; and the utricular portion, which forms the endolymphatic duct, the endolymphatic sac, the utricle, the semicircular duct, and the vestibular ganglion of cranial nerve VIII. The otic vesicle gives rise to all structures of the internal ear.

Answer A is incorrect. The six auricular hillocks give rise to the auricle, the outermost portion of the ear. The auricles are often malformed in chromosomal syndromes such as Down's syndrome (trisomy 21), Patau's syndrome (trisomy 13), and Edwards' syndrome (trisomy 18). However, this does not lead to deafness, and the auricles are not affected by congenital rubella infection.

Answer B is incorrect. The first pharyngeal arch gives rise to many structures of the ear, including the malleus, incus, and tensor tympani muscle (innervated by cranial nerve V). However, these structures are not commonly damaged by congenital rubella infection.

Answer C is incorrect. The optic cup is not an auditory structure. It is a neuroectoderm derivative that gives rise to the retina, iris epithelium, muscles of the iris, and ciliary body epithelium.

Answer E is incorrect. The stapes bone and the stapedius muscle are the ear structures that are derived from the second pharyngeal arch. Hyperacusis is commonly the result of stapedius muscle paralysis due to cranial nerve VII lesions. However, these structures are generally unaffected by congenital rubella infection.

CHAPTER 4

Microbiology and Immunology

1. A 30-year-old sexually active woman presents with painful vesicles on her external genitalia. The physician's suspicion is confirmed with a polymerase chain reaction test that is positive for herpes simplex virus type 2. Which of the following medications would be most helpful to this patient?

   (A) Acyclovir
   (B) Amantadine
   (C) Ribavirin
   (D) Rifampin
   (E) Vancomycin

2. A hepatitis panel is ordered for a 27-year-old woman as part of a routine workup for abdominal pain. Results of serologic testing are negative for HBeAg and HBsAg, but positive for HBsAb and IgG HBcAb. Which of the following is the appropriate conclusion?

   (A) The patient has been exposed to hepatitis B and has completely recovered
   (B) The patient has been exposed to hepatitis B and is in the acute disease phase
   (C) The patient has been exposed to hepatitis B and is in the window phase
   (D) The patient has been exposed to hepatitis B but is not infected
   (E) The patient has been exposed to hepatitis B and is now chronically infected

3. A 48-year-man with chronic renal failure undergoes a cadaveric renal transplant. One week later, the patient has an elevated creatinine level. The surgical team is concerned about the possibility of acute transplant rejection. The cell type shown in the image is believed to be an important mediator of this process. In which of the following locations does this cell type identified by the arrow complete maturation?

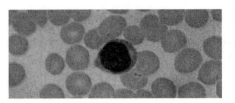

Reproduced, with permission, from Berman I. *Color Atlas of Basic Histology*, 3rd ed. New York, McGraw-Hill, 2003: Fig. 8-5.

   (A) Bone marrow
   (B) Lung
   (C) Spleen
   (D) Thymus
   (E) Yolk sac

4. A 43-year-old man living in Mexico presents to a clinic complaining of constipation and stomach pains for several months. On cardiac examination, the physician discovers a laterally displaced point of maximal impact. Radiological studies reveal pulmonary congestion, cardiomegaly, and megacolon. Sadly, the physician can offer the patient only symptomatic treatment. What insect is the most likely route of transmission for this patient's illness?

   (A) Anopheles mosquito
   (B) Ixodes tick
   (C) Reduviid bug
   (D) Sandfly
   (E) Tsetse fly

5. A patient in the hospital develops pleuritic chest pain, shortness of breath, fever, chills, productive cough, and colored sputum after 3 days of being in the hospital for major surgery. Blood and sputum cultures confirm gram-negative rods that ferment lactose, have a large mucoid capsule, and form viscous colonies. The patient subsequently dies from her infec-

tion. At autopsy, the lungs were sent for pathologic analysis. Which of the following is most likely to be found?

(A) Acute inflammatory infiltrates from bronchioles into adjacent alveoli
(B) Congestion, red hepatization, gray hepatization, and resolution
(C) Diffuse, patchy inflammation localized to the alveolar wall interstitium
(D) Intra-alveolar hyaline membranes without alveolar space exudates
(E) Predominantly intra-alveolar exudate resulting in consolidation

6. A 28-year-old male lawyer who lives in Manhattan visits his physician complaining of intermittent pain in his right elbow and left knee of 2 weeks' duration. He has also noticed a slight drooping of the left side of his face in the past 3 days. The patient reports that 2 months ago he spent 3 weeks at his summer home in Connecticut. While he was there, he noticed a rash on his right arm that was clear at the center. Upon examination, the physician notices several circular rashes with central clearing. Which pathogen is responsible for this patient's condition?

(A) *Borrelia burgdorferi*
(B) *Borrelia recurrentis*
(C) *Leptospira interrogans*
(D) *Rickettsia rickettsii*
(E) *Treponema pallidum*

7. A clinical researcher is studying how to make vaccines more effective. She combines an experimental vaccine with Freund's complete adjuvant in order to enhance the potency of the vaccine. Which of the following is the main mechanism by which this adjuvant is believed to enhance the immunity of this researcher's vaccine?

(A) The adjuvant activates antigen-presenting cells such as dendritic cells to promote phagocytosis and expression of costimulatory molecules
(B) The adjuvant activates antigen-presenting cells such as T lymphocytes to promote

phagocytosis and expression of costimulatory molecules
(C) The adjuvant allows for nonspecific activation of T lymphocytes within the local area of administration
(D) The adjuvant increases the half-life of the vaccine
(E) The adjuvant prevents activation-induced cell death of T and B lymphocytes systemically

8. A homeless 37-year-old woman with HIV infection comes to the clinic with a 4-week history of worsening hemiparesis, visual field deficits, and cognitive impairment. She has gone 2 years without antiretroviral therapy. The patient's CD4 count is 22/μL. An MRI shows several hyperintensities on T2-weighted images that do not enhance with contrast and are not surrounded by edema. A lumbar puncture shows a normal opening pressure, and cerebrospinal fluid analysis shows a mildly elevated protein level and the presence of myelin basic protein, with a mild mononuclear pleocytosis. Which of the following entities is most likely responsible for this patient's clinical picture?

(A) Cytomegalovirus encephalitis
(B) HIV encephalopathy
(C) JC virus
(D) Primary central nervous system lymphoma
(E) Toxoplasmosis

9. A 23-year-old man comes to the physician with a bacterial infection. On questioning, the patient reveals a history of recurrent bacterial, fungal, and viral infections. Blood is drawn and sent for laboratory analysis, which reveals all levels of immune cells (e.g., T lymphocytes, B lymphocytes) are low. Which of the following conditions is most likely to have caused the patient's symptoms?

(A) Ataxia-telangiectasia
(B) Chédiak-Higashi disease
(C) Job syndrome
(D) Severe combined immunodeficiency
(E) Wiskott-Aldrich syndrome

10. A sexually active 14-year-old boy comes to the physician because of a rash on his trunk and genital area. Physical examination shows multiple umbilicated nodules spread around his trunk and genitals. They are dome-shaped, waxy, and painless. Which of the following types of virus most likely caused this patient's rash?

(A) Herpes simplex virus type 1
(B) Human herpesvirus 8
(C) Poxvirus
(D) Rubeola virus
(E) Varicella-zoster virus

11. A 13-year-old boy is diagnosed with a hyperactive immune system. Normally, an antigen will activate the immune system to trigger a proinflammatory response. Following the proinflammatory response, anti-inflammatory signals then dampen the immune response to prevent it from causing damage. This patient has trouble dampening the immune response after it is no longer needed. Decreased activity in which of the following anti-inflammatory cytokines is most likely the basis for this boy's condition?

(A) Interferon-γ (IFN-γ)
(B) Interleukin-1 (IL-1)
(C) Transforming growth factor-β (TGF-β)
(D) Tumor necrosis factor-α (TNF-α)
(E) Tumor necrosis factor-β (TNF-β)

12. A 22-year-old man visits his college medical center complaining of flulike symptoms that have persisted for about a week. He reports low-grade fevers, night sweats, a painful sore throat, headaches, and increasing fatigue. He used to exercise 5 days a week but is no longer able to because of a "lack of energy." Physical examination reveals enlarged cervical lymph nodes and a spleen that is palpable 2 inches below the left costal margin. What is the structure of the virus that has infected this patient?

(A) Linear, double-stranded, DNA virus with an envelope
(B) Linear, double-stranded, DNA virus without an envelope
(C) Linear, double-stranded, RNA virus with an envelope

(D) Partially circular, double-stranded, DNA virus with an envelope
(E) Segmented, linear, single-stranded, negative-polarity, RNA virus with an envelope

13. A 36-year-old man comes to the physician complaining of an aching back, high fever, and vomiting of dark material. He is obviously ill and states that he has felt very poorly for approximately 1 week. Physical examination shows that the patient has a temperature of 39° C (102.2° F) and icteric sclera. The patient recently returned from a trip on safari in Africa. If a liver biopsy were done, it would show the following pathology. What are the names of the eosinophilic globules shown in this image?

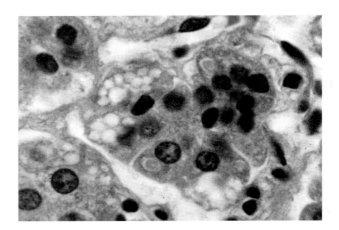

Image courtesy of PEIR Digital Library (http://peir.net).

(A) Councilman bodies
(B) Döhle bodies
(C) Negri bodies
(D) Pappenheimer bodies
(E) Weibel-Palade bodies

14. A 32-year-old woman comes to the physician complaining of a temperature, fatigue, cough, headache, and shaking chills. On physical examination, an inflamed area is found on her right leg. On closer examination, the inflammation appears to be a tick bite. Blood samples are sent for laboratory examination, and results show a Maltese cross–appearing parasite in the

patient's RBCs. This patient is most likely infected with which of the following protozoa?

(A) *Acanthamoeba* species
(B) *Babesia* species
(C) *Leishmania donovani*
(D) *Naegleria fowleri*
(E) *Trypanosoma cruzi*

15. Oncogenic viruses have different mechanisms by which they induce neoplasms. Neoplasia is defined as a clonal proliferation of cells that is uncontrolled and excessive. Which of the following viruses causes neoplasia by primarily destroying cells, and then subsequently stimulating repeated regeneration and subsequent aberrant cell growth?

(A) Epstein-Barr virus
(B) Hepatitis C virus
(C) Human immunodeficiency virus
(D) Human papillomavirus
(E) Human T-cell lymphoma virus type 1

16. A 19-year-old man comes to the physician with a bacterial infection. Without treatment, the patient's immune system will most likely be able to fight off the infection within a few days. One of the tools the patient's body uses against the organism is the membrane attack complex. The membrane attack complex functions as which of the following?

(A) A chemoattractant for neutrophils
(B) A scaffold to which antibodies can bind on the membrane of a cell
(C) A tube inserted into the lipid bilayer of the plasma membrane, increasing permeability
(D) An anaphylactic signal causing degranulation of mast cells and basophils
(E) An opsonization molecule, facilitating phagocytosis

17. In order to assess the risk of erythroblastosis fetalis occurring during the future pregnancy of an Rh-negative woman, a clinician sends a

sample of serum for detection of anti Rh-blood group antibodies. The laboratory performs an indirect Coombs' test as follows:

1. Isolate the patient's serum.
2. Mix the patient's serum with Rh-positive RBCs.
3. Wash off unbound antibody.
4. Add an anti-IgG antibody and observe for the presence or absence of agglutination.

The test results in agglutination. After receiving this test result, the clinician would be correct to conclude which of the following?

(A) The Coombs' test yielded a negative result, and therefore the mother does not have anti-Rh antibodies
(B) The laboratory performed the test incorrectly; they should have mixed the patient's serum with Rh-negative rather than Rh-positive RBCs
(C) The patient has had previous pregnancies and all of her children are Rh-negative
(D) The patient is currently pregnant with an Rh-positive fetus
(E) The presence of anti-Rh antibodies in the patient's serum suggests that she has been pregnant with an Rh-positive fetus

18. A newborn child is exposed to *Streptococcus agalactiae* and subsequently develops meningitis. Which of the following could have contributed to this child's bacterial infection?

(A) A defect in DNA repair enzymes with associated IgA deficiency
(B) An X-linked recessive defect in a tyrosine kinase gene
(C) Improper development of the thymus and parathyroid glands
(D) Improper transfer of IgG from the mother to the fetus
(E) Improper transfer of IgM from the mother to the fetus

19. Influenza virus type A usually produces a mild, self-limited febrile illness in the general population. However, worldwide epidemics have occurred at different times in history. Which of the following is the most important reason why these sporadic epidemics occur?

    (A) Antigenic drift
    (B) Antigenic shift
    (C) Hemagglutinin develops the ability to destroy a component of mucin, becoming more infectious
    (D) Neuraminidase develops the ability to attach to sialic acid receptors, becoming more infectious
    (E) RBCs agglutinate with certain strains

20. *Haemophilus influenzae* and *Neisseria meningitidis* both possess a polysaccharide outer capsule. Effective vaccination against these species results in the generation of antibodies that recognize this polysaccharide capsule. Which of the following best explains why the childhood vaccines for *Haemophilus influenzae* type B and *Neisseria meningitidis* serogroup C are composed of a polysaccharide coat conjugated to a protein carrier?

    (A) Polysaccharides are T-lymphocyte-independent antigens and therefore do not elicit effective immunity in infants; the protein is added in order to recruit T-lymphocyte help and increase antibody production
    (B) The protein carrier increases the half-life of the vaccine
    (C) The protein carrier increases the production of IgE immunoglobulins, which confer protection
    (D) The protein carrier makes the vaccine less virulent and thus decreases the risk of a child developing disease from the immunization
    (E) The protein carrier plays no role and is included only for ease of preparation

21. A type B blood group, Rh-positive recipient is mistakenly transplanted with a kidney from a type A blood group, Rh-negative donor. Which of the following best describes the mechanism of transplant rejection that is most likely to ensue in this recipient?

    (A) Acute rejection mediated by preformed recipient antibodies
    (B) Acute rejection mediated by recipient T lymphocytes
    (C) Graft-versus-host disease mediated by donor T lymphocytes
    (D) Hyperacute rejection mediated by preformed donor antibodies
    (E) Hyperacute rejection mediated by preformed recipient antibodies

22. A 30-year-old woman comes to the physician because of a fever of 38.4° C (101.1° F) and a diffuse macular rash on her torso. Her blood pressure is 91/51 mm Hg. The physician obtains a culture from her vagina that shows catalase-positive, gram-positive cocci. Over the next few days, the rash on her torso desquamates. Which of the following organisms is most likely responsible for this patient's symptoms?

    (A) *Actinomyces israelii*
    (B) *Clostridium perfringens*
    (C) *Proteus mirabilis*
    (D) *Staphylococcus aureus*
    (E) *Streptococcus pyogenes*

23. A young girl living in rural New Mexico is brought to her pediatrician with complaints of fever, cough, and fatigue for the past 2 weeks. The physician notices that the patient is having intermittent bouts of many coughs in a single breath followed by a deep inspiration. The parents report this pattern of cough has started in the past 2 days. The physician informs them that their daughter will most likely recover with only supportive care. However, he wants to confirm his diagnosis, so he sends a throat swab for culture. What type of medium should be used to grow the bacteria that are causing this patient's symptoms?

    (A) Bordet-Gengou medium
    (B) Charcoal yeast extract with iron and cysteine
    (C) Chocolate agar with factor V and X
    (D) Loffler's medium
    (E) Thayer-Martin medium

24. A 12-year-old girl is brought to the pediatrician by her mother because of a fever. The physician notes that the girl has features of albinism and the mother states that her daughter has always looked the way she does. The physician diagnoses the girl with a staphylococcal infection and prescribes a course of antibiotics. Three months later, the child returns to the pediatrician with another streptococcal infection. The patient's medical records indicate that she has had repeated bouts of staphylococcal and streptococcal infections for her entire life. This patient most likely has which of the following types of immune deficiency?

   (A) Chédiak-Higashi disease
   (B) Chronic granulomatous disease
   (C) Hyper-IgM syndrome
   (D) Selective IgA deficiency
   (E) Severe combined immunodeficiency

25. A 28-year-old man comes to the physician because of ascending symmetric muscle weakness that began after he had an episode of fever and diarrhea. Cerebrospinal fluid analysis shows an increased protein concentration, a normal cell count, and a normal glucose level. An infection with which of the following organisms can cause the nervous system syndrome described in this patient?

   (A) *Candida albicans*
   (B) *Haemophilus influenzae*
   (C) *Pseudomonas aeruginosa*
   (D) *Serratia marcescens*
   (E) *Staphylococcus saprophyticus*

26. A 70-year-old man presents with a shiny, beefy-looking tongue and numbness and tingling in the lower extremities. Biopsy of the stomach is significant for atrophy of chief cells and parietal cells. Which of the following findings would be expected on a peripheral blood smear from this patient?

   (A) A megaloblastic anemia with hypersegmented polymorphonuclear leukocytes
   (B) A microcytic anemia with hypersegmented polymorphonuclear leukocytes
   (C) A microcytic hypochromic anemia with decreased serum iron and increased total iron-binding capacity

   (D) A normochromic normocytic anemia with decreased serum iron and decreased total iron-binding capacity
   (E) Normal peripheral blood smear with normal serum iron and normal total iron-binding capacity

27. An elderly man recently visited his grandchildren in Arizona. Upon returning to his home in New York, he develops breathing difficulty, productive cough, and joint pain. He visits his physician, who orders an x-ray of the chest, which reveals infiltrates in the lungs with evidence of granulomas. A tissue specimen from biopsy reveals a fungus with endospores containing spherules when grown at 37° C and branched hyphae when grown at 25° C. What is the most likely cause of his symptoms?

   (A) *Aspergillus fumigatus*
   (B) *Blastomyces dermatitidis*
   (C) *Candida albicans*
   (D) *Coccidioides immitis*
   (E) *Histoplasma capsulatum*

28. Antigen processing and presentation within the context of a major histocompatibility complex (MHC) class I molecule is essential to generating a CD8+ T-lymphocyte response. Within which of the diagramed subcellular locations does self-peptide get loaded onto MHC class I molecules?

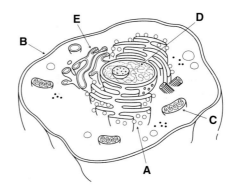

Reproduced, with permission, from USMLERx.com.

   (A) A
   (B) B
   (C) C
   (D) D
   (E) E

29. A number of theories have attempted to draw connections between vaccines and allergies or autoimmune diseases. One such theory suggests that vaccine administration may alter the helper T lymphocyte (Th) composition and/or immunoglobulin levels in the body. Which of the following statements accurately depicts the theoretical effects of vaccines on the immune system that may lead to allergies/autoimmune diseases?

(A) Decreased Th1 leads to increased Th2
(B) Decreased Th2 leads to increased Th1
(C) Increased Th1 leads to decreased Th2
(D) Increased Th1 leads to increased IgE
(E) Increased Th2 leads to increased IgE

30. After a long camping trip in the woods, a 29-year-old man comes to the physician complaining of fever and general malaise. His physical examination is significant for a well-demarcated skin lesion with a black base. On further questioning, the patient says that the lesion developed over a bite site. Which of the following organisms is most likely responsible for this patient's disease?

(A) *Brucella melitensis*
(B) *Francisella tularensis*
(C) *Nocardia asteroides*
(D) *Treponema pallidum*
(E) *Trichinella spiralis*

31. A 7-year-old boy presents to the clinic with a staphylococcal infection. He is well known at the clinic because he has had recurrent staphylococcal infections for most of his life. He is started on an antibiotic regimen and the infection subsides. Three weeks later, the boy is diagnosed with pruritic papulovesicular dermatitis. Which of the following immune deficiency syndromes would account for this patient's recurrent staphylococcal infections and pruritic papulovesicular dermatitis?

(A) Ataxia-telangiectasia
(B) Bruton's agammaglobulinemia
(C) Job syndrome
(D) Thymic aplasia (DiGeorge's syndrome)
(E) Wiskott-Aldrich syndrome

32. An obese 43-year-old white woman presents to the emergency department with epigastric pain, fever, and jaundice. Abdominal examination reveals right upper quadrant tenderness without peritoneal signs. Endoscopic retrograde cholangiopancreatography shows several stones in the common bile duct. Laboratory testing reveals a WBC count of 14,200/mm^3, with 74% segmented neutrophils, and a serum amylase level of 78 U/L. Which of the following is the most likely diagnosis for this patient?

(A) Acute appendicitis
(B) Acute pancreatitis
(C) Acute viral hepatitis
(D) Bacterial cholangitis
(E) Cholesterolosis

33. Hyper-IgM syndrome usually presents with severe pyogenic infections. The typical immunoglobulin profile in a patient with this disease shows an elevated level of IgM in contrast to the other immunoglobulin isotypes. Which of the following is the etiology behind the increased level of IgM in a patient with hyper-IgM syndrome?

(A) A defect in DNA repair enzymes
(B) A defect in LFA-1 adhesion proteins on phagocytes
(C) A defect in the CD40 ligand on CD4 T-helper cells
(D) Failure of interferon-γ production
(E) Failure of the thymus and parathyroid glands to develop

34. A 36-year-old man comes to the physician because he is experiencing abdominal pain, nausea, and a nonbloody diarrhea. He last ate about 18 hours ago at a Chinese restaurant. Which of the following treatments should this man receive?

(A) Bismuth subsalicylate, metronidazole, and amoxicillin
(B) Ciprofloxacin
(C) Erythromycin

(D) Prompt replacement of water and elec-trolytes; tetracyclines shorten the disease's course
(E) Supportive care only, without antibiotics

35. Which of the following pairs of vascular dis-eases is associated with production of perinu-clear antineutrophil cytoplasmic autoantibod-ies and circulating antineutrophil cytoplasmic autoantibodies, respectively?

(A) Kawasaki's disease, Buerger's disease
(B) Polyarteritis nodosa, Buerger's disease (thromboangiitis obliterans)
(C) Polyarteritis nodosa, Wegener's granulo-matosis
(D) Takayasu's arteritis, Wegener's granulo-matosis
(E) Temporal (giant cell) arteritis, Wegener's granulomatosis

36. An 87-year-old man is hospitalized after falling and breaking his hip. After 6 days in the hospi-tal, he develops burning on urination. Urinaly-sis shows leukocytosis and many gram-positive cocci. The patient is treated with trimetho-prim-sulfamethoxazole, but his fever persists. Two days later, the patient has a low-grade fever and new onset of a diastolic murmur that radiates to the axilla. Which of the following is the first-line treatment for the probable cause of this patient's infection?

(A) Ampicillin
(B) Gentamicin
(C) Piperacillin
(D) Quinupristin/dalfopristin
(E) Vancomycin

37. A 24-year-old woman comes to the physician complaining of recurrent upper abdominal pain that gets worse with food intake. She de-nies any history of vomiting, nausea, or diar-rhea. A urease breath test is positive. Which of the following organisms is most likely responsi-ble for this woman's symptoms?

(A) *Clostridium difficile*
(B) *Escherichia coli* O157:H7
(C) *Helicobacter pylori*
(D) *Proteus mirabilis*
(E) *Vibrio cholerae*

38. A 32-year-old man with Hodgkin's lymphoma is scheduled to undergo a bone marrow trans-plant. HLA typing of his immediate family shows that his identical twin brother is a suit-able match for harvesting an allogenic bone marrow graft. This type of graft can be classi-fied as which of the following?

(A) Autologous
(B) Combination graft
(C) Heterograft
(D) Syngeneic
(E) Xenogeneic

39. A 4-year-old boy presents to the pediatric emer-gency department with the classic meningitis triad of fever, headache, and nuchal rigidity. A lumbar puncture is performed and analysis of the fluid shows an increase in polymorphonu-clear cells (PMNs), an increased protein level, and a decreased glucose level. Which of the following is the most common cause of menin-gitis in a child of this age with this clinical pic-ture?

(A) Enteroviruses
(B) *Haemophilus influenzae* type B
(C) Herpes simplex virus
(D) *Listeria* species
(E) *Streptococcus pneumoniae*

40. A 32-year-old man presents to his doctor with painful urination and a purulent urethral discharge. The image shows cells that have been cultured from this discharge. Which of the following is the treatment of choice for this infection?

(A) Azithromycin
(B) Ceftriaxone
(C) Fluconazole
(D) Penicillin
(E) Vancomycin

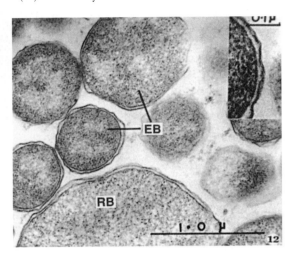

Reproduced, with permission, from Brooks GF, Butel JS, Morse SA. *Jawetz, Melnick, & Adelberg's Medical Microbiology*, 23rd ed. New York, McGraw-Hill, 2004: 358.)

41. Patients sharing similar clinical symptoms and disease pathology may nevertheless present differently based on age at disease onset. Which of the following represents an accurate distinction between juvenile rheumatoid arthritis (JRA) and adult-onset rheumatoid arthritis (RA)?

(A) Juvenile rheumatoid arthritis is simply the presence of RA that begins before the age of 21 years
(B) Patients with JRA are less likely to have systemic symptoms, but the likelihood of high levels of serum rheumatoid factor is the same
(C) Patients with JRA are more likely to have large joint involvement, but the likelihood of concurrent systemic symptoms is the same

(D) Patients with JRA are more likely to have systemic symptoms and high levels of serum rheumatoid factor
(E) Patients with JRA are more likely to have systemic symptoms and large joint involvement

42. A 43-year-old man presents with flulike symptoms, fevers, chills, and a productive cough. Physical examination is remarkable for pleuritic chest pain. On questioning, the patient says that he has just spent the last week on vacation in Central America. Cultures taken from the patient show a broad-based budding fungus. It is concluded that the man has systemic blastomycosis infection. Which of the following agents is the most appropriate treatment for this patient?

(A) Amphotericin B
(B) Fluconazole
(C) Itraconazole or potassium iodide
(D) Sodium stibogluconate only
(E) Topical miconazole or selenium sulfide

43. A 73-year-old woman steps on a rusty nail while gardening in her back yard. A neighbor drives her to the emergency department, where her wound is cleaned and bandaged. A complete history and review of her medical chart indicates that her vaccinations are not up to date, and she requires one vaccination and a shot of the appropriate immunoglobulin as prophylaxis against infection. What is the mechanism of toxicity of the organism for which she was vaccinated?

(A) ADP-ribosylation of a G protein, increasing chloride secretion
(B) ADP-ribosylation of an elongation factor, causing disrupted protein synthesis
(C) Binding to the MHC II receptor and T-lymphocyte receptor, causing cytokine synthesis
(D) Blocking release of the inhibitory neurotransmitter glycine
(E) Blocking the release of acetylcholine
(F) Lysis of RBCs
(G) Stimulation of guanylate cyclase

44. A 37-year-old man comes to the physician with recurrent viral infections. Blood studies show normal levels of circulating lymphocytes and neutrophils. A deficiency in which of the following cytokines would most likely lead to this man's condition?

    (A) Interleukin-2 (IL-2)
    (B) Interleukin-3 (IL-3)
    (C) Interleukin-4 (IL-4)
    (D) Interleukin-5 (IL-5)
    (E) Interleukin-8 (IL-8)

45. A 50-year-old man develops nonbloody watery diarrhea while working as an aid worker in a refugee camp in Central Africa. A stool smear shows no WBCs. He subsequently develops electrolyte abnormalities leading to cardiac and renal failure. Which of the following organisms is responsible for this man's enterocolitis?

    (A) *Bacillus cereus*
    (B) *Clostridium difficile*
    (C) *Helicobacter pylori*
    (D) *Salmonella* species
    (E) *Vibrio cholerae*

46. Which of the following glycoproteins are present on the cell surface of helper T lymphocytes, cytotoxic T lymphocytes, and B lymphocytes, respectively?

    (A) CD4, B7, CD19
    (B) CD4, CD8, CD19
    (C) CD8, CD4, CD19
    (D) CD19, CD4, CD8
    (E) CD19, CD8, CD4

47. Twenty-four hours after placement of a catheter, a hospitalized patient develops a fever and chills. Within 1 hour her systolic blood pressure falls 30 points and she develops swelling in her extremities. Despite valiant efforts by the hospital staff, the patient dies. The image shows an x-ray taken of the patient's lungs only hours before she passed away. Which of the following mediators of this patient's disease process is most likely responsible for the pathology depicted?

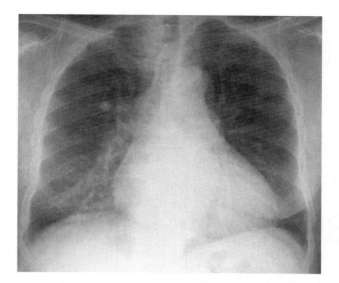

Reproduced, with permission, from Chen MYM, Pope TL, Ott DJ. *Basic Radiology*. New York, McGraw-Hill, 2004: Fig. 3-28A.

    (A) C3a
    (B) C5a
    (C) Hageman factor
    (D) Interleukin-1
    (E) Nitric oxide
    (F) Tumor necrosis factor

48. A 31-year-old pregnant woman comes to the physician because of painful lesions that have recently appeared on her genitalia. A positive result on which of the following diagnostic tests would mean that her baby is at risk for congenital anomalies?

    (A) Anti-HB surface antibody test
    (B) Giemsa stain
    (C) Monospot test
    (D) Tzanck smear
    (E) Weil-Felix test

49. A 2-year-old girl with a lifelong history of malabsorptive and foul-smelling diarrhea, weakness, and general failure to thrive has just undergone a small intestine biopsy (see image). Her parents believe her problems began at 6 months of age, when she started eating solid foods, but have significantly worsened over the past few months. The only recent change in her diet is that she eats a bowl of cereal every morning with her parents before they go to work. She tried a dairy-free diet a month ago, but it did not improve her symptoms. Which of the following is the most likely diagnosis?

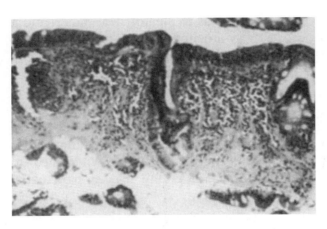

Reproduced, with permission, from Chandrasoma P, Taylor CR. *Concise Pathology*, 3rd ed. New York, McGraw-Hill, 1998: 590.

(A) Abetalipoproteinemia
(B) Celiac sprue
(C) Lactase deficiency
(D) Viral enteritis
(E) Whipple's disease

50. A pediatrician becomes concerned after learning the family and medical history of an infant who is currently suffering from pneumonia, with a presumed diagnosis of *Streptococcus pneumoniae* infection. Over the past year, the patient has suffered from erysipelas as well as a previous bout of pneumococcal pneumonia; both were treated successfully with antibiotics. The patient's mother says that her son's mater-

nal uncle also suffered from repeated bacterial infections and was successfully treated with antibiotics. On physical examination, it appears that the patient does not have tonsils. His mother denies a previous tonsillectomy. Analysis of the boy's serum would most likely yield which of the following results?

(A) < 200 CD4 T lymphocytes/μL
(B) Absence of T lymphocytes
(C) IgA, IgG, and IgM levels normal
(D) IgG and IgM levels markedly decreased, no IgA
(E) IgG and IgM levels normal, IgA markedly decreased

51. A 13-year-old girl who returned a few days ago from a school camping trip in North Carolina is home ill from school. She tells her parents that she has a headache and the chills. Over the next few days, she develops a rash that begins on her palms and soles, but spreads inward to her wrists and ankles and then to her trunk. Her worsening condition leads her parents to take her to the emergency department, where a blood test reveals antibodies that react with the *Proteus* antigen. This patient is most likely infected with which of the following?

(A) *Borrelia burgdorferi*
(B) *Coxiella burnetti*
(C) Coxsackievirus A
(D) *Rickettsia rickettsii*
(E) *Rickettsia typhi*
(F) *Treponema pallidum*

52. A 25-year-old man presents to his doctor with a 2-day history of blood in his urine. A kidney biopsy is obtained. When the tissue is stained with fluorescent IgG antibodies, the staining reveals a linear pattern. Which of the following is the most likely diagnosis?

(A) Acute poststreptococcal glomerulonephritis
(B) Alport's syndrome
(C) Goodpasture's syndrome
(D) IgA nephropathy
(E) Membranous glomerulonephritis

53. A clinician is concerned that an Rh-negative mother may be pregnant with an Rh-positive fetus. The potential pathology that the clinician is concerned about is classified as which of the following immune reactions?

(A) Graft-versus-host disease
(B) Type I hypersensitivity
(C) Type II hypersensitivity
(D) Type III hypersensitivity
(E) Type IV hypersensitivity

54. A 14-year-old boy presents to the physician with recurrent pyogenic infections. Physical examination shows that the boy has pruritic papulovesicular dermatitis. Blood is drawn and sent for laboratory evaluation of platelets and immunoglobulin levels. The results show a markedly low platelet count, a low serum IgM level, and an elevated IgA level. This patient most likely has which of the following conditions?

(A) Bruton's agammaglobulinemia
(B) Chédiak-Higashi disease
(C) Job syndrome
(D) Thymic aplasia (DiGeorge's syndrome)
(E) Wiskott-Aldrich syndrome

55. Infection with the *Malassezia furfur* organism causes skin hypopigmentation. It is found most frequently in hot, humid, tropical regions. It also is responsible for causing one of the cutaneous mycoses. Infection with *Malassezia furfur* also causes which of the following disorders?

(A) Tinea capitis
(B) Tinea cruris
(C) Tinea nigra
(D) Tinea pedis
(E) Tinea versicolor

56. A 32-year-old woman comes to the emergency department complaining of sudden blindness. On obtaining a thorough history, it is learned that the patient's right leg has "given out" from time to time, causing the patient to have episodes of weakness and falling. Periventricular white matter plaques are found on MRI. Which of the following cells are primarily damaged in this disease?

(A) Astrocytes
(B) Ependymal cells
(C) Oligodendrocytes
(D) Schwann cells
(E) T cells

57. A 22-year-old woman presents to the physician with vaginal itching and burning. On examination, she has a foul-smelling greenish discharge. A swab sample is taken and a wet mount slide is prepared. Results from the sample are shown in the image. Which of the following medications should be prescribed for this patient?

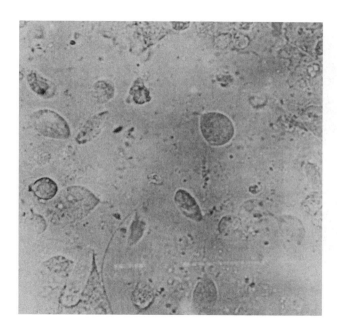

Reproduced, with permission, from Tintinalli JE, Kelen GD, Stapczynski JS, Ma OJ, Cline DM. *Tintinalli's Emergency Medicine: A Comprehensive Study Guide*, 6th ed. New York, McGraw-Hill, 2004: 694.

(A) Metronidazole
(B) Nifurtimox
(C) Quinine
(D) Sodium stibogluconate
(E) Sulfadiazine and pyrimethamine

58. Women have approximately a 2.7 times greater lifetime risk of developing at least one autoimmune disease than men. Which of the following statements, if true, would support the higher rate of systemic lupus erythematosus in women than in men?

    (A) Androgens such as testosterone have an inhibitory role in the process of clearing immune complexes
    (B) Both estrogens and androgens have the same potency in inhibiting the clearing of immune complexes
    (C) Estrogen has a stimulatory role in the process of clearing immune complexes
    (D) Estrogen has an inhibitory role in the process of antibody production of B cells
    (E) Estrogen has an inhibitory role in the process of clearing immune complexes

59. A 40-year-old man goes on a camping vacation with his family. One day after swimming in a freshwater lake near the camp site, he develops nausea and vomiting and starts to behave irrationally. His family takes him to the emergency department, where blood samples are taken and a spinal tap is performed. He is diagnosed with a rapidly progressing meningoencephalitis and dies shortly thereafter. Which of the following protozoa was most likely the cause of the man's illness?

    (A) *Cryptosporidium* species
    (B) *Entamoeba histolytica*
    (C) *Leishmania donovani*
    (D) *Naegleria fowleri*
    (E) *Plasmodium falciparum*

60. A 54-year-old man presents to the clinic with scleral icterus, hepatosplenomegaly, ascites, and a history of episodes of jaundice over the past 3 years. He was involved in an auto accident when he was 21, for which he required surgery and blood transfusions. His laboratory results are as follows:

    Aspartate aminotransferase (AST): 734 U/L
    Alanine aminotransferase (ALT): 846 U/L
    Direct bilirubin: 0.1 mg/dL
    Indirect bilirubin: 7.6 mg/dL

Assuming a viral etiology, which of the following is the most likely cause of this patient's illness?

(A) Hepatitis A
(B) Hepatitis C
(C) Hepatitis D
(D) Hepatitis E
(E) Hepatitis G

61. A 2-year-old boy is brought to the physician by his parents because of recurrent sinus infections. The parents also state that the boy has had multiple lung infections. Which of the following results would most likely be found on further testing?

    (A) A high IgE level and normal levels of all immunoglobulins
    (B) A low IgA level
    (C) A low IgM level, an elevated IgA level, and a normal IgG level
    (D) A normal immunoglobulin level
    (E) A normal immunoglobulin level and a negative nitroblue tetrazolium dye reduction test

62. A 19-year-old college student presents to his family physician with a 1-week history of fever, headache, and painful pharyngitis. Physical examination shows significant lymphadenopathy of the posterior auricular nodes and hepatosplenomegaly. Laboratory studies show an elevated leukocyte count of 15,000/mm^3 with 55% lymphocytes. A heterophile antibody test is positive. Which of the following is the most likely cause of this patient's symptoms?

    (A) Cytomegalovirus
    (B) Epstein-Barr virus
    (C) HIV infection
    (D) *Streptococcus pneumoniae*
    (E) *Toxoplasma gondii*

63. A 38-year-old man comes to the emergency department complaining of cyclic fevers and headaches. The fevers began about 1 week ago; 2 weeks ago, the patient returned from a trip to Africa. On examination, the patient is found to have splenomegaly, and brain imag-

ing studies show signs of significant cerebral involvement. Which of the following parasites most likely caused this patient's symptoms?

(A) *Giardia lamblia*
(B) *Plasmodium falciparum*
(C) *Plasmodium malariae*
(D) *Plasmodium ovale*
(E) *Plasmodium vivax*

64. Recombinant human granulocyte colony-stimulating factor is used clinically to mobilize hematopoietic progenitor and stem cells from bone marrow sites into circulating blood. Which of the following cell surface markers is used to select for these peripheral blood stem cells?

(A) B7
(B) CD4
(C) CD8
(D) CD28
(E) CD34
(F) Phosphatidylinositol glycan A

65. A 56-year-old man comes to the emergency department because of a sharp retrosternal pain that radiates to his back and arms. He states that the pain worsens on inspiration, as well as when he lies on his back. Physical examination reveals a high-pitched grating sound at the lower left sternal border. An ECG confirms the diagnosis. Which of the following viruses is a common cause of this condition?

(A) Coxsackievirus
(B) Cytomegalovirus
(C) Epstein-Barr virus
(D) Norwalk agent
(E) Rubella

66. A 50-year-old man was gardening outside his house recently and thinks that he may have been exposed to poison ivy. He presents to his clinician with bilateral itching, burning, and redness of the lower extremities. Which of the following statements is most correct?

(A) Goodpasture's syndrome is a disease with a similar reaction pathogenesis
(B) The pathogenesis implicates previously sensitized B lymphocytes
(C) The patient has never been exposed to poison ivy
(D) The patient is suffering from a type I hypersensitivity reaction
(E) The patient must have been exposed to the poison ivy plant prior to this instance

67. A 40-year-old man comes to the emergency department because of diplopia and dysphagia that developed after he consumed homemade strawberry jam. While in the emergency department, he develops general muscle weakness and requires intubation due to sudden respiratory muscle paralysis. Which of the following organisms is most likely responsible for this patient's condition?

(A) *Bacillus cereus*
(B) *Clostridium botulinum*
(C) *Clostridium perfringens*
(D) *Clostridium tetani*
(E) *Escherichia coli*

68. Antibodies are one of the major players in the adaptive immune response. All antibody molecules consist of two heavy chains and two light chains, and the specific type of heavy and light chain will determine the antigen binding site. In all antibodies, the two heavy chains and the two light chains are identical. Like most proteins, much of their functional capabilities and antigen binding characteristics stem from their three-dimensional structure. Which of the following holds the heavy and light chains together to make the three-dimensional structure of the antibody?

(A) Hydrogen bonds
(B) Intrachain disulfide bonds
(C) Ionic bonds
(D) Triple covalent bonds
(E) Van der Waals forces

69. A 55-year-old man comes to his physician with a tender, swollen, and red left knee. He has limited range of motion in his leg. On aspiration of the synovial fluid from his knee, the fluid is yellow and cloudy and has 150,000 neutrophils/mm³. A Gram's stain of the aspirate shows gram-positive cocci. The organisms most likely responsible for this patient's symptoms belong to which genus?

    (A) *Babesia*
    (B) *Bacillus*
    (C) *Clostridium*
    (D) *Pasteurella*
    (E) *Staphylococcus*

70. A family who recently emigrated from Romania brings their 7-year-old child to the pediatrician with complaints of conjunctivitis and periorbital swelling. The child has had coughing with a runny nose and high fever for 3 days. Small lesions with blue-white centers are seen in his oral cavity. Which of the following is the most likely cause of this child's symptoms?

    (A) Diphtheria
    (B) Pertussis
    (C) Roseola
    (D) Rubella
    (E) Rubeola

71. A 23-year-old woman comes to the physician for a routine checkup. She has generally been well over the past year, although she notes that she has "had a few falls lately." Physical findings on examination of her face are shown in the image. Blood is drawn for laboratory evaluation. The results show that the woman has very low levels of IgA. Based on her presentation, this patient will most likely also present with which of the following symptoms?

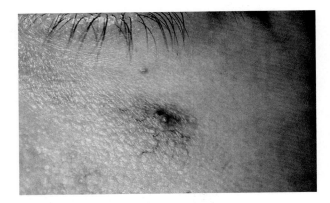

Reproduced, with permission, from Wolff K, Johnson RA, Suurmond D. *Fitzpatrick's Color Atlas & Synopsis of Clinical Dermatology*, 5th ed. New York, McGraw-Hill, 2005: 191.

    (A) Cerebellar problems
    (B) Granulomas
    (C) Low levels of all other immunoglobulin isotypes
    (D) Tetany
    (E) Visual hallucinations

72. A 34-year-old woman newly diagnosed with HIV is currently asymptomatic. She is not taking any medications yet, and she is skeptical about the impact medications might have on her fatal disease. She is aware that if left untreated, her disease will progress and make her susceptible to different infections. She inquires about the natural course her disease may take and the different infections she may acquire. Which of the following infections manifests with the lowest T-cell count?

    (A) Cryptococcal meningitis
    (B) Disseminated *Mycobacterium avium–intracellulare*
    (C) Herpes simplex
    (D) Herpes zoster

(E) Oral thrush
(F) *Pneumocystis carinii* pneumonia
(G) Toxoplasmosis brain lesion

73. A neonate who is born with a cleft palate and abnormal facies becomes cyanotic and hypoxic soon after birth. On physical examination, the neonatologist hears a crescendo-decrescendo murmur with a harsh systolic ejection. Further investigation shows tetralogy of Fallot. Laboratory tests show that the patient is hypocalcemic. This infant most likely has which of the following conditions?

(A) Bruton's agammaglobulinemia
(B) Job syndrome
(C) Severe combined immunodeficiency
(D) Thymic aplasia (DiGeorge's syndrome)
(E) Wiskott-Aldrich syndrome

74. An 8-year-old boy is brought to his pediatrician by his parents because of a fever and a sore throat. On examination, he has tonsillar exudates and swollen, tender anterior cervical nodes. His parents report no history of cough. Gram's stain of the tonsillar exudate reveals gram-positive cocci. Which of the following describes the organism most likely causing this patient's symptoms?

(A) Catalase-negative, β-hemolytic, bacitracin-resistant
(B) Catalase-negative, β-hemolytic, bacitracin-sensitive
(C) Catalase-negative, α-hemolytic, optochin-resistant
(D) Catalase-negative, α-hemolytic, optochin-sensitive
(E) Catalase-positive, coagulase-positive, novo-biocin-resistant
(F) Catalase-positive, coagulase-positive, novo-biocin-sensitive

75. A 50-year-old man comes to the physician with hemoptysis and diffuse joint pain. He states that both his father and cousin had similar symptoms and were diagnosed with microscopic polyangiitis, a disease affecting medium-to small-sized arteries that is believed to have an autoimmune component to its pathogenesis. Which of the following autoantibodies might be present in this patient?

(A) Anti-Smith antibodies
(B) Anti-SS-A (Ro) antibody
(C) Anti-SS-B (La) antibody
(D) Anticentromere antibodies
(E) Antineutrophil cytoplasmic autoantibodies

ANSWERS

1. **The correct answer is A.** Acyclovir has a high affinity for viral thymidine kinase. Once phosphorylated by this enzyme, these molecules inhibit herpes simplex virus (HSV) polymerase with 30–50 times the potency of human α-DNA polymerase. Acyclovir is thus concentrated in virus-infected cells. It is also effective against other herpesviruses, such as HSV-1, varicella-zoster virus, and Epstein-Barr virus. High doses of this drug can produce nephrotoxicity and neurologic symptoms.

   Answer B is incorrect. Amantadine prevents penetration and uncoating of viral particles, specifically influenza A. In Parkinson's disease, it causes the release of dopamine from nerve terminals via an unknown mechanism.

   Answer C is incorrect. Ribavirin is used to treat respiratory syncytial virus. It functions by inhibiting inosine monophosphate dehydrogenase, thus blocking the synthesis of guanine nucleotides.

   Answer D is incorrect. Rifampin is used to treat tuberculosis and as prophylaxis against meningococcal meningitis. It works by inhibiting the DNA-dependent RNA polymerase of these organisms.

   Answer E is incorrect. Vancomycin is a bactericidal antibiotic used for multidrug-resistant gram-positive organisms such as *Staphylococcus aureus* and *Clostridium difficile*. It functions by binding to mucopeptide precursors, preventing formation of the bacterial cell wall.

2. **The correct answer is A.** This patient has been exposed to hepatitis B and has completely recovered, as is demonstrated by her serologic markers. She does not carry the HB surface antigen (HBsAg), which is found on the surface of the hepatitis B virus and indicates a carrier state. She does carry the surface antibody, which indicates that she was exposed to hepatitis B and made antibodies to convey immunity. The fact that she also has IgG antibody to the core antibody (HBcAb) shows that she has recovered. HBcAb is also positive in

the chronic state, but in that case she would not also have HBsAb. To have both and not have HBsAg is an indication of complete recovery.

   Answer B is incorrect. The patient has completely recovered and is not in the acute disease phase.

   Answer C is incorrect. The patient has completely recovered and is not in the window phase.

   Answer D is incorrect. The patient has completely recovered but was once infected.

   Answer E is incorrect. The patient has completely recovered and is not now chronically infected.

3. **The correct answer is D.** Acute rejection is one complication of kidney transplantation. In acute rejection, the principal mediator is believed to be the cytotoxic T lymphocyte. Activated cytotoxic lymphocytes invade the tubular interstitium of the transplanted kidney, leading to tubulitis. In contrast, chronic rejection is mediated by antibody complex formation. Elevated creatinine levels allow early detection of acute rejection in the absence of clinical signs, which may include graft tenderness, oliguria, and fever. T lymphocytes mature in the thymus, where they undergo positive and negative selection. Thus, the correct answer is the thymus.

   Answer A is incorrect. B lymphocytes mature in the bone marrow.

   Answer B is incorrect. T lymphocytes do not undergo maturation in the lung.

   Answer C is incorrect. T lymphocytes are found in the periarterial lymphatic sheath in the white pulp of the spleen, but maturation occurs in the thymus.

   Answer E is incorrect. The yolk sac, the liver, and the spleen are important in RBC formation in utero but are not relevant in T-lymphocyte development.

4. **The correct answer is C.** This patient is presenting with Chagas' disease, which is caused by infection with *Trypanosoma cruzi*. Acute symptoms include chagomas (small dermal granulomas caused by local multiplication of the pathogen), myocarditis, and congestive heart failure as a severe, but rare, complication of myocarditis. More chronic symptoms include arrhythmias, dilated cardiomyopathy, megacolon, and megaesophagus as *T. cruzi* infects cardiac tissue and colonic nerves. Treatment is mainly symptomatic. Another form of infection occurs when the organism enters the body through the conjunctiva. In that case, eye edema known as Romana's sign occurs. Chagas' disease is mostly transmitted by the reduviid bug in Central and South America.

Answer A is incorrect. The *Anopheles* mosquito is responsible for transmission of the four plasmodia species that cause malaria.

Answer B is incorrect. The Ixodes tick transmits *Borrelia burgdorferi*, the cause of Lyme disease.

Answer D is incorrect. The sandfly is responsible for transmission of *Leishmania donovani*, also known as "kala-azar" or leishmaniasis.

Answer E is incorrect. The tsetse fly carries *Trypanosoma brucei gambiense* and *rhodesiense*, the two causes of African sleeping sickness. In this disease, patients complain of repeatedly falling asleep in addition to headaches and dizziness. Other symptoms include recurrent fevers and lymphadenopathy. *T. rhodesiense* causes a much more acute infection, while *T. gambiense* causes a more subacute, indolent, and progressive disease.

5. **The correct answer is A.** *Klebsiella pneumoniae* infection results in a bronchopneumonia, which is characterized by acute inflammatory infiltrates from bronchioles into adjacent alveoli.

Answer B is incorrect. Lobar pneumonia, most frequently due to *Streptococcus pneumoniae*, morphologically evolves through four stages without treatment: congestion, red hepatization, gray hepatization, and resolution.

Answer C is incorrect. Interstitial pneumonias, from mycoplasma and viruses, are characterized by diffuse patchy inflammation localized to interstitial areas at alveolar walls.

Answer D is incorrect. Interstitial pneumonias, from mycoplasma and viruses, are characterized by diffuse patchy inflammation localized to interstitial areas at alveolar walls. They also have no exudates in alveolar spaces, but have intra-alveolar hyaline membranes.

Answer E is incorrect. Lobar pneumonia, most frequently due to *Streptococcus pneumoniae*, characteristically has predominantly intra-alveolar exudates, resulting in consolidation.

6. **The correct answer is A.** This patient has Lyme disease caused by *Borrelia burgdorferi*. The vector is the *Ixodes* tick, which is found commonly in the Northeastern United States. The first phase of infection appears about 10 days after the initial tick bite and consists of a target-like rash (erythema migrans) with central clearing at the site of the bite. The initial rash resolves and the second phase begins weeks later. This phase is characterized by transient arthralgias, Bell's palsy, atrioventricular nodal block, secondary annular rashes, and carditis. The involvement of various systems in disseminated Lyme disease varies. Cardiac involvement is seen in 5% of patients, while neurological involvement is seen in 15%. The third phase can appear months to years later with signs of migratory joint paint, some evidence of chronic arthritis, encephalopathy, and acrodermatitis.

Answer B is incorrect. *Borrelia recurrentis* is spread by the human body louse and causes a disease that is characterized by relapsing fevers that last about 5 days, with about 1 week in between each episode. This relapse and remittance is attributed to the organism's ability to undergo antigenic variation. Arthralgias and rashes are not symptoms of this disease.

Answer C is incorrect. *Leptospira interrogans* causes leptospirosis and Weil's syndrome. The first phase is characterized by flulike symptoms and photophobia. In most cases it will present with abrupt onset of fever, myalgias, rigors, and headache. Nonproductive cough, nausea, vomiting, and diarrhea can also be seen in patients with acute leptospirosis. Weil's syndrome is a rare complication of leptospirosis. It is characterized by hemorrhagic vasculitis, infectious jaundice, renal dysfunction, and hepatic failure. Less than 10% of patients with leptospirosis progress to this state. This spirochete is carried by various animals and is shed in the urine.

Answer D is incorrect. *Rickettsia rickettsii* is the cause of Rocky Mountain spotted fever (RMSF), which occurs mostly on the east coast of the United States. The main symptoms of RMSF are headache, fever, and a rash that starts at the palms and soles and then progresses to include the wrists, ankles, and trunks. Bell's palsy and annular target lesions are not characteristic of RMSF.

Answer E is incorrect. *Treponema pallidum* is the cause of syphilis, a predominantly sexually transmitted disease. The primary phase consists of a painless chancre that develops within 6 weeks of exposure. Six weeks after the chancre heals, some patients progress to the secondary phase, which consists of condyloma lata, a maculopapular rash on the palms and soles, meningitis, hepatitis, and/or arthritis. If untreated, the disease can progress to tertiary syphilis, which is most often characterized by aortitis, ascending aortic aneurysm, and a variety of central nervous system symptoms.

7. **The correct answer is A.** Most adjuvants are believed to have their main effect on antigen-presenting cells (APCs) such as dendritic cells or macrophages. It has been suggested that they activate the APC through stimulation of pattern recognition receptors (such as toll-like receptors). This leads to increased costimulatory capacity and therefore makes it easier for the APC to activate T lymphocytes specific for the vaccine.

Answer B is incorrect. T lymphocytes are not antigen-presenting cells (APCs). The three types of professional APCs are dendritic cells,

macrophages, and B lymphocytes. Adjuvants most directly activate APCs, which can in turn activate T lymphocytes.

Answer C is incorrect. This is most likely not true.

Answer D is incorrect. While this may be true, it is not believed to be the main mechanism by which Freund's complete adjuvant (or any other adjuvant) acts.

Answer E is incorrect. This is not true.

8. **The correct answer is C.** The clinical picture and imaging are consistent with progressive multifocal leukoencephalopathy (PML) secondary to reactivation of latent JC virus infection, which can occur with CD4 counts below 50/μL. It typically presents with rapidly progressive focal neurologic deficits without signs of increased intracranial pressure. Ataxia, aphasia, and cranial nerve deficits may also occur. Lumbar puncture is nondiagnostic and frequently demonstrates mild elevations in protein and white blood cells. Cerebrospinal fluid (CSF) analysis can also reveal the presence of myelin basic protein, which is due to viral demyelination. PML typically presents as multiple nonenhancing T2-hyperintense lesions. When it is suspected, stereotactic biopsy is required for definitive diagnosis, but a positive CSF polymerase chain reaction for JC virus is diagnostic in the appropriate clinical setting. Although there is no definitive treatment, clearance of JC virus DNA can be observed with response to highly active antiretroviral therapy.

Answer A is incorrect. Cytomegalovirus (CMV) encephalitis can mimic the appearance of progressive multifocal leukoencephalopathy, but would be associated with enhancing periventricular white matter lesions in cortical and subependymal regions. CMV encephalitis is also typically associated with more systemic signs and symptoms; polymerase chain reaction analysis of cerebrospinal fluid would be positive for CMV.

Answer B is incorrect. HIV encephalopathy (HIVE) typically presents with the insidious onset of memory loss, gait disorder, and spasticity. It is the most common central nervous system complication of HIV-1 disease and also produces nonenhancing lesions without mass effect on imaging studies. Although variable in presentation, HIVE lesions are usually T2-hyperintense but are more symmetrical and less demarcated than progressive multifocal leukoencephalopathy (PML). Focal neurologic findings, as in PML, are uncommon until late in the course of disease.

Answer D is incorrect. Central nervous system (CNS) lymphoma typically also affects those with CD4 counts under 50/μL. MRI will demonstrate one or more enhancing lesions (50% multiple; 50% single) that are typically surrounded by edema and can produce mass effect. CNS lymphoma can present with polymerase chain reaction findings on cerebrospinal fluid as positive for Epstein-Barr virus.

Answer E is incorrect. Space-occupying lesions due to toxoplasmosis infection represent the most common cause of cerebral mass lesions in HIV-infected patients and typically present with multiple enhancing lesions on MRI. The lesions are typically located at the corticomedullary junction and are surrounded by edema that frequently produces mass effect and distinguishes its appearance from progressive multifocal leukoencephalopathy. Positive *Toxoplasma* serologies can assist in diagnosis, and clinical improvements will result from treatment with sulfadiazine and pyrimethamine.

9. **The correct answer is D.** Severe combined immunodeficiency is a defect in early stem-cell differentiation that can have many causes and leads to a total lack of a cellular immune system. The typical presentation of this disease includes recurrent bacterial, viral, protozoal, and fungal infections.

Answer A is incorrect. Ataxia-telangiectasia is a defect in DNA repair enzymes. The disease is associated with an IgA deficiency. The typical presentation of the disease is given away by the name, as symptoms include cerebellar problems (ataxia) and spider angiomas (telangiectasia).

Answer B is incorrect. Chédiak-Higashi disease is an autosomal recessive disease that presents with recurrent streptococcal and staphylococcal infections. A defect in lysosomal emptying of phagocytic cells due to microtubular dysfunction is the underlying cause of the disease.

Answer C is incorrect. Job syndrome involves the failure of helper T cells to produce interferon-γ (INF-γ). Since INF-γ is a potent activator of phagocytic cells, a decrease in its production leads to a failure of neutrophils to respond to chemotactic stimuli.

Answer E is incorrect. Wiskott-Aldrich syndrome is an X-linked defect associated with elevated IgA levels, elevated IgE levels, and low IgM levels. It involves a defect in the body's ability to mount an IgM response to bacteria. Recurrent pyogenic infections, eczema, and thrombocytopenia are the typical triad of symptoms that present with this disease.

10. **The correct answer is C.** This is a classic case of molluscum contagiosum caused by the poxvirus. The patient's physical examination indicates the presence of large cytoplasmic inclusions called molluscum bodies. Molluscum contagiosum is a benign skin disease transmitted by sexual contact, clothes, or towels. It may resolve spontaneously or be removed surgically.

Answer A is incorrect. Herpes simplex virus type 1 causes gingivostomatitis, herpetic keratitis of the eye, and encephalitis.

Answer B is incorrect. Human herpesvirus 8 is thought to be the causative factor of Kaposi's sarcoma. These lesions are purple/red/blue and are most common in patients with AIDS.

Answer D is incorrect. Rubeola virus is another name for the RNA virus that causes measles, an exanthematous disease that begins as Koplik's spots on the oral mucosa and progresses to a maculopapular rash.

Answer E is incorrect. Varicella-zoster virus is the causative agent in chickenpox. It is a highly contagious DNA herpesvirus that is self-limiting. It is transmitted by respiratory droplets or by direct contact and is characterized by a vesicular rash with macules, papules, and pustules over the head and trunk.

11. **The correct answer is C.** Mounting a strong immune response is crucial for the body to be able to fight off infections. However, reducing this response once the infection has been warded off is critical in order for the body to maintain its normal balance. TGF-β is the cytokine that is responsible for dampening the immune response after it is no longer needed.

Answer A is incorrect. INF-γ is secreted by helper T lymphocytes and helps stimulate macrophages.

Answer B is incorrect. IL-1 is secreted by macrophages and serves as one of the main cytokines involved in mounting an acute phase response.

Answer D is incorrect. TNF-α is one of the main cytokines involved in mounting an acute-phase response; it is secreted by macrophages.

Answer E is incorrect. TNF-β has functions similar to TNF-α in that it helps mount an acute-phase response. However, it is secreted by activated T lymphocytes instead of macrophages.

12. **The correct answer is A.** The question stem describes classic symptoms of infection with Epstein-Barr virus (EBV), including flulike symptoms, increasing fatigue, lymphadenopathy, and splenomegaly. EBV is a member of the herpes viral family with linear double-stranded, enveloped DNA. Herpes viruses are unique in that it is the only virus that obtains its envelope via budding from the nuclear membrane.

Answer B is incorrect. Linear, double-stranded DNA without an envelope describes the adenoviruses. This virus is mostly known for conjunctivitis or "pink eye." It can also

cause respiratory tract infections, hemorrhagic cystitis, and gastroenteritis.

Answer C is incorrect. The only double-stranded RNA viruses known to infect humans are the reoviruses. These includes *Reoviridae coltivirus*, which causes Colorado tick fever, and *Reoviridae rotavirus*, which causes gastroenteritis. Rotavirus infection is the principal cause of fatal diarrhea in children throughout the world. Colorado tick fever is transmitted via ticks carried by rodents and is found most commonly in hikers.

Answer D is incorrect. Partially circular, double-stranded DNA with an envelope describes the hepadnaviruses. The main infectious pathogen in this family is hepatitis B virus. Its main modes of transmission are blood and sexual contact. This patient does not present with signs of hepatitis.

Answer E is incorrect. The orthomyxoviruses are characterized by segmented, single-stranded RNA with negative polarity and an envelope. The principal disease caused by these viruses is influenza. Although this patient does have flulike symptoms, lymphadenopathy and splenomegaly are not characteristic of the flu.

13. **The correct answer is A.** The disease described is yellow fever, caused by a member of the Flaviviridae family. It presents with symptoms of jaundice, aching pain, and high fever. Its vector is the mosquito. Liver biopsy can reveal Councilman bodies—eosinophilic globules believed to be the result of apoptosis of individual hepatocytes.

Answer B is incorrect. Döhle bodies are oval bodies found in the neutrophils of patients with infections, trauma, pregnancy, or cancer.

Answer C is incorrect. Negri bodies are pathognomonic for the rabies virus. They are eosinophilic inclusion bodies found in the cytoplasm of nerve cells of infected individuals.

Answer D is incorrect. Pappenheimer bodies are found in RBCs in sideroblastic anemia and sickle cell disease. They are phagosomes containing ferruginous granules.

Answer E is incorrect. Weibel-Palade bodies can be seen by electron microscopy in vascular endothelial cells. They are collections of microtubules.

14. **The correct answer is B.** *Babesia* species infection presents with a malaria-like syndrome. Babesiosis is transmitted by the *Ixodes* tick. On microscopic examination, one observes no red blood cell pigment and the Maltese cross–appearing parasite. Quinine is used to treat babesiosis.

Answer A is incorrect. *Acanthamoeba* species infection presents with meningoencephalitis in immune-compromised patients. It can also cause keratitis through contaminated contact lens solution. On histologic examination, spiky trophozoites are found in the cerebrospinal fluid and brain tissue. Treatment is usually through multiple antibiotics and antifungals, and hospitalization is often needed.

Answer C is incorrect. *Leishmania donovani* infection presents with hepatomegaly and splenomegaly, malaise, anemia, and weight loss. *L. donovani* is transmitted via the sandfly. Microscopically, macrophages containing amastigotes are observed. Sodium stibogluconate is used to treat *L. donovani* infection.

Answer D is incorrect. *Naegleria fowleri* infection presents with meningoencephalitis that can progress to coma or death within 6 days. Other symptoms include nausea, vomiting, and irrational behavior. Transmission occurs through swimming in freshwater lakes. Microscopic analysis reveals amebas in the spinal fluid. Unfortunately, there is no treatment for *N. fowleri* infection.

Answer E is incorrect. *Trypanosoma cruzi* infection causes Chagas' disease, a condition in which the heart is enlarged and flaccid. *T. cruzi* is transmitted via the reduviid bug. Microscopic examination reveals flagellated trypomastigotes in the blood and nonmotile amastigotes in tissue culture. *T. cruzi* infection is treated with nifurtimox.

15. **The correct answer is B.** Both hepatitis C and hepatitis B infection are associated with an increased risk of developing hepatocellular carcinoma. The liver is the organ in the body with the most regenerative potential. If this ability is overused, the chance of an oncogenic mutation occurring during the regeneration of cells is higher.

Answer A is incorrect. Epstein-Barr virus (EBV) is associated with Burkitt's lymphoma (a B-lymphocyte lymphoma) and nasopharyngeal carcinoma. The t(8;14) translocation is consistently associated with Burkitt's lymphoma, but the translocation alone is not responsible for the neoplasm and is not found in nasopharyngeal carcinomas. The other factors that determine oncogenesis of EBV remain unclear.

Answer C is incorrect. HIV as a direct oncogenic agent is being intensely researched, but it is already known that immune suppression and dysregulation caused by HIV infection give rise to lymphomas and Kaposi's sarcoma.

Answer D is incorrect. Human papillomavirus causes carcinoma (usually cervical) by inactivating tumor suppressor genes such as *p*53 and *Rb*.

Answer E is incorrect. Human T-cell lymphoma virus causes adult T-cell leukemia, and although the mechanism of oncogenesis remains unclear, there is some evidence that integration into the host genome at locations near cellular growth genes may play a role.

16. **The correct answer is C.** The C5b, 6, 7, 8 complex guides the polymerization of C9 molecules into a tube, which is inserted into the lipid bilayer of the plasma membrane. This membrane attack complex allows the passage of ions and small molecules into the cell, causing the cell to lyse.

Answer A is incorrect. This answer choice refers to C5a, which is involved in neutrophil chemotaxis.

Answer B is incorrect. This is not the function of the membrane attack complex.

Answer D is incorrect. C3a and C5a are the molecules that are involved in anaphylaxis, not the membrane attack complex.

Answer E is incorrect. This answer choice refers to C3b, which is involved in opsonization.

17. **The correct answer is E.** When an Rh-negative mother gives birth to an Rh-positive fetus, fetal RBCs may enter the mother's circulation, and the body may recognize the Rh antigen as foreign and produce antibodies against it. As any maternal IgG may freely cross the placenta, any subsequent Rh-positive fetus is at risk for hemolytic disease. Thus, the indirect Coombs' test is an important laboratory tool to monitor for Rh incompatibilities that may complicate fetal health. The test result given in this question indicates that the patient does possess anti-Rh antibodies within her serum. Therefore, it would be logical for the clinician to suspect previous pregnancy with an Rh-positive fetus.

Answer A is incorrect. The test yielded a positive result. Agglutination occurs when the anti-IgG antibody secondary antibody binds to the anti-Rh antibodies and cross-links the RBCs.

Answer B is incorrect. The laboratory protocol described in the question stem is correct. Rh-positive RBCs must be added because the test is assaying for the presence anti-Rh antibodies, which will bind the Rh antigen on the RBCs.

Answer C is incorrect. The presence of anti-Rh antibodies within the patient's serum suggests that she delivered at least one Rh-positive fetus.

Answer D is incorrect. The results of the Coombs' test cannot be used to determine current pregnancy status.

18. **The correct answer is D.** Circulating IgG that is passed from the mother to the newborn through the placenta protects the newborn from many microorganisms for the first 6 months of life. Thus, improper transfer of IgG from the mother to the fetus can leave the newborn sus-

ceptible to infections. While IgA is found in breast milk, a neonate will have access only to antenatal antibodies, and IgG is the only antibody isotype that can cross the placenta.

Answer A is incorrect. Ataxia-telangiectasia is caused by a defect in DNA repair enzymes with associated IgA deficiency. This usually presents with cerebellar problems (ataxia) and spider angiomas (telangiectasia). It would not cause a neonate to be immunocompromised, because for the first 6 months of life the infant relies on IgG from the mother.

Answer B is incorrect. An X-linked recessive defect in a tyrosine kinase gene is seen in Bruton's agammaglobulinemia. This is associated with low levels of all classes of immunoglobulins. However, with Bruton's agammaglobulinemia, bacterial infections tend to occur after 6 months of age, when levels of maternal IgG antibody start to decline to levels insufficient to provide host defense.

Answer C is incorrect. Improper development of the thymus and parathyroid glands is seen in thymic aplasia (DiGeorge's syndrome). This leads to recurrent viral and fungal infections due to a T-lymphocyte deficiency. It would not have any effect on susceptibility to bacterial infections.

Answer E is incorrect. The only antibody isotype that can cross the placenta is IgG. Therefore, IgM would not play a role in an infant's immunity until an infant can produce it themselves, at the age of 6 months.

19. **The correct answer is B.** Influenza virus has both hemagglutinin (HA) and neuraminidase (NA) molecules on its surface. These two molecules are responsible for the ability of the virus to be absorbed and penetrate the host cells. After a human is infected with the influenza virus, that person will be immune to infection by the same virus because of antibodies created against HA and NA. If either HA or NA is changed, as can be the case if two different influenza viruses infect the same cell and exchange RNA, antigenic shift can occur. This creates a new virus that has never been ex-

posed to the human immune system before, with potentially catastrophic consequences. This type of mixing is most commonly thought to be between a human and an avian strain mixing in an intermediary porcine host—leading to the term *avian flu*.

Answer A is incorrect. Antigenic drift describes mutations that can occur in hemagglutinin and neuraminidase, making them less antigenic to the preexisting antibodies in the human host. Since this results in small changes in viral toxicity, it will lead to a slightly different strain, but it is not likely to lead to a global epidemic.

Answer C is incorrect. Hemagglutinin has the ability to attach to sialic acid receptors, which activates fusion of the virus to the cell. All infectious influenza viruses have this molecule.

Answer D is incorrect. Neuraminidase has the ability to destroy neuraminic acid, a component of mucin. This helps break down the barrier to the upper airways and aids in infectivity.

Answer E is incorrect. RBCs agglutinate in the presence of hemagglutinin; hence the name. This does not affect the infection rate of the influenza virus.

20. **The correct answer is A.** Helper T lymphocytes can assist in the activation of B cells as long as the epitopes they recognize are linked (they do not have to be identical). Polysaccharides are very poor T-lymphocyte epitopes and thus do not by themselves elicit a T-lymphocyte response. Conjugating the polysaccharide to a protein carrier links the two epitopes and allows a B lymphocyte that recognizes the polysaccharide to be activated by a T-helper cell that recognizes epitopes present within the protein carrier.

Answer B is incorrect. Even if the protein carrier does increase the half-life of the vaccine, it is not the reason the vaccine is conjugated to a protein carrier.

Answer C is incorrect. IgE mediates allergic and type I hypersensitivity responses. It is not

expected to be an important immunoglobulin isotype produced in response to this vaccination.

Answer D is incorrect. The polysaccharide coat is not capable of causing disease. It is not a live or attenuated bacterium.

Answer E is incorrect. This is not true; see answer explanation above.

21. **The correct answer is E.** This clinical scenario would result in hyperacute rejection (within minutes of transplantation; clinical presentation within minutes to hours) mediated by preformed recipient antidonor antibodies in the recipient. The recipient would possess anti–type A antibodies, which react to the A antigen present not only on RBCs but on most other cell types. Hyperacute rejection occurs almost immediately, as the antidonor antibodies bind directly to vascular endothelial cells, initiating complement and clotting cascades and resulting in hemorrhage and necrosis of the transplanted kidney. It should be noted that it is not only ABO blood group mismatches but any antidonor antibodies possessed by the recipient that can lead to hyperacute rejection; thus it is important to carefully cross-match donor and recipient.

Answer A is incorrect. Acute rejection is cell-mediated and occurs within weeks following major histocompatibility complex (MHC)-mismatched transplant as a result of cytotoxic T lymphocytes reacting to foreign MHC molecules. It is reversible with cyclosporine.

Answer B is incorrect. Acute rejection is cell-mediated and occurs within weeks following major histocompatibility complex (MHC)-mismatched transplant as a result of CTLs reacting to foreign MHC molecules. In this scenario, hyperacute rejection would be expected to occur first (within the first few hours after transplant).

Answer C is incorrect. Graft-versus-host disease (GVHD) is a serious side effect of bone marrow transplantation mediated by donor-derived T lymphocytes. Acute GVHD usually occurs within the first 3 months following an allogeneic bone marrow transplantation, whereas chronic GVHD usually develops after the third month posttransplant.

Answer D is incorrect. Hyperacute rejection is typically mediated by preformed antidonor antibodies that are possessed by the recipient.

22. **The correct answer is D.** *Staphylococcus aureus* is a gram-positive, catalase-positive coccus. It produces a superantigen called toxic shock syndrome toxin (TSST-1). The toxin causes a disease characterized by fever, hypotension, and a diffuse macular rash that desquamates after a few days.

Answer A is incorrect. *Actinomyces israelii* is a filamentous organism that is part of the normal flora of the mouth and gastrointestinal tract. It does not cause toxic shock syndrome.

Answer B is incorrect. *Clostridium perfringens* is the organism responsible for the development of gas gangrene. This organism is associated with contaminated wounds and not with toxic shock syndrome.

Answer C is incorrect. *Proteus mirabilis* is a common cause of urinary tract infections and is not associated with toxic shock syndrome.

Answer E is incorrect. *Streptococcus pyogenes*, a gram-positive coccus, can also cause toxic shock syndrome. Unlike *S. aureus*, it is catalase-negative.

23. **The correct answer is A.** This patient is presenting with a classic case of whooping cough caused by *Bordetella pertussis*. The initial phase is characterized by flulike symptoms for the first 1–2 weeks. During this time, erythromycin is an effective treatment. The second phase, the paroxysmal stage, is marked by bouts of multiple coughs in a single breath followed by a deep inspiration (the classic whooping cough). Treatment during this phase does not change the disease course, so only supportive care is indicated and the infection ought to pass in otherwise healthy individuals. In the United States, the DTaP vaccine is supposed to be given to all infants and protects them against diphtheria, tetanus, and pertussis. In-

fants who are not vaccinated are at risk for infection. *B. pertussis* can only be cultured on Bordet-Gengou medium.

Answer B is incorrect. Charcoal yeast extract when buffered with increased levels of iron and cysteine is used to culture *Legionella pneumophila*.

Answer C is incorrect. Chocolate agar with factor V and X is used to culture *Haemophilus influenzae*.

Answer D is incorrect. Loffler's medium is needed to culture *Corynebacterium diphtheriae*.

Answer E is incorrect. Thayer-Martin medium is used to culture *Neisseria gonorrhoeae*.

24. **The correct answer is A.** Chédiak-Higashi disease is an inherited autosomal recessive disease. It is caused by a deficiency in lysosomal emptying of phagocytic cells due to a defect in microtubular function. Chédiak-Higashi disease often presents with recurrent streptococcal and staphylococcal infections. Partial albinism may be present, as melanosomes are derivatives of lysosomes.

Answer B is incorrect. Chronic granulomatous disease presents with an increased susceptibility to opportunistic bacterial infections. It results from defective neutrophil phagocytosis due to a lack of NADPH oxidase (or similar enzymes) activity. A negative nitroblue tetrazolium dye reduction test confirms the diagnosis of chronic granulomatous disease.

Answer C is incorrect. Hyper-IgM syndrome is caused by a defect in the CD40 ligand on CD4 T-helper cells. This defect leads to an inability to class switch between the different immunoglobulin isotypes. Since IgM is initially created and subsequently switched to the other isotypes, an inability to do so leads to elevated IgM levels and low levels of all other isotypes.

Answer D is incorrect. Selective immunoglobulin deficiency is a deficit in a specific class of immunoglobulins. IgA deficiency is the most common of these diseases. Since IgA is the most prominent immunoglobulin found in mucous membranes, patients suffering from a deficiency of it often present with sinus and lung infections.

Answer E is incorrect. Severe combined immunodeficiency is a defect in early stem cell differentiation that can have many causes. The typical presentation of this disease includes recurrent bacterial, viral, protozoal, and fungal infections.

25. **The correct answer is B.** The syndrome described is Guillain-Barré syndrome (GBS), a common cause of acute peripheral neuropathy that results in progressive weakness over a period of days. Although one-third of patients report no history of an antecedent infection, the other two-thirds have recently experienced an acute gastrointestinal or influenzalike illness prior to developing the neuropathy. The most common epidemiologic associations involve infections with *Campylobacter jejuni*, *Haemophilus influenzae*, cytomegalovirus, Epstein-Barr virus, *Mycoplasma pneumoniae*, and varicella-zoster virus. Laboratory abnormalities associated with GBS include elevated gamma globulin, decreased nerve conduction velocity indicative of demyelination, and albuminocytologic dissociation or increased cerebrospinal fluid protein concentration without cellular increase in the setting of normal glucose. Although the organisms listed frequently precede the syndrome, there has never been any consistent demonstration of any single infectious agent in the peripheral nerves of these patients, and the disease is thought to be immunologically mediated.

Answer A is incorrect. Although immunocompromised patients may be at greater risk for the organisms that are commonly associated with Guillain-Barré syndrome, *Candida albicans* does not have any association with the syndrome.

Answer C is incorrect. *Pseudomonas aeruginosa* is not an organism that has a relationship to Guillain-Barré syndrome.

Answer D is incorrect. There are currently no reports demonstrating a link between *Serratia marcescens* and Guillain-Barré syndrome.

Answer E is incorrect. *Staphylococcus saprophyticus* infections are not associated with Guillain-Barré syndrome.

26. **The correct answer is A.** This patient most likely has pernicious anemia, a chronic progressive anemia that is caused by a failure to absorb vitamin B_{12} due to a lack of availability of intrinsic factor. The disease process is thought to occur via autoantibodies that block a step in the vitamin B_{12}/intrinsic factor absorption pathway and/or autoimmune destruction of intrinsic factor–secreting gastric parietal cells. One test sometimes used to diagnose this disease is the Schilling test. Patients who receive a Schilling test (patients are given radiolabeled vitamin B_{12} orally; absorption from the intestines is measured based on how much of the radiolabeled vitamin B_{12} is found in the urine) reveal an insignificant amount of radiolabeled vitamin B_{12} in their urine (absorption of the radiolabeled vitamin B_{12} may increase if exogenous intrinsic factor is given at the same time). Gastrointestinal manifestations include atrophic glossitis (shiny, beefy-looking tongue) and atrophy of the fundic glands of the stomach, particularly affecting chief cells and parietal cells. Changes in the blood include a megaloblastic anemia with hypersegmented polymorphonuclear leukocytes.

Answer B is incorrect. The findings in this choice are not consistent with pernicious anemia, the condition described in the question stem.

Answer C is incorrect. The findings in this choice are often found in iron deficiency anemia, not pernicious anemia.

Answer D is incorrect. The findings in this choice are often found in anemia of chronic disease, not pernicious anemia, the condition described in the question stem.

Answer E is incorrect. The findings in this answer choice are not consistent with pernicious anemia, the condition described in the question stem.

27. **The correct answer is D.** The patient presents with pneumonia. The presence of a single-celled yeast endospore containing spherules is indicative of *Coccidioides immitis* infection. *Coccidioides* is characterized by endospores containing spherules when cultured at 37° C and branched hyphae when the organism is cultured at 25° C. *Coccidioides* infection is most commonly seen in immunocompromised patients or the elderly, and is most prevalent in the Southwest United States. While normal hosts are susceptible to infection, they usually do not present with symptoms. This patient's recent travel to Arizona makes *C. immitis* the most likely candidate.

Answer A is incorrect. *Aspergillus* infection is also seen almost exclusively in the immunocompromised patient; exceptions include allergic bronchopulmonary aspergillosis, an allergic disease that occurs in otherwise healthy individuals. *Aspergillus* most often causes fever, hemoptysis, and pneumonia. A tissue biopsy will show branching hyphae with septae, but a sputum culture will show radiating chains of spores.

Answer B is incorrect. *Blastomyces* grows as thick-walled budding yeasts at 37° C and hyphae with small conidia at 25° C. It is mostly seen along the Mississippi River and in Central America. It also causes a pneumonia that can progress to disseminated granulomatous disease.

Answer C is incorrect. *Candida* is the cause of thrush and is seen most often in the immunocompromised patient, such as those with HIV infection. In a tissue biopsy it will be seen as pseudohyphae and budding yeast. Candidal infection, however, is more likely to affect the esophagus than the airways and lungs.

Answer E is incorrect. *Histoplasma* grows as branched hyphae at 25° C and as full yeast cells at 37° C that are 2–5 μm in diameter and live within macrophages. *Histoplasma* infection causes both a pulmonary disease similar to a pneumonia and a severe granulomatous disease throughout the body, especially in the adrenals, liver, and spleen. It is prevalent in the Mississippi and Ohio River valleys.

28. **The correct answer is A.** Self- and virally derived cytosolic proteins are targeted for degradation by the proteasome. After degradation, peptides enter the rough endoplasmic reticulum (RER) by ATP-dependent transport via TAP (transporters associated with antigen processing) proteins. These peptides may then bind within the peptide-binding groove of a newly folded major histocompatibility complex (MHC) class I molecule. The MHC class I molecule can now exit the RER and travel via the Golgi apparatus to the cell surface, where it may interact with the T-lymphocyte receptor and CD8 coreceptor.

Answer B is incorrect. Self-peptide is loaded onto class I in the rough endoplasmic reticulum. The major histocompatibility complex molecule does not travel to the cell surface unless peptide is bound within the peptide-binding groove.

Answer C is incorrect. Mitochondria are not directly involved in antigen processing or presentation.

Answer D is incorrect. The nucleus is not directly involved in antigen processing or presentation.

Answer E is incorrect. The Golgi apparatus is not the site of self-peptide loading onto the major histocompatibility complex molecule.

29. **The correct answer is A.** Helper T2 (Th2)-lymphocyte production, which can be stimulated by exposure to environmental allergens, facilitates production of allergen-specific IgE by B cells. This IgE binds to and stimulates mast cells to release inflammatory mediators such as histamine. Some theorize that since Th1-lymphocyte production is stimulated by bacteria and viruses, childhood vaccinations will lead to less stimulation of Th1 lymphocytes (i.e., vaccination leads to fewer bacterial/viral infections, which leads to less Th1-lymphocyte production). This causes a relative overproduction of Th2 lymphocytes and leads to an increase of allergen-specific IgE, which leads to allergies. Furthermore, Th1 lymphocytes decrease production of IgE.

Answer B is incorrect. Th1 lymphocytes, not Th2 lymphocytes, are predominantly stimulated by bacteria and viruses, so the effect of vaccines is seen first there, and it is a decrease.

Answer C is incorrect. Vaccination causes a decrease in Th1 lymphocytes.

Answer D is incorrect. Vaccination causes a decrease in Th1 lymphocytes.

Answer E is incorrect. A decrease in Th2-lymphocyte levels and an increase in Th1-lymphocyte levels do not draw an accurate link to predisposition to allergies. See the correct answer for an explanation.

30. **The correct answer is B.** One of the diseases caused by *Francisella tularensis* is ulceroglandular tularemia. This disease is characterized by a well-demarcated skin lesion with a black base following a tick or deerfly bite or contact with the body fluids or fur of an infected rabbit. Over the next few days, systemic symptoms develop and the local lymph nodes may become swollen and painful.

Answer A is incorrect. *Brucella* species enter the body after the ingestion of contaminated milk products or following direct contact with contaminated livestock. It is an intracellular bacterium that causes undulating fever, weakness, and loss of appetite.

Answer C is incorrect. *Nocardia asteroides* is an acid-fast aerobe found in soil. This organism causes pulmonary infections, primarily in immunocompromised individuals.

Answer D is incorrect. *Treponema pallidum* causes syphilis. Primary syphilis typically presents with a painless chancre, not a lesion on a black base.

Answer E is incorrect. A person infected with *Trichinella spiralis* presents with fever, periorbital and facial edema, myalgia, and eosinophilia.

31. **The correct answer is C.** Job syndrome involves the failure of helper T lymphocytes to produce interferon-γ (INF-γ). Since INF-γ is a potent activator of phagocytic cells, a decrease in its production leads to a failure of neu-

trophils to respond to chemotactic stimuli. Job syndrome presents with recurrent staphylococcal abscesses, eczema, and high levels of IgE.

Answer A is incorrect. Ataxia-telangiectasia is caused by a defect in DNA repair enzymes. The disease is associated with an IgA deficiency. The typical presentation of the disease is given away by the name, as symptoms include cerebellar problems (ataxia) and spider angiomas (telangiectasia).

Answer B is incorrect. Bruton's agammaglobulinemia is an X-linked defect and therefore presents in males. It is caused by a defect in tyrosine kinase associated with low levels of all classes of immunoglobulins. After 6 months of age, when the levels of maternal antibodies have declined, patients with the disease tend to present with recurrent bacterial infections.

Answer D is incorrect. The third and fourth pharyngeal pouches, and thus the thymus and parathyroid glands, fail to develop in patients with thymic aplasia (DiGeorge syndrome). The disease often presents with many congenital defects, such as cardiac abnormalities, cleft palate, and abnormal facies. Thymic aplasia can also present with tetany due to hypocalcemia.

Answer E is incorrect. Wiskott-Aldrich syndrome is an X-linked defect associated with elevated IgA levels, elevated IgE levels, normal IgG levels, and low IgM levels. It involves a defect in the body's ability to mount an IgM response to bacteria. Recurrent pyogenic infections, eczema, and thrombocytopenia are the typical triad of symptoms. It does not present with any specific enzyme abnormality.

32. **The correct answer is D.** Bacterial cholangitis is defined as bacterial infection of the bile ducts. Cholangitis can result from any condition obstructing the bile flow, most commonly choledocholithiasis. The bacteria are usually enteric gram-negative rods such as *Escherichia coli*, *Klebsiella* species, *Bacteroides* species, or *Enterobacter* species that enter the bile duct via the sphincter of Oddi. Charcot's classic triad of pain, jaundice, and fever is typically found in patients with cholangitis. Leukocyto-

sis with neutrophilia and bandemia is commonly present as well. This patient satisfies the described classical criteria and findings for bacterial cholangitis. The endoscopic retrograde cholangiopancreatography results further support this diagnosis.

Answer A is incorrect. Acute appendicitis generally presents with right lower quadrant pain and not right upper quadrant pain, as seen in this patient. Moreover, the presence of jaundice, the normal endoscopic retrograde cholangiopancreatography findings make this diagnosis even more unlikely.

Answer B is incorrect. In contrast to the normal amylase levels in this patient, acute pancreatitis usually presents with radiating epigastric pain and increased serum amylase levels. Moreover, jaundice is not a classical finding in acute pancreatitis.

Answer C is incorrect. Acute viral hepatitis also presents with jaundice and fever. However, findings of positive blood cultures with neutrophilia, in addition to endoscopic retrograde cholangiopancreatography results, argue against the diagnosis of acute viral hepatitis.

Answer E is incorrect. Cholesterolosis or strawberry gallbladder is characterized by yellow cholesterol-containing flecks in the mucosal surface. In contrast to this patient's diagnosis, it is not associated with elevated WBC count, sepsis, jaundice, and choledocholithiasis.

33. **The correct answer is C.** Hyper-IgM syndrome is caused by a defect in the CD40 ligand on CD4 T-helper cells. This defect leads to an inability to class switch between the different immunoglobulin isotypes. Since IgM is initially created and subsequently switched to the other isotypes, an inability to do so leads to elevated IgM levels and low levels of all other isotypes.

Answer A is incorrect. Ataxia-telangiectasia is caused by a defect in DNA repair enzymes. The disease is associated with an IgA deficiency. The typical presentation of the disease is given away by the name, as symptoms include cerebellar problems (ataxia) and spider angiomas (telangiectasia).

Answer B is incorrect. Leukocyte adhesion deficiency syndrome is caused by a defect in the LFA-1 adhesion protein on the surface of neutrophils. The disease usually presents with marked leukocytosis and localized bacterial infections that are difficult to detect until they have progressed to an extensive life-threatening level. Since neutrophils are unable to adhere to the endothelium and transmigrate into tissues, infections in patients with leukocyte adhesion deficiency syndrome act similarly to those observed in neutropenic patients.

Answer D is incorrect. Job syndrome involves the failure of helper T lymphocytes to produce interferon-γ (INF-γ). Since INF-γ is a potent activator of phagocytic cells, a decrease in its production leads to a failure of neutrophils to respond to chemotactic stimuli. Job syndrome presents with recurrent staphylococcal abscesses, eczema, and high levels of IgE.

Answer E is incorrect. In thymic aplasia (DiGeorge's syndrome), the third and fourth pharyngeal pouches, and thus the thymus and parathyroid glands, fail to develop. The disease often presents with many congenital defects, such as cardiac abnormalities, cleft palate, and abnormal facies. Thymic aplasia can also present with tetany due to hypocalcemia.

34. **The correct answer is E.** *Bacillus cereus* causes food poisoning after eating contaminated reheated rice. This bacterium can produce two types of enterotoxins, one of which can cause food poisoning similar to that caused by *Escherichia coli*. Since the food poisoning is caused by preformed enterotoxins, antibiotic treatment will not help.

Answer A is incorrect. Bismuth subsalicylate, metronidazole, and amoxicillin are used in the treatment of *Helicobacter pylori* infection.

Answer B is incorrect. Fluoroquinolones can be used in the treatment of severe *Shigella* species infection.

Answer C is incorrect. *Campylobacter jejuni* enterocolitis can be treated with erythromycin or ciprofloxacin. Infection with this organism is not associated with eating reheated rice.

Answer D is incorrect. *Vibrio cholerae* causes large-volume, watery diarrhea. Treatment involves prompt replacement of water and electrolytes. Although antibiotics are not needed for treatment, tetracyclines have been shown to reduce the course of the disease.

35. **The correct answer is C.** Polyarteritis nodosa (PAN) is characterized by immune complex–mediated destruction of small to medium-sized vessels—particularly affecting the renal and visceral vasculature. Patients suffering from PAN often have P-ANCA (perinuclear antineutrophil cytoplasmic autoantibodies) present in their serum. Wegener's granulomatosis is also a vasculitis, but it is characterized by necrotizing granuloma formation in the lung and kidneys. Patients suffering from Wegener's granulomatosis often have circulating antineutrophil cytoplasmic autoantibodies (C-ANCA) present in their serum. Interestingly, in both of these diseases, the patient's autoantibody titer is usually a good indicator of disease severity.

Answer A is incorrect. Kawasaki disease is not associated with serum perinuclear antineutrophil cytoplasmic autoantibodies, and Buerger's disease is not associated with serum circulating antineutrophil cytoplasmic autoantibodies.

Answer B is incorrect. Buerger's disease is not associated with serum circulating antineutrophil cytoplasmic autoantibodies.

Answer D is incorrect. Takayasu's arteritis is not associated with serum perinuclear antineutrophil cytoplasmic autoantibodies.

Answer E is incorrect. Temporal (giant cell) arteritis is not associated with serum perinuclear antineutrophil cytoplasmic autoantibodies.

36. **The correct answer is A.** Enterococcus is a common cause of nosocomial urinary tract infection and subacute endocarditis. Ampicillin is the standard treatment for susceptible enterococcal infections. For those strains that are not susceptible, vancomycin is the treatment of choice. For vancomycin-resistant strains, other therapies (such as quinupristin/dalfopristin) are available, but extensive knowledge of the indications for each is beyond the scope of knowledge necessary for the USMLE Step 1 examination.

Answer B is incorrect. Gentamicin is an aminoglycoside antibiotic. It inhibits the 30S subunit by inhibiting the formation of the initiation complex. It is not an effective monotherapy for enterococci, but it can be used in combination with other therapies to increase efficacy.

Answer C is incorrect. Piperacillin is an extended-spectrum penicillin agent. In addition to gram-positive organisms, it is particularly active against *Pseudomonas aeruginosa* and the Enterobacteriaceae viruses. It is not first-line therapy for enterococcus infections.

Answer D is incorrect. Quinupristin/dalfopristin (Synercid) is a new therapy that may be effective for vancomycin-resistant enterococcus endocarditis. It is not first-line treatment for enterococcus infections.

Answer E is incorrect. Vancomycin is an antibiotic that is effective only against gram-positive cocci. It binds tightly to a cell wall precursor containing the amino acid sequence D-ala D-ala, preventing cell wall synthesis. It is indicated for ampicillin-resistant enterococcal infection.

37. **The correct answer is C.** *Helicobacter pylori* infection causes gastritis characterized by recurrent abdominal pain that is not relieved by food intake. It produces ammonia from urea, and therefore the urease breath test (which detects the presence of ammonia) is positive in the presence of *H. pylori*.

Answer A is incorrect. *Clostridium difficile* causes pseudomembranous colitis and is not thought to be associated with gastritis.

Answer B is incorrect. *Escherichia coli* O157:H7 causes acute food poisoning. This patient does not report any vomiting or bloody diarrhea, and therefore this organism is unlikely to be causing her symptoms.

Answer D is incorrect. *Proteus mirabilis*, like *Helicobacter pylori*, is able to cleave urea into ammonia. However, it is a common cause of urinary tract infections and not gastritis.

Answer E is incorrect. *Vibrio cholerae* causes food poisoning that is characterized by watery diarrhea (rice-water stools). This patient reports no such symptoms.

38. **The correct answer is D.** Allogenic grafts, or homografts, are harvested from another individual of the same species. An allogenic graft from a patient's identical twin sibling is called a syngeneic graft.

    Answer A is incorrect. An autologous bone marrow graft, or self-graft, would be a transplantation from the patient's own tissue.

    Answer B is incorrect. A combination graft is usually composed of a mixture of autogenous and allogenic tissue.

    Answer C is incorrect. A heterograft (also called a xenogeneic graft) is a graft taken from a different species.

    Answer E is incorrect. A xenogeneic graft, or heterograft, is a graft taken from a different species.

39. **The correct answer is E.** The results of the fluid analysis are consistent with a bacterial meningitis (increased PMNs, high protein, low glucose). The most common cause of meningitis in children ages 6 months to 6 years is *Streptococcus pneumoniae*.

    Answer A is incorrect. Results of the fluid analysis are not consistent with a viral meningitis. One would expect to see increased lymphocyte counts, normal protein levels, and normal sugar levels in this type of infection.

    Answer B is incorrect. *Haemophilus influenzae* meningitis is a less common cause of meningitis in children of this age group. Since the introduction of the *Haemophilus* flu vaccine, the incidence of this cause of meningitis has greatly decreased.

Answer C is incorrect. The clinical picture does not fit with a viral meningitis. In a viral meningitis, one would expect the fluid analysis to come back with increased lymphocytes, normal protein, and normal sugar.

Answer D is incorrect. *Listeria* species is not a common cause of meningitis in this age group. It is much more commonly seen in newborns age 0–6 months and in the elderly.

40. **The correct answer is A.** These symptoms are typical of urethritis. The most common causes of urethritis in males are *Chlamydia trachomatis* and *Neisseria gonorrhoeae*. The image shows intracellular inclusions that indicate that this man is infected with *C. trachomatis*; in the image, *EB* indicates the elementary body particles with cell walls and *RB* indicates the reticular body. *N. gonorrhoeae* is a gram-negative coccus, not an intracellular parasite. The treatment of choice for *Chlamydia* urethritis is azithromycin or doxycycline.

    Answer B is incorrect. Ceftriaxone is an effective treatment for gonorrhea, but the cephalosporins are relatively ineffective against *Chlamydia trachomatis*.

    Answer C is incorrect. Fluconazole inhibits fungal steroid synthesis. It is used in the treatment of fungal infections, such as *Candida albicans*.

    Answer D is incorrect. Penicillin has been shown to suppress chlamydial multiplication. However, it does not eradicate the organism and thus is not the best treatment for this type of infection. Penicillin is the treatment of choice for syphilis.

    Answer E is incorrect. Vancomycin has not been shown to be effective in the treatment of chlamydial infection. It is used to treat drug-resistant *Staphylococcus aureus* and *Clostridium difficile*.

41. **The correct answer is E.** JRA may appear with a different presentation than adult-onset RA. By definition, JRA begins before age 16 years and must include arthritis in at least one

joint for at least 6 weeks. Additionally, the morphologic joint pathology is similar to that of adult-onset RA. However, there are several signs and symptoms that occur more commonly in JRA than in adult-onset RA; these include increased likelihood of systemic onset (with symptoms including high fevers, lymphadenopathy, and hepatomegaly), increased likelihood of large joint involvement, and increased likelihood of antinuclear antibody seropositivity. Furthermore, JRA patients are less likely to have rheumatoid nodules and rheumatoid factor.

Answer A is incorrect. There are several signs and symptoms that occur more commonly in JRA than in adult-onset RA, including increased likelihood of systemic onset, increased likelihood of large joint involvement, and increased likelihood of antinuclear antibody seropositivity.

Answer B is incorrect. Systemic symptoms are more likely, but high levels of serum rheumatoid factor are less likely, in patients with JRA.

Answer C is incorrect. Both systemic symptoms and large joint involvement are more likely in patients with JRA.

Answer D is incorrect. Systemic symptoms are more likely, but high levels of serum rheumatoid factor are less likely, in patients with JRA.

42. **The correct answer is A.** Blastomycosis can present with flulike symptoms, fevers, chills, productive cough, myalgia, arthralgia, and pleuritic chest pain. Some patients will fail to recover from an acute infection and progress to develop chronic pulmonary infection or widespread disseminated infection. Fluconazole or ketoconazole is used for the treatment of local blastomycosis infections, and amphotericin B is used for the treatment of systemic infections.

Answer B is incorrect. Fluconazole or ketoconazole are effective treatments for local blastomycosis infections but are ineffective if the infection is systemic. Systemic infections require amphotericin B.

Answer C is incorrect. Itraconazole or potassium iodide is used for the treatment of *Sporothrix schenckii*. *S. schenckii* is the cause of sporotrichosis. When *S. schenckii* is introduced into the skin, usually by a thorn prick, it causes a local pustule or ulcer with nodules along draining lymphatics (ascending lymphangitis). *S. schenckii* is a dimorphic fungus that has cigar-shaped budding yeast visible in pus.

Answer D is incorrect. Sodium stibogluconate is used to treat *Leishmania donovani* infection. *L. donovani* presents with hepatomegaly and splenomegaly, malaise, anemia, and weight loss. *L. donovani* is transmitted via the sandfly. Microscopically, macrophages containing amastigotes are observed.

Answer E is incorrect. Topical miconazole or selenium sulfide (Selsun) is used to treat *Malassezia furfur*. *M. furfur* is the cause of tinea versicolor. Symptoms of this infection include hypopigmented skin lesions that occur in hot and humid conditions.

43. **The correct answer is D.** The penetrating wound from the rusty nail puts this patient at risk for infection with *Clostridium tetani*, whose symptoms are caused by the tetanus toxin. This toxin blocks the release of glycine from Renshaw cells in the spinal cord and results in "lockjaw" and other similar symptoms. Tetanus revaccination is required approximately every 10 years to ensure adequate blood levels of protective antibodies.

Answer A is incorrect. The *Vibrio cholera* toxin ADP ribosylates a G protein in the intestine, increasing adenylate cyclase activity and causing pumping of water and chloride ions into the gut lumen. Its most characteristic symptom is voluminous "rice-water" diarrhea. The heat-labile toxin of *Escherichia coli* has the same mechanism of action.

Answer B is incorrect. The *Corynebacterium diphtheriae* toxin inactivates the elongation factor EF-2 by ADP ribosylation, disrupting protein synthesis. It causes pharyngitis and "pseudomembrane" in the throat. Although the patient's prior vaccinations most likely included vaccination for diphtheria as well, this infection is less likely than tetanus to occur with a penetrating wound.

Answer C is incorrect. Superantigens such as the *Staphylococcus aureus* toxin and the *Streptococcus pyogenes* erythrogenic toxin bind to the MHC class II receptor and the T-lymphocyte receptor, resulting in cytokine release and sometimes toxic shock syndrome.

Answer E is incorrect. The *Clostridium botulinum* toxin inhibits the release of acetylcholine, resulting in anticholinergic symptoms and even central nervous system paralysis. *C. botulinum* is most often found in canned food and honey (resulting in "floppy baby" syndrome when consumed by young children).

Answer F is incorrect. The streptolysin O toxin of *Streptococcus pyogenes* is a hemolysin.

Answer G is incorrect. The heat-stable toxin of *Escherichia coli* stimulates guanylate cyclase.

44. **The correct answer is A.** Recurrent viral infections are a sign of T-lymphocyte dysfunction. Particularly important in the response to viral infections are cytotoxic (CD8) T lymphocytes. IL-2 is a cytokine secreted by helper T lymphocytes that stimulates the growth of helper and cytotoxic T lymphocytes. Therefore, even though this patient may have an adequate number of T lymphocytes, a deficiency in IL-2 could lead to impaired cytotoxic T-lymphocyte differentiation and activation. This would result in an increased susceptibility to viral infections.

Answer B is incorrect. IL-3 is secreted by activated T lymphocytes and has functions similar to granulocyte macrophage colony-stimulating factor.

Answer C is incorrect. IL-4 is secreted by helper T lymphocytes and promotes the growth of B lymphocytes.

Answer D is incorrect. IL-5 is secreted by helper T lymphocytes and promotes the differentiation of B lymphocytes.

Answer E is incorrect. IL-8 is the major chemotactic factor for neutrophils.

45. **The correct answer is E.** *Vibrio cholerae* causes watery stools, often called rice-water stool. This illness is not accompanied by abdominal pain, but the symptoms are due to dehydration leading to electrolyte imbalances. Cholera toxin causes uncontrolled stimulation of adenylate cyclase; the resulting excess of cAMP causes uncontrolled secretion of chloride and water (due to the osmotic gradient), resulting in extremely watery diarrhea accompanied by electrolyte imbalances.

Answer A is incorrect. *Bacillus cereus* also causes nonbloody diarrhea, but it is less severe than the diarrhea caused by *Vibrio cholerae*. Infection is associated with eating reheated rice.

Answer B is incorrect. *Clostridium difficile* causes severe nonbloody diarrhea associated with pseudomembranes. It is associated with previous antibiotic treatment.

Answer C is incorrect. *Helicobacter pylori* infection causes gastritis and would not cause the symptoms described in this patient.

Answer D is incorrect. *Salmonella* species cause bloody diarrhea and can be acquired from poultry, meat, and eggs.

46. **The correct answer is B.** CD4 and CD8 are glycoproteins present on the surface of helper T lymphocytes (CD4) or cytotoxic T lymphocytes (CD8). CD4 binds to an invariant region of the class II major histocompatibility complex (MHC) molecule, while CD8 binds to an invariant region of the class I MHC molecule. Thus, these molecules are termed *coreceptors*. CD19 is a glycoprotein present on the surface of B cells. CD19 is a member of the B-lymphocyte coreceptor signaling complex and plays a role in B-lymphocyte development.

Answer A is incorrect. CD4 is indeed present on helper T lymphocytes, and CD19 is indeed present on B lymphocytes. However, B7 is a cell surface molecule present on activated antigen-presenting cells, not on T or B lymphocytes. It binds to CD28 and CTLA-4 present on the surface of T lymphocytes, which delivers a costimulatory and inhibitory signal, respectively.

Answer C is incorrect. CD4 is present on the surfaces of helper (rather than cytotoxic) T lymphocytes, while CD8 is present on the surfaces of cytotoxic (rather than helper) T lymphocytes.

Answer D is incorrect. CD19 is present on B lymphocytes, CD4 is present on helper T lymphocytes, and CD8 is present on cytotoxic T lymphocytes.

Answer E is incorrect. CD19 is present on B lymphocytes, CD8 is present on cytotoxic T lymphocytes, and CD4 is present on helper T lymphocytes.

47. **The correct answer is A.** This patient suffered from shock, most likely endotoxic shock due to gram-negative bacteremia. The endotoxin lipopolysaccharide (LPS) is found in the cell wall of gram-negative bacteria. LPS activates the alternative pathway of the complement cascade. The x-ray shows pulmonary edema, which contributes to the acute respiratory distress syndrome that accompanies septic shock. The C3a component of the complement cascade contributes to the hypotension and edema seen in endotoxic shock.

Answer B is incorrect. The C5a component of the complement cascade, activated by endotoxin, functions in neutrophil chemotaxis.

Answer C is incorrect. Endotoxin can directly activate Hageman factor, activating the coagulation cascade and leading to disseminated intravascular coagulation.

Answer D is incorrect. The cytokine interleukin-1, released by macrophages activated by endotoxin, causes fever.

Answer E is incorrect. Nitric oxide, released by macrophages activated by endotoxin, causes hypotension (shock).

Answer F is incorrect. The cytokine tumor necrosis factor, released by macrophages acti-

vated by endotoxin, causes fever and hemorrhagic tissue necrosis.

48. **The correct answer is D. ToRCHeS** is an acronym for organisms that can cross the placenta and cause congenital anomalies: **To**xoplasmosis, **R**ubella, **C**ytomegalovirus, **H**IV/**H**erpes, and **S**yphilis. Genital lesions suggest a sexually transmitted disease. The Tzanck test is a smear of an opened skin vesicle that detects multinucleated giant cells, indicative of herpes simplex virus (HSV) types 1 and 2 or varicella zoster (VZV). HSV-1, HSV-2, and VZV may all be transmitted vertically to the fetus. Remember: "**Tzanck** heaven I don't have **herpes!**"

Answer A is incorrect. The presence of anti-HB surface antibody indicates immunity to the hepatitis B virus, either by previous exposure or by vaccination. While active or chronic hepatitis B can be vertically transmitted to the fetus, it does not cause congenital anomalies. Furthermore, hepatitis B is not associated with genital lesions.

Answer B is incorrect. Cytoplasmic inclusions seen on Giemsa or fluorescent antibody–stained smear suggest *Chlamydia trachomatis*. Although *Chlamydia* can be vertically transmitted to the fetus at delivery, it is not associated with congenital anomalies. It can, however, cause blindness and pneumonia in the newborn and should be treated during pregnancy.

Answer C is incorrect. The monospot test uses heterophilic Paul-Bunnell antibodies to detect agglutination of sheep RBCs, indicative of Epstein-Barr virus (EBV). While EBV can cause mononucleosis and Burkitt's lymphoma, it is not one of the TORCHeS organisms and does not transmit vertically to the fetus. Moreover, EBV does not produce genital lesions.

Answer E is incorrect. The Weil-Felix test uses *Proteus* antigen to test for antirickettsial antibodies, indicative of typhus or Rocky Mountain spotted fever. *Rickettsia* species can cause headache, fever, and rash; however, they do not produce genital lesions.

49. The correct answer is B. The correct answer is celiac sprue. This condition is also known as gluten-sensitive enteropathy, nontropical sprue, and celiac disease. It is due to a sensitivity to gluten, which is found in wheat, grains, and many cereals. Biopsy shows marked atrophy, total loss, or flattening of the villi of the small bowel.

Answer A is incorrect. Abetalipoproteinemia is an autosomal recessive disease that causes a defect in the synthesis and export of mucosal cells because of the inability to synthesize apolipoprotein B. These patients usually have burr cells (red cells that have spiny projections) and do not have any characteristic features of the intestine found in celiac disease.

Answer C is incorrect. Lactase deficiency causes osmotic diarrhea from the inability to break down lactose into glucose and galactose.

Answer D is incorrect. Viral enteritis, usually caused by a rotavirus, is common in children and can cause diarrhea. However, the clinical time course, suggested gluten sensitivity, and findings on biopsy make viral enteritis unlikely.

Answer E is incorrect. Whipple's disease usually presents in middle-aged men who have malabsorptive diarrhea, and the hallmark is the presence of periodic acid-Schiff–positive macrophages in the intestinal mucosa. Rod-shaped bacilli of the causal agent, *Tropheryma whippelii*, are found on electron microscopy.

50. The correct answer is D. The infant's family history is suggestive of a trait with X-linked inheritance, and the preponderance of bacterial infections suggests a defect in the humoral (antibody-mediated) immune response. These two clues are most suggestive of a diagnosis of Bruton's X-linked agammaglobulinemia. The molecular defect occurs in a signaling molecule named Btk (Bruton's tyrosine kinase), leading to maturing arrest of developing B cells at the pre-B-cell stage. Arrest at the pre-B-cell stage would result in an inability to produce immunoglobulins, and thus the patient would have very low levels of all immunoglobulins in his serum. Indeed, it should be noted that these patients are particularly susceptible to extracellular pyogenic bacterial infections with organisms such as *Haemophilus influenzae*, *Streptococcus pyogenes*, *Staphylococcus aureus*, and *Streptococcus pneumoniae*.

Answer A is incorrect. A CD4 T-lymphocyte count < 200/µL suggests a diagnosis of AIDS, not an inherited genetic defect, and one that results in a defect in cell-mediated immunity.

Answer B is incorrect. Absence of T lymphocytes would result in a defect in cell-mediated immunity, and the patient would be more highly susceptible to viral and intracellular bacterial pathogens.

Answer C is incorrect. The physical examination and family and patient history are all highly suggestive of an immunoglobulin deficiency.

Answer E is incorrect. Low serum IgA levels are suggestive of selective IgA deficiency, the most common inherited immunodeficiency in the European population and, interestingly enough, one that appears to have no striking disease associations.

51. The correct answer is D. This patient most likely has Rocky Mountain spotted fever, as indicated by the rash on her palms and soles and the inward, "centripetal" pattern of spread. Other supporting evidence are the accompanying headache and fever, and a positive Weil-Felix reaction, which is a cross-reaction of certain antirickettsial antibodies with the *Proteus* antigen. Rocky Mountain spotted fever is caused by the rickettsial organism *Rickettsia rickettsii*, and is endemic to the east coast of the United States. It is transmitted by the Ixodes tick, thus the patient probably acquired it during her recent camping trip.

Answer A is incorrect. *Borrelia burgdorferi* causes Lyme disease. The rash of Lyme disease is typically a bull's-eye type rash, with negative Weil-Felix reaction.

Answer B is incorrect. *Coxiella burnetii* is also a rickettsial organism. It is transmitted by aerosols, causes Q fever, and has no associated rash or positive Weil-Felix reaction.

Answer C is incorrect. Coxsackie A is an RNA virus that causes hand, foot, and mouth disease, which can also present with a rash on the palms and soles, in addition to oral and occasionally genital lesions. However, the positive Weil-Felix reaction in this case and recent history of a camping trip point to *Rickettsia rickettsiae* as a more likely causative organism in this case.

Answer E is incorrect. *Rickettsia typhi* causes endemic typhus, and is transmitted by fleas. The rash of typhus is centrifugal—it spreads outward, not inward as in this case.

Answer F is incorrect. *Treponema pallidum* is the spirochete that causes syphilis, a sexually transmitted disease. Although syphilis can also present with a rash on the palms and soles, this patient has no history of a sexual encounter that would put her at risk for this disease.

52. **The correct answer is C.** Goodpasture's syndrome is characterized by autoantibodies forming against the glomerular basement membrane. Forming against a tissue, as opposed to something in the blood, constitutes a type II sensitivity reaction. This produces linear immunofluorescent staining. Renal involvement in Goodpasture's syndrome leads to hematuria, anemia, and crescentic glomerulonephritis. Along with the kidney, this syndrome may include pulmonary involvement, leading to hemoptysis.

Answer A is incorrect. Acute poststreptococcal glomerulonephritis occurs 1–4 weeks after a β-hemolytic streptococci infection; it is classified as a type III sensitivity reaction in which deposits of IgG, IgM, and C3 form in the mesangium along the basement membrane. On immunofluorescent staining, a granular pattern is seen, rather than a linear one.

Answer B is incorrect. Alport's syndrome is not an immune reaction against the glomerular basement membrane. It is an X-linked disorder characterized by absent or mutated collagen IV, affecting kidney, nerve, and ocular function.

Answer D is incorrect. IgA nephropathy, also known as Berger's disease, produces mesangial deposits of IgA antibodies. It does not produce a linear pattern, and the staining will require anti-IgA antibodies rather than IgG.

Answer E is incorrect. Membranous glomerulonephritis is an immune-mediated kidney disease that leads to sub-epithelial deposits of IgG and complement. With immunofluorescent staining, it produces a granular pattern along the glomerular basement membrane.

53. **The correct answer is C.** This clinician is concerned that the fetus may have erythroblastosis fetalis (hemolytic disease of the newborn). This disease is mediated by maternally derived IgG anti-Rh antibodies developed in Rh-negative mothers that are directed at the Rh antigen present on the fetal RBCs of a Rh+ fetus in a previous pregnancy. If the mother possesses the antibodies developed from a previous exposure to an Rh+ fetus, they may cross the placenta (antibodies of the IgG isotype readily cross the placenta) and coat the fetal RBCs of a Rh+ fetus if the mother is now pregnant with another Rh+ child. Antibody coating of the RBCs leads to phagocytosis of RBCs (via Fc receptors) and/or destruction of the RBCs by the complement system and potentially fatal anemia. This antibody-mediated cytotoxic reaction is an example of a type II hypersensitivity reaction.

Answer A is incorrect. Graft-versus-host disease is a potentially lethal side effect of bone marrow transplantation.

Answer B is incorrect. Type I hypersensitivity reactions are antibody-mediated but require antigen binding to IgE, which is prebound to the surface of mast cells. Mast cell degranulation then ensues. Examples include anaphylaxis, asthma, hives, and local wheal and flare.

Answer D is incorrect. Type III hypersensitivity reactions are immune complex–mediated. Examples include polyarteritis nodosa, glomerulonephritis, rheumatoid arthritis, and systemic lupus erythematosus.

Answer E is incorrect. Type IV hypersensitivity reactions are a group of T cell–mediated pathologies. Examples include the tuberculin skin test, transplant rejection, and contact dermatitis.

54. **The correct answer is E.** Wiskott-Aldrich syndrome is an X-linked defect associated with elevated IgA levels, elevated IgE levels, normal IgG levels, and low IgM levels. It involves a defect in the body's ability to mount an IgM response to bacteria. Recurrent pyogenic infections, eczema, and thrombocytopenia are the typical triad of symptoms. It does not present with any specific enzyme abnormality.

Answer A is incorrect. Bruton's agammaglobulinemia is an X-linked deficit and therefore presents in males. It is a defect in a tyrosine kinase associated with low levels of all classes of immunoglobulins. After 6 months of age, when the levels of maternal antibodies have declined, patients with the disease tend to present with recurrent bacterial infections.

Answer B is incorrect. Chédiak-Higashi disease is an autosomal recessive disease that presents with recurrent streptococcal and staphylococcal infections. A defect in lysosomal emptying of phagocytic cells due to microtubular dysfunction is the underlying cause of the disease.

Answer C is incorrect. Job syndrome involves the failure of helper T lymphocytes to produce interferon-γ (INF-γ). Since INF-γ is a potent activator of phagocytic cells, a decrease in its production leads to a failure of neutrophils to respond to chemotactic stimuli.

Answer D is incorrect. The third and fourth pharyngeal pouches, and thus the thymus and parathyroid glands, fail to develop in patients with thymic aplasia (DiGeorge syndrome). The disease often presents with congenital defects such as cardiac abnormalities, cleft palate, and abnormal facies. Thymic aplasia can also present with tetany due to hypocalcemia.

55. **The correct answer is E.** *Malassezia furfur* infection is the cause of tinea versicolor. Symptoms of this infection include hypopigmented skin lesions that occur in the hot and humid conditions of the tropics. *M. furfur* is treated with topical miconazole or selenium sulfide (Selsun).

Answer A is incorrect. Microsporum canis is the organism responsible for causing tinea capitis and tinea corporis. These diseases are usually acquired from domestic cats and dogs. Microscopically, *M. canis* produces macroconidia, microconidia, and septate hyphae.

Answer B is incorrect. Tinea cruris is more commonly known as "jock itch." Its incidence in men vastly outnumbers that in women. Tinea cruris is most frequently caused by *Trichophyton rubrum*. The patient's sweat provides a culture media for the fungus. Potassium hydroxide mounts will reveal segmented hyphae and arthrospores.

Answer C is incorrect. The causative agent for tinea nigra, a superficial infection of the stratum corneum, is *Hortaea werneckii*. The fungus is most often acquired through direct contact with soil, wood, and decaying vegetation.

Answer D is incorrect. *Trichophyton* causes approximately 90% of the dermatophyte hair infections in the United States. Typically, it is this genus of fungi that causes tinea pedis, tinea cruris, and tinea unguium. This fungus does not fluoresce, and thus ultraviolet examination should not be relied on for diagnosis.

56. **The correct answer is C.** Multiple sclerosis is a central nervous system (CNS) demyelinating disorder characterized by lesions that are separated by both time and anatomic location in the CNS. The exact etiology is unknown, but there is evidence supporting a role of autoimmune antibody attack to the CNS myelin-secreting oligodendrocytes. Oligodendrocytes, which are found in the CNS, are involved in myelination of axons.

Answer A is incorrect. Astrocytes are found in the central nervous system and are involved in regulating the metabolic and structural environment of neurons, including repair and scar formation. Astrocytes are not the primary cells affected in multiple sclerosis, but they may proliferate in areas of multiple sclerosis lesions in an effort to repair inflammatory damage.

Answer B is incorrect. Ependymal cells line the ventricles. Disruptions in this cell barrier can cause proliferation of astrocytes nearby, but is not thought to be related to multiple sclerosis.

Answer D is incorrect. Schwann cells are found in the peripheral nervous system and are involved in myelination of axons. Schwann cells are not the primary cells affected in multiple sclerosis. The morphologic changes in this disease are limited to the central nervous system.

Answer E is incorrect. T cells are the primary cells responsible for cellular immunity. It is likely that they are involved in the putative autoimmune attack on the central nervous system in multiple sclerosis, but they are not the cells primarily damaged in this disease.

57. **The correct answer is A.** *Trichomonas vaginalis* is the cause of vaginitis. Symptoms of vaginitis include a foul-smelling greenish discharge, itching, and burning. *T. vaginalis* is transmitted sexually. On microscopic wet mount, one finds trophozoites. Metronidazole is used to treat *T. vaginalis* infection.

Answer B is incorrect. Nifurtimox is used to treat *Trypanosoma cruzi*. *T. cruzi* infection causes Chagas' disease, a condition in which the heart is enlarged and flaccid. *T. cruzi* is transmitted via the reduviid bug. Microscopic examination reveals flagellated trypomastigotes in the blood and nonmotile amastigotes in tissue culture.

Answer C is incorrect. Quinine is used to treat babesiosis. *Babesia* species present with a malaria-like syndrome. Babesiosis is transmitted by the *Ixodes* tick. On microscopic examination, one observes no red blood cell pigment and the Maltese cross–appearing parasite.

Answer D is incorrect. Sodium stibogluconate is used to treat *Leishmania donovani* infection. *L. donovani* presents with hepatomegaly and splenomegaly, malaise, anemia, and weight loss. *L. donovani* is transmitted via the sandfly. Microscopically, macrophages containing amastigotes are observed.

Answer E is incorrect. Sulfadiazine and pyrimethamine are used to treat toxoplasmosis. *Toxoplasma gondii* infection presents with brain abscesses in HIV-positive patients and with birth defects. *T. gondii* is transmitted via cysts in raw meat or cat feces. The definitive stage (sexual stage) occurs in cats. Microscopically, acid-fast staining cysts are found.

58. **The correct answer is E.** This statement supports the notion that there is a higher occurrence of systemic lupus erythematosus (SLE) among women than among men. SLE is a type III hypersensitivity disease. Autoantibodies bind to self-antigens to form immune complexes that activate complement, leading to the activation of neutrophils. Since estrogen plays an inhibitory role on the process of clearing immune complexes, women have a higher risk than men of developing pathologically high levels of immune complexes, a number of which can lead to autoimmune diseases such as SLE.

Answer A is incorrect. If this statement were true, then men, who have higher levels of androgens than women, would be at an increased risk of developing pathologically high levels of immune complexes (see the explanation of the correct answer). Note that androgens actually accelerate the clearance of circulating immune complexes.

Answer B is incorrect. This statement does not support the epidemiologic phenomenon that women have a higher occurrence of systemic lupus erythematosus than men.

Answer C is incorrect. This statement is the exact opposite of the correct answer choice. See the explanation for the correct answer.

Answer D is incorrect. This statement does not support the higher occurrence of systemic lupus erythematosus (SLE) in women than in men. As stated in the explanation of the correct answer choice, antibodies (particularly certain antibodies against self-antigens) are needed to form immune complexes. Estrogen actually stimulates the process of antibody production by B cells, which contributes to the higher risk of developing SLE among women than among men.

59. **The correct answer is D.** *Naegleria fowleri* presents with a rapidly progressing meningoencephalitis that can progress to coma or death within 6 days. Other symptoms include nausea, vomiting, and irrational behavior. Transmission occurs through swimming in freshwater lakes. Microscopic analysis will reveal amebas in the spinal fluid. Unfortunately, there is no treatment for *N. fowleri*.

Answer A is incorrect. *Cryptosporidium* species infection presents with severe diarrhea in HIV-positive patients and mild watery diarrhea in HIV-negative patients. *Cryptosporidium* species are transmitted via cysts in water (fecal-oral transmission). Microscopically, acid-fast staining cysts are found. Unfortunately, there is no treatment available for *Cryptosporidium* species infection; however, in healthy patients, cryptosporidiosis is self-resolving.

Answer B is incorrect. *Entamoeba histolytica* infection presents with bloody diarrhea (dysentery), abdominal cramps with tenesmus, and pus in the stool. It can also cause right upper quadrant pain and liver abscesses. *E. histolytica* is transmitted via cysts in water (fecal-oral transmission). On microscopy, one observes amebas with ingested RBCs. Treatment for *E. histolytica* infection includes metronidazole and iodoquinol.

Answer C is incorrect. *Leishmania donovani* infection presents with hepatomegaly and splenomegaly, malaise, anemia, and weight loss. *L. donovani* is transmitted via the sandfly. Microscopically, macrophages containing amastigotes are observed. Sodium stibogluconate is used to treat *L. donovani* infection.

Answer E is incorrect. The *Plasmodium falciparum* parasite is responsible for causing malaria. It is spread by the *Anopheles* mosquito. Diagnosis of *Plasmodium falciparum* infection is made through a blood smear.

60. **The correct answer is B.** This is a classic presentation of chronic hepatitis C infection. It is a common cause of post-transfusion viral hepatitis. Hepatitis C is a blood-borne pathogen that can ultimately cause cirrhosis of the liver. Hepatitis B, C, and D may also cause chronic hepatitis.

Answer A is incorrect. Hepatitis A is transmitted via the fecal-oral route and does not cause chronic infection.

Answer C is incorrect. Hepatitis D is transmitted parenterally and can cause infection only if its host is coinfected with hepatitis B.

Answer D is incorrect. Hepatitis E is transmitted via the fecal-oral route and does not cause chronic infection.

Answer E is incorrect. Hepatitis G is a transmissible flavivirus that has not been shown to cause liver disease.

61. **The correct answer is B.** Selective immunoglobulin deficiency is a deficit in a specific class of immunoglobulins. IgA deficiency is the most common of these diseases. Since IgA is the most prominent immunoglobulin found in mucous membranes, patients suffering from a deficiency of it can present with sinus and lung infections.

Answer A is incorrect. A very high IgE level and normal levels of all immunoglobulins are characteristics of Job syndrome. Job syndrome is a disorder of the immune system that involves the failure of helper T lymphocytes to produce interferon-γ. It presents with multiple "cold," or noninflamed, skin lesions and high IgE levels.

Answer C is incorrect. A low IgM level with an elevated IgA level and a normal IgG level is characteristic of Wiskott-Aldrich syndrome. Wiskott-Aldrich syndrome involves a defect in the body's ability to mount an IgM response to encapsulated bacteria. The triad of symptoms consists of recurrent pyogenic infections, eczema, and thrombocytopenia.

Answer D is incorrect. Normal immunoglobulin levels can be seen in thymic aplasia (Di-

George's syndrome). Thymic aplasia presents with recurrent viral and fungal infections. It results from a congenital problem with the migration of the pharyngeal pouches that form the thymus and parathyroid glands. It results in a total lack of T lymphocytes and tetany due to hypocalcemia. It often presents with disorders of the great vessels and heart.

Answer E is incorrect. Normal immunoglobulin levels and a negative nitroblue tetrazolium dye reduction test indicate a diagnosis of chronic granulomatous disease. Chronic granulomatous disease involves a defect in the phagocytic ability of neutrophils and does not present with low levels of immunoglobulins. The definitive test for this disorder is a negative nitroblue tetrazolium dye reduction test.

62. **The correct answer is B.** Epstein-Barr virus (EBV) causes infectious mononucleosis and is a member of the Herpesviridae family. Mononucleosis typically presents with a high fever, an elevated white blood cell count, a painful pharyngitis, and enlarged lymph nodes. The difference between EBV mononucleosis and one caused by another virus, such as cytomegalovirus, is the heterophile antibody test, which is pathognomonic for EBV infection.

Answer A is incorrect. Cytomegalovirus causes mononucleosis, pneumonia, and birth defects if transmitted congenitally. Cytomegalovirus can reactivate and cause a variety of illnesses in the immunocompromised but is usually asymptomatic in healthy individuals.

Answer C is incorrect. HIV is the virus that causes AIDS. AIDS is a syndrome characterized by a decline in CD4 count and corresponding immunosuppression. As the T-lymphocyte count drops below 200 cells/mm^3, the infected individual is more susceptible to opportunistic infections. An acute HIV infection would present in a very similar fashion to Epstein-Barr virus and can result in either an elevated or a depressed white blood cell count. It would not, however, have a positive heterophile test.

Answer D is incorrect. *Streptococcus pneumoniae* is a gram-positive diplococcus and the most common cause of lobar pneumonia worldwide. It would not result in a positive heterophile antibody test.

Answer E is incorrect. Toxoplasmosis is caused by protozoa that are transmitted by ingestion of undercooked meat or food contaminated by cat feces. It is usually asymptomatic in immune competent individuals but can present as a brain lesion with focal neurologic deficits in immunocompromised individuals.

63. **The correct answer is B.** The *Plasmodium falciparum* parasite is responsible for causing malaria. It is spread by the *Anopheles* mosquito. Diagnosis of *Plasmodium falciparum* infection is made through a blood smear. The only species of *Plasmodium* that causes cerebral malaria is *P. falciparum*.

Answer A is incorrect. *Giardia lamblia* infection presents with bloating, flatulence, foul-smelling diarrhea, and light-colored fatty stools. *G. lamblia* is transmitted via cysts in water (fecal-oral transmission). On microscopy, one observes teardrop-shaped trophozoites with a ventral sucking disc or cysts. *G. lamblia* does not cause cerebral malaria.

Answer C is incorrect. *Plasmodium malariae* infection has a 72-hour cyclic fever. *P. malariae*, like *P. vivax* and *P. ovale*, does not cause cerebral malaria.

Answer D is incorrect. *Plasmodium ovale* infection has a 48-hour cyclic fever. A unique feature of *P. vivax* and *P. ovale* organisms is that they can form hypnozoites that can remain dormant in the liver for long periods of time, only to resurface later. However, *P. ovale* does not cause cerebral malaria.

Answer E is incorrect. *Plasmodium vivax* infection has a 48-hour cyclic fever. A unique feature of both *P. vivax* and *P. ovale* organisms is that they can form hypnozoites that can remain dormant in the liver for long periods of time, only to resurface later. However, *P. vivax* does not cause cerebral malaria.

64. **The correct answer is E.** CD34 is a surface antigen found in pluripotent stem cells. CD34+ cells can form pluripotent colonies in vitro.

    Answer A is incorrect. The antigen-presenting cell phagocytoses foreign material (for example, through Toll-like receptors) and processes foreign proteins into antigens that are presented on MHC class II surface proteins. This MHC class II/antigen complex then interacts with T-lymphocyte receptors on the helper T lymphocyte. Concurrently, B7 protein is expressed on the surface of the antigen-presenting cell, which interacts with its cognate receptor CD28 found on the helper T lymphocyte; this, in turn, provides the necessary costimulatory signal leading to T-lymphocyte activation.

    Answer B is incorrect. Helper T lymphocytes are CD4+.

    Answer C is incorrect. Cytotoxic killer T lymphocytes are CD8+.

    Answer D is incorrect. The CD28 receptor is found on the helper T lymphocyte and binds to B7 expressed on the surface of the antigen-presenting cell. The CD28/B7 interaction is necessary for the costimulatory signal required to activate the helper T lymphocyte.

    Answer F is incorrect. Phosphatidylinositol glycan A is required for GPI anchoring of decay-accelerating factor, which blocks complement activation on RBCs. Loss of this enzyme results in episodic acute intravascular hemolysis and thrombosis, presenting clinically as paroxysmal nocturnal hemoglobinuria.

65. **The correct answer is A.** This patient's symptoms are the typical presentation for pericarditis, which is inflammation of the pericardial membrane. The high-pitched grating sound is descriptive of a pericardial friction rub, a common finding in pericarditis. Coxsackievirus A or B is a common cause of viral pericarditis. Pain is usually severe, although the presentation can vary.

    Answer B is incorrect. Cytomegalovirus can cause retinitis, pneumonitis, and systemic diseases in immunocompromised patients, but otherwise causes heterophil-negative mononucleosis.

    Answer C is incorrect. Epstein-Barr virus causes heterophil-positive mononucleosis with fever, fatigue, lymphadenopathy, and splenomegaly.

    Answer D is incorrect. Norwalk virus is not a cause of infectious pericarditis. It usually causes gastroenteritis in school-aged children and adults.

    Answer E is incorrect. Rubella does not cause viral pericarditis and is rare in the United States because of extensive vaccination.

66. **The correct answer is E.** The patient is suffering from a type IV hypersensitivity reaction, also known a delayed-type hypersensitivity (DTH). More specifically, the patient is suffering from contact dermatitis after reexposure to the poison ivy plant. DTH is mediated by T-helper 1 cells that were previously sensitized to the antigen. When reexposed, these cells are quickly activated to secrete cytokines, which mediate the local inflammatory response that takes place in the skin. On first exposure, this reaction is primed but does not take place until reexposure.

    Answer A is incorrect. Goodpasture's syndrome is a type II hypersensitivity reaction and usually affects the lungs and kidneys.

    Answer B is incorrect. Type IV hypersensitivity reactions are mediated by previously sensitized T lymphocytes, not B lymphocytes.

    Answer C is incorrect. The patient must have been previously exposed in order to activate the cytokines to mediate the dermatitis.

    Answer D is incorrect. Contact dermatitis is a type IV hypersensitivity reaction, not a type I hypersensitivity reaction.

67. **The correct answer is B.** Adult botulism is characterized by the development of diplopia and dysphagia. This is followed by the development of general muscle weakness, respiratory muscle failure, and even death. The organism responsible for this disease is *Clostridium botu-*

linum, and it can be found in contaminated homemade canned goods and smoked fish.

Answer A is incorrect. *Bacillus cereus* causes food poisoning, and the patient typically presents with vomiting and diarrhea. It is most often associated with eating reheated rice.

Answer C is incorrect. *Clostridium perfringens* is the organism responsible for the development of gas gangrene. This organism is associated with contaminated wounds.

Answer D is incorrect. *Clostridium tetani* causes tetanus, which presents with severe muscle spasms and not muscle weakness. The disease usually follows a puncture wound (as the bacteria involved are anaerobic) and is not associated with eating canned goods.

Answer E is incorrect. *Escherichia coli* is not associated with botulism. *E. coli* O157:H7 causes food poisoning that presents with bloody diarrhea and vomiting after eating undercooked meat.

68. **The correct answer is B.** Antibody molecules consist of two heavy chains and two light chains. Intrachain disulfide bonds connect both the heavy chains and the light chains.

Answer A is incorrect. Hydrogen bonds are weaker than disulfide bonds and do not connect the antibody chains.

Answer C is incorrect. Ionic bonds are found in chemicals such as sodium chloride but are not responsible for holding antibody chains together.

Answer D is incorrect. Triple covalent bonds are seen between some atoms, such as nitrogen, but are not responsible for holding the chains of antibody molecules together.

Answer E is incorrect. Van der Waals forces are weak attraction forces and do not hold antibody chains together.

69. **The correct answer is E.** This man is suffering from septic arthritis, commonly characterized by a swollen, tender, and erythematous joint. The organism most commonly responsible for this infection is *Staphylococcus aureus*.

The infection results from the invasion of the bacteria into the synovial fluid. The diagnosis of septic arthritis requires the aspiration of the synovial fluid, which appears yellow and turbid with a predominance of neutrophils. Gram's stain and culture of the fluid show gram-positive cocci in clusters.

Answer A is incorrect. Septic arthritis is most commonly caused by *Staphylococcus aureus*, which is not in the *Babesia* genus.

Answer B is incorrect. Septic arthritis is most commonly caused by *Staphylococcus aureus*, which is not in the *Bacillus* genus.

Answer C is incorrect. Septic arthritis is most commonly caused by *Staphylococcus aureus*, which is not in the *Clostridium* genus.

Answer D is incorrect. Septic arthritis is most commonly caused by *Staphylococcus aureus*, which is not in the *Pasteurella* genus.

70. **The correct answer is E.** Rubeola, also called measles, is a relatively rare illness in the United States because of the ubiquity of the measles/mumps/rubella (MMR) vaccine. It presents with the prodrome described in this patient. The rash that spreads from head to toe over a 3-day period develops 1 or 2 days after the appearance of Koplik's spots, which are red oral lesions with blue-white centers.

Answer A is incorrect. Diphtheria is an illness virtually unknown in the United States because of the prevalence of the diphtheria/tetanus/pertussis (DTP) vaccine. It is caused by *Corynebacterium diphtheriae* and is characterized by a membranous pharyngitis.

Answer B is incorrect. Pertussis, or whooping cough, is also rare due to widespread vaccinations. It is a respiratory infection of children that characteristically produces coughing spasms followed by a loud inspiratory whoop.

Answer C is incorrect. Roseola is a febrile disease of very young children that begins with a high fever and progresses to a rash similar to measles. Infants and young children are most at risk. It is believed to be caused by human herpesvirus 6.

Answer D is incorrect. Rubella, also known as German measles, is a less severe viral exanthem. Many infections are subclinical, but rubella can cause severe birth defects when infection occurs during the prenatal period.

71. **The correct answer is A.** Ataxia-telangiectasia involves a defect in DNA repair enzymes. The image shows spider angiomas, which are a common symptom in patients with this condition. Ataxia-telangiectasia is associated with an IgA deficiency and cerebellar problems leading to ataxia and, in this case, multiple falls.

Answer B is incorrect. Granulomas are collections of cells seen in (among other things) chronic granulomatous disease. This disease is caused by an inability of neutrophils to kill bacteria once they have phagocytosed them.

Answer C is incorrect. Bruton's agammaglobulinemia is an X-linked deficit and therefore presents in males. It is a defect in a tyrosine kinase associated with low levels of all classes of immunoglobulins. After 6 months of age, when the levels of maternal antibodies have declined, patients with the disease tend to present with recurrent bacterial infections. Patients also present with uniformly low antibody titers of all classes.

Answer D is incorrect. The third and fourth pharyngeal pouches, and thus the thymus and parathyroid glands, fail to develop in patients with thymic aplasia (DiGeorge's syndrome). The disease often presents with many congenital defects such as, cardiac abnormalities, cleft palate, and abnormal facies. Thymic aplasia can also present with tetany due to hypocalcemia.

Answer E is incorrect. Visual hallucinations are not a symptom of any of the known immune deficiencies.

72. **The correct answer is B.** Disseminated *Mycobacterium avium–intracellulare* usually infects birds and other animals. It can infect humans when their T-cell count is below approximately 50/mm³. It presents as a chronic wasting illness as the bacteria proliferate throughout the body.

Answer A is incorrect. Cryptococcal meningitis can present when the T-cell count is below 200/mm³. It presents with fever, nausea, and vomiting. Unfortunately, because the immune system is impaired, signs of meningeal inflammation may not be present.

Answer C is incorrect. Herpes simplex infection often occurs severely with a T-cell count below 400/mm³ or before. While herpes simplex can affect individuals with a normal immune system, infection in immunocompromised patients will be more severe, with more oral and genital ulcers.

Answer D is incorrect. Herpes zoster infection can present when the T-cell count is below 400/mm³ or before. It is characterized as a painful collection of vesicles in a dermatomal pattern.

Answer E is incorrect. Oral thrush can present when the T-cell count is below 400/mm³ or before. It presents with white patches and plaques on the oral mucosa.

Answer F is incorrect. *Pneumocystis carinii* pneumonia can present when the T-cell count is below 200/mm³. It presents with hypoxia and cough and is one of the most common opportunistic infections.

Answer G is incorrect. Toxoplasmosis brain lesions usually present with focal neurologic deficits. A CT scan will show a ring-enhancing lesion. Toxoplasmosis prophylaxis is started when the T-cell count is below 100/mm³.

73. **The correct answer is D.** The third and fourth pharyngeal pouches, and thus the thymus and parathyroid glands, fail to develop in patients with thymic aplasia (DiGeorge syndrome). This disease often presents with congenital defects such as cardiac abnormalities, cleft palate, and abnormal facies. Thymic aplasia can also present with tetany due to hypocalcemia.

Answer A is incorrect. Bruton's agammaglobulinemia is an X-linked defect in tyrosine kinase associated with low levels of all classes of immunoglobulins. After 6 months of age, when the levels of maternal antibodies have declined, patients with the disease tend to present with recurrent bacterial infections.

Answer B is incorrect. Job syndrome is a disorder of the immune system that involves the failure of helper T lymphocytes to produce interferon-γ. It presents with multiple "cold," or noninflamed, skin lesions and high IgE levels.

Answer C is incorrect. Severe combined immunodeficiency presents with recurrent viral, bacterial, fungal, and protozoal infections due to a total lack of cellular immunity secondary to a stem cell deficit in the bone marrow. It does not present with the congenital defects described.

Answer E is incorrect. Wiskott-Aldrich syndrome is an X-linked defect associated with elevated IgA levels, elevated IgE levels, normal IgG levels, and low IgM levels. It involves a defect in the body's ability to mount an IgM response to bacteria. Recurrent pyogenic infections, eczema, and thrombocytopenia are the typical triad of symptoms. It does not present with any specific enzyme abnormality.

74. **The correct answer is B.** This patient has a classic presentation (fever, sore throat, anterior cervical lymphadenopathy, lack of cough) of streptococcal pharyngitis, or strep throat. Strep throat is caused by *Streptococcus pyogenes*, or group A strep. Diagnosis is confirmed with a rapid strep test or with throat swab culture. The treatment of choice is penicillin. To differentiate this organism from other gram-positive organisms, several tests can be performed in the lab. For example, when cultured on blood agar, *S. pyogenes* creates a clear halo (β-hemolysis) around the colonies due to damage of the RBCs. To further differentiate strep species, sensitivity to different antibiotics is measured. *S. pyogenes* is sensitive to bacitracin.

Answer A is incorrect. Catalase-negative, β-hemolytic, bacitracin-resistant describes *Streptococcus agalactiae*, or group B strep. *S. agalactiae* is a significant cause of serious bacterial infection in neonates.

Answer C is incorrect. Catalase-negative, α-hemolytic, optochin-resistant describes *Strep-*

tococcus viridans. S. mutans is associated with the formation of dental caries.

Answer D is incorrect. Catalase-negative, α-hemolytic, optochin-sensitive describes *Streptococcus pneumoniae*. This organism causes pneumonia and otitis media. Rates of *S. pneumoniae* meningitis have decreased with the advent of the pneumococcal vaccine.

Answer E is incorrect. Catalase-positive, coagulase-positive, novobiocin-resistant describes *Staphylococcus saprophyticus*. This is the second most common cause of urinary tract infection in young, healthy women.

Answer F is incorrect. Catalase-positive, coagulase-positive, novobiocin-sensitive describes *Staphylococcus epidermidis*. Infection with *S. epidermidis* is associated with skin penetration by implanted prosthetic devices such as prosthetic heart valves, intravenous lines, and intraperitoneal catheters.

75. **The correct answer is E.** Microscopic polyangiitis is one of the trio of diseases (with Wegener's granulomatosis and Churg-Strauss syndrome) that are referred to as the ANCA (antineutrophil cytoplasmic antibody)–associated vasculitides. Over 80% of patients with this disease have ANCA, usually the perinuclear pattern of staining (p-ANCA) type. Inflammation of the pulmonary capillaries, which can lead to hemoptysis, is common in these patients, and 90% of patients have necrotizing glomerulonephritis (leading to hematuria). Other common symptoms include intestinal pain/bleeding, muscle pain, and weakness. The pathologic lesions are similar to those found in classic polyarteritis nodosa (PAN), but unlike PAN, large and muscular arteries as well as those in the pulmonary circulation are spared. The term *classic* is now often added to the term *PAN* to differentiate classic polyarteritis nodosa from other small-vessel vasculitides (such as microscopic polyangiitis), which are now thought to represent distinct entities. Classic polyarteritis nodosa has little association with ANCA.

Answer A is incorrect. Anti-Smith antibodies are found in 20–30% of patients with systemic lupus erythematosus and are not particularly associated with microscopic polyangiitis. "Smith antigen" describes certain core proteins of small nuclear ribonucleoprotein particles. Nonspecific antinuclear antibodies and/or rheumatoid factor may be found in patients with microscopic polyangiitis, but anti-Smith antibodies are more specific for systemic lupus erythematosus.

Answer B is incorrect. Anti-ribonucleoprotein (anti-RNP) antibody SS-A (Ro), which is present in 70–95% of patients with Sjögren's syndrome, is not particularly associated with microscopic polyangiitis. Anti-RNP SS-A is more specific for Sjögren's syndrome.

Answer C is incorrect. Anti-ribonucleoprotein (anti-RNP) antibody SS-B (La), which is present in 60–90% of patients with Sjögren's syndrome, is not particularly associated with microscopic polyangiitis. Anti-RNP SS-B is more specific for Sjögren's syndrome.

Answer D is incorrect. Anticentromere antibodies, which are found in 90% of patients with the CREST variant of scleroderma, are not particularly associated with microscopic polyangiitis. Anticentromere antibodies are more specific for the CREST variant of scleroderma.

CHAPTER 5

Pharmacology

QUESTIONS

1. A 37-year-old man who is HIV-positive recently started on a highly active antiretroviral regimen. The patient's CD4 cell count subsequently fell below 200/mm^3. Over the course of the next 3 months, he develops diarrhea and notices a redistribution of fat on his body. Which of the following agents is most likely causing this patient's symptoms?

   (A) Fusion inhibitor
   (B) Non-nucleoside reverse transcriptase inhibitor
   (C) Nucleoside reverse transcriptase inhibitor
   (D) Nucleotide reverse transcriptase inhibitor
   (E) Protease inhibitor

2. A patient is being treated with β-blockers for hypertension. Which of the following describes the effects of β-blockers on end-diastolic volume (EDV), blood pressure (BP), contractility, heart rate (HR), and ejection time?

CHOICE	EDV	BP	CONTRACTILITY	HR	EJECTION TIME
A	None or ↓	↓	Little/no effect	↓	Little/no effect
B	↓	↓	↓	↑	↓
C	↓	↓	↓	↓	↓
D	↑	↓	↓	↓	↑
E	↓	↓	↑	↑	↓

   (A) A
   (B) B
   (C) C
   (D) D
   (E) E

3. A 68-year-old woman with scleroderma presents to the physician with a 6-month history of nausea and bloating. Symptoms are most prominent following a meal. The best treatment option for this patient is which of the following?

   (A) Esophageal resection
   (B) Metoclopramide
   (C) Omeprazole
   (D) Ondansetron
   (E) Vagotomy

4. A 33-year-old woman with a history of Graves' disease is brought to the emergency department unresponsive following a bout of confusion and agitation. On physical examination her temperature is 39.2° C (102.5° F), her blood pressure is 100/70 mm Hg, and her pulse is 165/min. A systolic ejection murmur is heard at the apex, and the patient has 3+ pitting edema at the ankles. Following primary stabilization, which of the following would constitute appropriate pharmacotherapy for this patient's underlying condition?

   (A) Aspirin
   (B) Dobutamine
   (C) Iodine
   (D) Levothyroxine
   (E) Propylthiouracil

5. A 28-year-old woman comes to the physician concerned about an excessive amount of bleeding from her gums when she brushes her teeth. Her laboratory results show an increased partial thromboplastin time (PTT) and an increased bleeding time, but are otherwise unremarkable. Which of the following treatments will most likely alleviate this patient's symptoms?

   (A) Cryoprecipitate
   (B) Factor VIII concentrate
   (C) Fresh frozen plasma
   (D) Low-molecular-weight heparin
   (E) Protamine sulfate

6. A 32-year-old woman presents to her primary care physician complaining of overwhelming fear and apprehension. On further question-

ing, the patient states that she feels anxious and worried about many things and has difficulty concentrating because she "can't seem to keep her mind off of the everyday issues of life." She states that often she feels tense and restless, and feels as though her heart is going to "beat right out of my chest." Which of the following drugs would be considered first-line treatment for her illness?

(A) Amitriptyline
(B) Diazepam
(C) Flumazenil
(D) Haloperidol
(E) Thiopental

7. A 40-year-old man has been diagnosed with glioblastoma multiforme. The patient's neurologist must choose an appropriate cancer drug to treat this tumor. Which of the following classes of oncologic drugs or drug classes can cross the blood-brain barrier for effective treatment of brain tumors?

(A) Cytarabine
(B) Etoposide
(C) Nitrosoureas
(D) Selective estrogen receptor modulators
(E) Vinca alkaloids

8. A 5-year-old white boy presents to the physician's office for treatment of chronic recurrent pulmonary infections and bronchitis. The boy's history is significant for ileus as a newborn and chronic floating, foul-smelling diarrhea. Analysis of the child's sweat reveals an increased concentration of Cl^- ions. Which of the following pharmacologic treatments is used to treat the underlying symptoms of the disease that is responsible for this patient's overall pathology?

(A) Ceftriaxone
(B) Granulocyte colony-stimulating factor
(C) N-acetylcysteine
(D) Prednisone
(E) Terbutaline

9. A 70-year-old man presents to his cardiologist with shortness of breath, crackles along both lung bases, and 1+ pitting edema in his lower

extremities. His cardiologist diagnoses him with mild congestive heart failure and places him on a thiazide diuretic. Two days later, the patient comes to the emergency department obtunded and oliguric, with a highly elevated creatinine level of 8.3 mg/dL. His wife reports that the only medication that he took besides his diuretic was "some ibuprofen for his headache." Which of the following is the most likely reason for this patient's sudden renal failure?

(A) Decrease of prostaglandin E_2 production in both arterioles of the kidney
(B) Decrease of prostaglandin E_2 production in the afferent arterioles of the kidney
(C) Decrease of prostaglandin E_2 production in the efferent arterioles of the kidney
(D) Excessive diuresis
(E) Inadequate diuresis

10. A 74-year-old man comes to the physician complaining of increased urinary frequency along with difficulty starting and stopping urination. Assuming a benign underlying cause, which of the following is the mechanism of action of a common medication used to treat this condition?

(A) Formation of superoxide radicals that attack DNA bonds
(B) Gonadotropin-releasing hormone analog
(C) Inhibition of 5-α-reductase
(D) Inhibition of cytochrome P450 enzymes
(E) Inhibition of testosterone's negative feedback on gonadotropin secretion

11. A 56-year-old stabbing victim has been in the hospital for 4 days with an infected wound that presented with crepitus on palpation. The wound was debrided and treated with antibiotics. The wound showed improvement, but on hospital day 5, the patient has a fever, an increased WBC count, and diarrhea. Which of the following is the agent most likely causing this patient's symptoms?

(A) Amantadine
(B) Clindamycin
(C) Metronidazole
(D) Tetracycline
(E) Vancomycin

12. The targets of multiple lipid-lowering agents are labeled in the image. Which of the targets corresponds to the therapy associated with the most significant decrease in triglyceride levels?

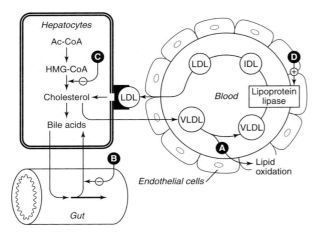

Reproduced, with permission, from USMLERx.com.

(A) A
(B) B
(C) C
(D) D

13. A 72-year-old man comes to the emergency department because of shortness of breath and dyspnea on exertion for the past few days. Physical examination reveals pitting edema bilaterally in the lower extremities. The patient is given a combination drug therapy for his condition. Which of the following effective therapies have possible toxic interactions?

(A) Acetylsalicylic acid and a thiazide diuretic
(B) Acetylsalicylic acid and nitroprusside
(C) β-Blocker and a thiazide diuretic
(D) β-Blocker and spironolactone
(E) Digoxin and furosemide
(F) Digoxin and spironolactone

14. A 68-year-old man comes to the emergency department because of a 5-hour history of palpitations and light-headedness. He states that he has experienced shorter episodes of palpitations before, but nothing so severe. After admission to the hospital, the patient receives a full cardiac workup and is diagnosed with rapid atrial fibrillation, likely secondary to a moderately stenosed mitral valve. Medical treatment to convert him to sinus rhythm is unsuccessful. However, his heart rate is well controlled with various atrioventricular node blocking agents. The patient is prescribed a regimen of daily medications. Along with his heart rate control medications, which of the following is another medication he will likely be taking on a daily basis?

(A) Aspirin
(B) Protamine sulfate
(C) Streptokinase
(D) Unfractionated heparin
(E) Warfarin

15. The plasma concentration of drug Y is 50 mg/L, and it is eliminated at a rate of 2 mg/min. Which of the following is the clearance rate of drug Y?

(A) 0.04 L/min
(B) 0.1 L/min
(C) 4 L/min
(D) 10 L/min
(E) 400 L/min

16. A 33-year-old immigrant from Peru comes to a women's health clinic because she has missed her period for the past 2 months. Already a mother of four, she explains that she can't afford to have another child. When her pregnancy test comes back positive, she becomes obviously distraught, saying that she has been on the pill for the past year and has not missed a single dose. As she starts to cry, her tears are noted to have an orange tint. The physician tells her that the most likely reason her oral contraceptives were ineffective was an interaction with one of her other medications. She is most probably being treated for which of the following?

(A) Breast cancer
(B) Epilepsy
(C) *Giardia* infection
(D) Refractory atrial fibrillation
(E) Tuberculosis

17. A 43-year-old man with a 7-year history of chronic renal disease comes to the emergency

department with a 5-day history of productive cough and shortness of breath. On physical examination, he is found to have rales in the middle lobe of his right lung. An x-ray film of the chest shows consolidation in the same area, and he is started on levofloxacin. Which of the following indicates how the dosing of the levofloxacin would be different in this patient as compared to an otherwise healthy patient?

(A) Higher loading dose, higher maintenance dose
(B) Higher loading dose, same maintenance dose
(C) Lower loading dose, lower maintenance dose
(D) Lower loading dose, same maintenance dose
(E) Same loading dose, higher maintenance dose
(F) Same loading dose, lower maintenance dose
(G) Same loading dose, same maintenance dose

18. A 64-year-old man with an extensive past medical history develops chronic renal failure. After a kidney biopsy is taken (see image), his physician immediately starts him on a new medication. What pharmacologic treatment has been shown to most effectively delay the progression of the pathology shown in this photomicrograph?

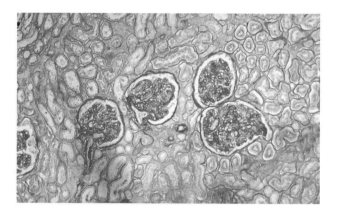

Image courtesy of PEIR Digital Library (http://peir.net).

(A) Angiotensin-converting enzyme inhibitors
(B) β-Blockers
(C) Cyclophosphamide
(D) Gold therapy
(E) Prednisone

19. A 24-year-old law student has been experiencing frequent headaches for which he has been taking increasingly large doses of aspirin for 3 months. One night he takes a particularly large dose, becomes confused, and falls into a seizure. He presents to the emergency department with a serum salicylate level of 130 mg/dL. Which of the following is the most appropriate treatment?

(A) Bicarbonate
(B) Glucagon
(C) N-acetylcysteine
(D) Protamine
(E) Vitamin K

20. A 55-year-old man who has smoked for 30 years comes to the physician because of a 3-month history of a cough with sputum production. The man says that over the past 2 years he has had the same cough five or six times, and it usually lasts for several months. On physical examination, the patient is afebrile. An x-ray film of his chest shows bilateral hyperinflated lungs and flattened diaphragms. The physician tells him that he has chronic obstructive pulmonary disease and prescribes inhaled steroids, a β₂ agonist, and ipratropium bromide. Ipratropium bromide will produce bronchodilation through which of the following mechanisms?

(A) Blockage of acetylcholine at muscarinic receptors
(B) Inhibiting the degranulation of mast cells
(C) Inhibiting the synthesis of cytokines
(D) Inhibition of phosphodiesterase resulting in increased cAMP levels
(E) Stimulation of adenylyl cyclase resulting in increased cAMP levels

21. A 4-year-old girl is brought to the emergency department with abdominal pain after eating 10–15 sugar-coated iron tablets. Soon after arriving she begins to vomit, and the emesis has blood in it. Physical examination shows hypotension and tachycardia. Which of the following is the best treatment for this patient's elevated blood iron levels?

   (A) Aminocaproic acid
   (B) Deferoxamine
   (C) Dimercaprol
   (D) Ethylenediaminetetraacetic acid
   (E) Oral bicarbonate

22. A 52-year-old man with end-stage renal disease presents to his renal clinic with a hemoglobin concentration of 8 g/dL and an absolute reticulocyte count of < 25,000 cells/μL. His WBC count is 11,000/mm³ and the differential is within normal limits. A peripheral blood smear shows hypochromic, microcytic RBCs. Iron staining of a bone marrow aspirate shows macrophages positive and RBCs negative for iron within the cytoplasm. Which of the following is the most likely cause of this patient's condition?

   (A) An overdose of tacrolimus
   (B) Anti-Rh D immunoglobulin
   (C) Low erythropoietin
   (D) Myelodysplastic syndrome
   (E) Tissue plasminogen activator

23. The following illustration contains the dose-response curves for drug X as well as two other agents. Which of the following curves represents drug X plus a noncompetitive antagonist?

   (A) Curve A
   (B) Curve B
   (C) Curve C
   (D) Curve D
   (E) Curve E

24. Class I antiarrhythmics are Na+ channel blockers that slow or block cardiac conduction, especially in depolarized cells. Which of the following Class I antiarrhythmics will increase both the action potential and the effective refractory period (ERP)?

   (A) Encainide
   (B) Mexiletine
   (C) Procainamide
   (D) Propafenone
   (E) Tocainide

25. A 74-year-old woman comes to the clinic complaining of fever and a productive cough. Physical examination shows dullness to percussion and bronchial breath sounds on the lower right side. A stain of her yellow-brown sputum shows gram-positive diplococci. In light of her history of penicillin allergy, she is started on erythromycin. What is the mechanism of action of erythromycin?

   (A) Binds to the 30S ribosomal subunit of bacteria
   (B) Inhibits binding of aminoacyl tRNA to the A site of the ribosome
   (C) Inhibits elongation factor 2
   (D) Inhibits eukaryotic initiation factor 2
   (E) Inhibits translocation of the tRNA

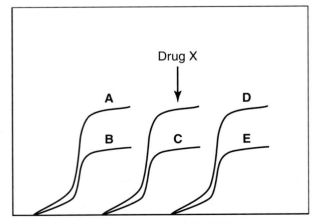

Reproduced, with permission, from USMLERx.com.

ANSWERS

1. The correct answer is E. Protease inhibitors such as lopinavir/ritonavir (Kaletra), amprenavir, nelfinavir, indinavir, and saquinavir can cause gastrointestinal intolerance and fat redistribution. Lopinavir/ritonavir is one of the main combinations forming the basis of highly active antiretroviral therapy (HAART). Two nucleotide reverse transcriptase inhibitors are added to form the backbone.

Answer A is incorrect. The only fusion inhibitor currently available, enfuvirtide, is not recommended for inclusion in the initial highly active antiretroviral therapy (HAART) regimen. It is associated with reactions at the injection site, but not fat distribution.

Answer B is incorrect. Non-nucleoside reverse transcriptase inhibitors such as nevirapine, delavirdine, and efavirenz cause a variety of adverse effects such as rash and hepatitis, but they do not cause fat redistribution.

Answer C is incorrect. Some of the nucleoside reverse transcriptase inhibitors (zidovudine, stavudine, didanosine, zalcitabine, abacavir, and lamivudine) can cause peripheral neuropathies, gastrointestinal intolerance, and pancreatitis, but they are not known to cause fat redistribution.

Answer D is incorrect. The nucleotide reverse transcriptase inhibitor tenofovir is usually well tolerated. It is recommended that it be taken with meals. The Department of Health and Human Services recommends that it be used in one of its treatment regimens.

2. The correct answer is D. β-Blockers decrease the contractility and rate of the heart (resulting in decreased oxygen consumption) and decrease the secretion of renin, thus diminishing the renin-angiotensin cascade. Rate and contractility is reduced by a blockade of the β_1 receptors located in the sinoatrial node, atrioventricular node, and the ventricular muscle of the heart. By reducing the contractility of the heart, the ejection time is increased. In addition to this, the EDV increases because filling time is lengthened (negative chronotropic, dromotropic, and ionotropic effects). The effects of β-blockers result in an overall decrease in blood pressure and afterload.

Answer A is incorrect. Answer A reflects the physiologic effects of a combination of nitrates and β-blockers.

Answer B is incorrect. Answer B is incompatible with antihypertensives.

Answer C is incorrect. Answer C is incompatible with antihypertensives.

Answer E is incorrect. Answer E is compatible with the effects of nitrates alone. Nitrates serve to decrease the preload on the heart by vasodilation. EDV decreases as a result and thus the ejection time decreases. Nitrates have no direct chronotropic, dromotropic, or ionotropic effects. However, because of the vasodilation, there is a reflex increase in both contractility and HR.

3. The correct answer is B. This patient presents with esophageal dysmotility secondary to scleroderma. Other causes of esophageal dysmotility include diabetic gastroparesis, Chagas' disease, lupus, and other collagen vascular diseases. Initial treatment consists of promotility agents, with metoclopramide, an anticholinergic and dopamine agonist, being first-line therapy.

Answer A is incorrect. Esophageal resection is the treatment for squamous cell carcinoma or adenocarcinoma of the esophagus or for high-grade Barrett's esophagus.

Answer C is incorrect. Omeprazole is a proton pump inhibitor used to treat gastroesophageal reflux disease, peptic ulcer disease, and acid hypersecretion.

Answer D is incorrect. Ondansetron is a 5-HT_3 receptor antagonist used to treat refractory or severe nausea and vomiting.

Answer E is incorrect. Vagotomy is a treatment option for peptic ulcer disease or acid hypersecretion states such as in Zollinger-Ellison syndrome.

4. **The correct answer is E.** This patient is presenting with a medical emergency: an extreme form of thyrotoxicosis known as "thyroid storm." The symptoms of this syndrome are due primarily to increased β-adrenergic outflow stimulated by thyroid hormones. After primary stabilization (airway, breathing, and circulation), propylthiouracil or methimazole is the most appropriate pharmacologic treatment for this condition. These agents inhibit the endogenous synthesis of thyroxine, which can cause or worsen this condition.

Answer A is incorrect. Aspirin displaces thyroxine from thyroid-binding globulin and can thus worsen the symptoms of thyrotoxicosis. In contrast, acetaminophen is useful as an antipyretic in the treatment of thyrotoxicosis and thyroid storm.

Answer B is incorrect. Dobutamine is a β-adrenergic agonist that is useful in the treatment of acute congestive heart failure but would exacerbate the adrenergic effects of high-output congestive heart failure secondary to thyrotoxicosis. A β-adrenergic antagonist such as propranolol would be more appropriate in the treatment of thyrotoxicosis.

Answer C is incorrect. Iodine, which decreases the release of preformed thyroxine, can be used as an adjunct to propylthiouracil or methimazole but should not be used until one of these agents is allowed to take effect. Iodine can stimulate the endogenous synthesis of thyroxine and thus exacerbate this condition.

Answer D is incorrect. Levothyroxine, a synthetic form of thyroid hormone, is contraindicated in the treatment of thyrotoxicosis. The addition of more thyroid hormone to a patient with a condition of symptomatic hyperthyroidism would only worsen the condition.

5. **The correct answer is A.** This woman suffers from von Willebrand's disease, the most common inherited bleeding disorder; it results from a malfunction of von Willebrand factor. Von Willebrand factor (vWF) has two func-

tions: it serves as the ligand for platelet adhesion to a damaged vessel wall, and it is the plasma carrier of factor VIII. Due to platelet dysfunction and lack of a carrier for factor VIII, the unique lab finding in this disease consists of an increased bleeding time and an increased partial thromboplastin time. Cryoprecipitate contains sufficient normal vWF to correct the bleeding dyscrasia.

Answer B is incorrect. Factor VIII concentrate is used to treat individuals with hemophilia A, an inherited condition that results in factor VIII deficiency.

Answer C is incorrect. Fresh frozen plasma (FFP) is used to treat several factor deficiencies, including V, VII, X, and XI. FFP administration will replace several factor deficiencies, although factor concentrations in FFP tend to vary.

Answer D is incorrect. Low-molecular-weight heparin (LMWH) is a newer anticoagulant that acts predominantly on factor Xa. LMWH can be administered subcutaneously. Partial thromboplastin time does not need to be monitored with this drug.

Answer E is incorrect. Protamine sulfate is used for reversal of heparinization. It is a positively charged molecule that acts by binding to heparin, a negatively charged molecule. Protamine would have no therapeutic benefit for this patient.

6. **The correct answer is B.** This patient suffers from generalized anxiety disorder, which is marked by symptoms of excessive worry and anxiety about every aspect of one's life. Patients tend to manifest difficulty concentrating, feelings of being tense, and signs of autonomic arousal such as rapid heartbeat and/or sweating. Benzodiazepines are first-line agents in the treatment of such anxiety disorders due to their sedative properties. Longer-acting agents such as diazepam are preferred in those patients with anxiety who require treatment for long periods of time. These agents should be used only for short periods of time because of their potential for tolerance and dependence.

Answer A is incorrect. Amitriptyline, a tricyclic antidepressant, may be effective for the treatment of anxiety disorder but is not considered a first-line agent. Agents in this class are better suited for the treatment of endogenous depression.

Answer C is incorrect. Flumazenil is a competitive γ-aminobutyric acid–receptor antagonist that is used to reverse the effects of benzodiazepines; it is indicated for use in cases of acute benzodiazepine overdose.

Answer D is incorrect. Haloperidol is indicated for the treatment of psychotic disorders such as schizophrenia and plays no role in the treatment of generalized anxiety disorder.

Answer E is incorrect. Thiopental, a barbiturate, has some sedative properties that may be helpful in patients with anxiety disorder. However, this agent is more commonly given for the induction of anesthesia. Barbiturates have largely been replaced by benzodiazepines as first-line agents for the treatment of anxiety because of the significant side effect profile of barbiturates.

7. **The correct answer is C.** The lipophilic nitrosoureas, such as carmustine and lomustine, are alkylating agents that can penetrate the blood-brain barrier, making them excellent drugs for the treatment of brain tumors. The nitrosoureas are metabolized to active products and excreted in the urine.

Answer A is incorrect. Cytarabine inhibits DNA polymerase and is used in the treatment of acute myelogenous leukemia. Cytarabine cannot penetrate the blood-brain barrier.

Answer B is incorrect. Etoposide is noted for poor penetration into the cerebrospinal fluid.

Answer D is incorrect. Selective estrogen receptor modulators (SERMs), such as raloxifene, block estrogen from binding to estrogen receptors on estrogen receptor–positive cells. SERMs do not penetrate the blood-brain barrier.

Answer E is incorrect. Vinca alkaloids, given intravenously, are concentrated in the liver and excreted through bile in the feces. Vinca alkaloids do not cross the blood-brain barrier.

8. **The correct answer is C.** This is the classic presentation of a child with cystic fibrosis (CF), an autosomal recessive defect in the cystic fibrosis transmembrane conductance regulator (*CFTR*) gene on chromosome 7 that results in a defective Cl⁻ channel, leading to the secretion of abnormally thick mucus in the lungs, pancreas, and liver. Pharmacologic treatment for CF includes N-acetylcysteine, which serves to loosen mucous plugs and restore pulmonary and pancreatic functions.

Answer A is incorrect. Ceftriaxone, a third-generation cephalosporin, may be used to treat infections in cystic fibrosis (CF) patients, but it does not treat CF itself.

Answer B is incorrect. Granulocyte colony-stimulating factor, a stimulator for the production of granulocytes, is used in the treatment of neutropenic states such as those associated with leukemia, chemotherapy, and bone marrow disorders.

Answer D is incorrect. Prednisone, a steroid, is not used in the treatment of cystic fibrosis.

Answer E is incorrect. Terbutaline, an asthma treatment, is not used in the treatment of cystic fibrosis.

9. **The correct answer is B.** Renal failure is a very dangerous adverse event associated with nonsteroidal anti-inflammatory drugs (NSAIDs). The patient was in congestive heart failure when he first presented. His cardiologist consequently treated him with a diuretic, intending to reduce his total body fluids. When the amount of fluids in the body contracts, the body attempts to compensate by releasing angiotensin II, a potent vasoconstrictor. In order to protect the kidney from losing its perfusion due to this vasoconstriction, the kidney simultaneously releases prostaglandins at both the afferent and efferent arterioles, where they act as vasodilators. By taking an NSAID like ibuprofen and inhibiting the cyclooxygenase (COX)-1 and COX-2 enzymes, this patient blocked the pathway producing the prosta-

glandins that were keeping the afferent arterioles dilated and thus keeping his kidneys perfused. His renal failure is prerenal in origin, resulting from the constriction of these arterioles.

Answer A is incorrect. The nonsteroidal anti-inflammatory drugs will block the production of prostaglandin E_2 at both arterioles, but the constriction of the afferent arteriole is the primary cause of this man's renal failure.

Answer C is incorrect. While the nonsteroidal anti-inflammatory drug would also have blocked the production of prostaglandin E_2 at the efferent arteriole, this would not cause renal failure, it would actually increase glomerular filtration rate (blocking the outflow without blocking the inflow will increase filtration). This would not cause the patient to present with oliguria or a rising creatinine level.

Answer D is incorrect. Excessive diuresis could lead to a loss of perfusion in the kidneys in extreme cases; however, thiazide diuretics are unlikely to cause such a severe diuresis. A more potent diuretic, such as furosemide, could cause prerenal failure due to volume contraction if it is not administered carefully.

Answer E is incorrect. Inadequate diuresis would lead to volume expansion, but this alone would not cause renal failure to develop.

10. **The correct answer is C.** This man has the symptoms of benign prostatic hypertrophy, which include difficulty starting and maintaining a urine stream, feeling as though the bladder is never emptied, having the urge to urinate again soon after voiding, and pain on urination or dysuria. Finasteride is most commonly used to treat this condition. Finasteride acts by inhibiting the conversion of testosterone to dihydrotestosterone by inhibiting 5-α-reductase. This leads to a reduction in the size of the prostate, providing symptomatic relief.

Answer A is incorrect. Bleomycin acts by chelating mechanisms to attack the phosphodiester bonds of DNA. It is used to treat testicular tumors, not benign prostatic hypertrophy.

Answer B is incorrect. Leuprolide is a gonadotropin-releasing hormone analog that binds the luteinizing hormone (LH)-releasing hormone receptor in the pituitary. This leads to desensitization of the receptor and, subsequently, to reduced release of LH. Leuprolide is used to treat metastatic carcinoma of the prostate, not benign prostatic hypertrophy.

Answer D is incorrect. Ketoconazole is an antifungal with antiandrogenic properties that acts by inhibiting cytochrome P450 enzymes. It is not used in the treatment of benign prostatic hypertrophy.

Answer E is incorrect. Flutamide is a potent androgen receptor antagonist that has limited efficacy when used alone because the increased luteinizing hormone secretion stimulates higher serum testosterone levels. This drug is used primarily in conjunction with a gonadotropin-releasing hormone analog in the treatment of metastatic prostate cancer.

11. **The correct answer is B.** The patient most likely had an anaerobic infection at the wound site, probably with *Clostridium perfringens*, which would have responded well to clindamycin. Unfortunately, one of the adverse effects of clindamycin is superinfection (i.e., an infection on top of another infection) caused by destruction of most colonic bacteria and an overgrowth of *Clostridium difficile*, which is resistant to clindamycin.

Answer A is incorrect. Amantadine is an antiviral agent associated with ataxia, dizziness, and slurred speech.

Answer C is incorrect. Metronidazole is associated with a disulfiramlike reaction with alcohol.

Answer D is incorrect. Tetracycline is associated with tooth discoloration in children.

Answer E is incorrect. Vancomycin is associated with "red man" syndrome when given rapidly through an intravenous line.

12. **The correct answer is D.** Fibrates like gemfibrozil act at point D. They are ligands for the peroxisome proliferator-activated receptor-α (PPAR-α) protein, a receptor that regulates the

transcription of genes involved in lipid metabolism. Increased expression of the PPAR-α protein results in increased activity of lipoprotein lipase and thus increased clearance of triglyceride-rich lipoproteins.

Answer A is incorrect. Nothing acts at point A.

Answer B is incorrect. Resins act at point B by reducing the absorption of dietary cholesterol and cholesterol-containing bile acids.

Answer C is incorrect. 3-Hydroxy-3-methylglutaryl coenzyme A (HMG-CoA) reductase inhibitors act at point C by competitively inhibiting the synthesis of mevalonate by HMG-CoA reductase, an essential step in the production of cholesterol in the liver.

13. **The correct answer is E.** This patient has congestive heart failure. Decreased cardiac contractility results in a backup of the cardiac circuit, leading to pulmonary edema followed by peripheral edema. Digoxin and diuretics are often given to increase cardiac output and reduce edema, respectively. Diuretics cause a fluctuation in potassium levels. Potassium and digoxin compete for ATPase, leading to toxicity in hypokalemic states caused by thiazides, furosemide, and ethacrynic acid.

Answer A is incorrect. Acetylsalicylic acid (aspirin) and thiazides together do not constitute an effective therapy for congestive heart failure and do not result in a toxic interaction.

Answer B is incorrect. Acetylsalicylic acid (aspirin) and nitroprusside together do not constitute an effective therapy for congestive heart failure and do not result in a toxic interaction.

Answer C is incorrect. β-Blockers and thiazides may interact to produce an increased β-blocker effect, but the resulting effect is not toxic.

Answer D is incorrect. β-Blockers and spironolactone together do not cause a toxic interaction.

Answer F is incorrect. Digoxin and spironolactone result in reduced digoxin effectiveness due to hyperkalemic states caused by potassium-sparing diuretics, not toxicity.

14. **The correct answer is E.** Chronic atrial fibrillation is a risk factor for clot formation and systemic embolization. This man needs ongoing anticoagulation to prevent possible complications, such as cerebrovascular accidents or mesenteric infarction. Warfarin inhibits gamma-carboxylation of vitamin K–dependent clotting factors and is used for chronic anticoagulation. It is taken orally and has a long half-life. The degree of anticoagulation must be followed by measuring the International Normalized Ratio (INR).

Answer A is incorrect. Aspirin works by irreversibly inhibiting cyclooxygenase, thereby preventing the conversion of arachidonic acid to prostaglandins. The four effects of aspirin are antiplatelet (thereby inhibiting thrombus formation), antipyretic, analgesic, and anti-inflammatory. Aspirin is not used to prevent clot formation in the setting of atrial fibrillation, but rather to prevent myocardial infarction.

Answer B is incorrect. Protamine sulfate is used for rapid reversal of heparinization in the setting of overzealous anticoagulation.

Answer C is incorrect. Streptokinase is a thrombolytic used to break down existing clots. This could be used in the setting of a myocardial infarction. It would not be used prophylactically to prevent clot formation in atrial fibrillation.

Answer D is incorrect. Heparin is taken parenterally and is used for immediate, not long-term, anticoagulation. This patient was likely given heparin on admission to the hospital and was then converted to warfarin for chronic anticoagulation before his discharge.

15. **The correct answer is A.** Clearance is calculated as: (rate of drug elimination / plasma drug concentration) = (2 mg/min) / (50 mg/L) = 0.04 L/min.

Answer B is incorrect. Calculation error.

Answer C is incorrect. Calculation error.

Answer D is incorrect. Calculation error.

Answer E is incorrect. Calculation error.

16. The correct answer is E. Rifampin is an antibiotic used to treat tuberculosis. It works by suppressing RNA synthesis. One major adverse effect of rifampin is that it is metabolized by and induces the cytochrome P450 system; thus drugs such as oral contraceptives, warfarin, and ketoconazole may need to be given in higher concentrations in order to be therapeutic. This is probably the reason why this woman's oral contraceptive pills failed. Another well-known adverse effect that can be frightening to patients is that rifampin turns all bodily fluids (tears, sweat, urine) orange. Note that isoniazid, another drug that is used to treat tuberculosis, is also a P450 inhibitor, but the orange tears in this case clearly point to rifampin.

Answer A is incorrect. Chemotherapeutic agents used to treat breast cancer have a number of adverse effects, but are not associated with orange body fluids. Chronic pain often associated with cancer is a difficult entity to treat. Frequently, patients depend on nonsteroidal anti-inflammatory drugs (NSAIDs) to help control their pain. Chronic use of NSAIDs can cause epigastric distress and even ulcers. NSAIDs also decrease platelet aggregation ability and can cause bleeding problems, thus they should be discontinued before surgery.

Answer B is incorrect. Phenytoin is one of the drugs used to treat epilepsy, particularly tonic-clonic and partial seizures. It has many adverse effects, including induction of the P450 cytochrome system, and thus would interact with oral contraceptive pills. However, phenytoin does not cause red-orange body fluids. Some other adverse effects of phenytoin include gingival hyperplasia, megaloblastic anemia secondary to folate deficiency, and central nervous system depression. Phenytoin is also teratogenic and causes fetal hydantoin syndrome (prenatal growth deficiency, mental retardation, and congenital malformations).

Answer C is incorrect. *Giardia* infection is treated with metronidazole, an antibiotic effective against amoebae and anaerobes. One of metronidazole's famous adverse effects is a disulfiramlike reaction with ethanol. Metronidazole is also highly teratogenic and should not be given to pregnant women.

Answer D is incorrect. Amiodarone is an antiarrhythmic drug that has properties of both class I and class IV antiarrhythmics and is most often used to treat refractory atrial fibrillation and ventricular tachyarrhythmias. Amiodarone is infamous for its many adverse effects including interstitial pulmonary fibrosis, thyroid dysfunction (both hyper- and hypothyroidism), and hepatocellular necrosis. Thus, before starting amiodarone therapy, patients must have liver function tests, pulmonary function tests, and thyroid function tests. Amiodarone and other antiarrhythmic drugs do not cause orange bodily fluids.

17. The correct answer is F. The most important concept in this answer is that the loading dose is independent of renal or liver disease; the loading dose has more to do with volume of distribution, since excretion and metabolism have not yet occurred. The maintenance dose will be lower, since this patient has a history of renal disease and levofloxacin is excreted in the urine.

Answer A is incorrect. A higher loading dose is unnecessary and may lead to elevated drug levels, which can cause elongated QT intervals. A higher maintenance dose would also lead to elevated drug levels.

Answer B is incorrect. A higher loading dose is unnecessary and may lead to elevated drug levels, which can cause elongated QT intervals. Keeping the maintenance dose the same may also lead to elevated drug levels.

Answer C is incorrect. A lower loading dose would lead to subtherapeutic drug levels; however, adjusting for the compromised renal excretion and lowering the maintenance dose would be appropriate.

Answer D is incorrect. A lower loading dose would lead to subtherapeutic drug levels; keeping the maintenance dose the same may also lead to elevated drug levels.

Answer E is incorrect. Keeping the same loading dose is the correct choice; however, a higher maintenance dose would lead to elevated drug levels.

Answer G is incorrect. Keeping the same loading dose is the correct choice; however, keeping the maintenance dose the same may also lead to elevated drug levels.

18. **The correct answer is A.** The photomicrograph shows Kimmelstiel-Wilson nodules, which are pathognomonic for diabetic nephropathy. Angiotensin-converting enzyme (ACE) inhibitors are the drugs of choice in the control of diabetes-induced renal disease because they reduce systemic blood pressure, reduce the effects of angiotensin II (AT II) on efferent arterioles, and attenuate the stimulatory effect of AT II on glomerular cell growth and matrix production. ACE inhibitors have been conclusively shown to delay the time to end-stage renal disease by 50% in type 1 diabetics and to significantly delay progression of renal disease in type 2 diabetics. All diabetics should begin ACE inhibitor therapy at the onset of microalbuminuria, even in the absence of hypertension.

Answer B is incorrect. β-Blockers are used to control essential hypertension, not diabetic nephropathy.

Answer C is incorrect. Cyclophosphamide is often used in conjunction with prednisone to treat immunologically mediated kidney disease.

Answer D is incorrect. Gold therapy, used in the treatment of rheumatoid arthritis, is known to cause glomerular disease.

Answer E is incorrect. Prednisone is used in the treatment of immune-mediated nephropathy, not diabetic nephropathy.

19. **The correct answer is A.** Administration of bicarbonate will alkalinize the urine, thereby allowing the acidic toxin to be excreted and not reabsorbed. Alkalinization of the urine will lead to ionization of acids (such as salicylates) within the renal tubules. In general, charged molecules cannot be reabsorbed, while uncharged molecules are easily reabsorbed from the tubules. Thus, bicarbonate administration is indicated because it promotes "trapping" and hence excretion of salicylate molecules. Note that the concept can only be applied in reverse order to promote excretion of basic drugs: the goal is to acidify the urine so as to promote retention of the charged basic drug molecules within the urine.

Answer B is incorrect. Glucagon is used to treat β-blocker toxicity.

Answer C is incorrect. N-acetylcysteine is used to treat acetaminophen toxicity.

Answer D is incorrect. Protamine is used to treat heparin toxicity.

Answer E is incorrect. Vitamin K is used to treat warfarin toxicity.

20. **The correct answer is A.** Ipratropium bromide is a muscarinic antagonist used in both chronic obstructive pulmonary disease and asthma. It competitively blocks muscarinic receptors, preventing acetylcholine-mediated bronchoconstriction. It is administered directly to the airway and is minimally absorbed, leading to few adverse events. At high doses, atropine-like toxicity may occur. Tiotropium is a new and longer-acting muscarinic antagonist.

Answer B is incorrect. Cromolyn prevents the release of mediators such as leukotrienes and histamine from mast cells. It has no effect on bronchodilation and is used prophylactically to prevent asthma attacks.

Answer C is incorrect. Corticosteroids such as beclomethasone and prednisone inhibit the synthesis of cytokines. They inactivate NF-κB, which is the transcription factor that induces TNF-α production.

Answer D is incorrect. Methylxanthines such as theophylline are purine derivatives used in asthma. They inhibit phosphodiesterase, causing increased cAMP levels and leading to bronchodilation.

Answer E is incorrect. β agonists such as albuterol and salmeterol relax bronchial smooth muscle. They act on β-2-adrenergic receptors, stimulating adenylyl cyclase and causing increased cAMP levels.

21. **The correct answer is B.** Deferoxamine is a chelating agent specific for iron and will reduce effective blood iron levels.

    Answer A is incorrect. Aminocaproic acid is used in the treatment of tissue plasminogen activator or streptokinase overdose.

    Answer C is incorrect. Dimercaprol is used to treat poisoning by arsenic, mercury, and gold.

    Answer D is incorrect. Ethylenediaminetetraacetic acid is used to treat lead poisoning.

    Answer E is incorrect. Bicarbonate would be used to inactivate iron in the gastrointestinal tract.

22. **The correct answer is C.** Erythropoietin is a hormone that is produced in the kidney, and hence low levels are seen in the setting of kidney failure. Low levels of erythropoietin could cause anemia, which this patient is experiencing. Erythropoietin acts by increasing RBC proliferation and differentiation in the bone marrow. Lack of erythropoietin causes a microcytic anemia with iron sequestration in the bone marrow, as shown on the slide. Human recombinant erythropoietin (epoetin) is used in patients with severe anemias, which often occur in the setting of renal failure.

    Answer A is incorrect. Tacrolimus is an immunosuppressive agent used in organ transplant recipients. It does not cause microcytic anemia.

    Answer B is incorrect. Anti-Rh D immunoglobulin is administered to Rh-negative mothers with Rh-positive fetuses to prevent the development of erythroblastosis fetalis (fetal hydrops). It does not cause anemia and in fact prevents the development of the immune-mediated fetal anemia that can occur in the context of Rh-incompatibility.

    Answer D is incorrect. Patients with myelodysplastic syndrome typically present with a pancytopenia, not an isolated anemia, as

is seen in this case. Isolated anemia in the context of chronic renal failure is much more likely to be due to erythropoietin deficiency than to a concurrent myelodysplastic syndrome.

    Answer E is incorrect. Tissue plasminogen activator is a thrombolytic agent that produces fibrinolysis and is utilized in thromboembolic disease. It does not cause anemia.

23. **The correct answer is C.** A noncompetitive antagonist, or an irreversible antagonist, can bind to the active site of the receptor or to other sites on the receptor. However the binding occurs, it results in the same potency, but with a decreased maximum response, or efficacy, that cannot be overcome by the addition of more agonist.

    Answer A is incorrect. Curve A represents a dose-response curve with the same efficacy but increased potency. The addition of any antagonist would be unlikely to cause this response.

    Answer B is incorrect. Curve B represents a drug with a lower efficacy but a greater potency than drug X. This could occur with the addition of a partial agonist.

    Answer D is incorrect. Curve D represents a drug with a decreased potency but the same efficacy. This could occur with the addition of a competitive antagonist.

    Answer E is incorrect. Curve E represents a drug with a lower efficacy and potency. This could occur with the addition of a partial agonist.

24. **The correct answer is C.** Class IA antiarrhythmics, such as procainamide, affect both atrial and ventricular arrhythmias. They block sodium channels and thus slow conduction velocity in the atria, ventricles, and Purkinje fibers. This decreased conduction velocity slows phase 0 of the action potential (AP) and is manifested as an increased QRS duration on ECG. In addition to blocking sodium channels, Class IA antiarrhythmics also block potassium channels and thus increase the AP duration and ERP.

Answer A is incorrect. Encainide is a Class IC antiarrhythmic.

Answer B is incorrect. Mexiletine is a Class IB antiarrhythmic.

Answer D is incorrect. Class IC antiarrhythmics, such as propafenone, slow phase 0 of the action potential (AP), but have no effect on the AP duration. These antiarrhythmics have no affect on the ERP.

Answer E is incorrect. Class IB antiarrhythmics, such as tocainide, slow phase 0 of the action potential (AP), but decrease the AP duration. These antiarrhythmics affect ischemic or depolarized Purkinje and ventricular tissues. These antiarrhythmics have no affect on the ERP.

25. **The correct answer is E.** Erythromycin and other macrolides bind to the 50S subunit of ribosomes and prevent translocation of the tRNA.

Answer A is incorrect. Aminoglycosides and tetracycline act by binding to the ribosomal 30S subunit, thus preventing the binding of aminoacyl tRNA to the A site of the ribosome.

Answer B is incorrect. Aminoglycosides and tetracycline act by binding to the ribosomal 30S subunit, thus preventing the binding of aminoacyl tRNA to the A site of the ribosome.

Answer C is incorrect. Diphtheria toxin inhibits elongation factor 2.

Answer D is incorrect. Erythromycin does not inhibit eukaryotic initiation factor 2.

Organ Systems

CHAPTER 6

Cardiovascular

1. A physician decides to place a patient on a calcium channel blocker for treatment of her angina. Calcium channel blockers can relax the smooth muscle of blood vessels and can also have various effects on cardiac contractility, conduction, and heart rate. Which of the following calcium channel blockers would be most effective in reducing heart rate and contractility?

   (A) Dihydropyridine
   (B) Diltiazem
   (C) Nifedipine
   (D) Nimodipine
   (E) Verapamil

2. A 28-year-old African-American man presents to the physician with fever, weight loss, and abdominal pain. His blood pressure is 168/92 mm Hg, his pulse is 83/min, and his respiratory rate is 18/min. On physical examination, there is palpable purpura on his lower extremities; a funduscopic examination shows cotton-wool spots. His past medical history is significant for a previous hepatitis B infection. Laboratory values reveal an elevated erythrocyte sedimentation rate and positive perinuclear antineutrophil cytoplasmic autoantibodies. An arterial biopsy is shown in the image. Which of the following is the most prominent morphologic feature of the affected arteries in this patient's disease process?

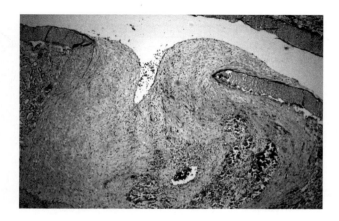

Image courtesy of PEIR Digital Library (http://peir.net).

   (A) Caseating necrosis
   (B) Eosinophilic infiltrate
   (C) Fibrinoid necrosis
   (D) Granulomatous inflammation
   (E) Langhans' giant cells

3. Epidemiologic evidence indicates that elevated serum cholesterol levels increase a patient's risk of developing coronary disease. The relative risk of coronary heart disease is eight times greater in an individual with a plasma cholesterol level of 300 mg/dL than it is in an individual with a level of only 150 mg/dL. In patients for whom pharmacologic treatment is indicated in addition to lifestyle changes, a variety of agents are available. In particular, the statins have been shown to significantly reduce overall mortality as well as serious cardiovascular events in these patients. Which of the following mechanisms describes the action of statins in reducing serum levels of LDL cholesterol?

   (A) Competitive inhibition of 3-hydroxy-3-methylglutaryl coenzyme A reductase
   (B) Inactivation of 3-hydroxy-3-methylglutaryl coenzyme A synthase
   (C) Negative feedback to decrease thiolase activity
   (D) Noncompetitive inhibition of citrate synthase
   (E) Positive feedback to increase 3-hydroxy-3-methylglutaryl coenzyme A lyase activity

4. A 45-year-old man who takes spironolactone and digoxin for his congestive heart failure is admitted to the hospital because he is experiencing an altered mental status. The ECG changes shown in the image are noted on testing. An analysis of urine electrolytes in this patient would most likely reveal which of the following?

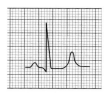

Reproduced, with permission, from USMLERx.com.

(A) High K^+, high Na^+, normal volume
(B) High K^+, low Na^+, low volume
(C) High K^+, low Na^+, normal volume
(D) Low K^+, high Na^+, normal volume
(E) Low K^+, low Na^+, normal volume

5. While many congenital cardiac defects can be discovered and monitored before birth, some present in a delayed fashion. Pediatric clinics see patients with an unknown cardiac history who present with early cyanosis, which is later found to exist in the context of a congenital heart defect. Which of the following is the most common cause of early cyanosis?

(A) Atrial septal defect
(B) Patent ductus arteriosus
(C) Tetralogy of Fallot
(D) Transposition of the great vessels
(E) Ventricular septal defect

6. The following image is a trace of a nodal action potential. The plateau (phase 2) is a result of which of the following actions?

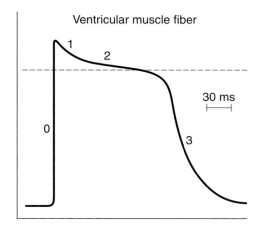

Reproduced, with permission, from USMLERx.com.

(A) Ligand-gated Ca^{2+} channels opening
(B) Ligand-gated Na^+ channels opening

(C) Voltage-gated Ca^{2+} channels opening
(D) Voltage-gated Na^+ channels closing
(E) Voltage-gated Na^+ channels opening

7. A 48-year-old man presents to the emergency department 1.5 hours after having severe substernal chest pain radiating to his left arm with diaphoresis and shortness of breath. His blood pressure is 165/94 mm Hg, pulse is 82/min, and respirations are 18/min. On further questioning, he states that he smokes two packs of cigarettes per day and that his brother died of a heart attack at the age of 45. Measurements using which of the following would be the best first indicator in determining if this patient is having a myocardial infarction?

(A) Aspartate aminotransferase
(B) Creatine kinase-myocardial bound
(C) ECG
(D) Lactate dehydrogenase
(E) Troponin I

8. This image depicts the administration of drug X, which produces an increase in systolic, diastolic, and mean arterial pressure. Drug Y is then added, resulting in little or no change to the blood pressure. Drug X is then readministered, causing a net decrease in blood pressure. Which of the following drug combinations are drug X and drug Y, respectively?

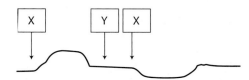

Reproduced, with permission, from USMLERx.com.

(A) Epinephrine, phentolamine
(B) Isoproterenol, clonidine
(C) Norepinephrine, propranolol
(D) Phenylephrine, metoprolol
(E) Phenylephrine, phentolamine

9. Viral myocarditis most often presents as biventricular heart failure in young people who do not have valvular, rheumatic, or congenital heart disease. It is characterized by diffuse myocardial degeneration and necrosis with an inflammatory infiltrate.

   (A) Coxsackievirus B
   (B) Hepatitis B
   (C) Polio
   (D) Rubella
   (E) Streptococcus

10. During periods of stress such as exercise, increased contractility, or pregnancy in women, there is an increase in oxygen demand on the heart. In response to an increase in oxygen demand, which of the following physiologic mechanisms will the heart employ?

    (A) Decreased coronary blood flow
    (B) Decreased metabolite production
    (C) Decreased oxygen extraction
    (D) Increased coronary blood flow
    (E) Increased oxygen extraction

11. A 16-year-old Asian girl presents to the physician with a history of fevers, joint pain, night sweats, and muscle pains. On physical examination, the patient is found to have extremely weak pulses in her upper extremities with normal pulses in her lower extremities. Laboratory studies reveal an elevated erythrocyte sedimentation rate. Which of the following is this individual most likely suffering from?

    (A) Buerger's disease
    (B) Giant cell arteritis
    (C) Polyarteritis nodosa
    (D) Takayasu's arteritis
    (E) Wegener's granulomatosis

12. A 72-year-old African-American man who had a bilateral hip replacement 7 days ago is experiencing chest pain, tachycardia, tachypnea, dyspnea, and a low-grade fever. The man codes, and efforts to resuscitate him are unsuccessful. The gross specimen of his lung shown in this image is from the autopsy. Which of the following most likely predisposed this patient to this event?

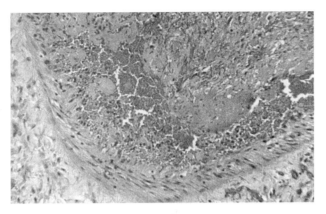

Image courtesy of PEIR Digital Library (http://peir.net).

   (A) Factor VIII deficiency
   (B) Hypocoagulability
   (C) Intact endothelial surface
   (D) Thrombocytopenia
   (E) Venous stasis

13. A 70-year-old woman with a history of type 2 diabetes mellitus, a body mass index of 30 kg/m^2, and a myocardial infarction (MI) 10 years prior presents to the emergency department with crushing substernal chest pain radiating to her neck and jaw. Emergency cardiac catheterization with percutaneous coronary intervention (PCI) shows a 99% occlusion of her left anterior descending artery, and an ECG reveals an anterior wall ST-segment elevation MI. The patient remains stable after PCI, and echocardiography shows a mildly impaired ejection fraction (EF) of 45%. Three days later, the patient becomes acutely hypotensive and dyspneic, and physical examination reveals a high-pitched holosystolic murmur, loudest at the apex and radiating to the axilla, that had not been heard on previous exams. An emergency echocardiogram shows an EF of 25%. This patient has developed which of the following?

   (A) Aortic stenosis
   (B) Dressler's syndrome
   (C) Ruptured interventricular septum
   (D) Ruptured left ventricular free wall
   (E) Ruptured papillary muscle
   (F) Ventricular aneurysm

14. A 67-year-old woman presents to the emergency department with symptoms of dizziness, syncope, and palpitations. Her past medical history is significant for supraventricular arrhythmias and congestive heart failure. An ECG is taken and the result is shown. Which of this patient's current medications might have caused this abnormal ECG pattern?

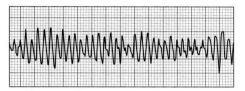

Reproduced, with permission, from USMLERx.com.

(A) Adenosine
(B) Bretylium
(C) Propranolol
(D) Quinidine
(E) Verapamil

15. A 42-year-old man with a known bicuspid aortic valve presents to his primary care physician for his annual checkup. His blood pressure is 142/78 mm Hg, his pulse is 78/min, and his respiratory rate is 18/min. His physical examination is remarkable for a weak peripheral pulse that is slow and prolonged and a crescendo-decrescendo systolic ejection murmur over his right second intercostal space that radiates to his carotid arteries. This patient's murmur is most likely caused by which of the following?

(A) Aortic regurgitation
(B) Aortic stenosis
(C) Mitral regurgitation
(D) Mitral stenosis
(E) Mitral valve prolapse

16. A 25-year-old pregnant woman goes to her gynecologist for her 36-week checkup. She complains of light-headedness when she goes to bed at night. In the office, her blood pressure is 120/70 mm Hg while sitting upright and 90/50 mm Hg while lying supine. Which of the following is the most likely cause of this hypotension?

(A) Cardiogenic shock
(B) Inferior vena cava compression
(C) Neurogenic shock
(D) Third spacing of fluid
(E) Vasodilation

17. A 48-year-old obese man presents to his primary care physician with complaints of lower leg pain that occurs after he walks a few city blocks and is relieved with rest. He has no other complaints. His blood pressure is 165/85 mm Hg, his pulse is 83/min, and his respirations are 18/min. After further questioning, he admits to smoking two packs of cigarettes per day. Which of the following types of vessels is most likely involved in the pathologic process surrounding this patient's symptoms?

(A) Arteries
(B) Arterioles
(C) Capillaries
(D) Veins
(E) Venules

18. Jugular venous pressure (JVP) curves are designed to show the pressure changes that normally take place in the right atrium throughout the cardiac cycle. A JVP curve consists of two, or sometimes three, positive waves and two negative troughs. A normal JVP curve is shown. Which of the following points on the normal jugular venous tracing below would be most prominently affected in tricuspid regurgitation?

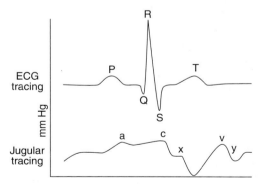

Reproduced, with permission, from USMLERx.com.

(A) A and C
(B) A and Y
(C) C and X
(D) V and Y

19. A 62-year-old breast cancer survivor visits her physician because of weakness, fatigue, and weight gain. The physician also elicits complaints about abdominal discomfort and exertional dyspnea. Physical examination reveals jugular venous distention that fails to subside on inspiration. A CT scan and an MRI show a normal-sized heart with no apparent hypertrophy of the ventricular walls. Which of the following is the most likely diagnosis of this patient?

(A) Cardiac tamponade
(B) Congestive heart failure
(C) Constrictive pericarditis
(D) Recurrence of breast cancer
(E) Restrictive cardiomyopathy

20. The most common location for an abdominal aortic aneurysm is inferior to the renal arteries and extending to the bifurcation of the common iliac arteries. Repair involves resecting the diseased portion of the aorta and replacing it with a synthetic graft. Which of the following arteries would likely be sacrificed during the repair of an infrarenal abdominal aortic aneurysm?

(A) Gastroduodenal artery
(B) Hepatic artery
(C) Inferior mesenteric artery
(D) Left gastric artery
(E) Splenic artery
(F) Superior mesenteric artery

21. A 52-year-old African-American man is brought to the emergency department unresponsive, and efforts to resuscitate him are unsuccessful. On autopsy, it is found that he suffered from a ruptured aneurysm of the aortic root. His dilated aorta, as seen on autopsy, is shown here. In addition, inspection of the man's skin revealed several ulcerated lesions. Which of the following is most likely associated with the underlying etiology of this patient's aneurysm?

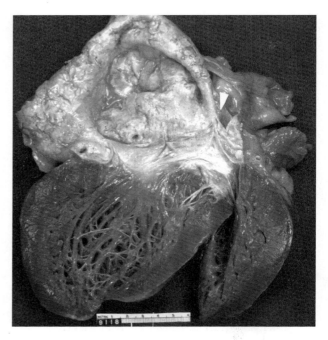

Image courtesy of PEIR Digital Library (http://peir.net).

(A) Atherosclerosis
(B) Congenital medial weakness
(C) Cystic medial necrosis
(D) Disruption of the vasa vasorum
(E) Hypertension

22. A baby was observed at birth to be noncyanotic. The mother was known to have been infected with rubella during the pregnancy. On examination, the patient is found to have a continuous murmur that is present in both systole and diastole. The patient also seems to have some digital cyanosis. A nonsteroidal anti-inflammatory drug was prescribed, and on follow-up, the murmur was found to have disappeared. Which of the following is the most likely congenital lesion?

(A) Patent ductus arteriosus
(B) Tetralogy of Fallot
(C) Transposition of the great vessels
(D) Truncus arteriosus
(E) Ventricular septal defect

23. A 25-year-old white woman with no past medical history presents to the emergency department for "a racing heartbeat." It is determined that she has paroxysmal supraventricular tachycardia. Which of the following is the drug of choice used for diagnosing and abolishing atrioventricular nodal arrhythmias by virtue of its effectiveness and its low toxicity?

    (A) Adenosine
    (B) Bretylium
    (C) Encainide
    (D) Lidocaine
    (E) Sotalol

24. As a sympathomimetic, norepinephrine exerts multiple actions. For a patient who is in septic shock, norepinephrine can be given intravenously. Which of the following is the main function of this adrenergic agonist in this clinical scenario?

    (A) Bradycardia
    (B) Bronchoconstriction
    (C) Decreased inotropy
    (D) Vasoconstriction
    (E) Vasodilation

25. An 85-year-old man dies from aspiration pneumonia as a complication of Alzheimer's disease. Autopsy reveals a small (230-g) heart that appears grossly dark brown in color. Hematoxylin and eosin staining of cardiac muscle cells reveals brownish perinuclear pigmentation. The pathologist determines this phenomenon to be a consequence of age and not a causative agent in the patient's death. Accumulation of which of the following substances is the most likely cause of the brown pigmentation seen most often in the heart, liver, or spleen of the elderly?

    (A) Bilirubin
    (B) Calcium
    (C) Cholesterol
    (D) Glycogen
    (E) Iron
    (F) Lipofuscin

26. A 72-year-old woman presents to the emergency department with sudden onset of vision loss in her left eye. She says that she has recently been having left-sided jaw pain when chewing food. Laboratory studies reveal an elevated erythrocyte sedimentation rate. A high-power view of her arterial biopsy is shown in the image. Which of the following is the most frequently involved artery in this disease process?

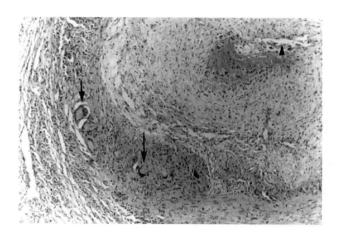

Reproduced, with permission, from Dean RH, Yao JST, Brewster DC, eds. *Current Diagnosis & Treatment in Vascular Surgery.* Originally published by Appleton & Lange. Copyright © 1995 by The McGraw-Hill Companies, Inc.

    (A) Carotid artery
    (B) Middle cerebral artery
    (C) Ophthalmic artery
    (D) Subclavian artery
    (E) Temporal artery

27. A 56-year-old obese man comes to the emergency department because of crushing chest pain that has been present for 3 hours. The pain radiates to his left arm and neck. He also complains of nausea. On physical examination, the patient is found to be sweating and his blood pressure is 164/122 mm Hg. Laboratory analysis reveals that his cardiac enzyme levels are elevated. His ECG is abnormal with an ST-segment depression. Which of the following is the pathophysiology underlying the correct diagnosis?

    (A) Complete occlusion of the coronary arteries by a mural thrombus
    (B) Coronary artery vasospasm caused by cigarettes and cocaine
    (C) Increased cardiac demand with coronary arteries that are > 75% occluded
    (D) Ischemic necrosis of 30% of the ventricle wall
    (E) Ischemic necrosis of 70% of the ventricle wall

28. A 75-year-old woman arrives at the emergency department and states that her left arm is numb. She is diaphoretic. Laboratory studies show an elevated troponin I level. An echocardiogram indicates an abnormality of the anterior interventricular septum. Stenosis of which of the following arteries would most likely cause this condition?

    (A) Acute marginal artery
    (B) Circumflex artery
    (C) Left anterior descending artery
    (D) Posterior descending artery
    (E) Right coronary artery

29. A 24-year-old man presents to the emergency department with a fever, chills, night sweats, malaise, and fatigue that started 3 days ago. In the past day he has also become short of breath. He admits to using intravenous drugs regularly. At presentation, the patient is shaking and appears pale. Physical examination is remarkable for a temperature of 39.4° C (103° F), hypoxia to 88% on room air, jugular venous distention, bilaterally decreased breath sounds at the bases with dullness to percussion at the bases, and a grade III/VI systolic murmur heard best at the lower left sternal border. The patient states that he never had anything wrong with his heart before. Which pathogen is most likely responsible for this patient's condition?

    (A) *Enterococcus faecalis*
    (B) *Haemophilus aphrophilus*
    (C) *Staphylococcus aureus*
    (D) *Streptococcus bovis*
    (E) Viridans streptococci

30. Drugs such as cholestyramine and colestipol have been shown to decrease circulating serum LDL cholesterol and to slightly elevate triglycerides. These drugs work by which of the following mechanisms?

    (A) Binding and excreting of bile-soluble lipids
    (B) Decreasing peripheral lipolysis
    (C) Increasing lipoprotein lipase activity
    (D) Inhibiting cholesterol absorption at the small intestine brush border
    (E) Inhibiting of the rate-limiting enzyme of cholesterol formation
    (F) Sequestering bile acid resins in hepatocytes

31. A 30-year-old patient comes to an ophthalmologist with complaints of decreased vision. On examination, angiomatous lesions are visible in the retina. The patient also has documented cerebellar and spinal hemangioblastomas, bilateral renal cysts, and pancreatic microcystic adenomas. A previous chromosomal analysis on this patient showed a deleted tumor suppressor gene. A detailed family history shows similar problems in the patient's brother, father, aunt, and grandfather. Which of the following is the inheritance pattern of this patient's disease?

    (A) Autosomal dominant
    (B) Autosomal recessive
    (C) Mitochondrial
    (D) Spontaneous
    (E) X-linked recessive

32. A 23-year-old white woman is brought to the emergency department after she is involved in a motor vehicle crash. Her blood pressure is 92/45 mm Hg, her pulse is 128/min, and her respiratory rate is 28/min. On physical examination, she is found to have bilateral femur fractures. Which of the following types of emboli are most likely to develop in this patient?

(A) Air emboli
(B) Amniotic fluid emboli
(C) Bacteria emboli
(D) Fat emboli
(E) Thrombus emboli

33. A 57-year-old white man presents to his primary care physician with dyspnea after attempting to mow his lawn. He says that he likes to maintain his yard and garden himself, but recently he has had increasing trouble doing the work, and even gets short of breath walking up the one flight of stairs in his house. On further questioning, he says that sometimes he wakes up short of breath in the middle of the night. Physical examination demonstrates ankle edema. Which of the following findings would also be expected in this patient?

(A) Decreased sympathetic outflow
(B) Decreased venous pressure
(C) Increased aldosterone secretion
(D) Increased effective arterial blood volume
(E) Increased glomerular filtration rate

34. A number of tests are used to diagnose a myocardial infarction. Measuring an elevation in the cardiac enzymes aspartate aminotransferase (AST), creatine kinase-MB fraction (CK-MB), lactate dehydrogenase (LDH), and troponin is one indication that a myocardial infarction (MI) has occurred. The diagram shown is a representation of the average length of time it takes to see an elevation in these four enzymes [labeled (1) through (4)]. What is the correct order of cardiac enzyme elevation after an MI?

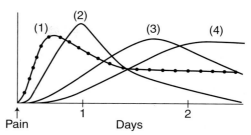

Reproduced, with permission, from USMLERx.com.

(A) AST, CK-MB, troponin, LDH
(B) AST, LDH, troponin, CK-MB
(C) CK-MB, AST, troponin, LDH
(D) CK-MB, troponin, AST, LDH
(E) LDH, CK-MB, troponin, AST
(F) LDH, troponin, CK-MB, AST
(G) Troponin, CK-MB, AST, LDH

35. A 73-year-old man with a history of hypertension and type 2 diabetes mellitus presents with the sudden onset of right-sided paralysis. An ultrasound study shows significant atherosclerosis in a major artery that is embryologically derived from one of the aortic arches. The artery that is most likely involved in this patient's paralysis is derived from which of the following aortic arches?

(A) First aortic arch
(B) Second aortic arch
(C) Third aortic arch
(D) Fourth aortic arch
(E) Sixth aortic arch

36. A 76-year-old female visits her physician with complaints of increased fatigue. She states that she tires easily even with very low levels of activity. The woman has a history of coronary artery disease and diabetes. On physical examination, her doctor notices a disappearing arterial pulse on inspiration. The doctor orders an echocardiogram to confirm the diagnosis. What invasive procedure will be necessary to treat this patient?

(A) Angioplasty
(B) Aortic valve replacement
(C) Mitral valve replacement
(D) Pericardiocentesis
(E) Surgical reduction of an aortic aneurysm

37. A 60-year-old woman dies in a car accident. On autopsy, the cause of death is determined to be a massive brain hemorrhage due to a skull fracture. An additional abnormality, shown below in the image of the opened left atrium, is also found and determined to be unrelated to the cause of death. This abnormality could have led to which of the following physical examination findings when the woman was alive?

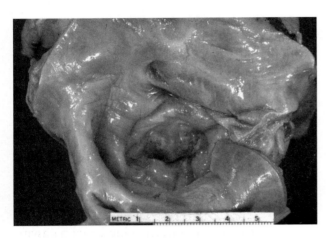

Image courtesy of PEIR Digital Library (http://peir.net).

(A) Continuous murmur throughout both diastole and systole, loudest at the end of ventricular systole
(B) Decrescendo murmur in early ventricular diastole
(C) Sharp, high-pitched sound in early ventricular diastole, followed by a decrescendo, crescendo murmur
(D) Sharp, high-pitched sound in early ventricular systole, followed by a crescendo, decrescendo murmur
(E) Sharp, high-pitched sound in mid ventricular systole, followed by a uniform murmur

38. A 3-year-old boy comes to the pediatrician with fever, conjunctivitis, erythema in the oral mucosa, and cervical lymphadenopathy. The boy suddenly becomes hypotensive and goes into cardiac arrest and dies shortly thereafter. Autopsy shows aneurysmal dilations of the left circumflex and right coronary arteries. The boy's disease is characterized as a self-limiting disease that most commonly affects the coronary arteries. Which of the following diseases is the correct diagnosis?

(A) Buerger's disease
(B) Kawasaki's disease
(C) Polyarteritis nodosa
(D) Takayasu's arteritis
(E) Wegener's granulomatosis

39. A 54-year-old woman comes to the physician 3 months after a undergoing a root canal because of persistent general malaise and fever. The symptoms came on slowly over the weeks following her root canal, but have not let up since they started. On physical examination, the patient is found to have a temperature of 38.3° C (101° F). Ophthalmic examination reveals retinal hemorrhages with clear central regions. Examination of the extremities reveals painful red nodules on her digits and dark macules on her palms and soles. On cardiac examination, a click and a systolic murmur are easily auscultated over the mitral valve. She tells the physician that the click is due to a mechanical valve replacement done 4 years ago due to rheumatic fever as a child. Given this history, which of the following is the most appropriate treatment for this patient?

(A) Caspofungin
(B) Clindamycin
(C) Mebendazole
(D) Metronidazole
(E) Nafcillin
(F) Penicillin
(G) Pentamidine

40. A 67-year-old woman who has recently begun to take a new antihypertensive medication presents to her primary care physician with complaints of new-onset fatigue and depressed mood. Her physical examination is unremarkable except for a blood pressure of 120/82 mm Hg. Her laboratory studies show the following results:

Na^+: 137 mEq/L
K^+: 4.1 mEq/L
Blood urea nitrogen: 12 mg/dL
Creatinine: 0.5 mg/dL
Glucose: 82 mg/dL

Which of the following is most likely the new medication that this patient has started?

(A) Enalapril
(B) Furosemide
(C) Hydrochlorothiazide
(D) Losartan
(E) Metoprolol
(F) Nifedipine
(G) Prazosin

41. A dysfunctional myocardial endothelium underlies one common form of heart disease. In patients experiencing symptoms of this type of heart disease, there is a paradoxical lack of coronary artery vasodilation needed to provide increased blood flow in states of increased physical exertion or emotional stress. What is the predominant sign or symptom associated with this condition?

(A) Arrhythmia
(B) Bradycardia
(C) Hypertension
(D) Tachycardia
(E) Transient chest pain

42. The image below depicts the relationship of ventricular pressure and volume in the cardiac cycle. The various phases of the cardiac cycle are labeled I through IV. Which of the following phases occurs between aortic valve closing and mitral valve opening?

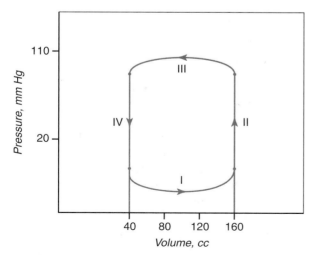

Reproduced, with permission, from USMLERx.com.

(A) Atrial contraction
(B) Isovolumetric contraction
(C) Isovolumetric relaxation
(D) Ventricular ejection
(E) Ventricular filling

43. A 32-year-old man with diabetes presents to his physician with orthostatic hypotension. This suggests a deficiency in the normal physiologic response carried out by arterial baroreceptors located in the aortic arch and the carotid sinus. What is the normal physiological response to hypotension?

(A) Decreased baroreceptor afferent firing in the aortic arch leads to increased sympathetic efferents
(B) Decreased baroreceptor afferent firing in the carotid sinus leads to increased parasympathetic efferents
(C) Decreased baroreceptor afferent firing in the carotid sinus leads to increased sympathetic efferents
(D) Increased baroreceptor afferent firing in the aortic arch leads to increased parasympathetic efferents
(E) Increased baroreceptor afferent firing in the carotid sinus leads to increased parasympathetic efferents

44. A 56-year-old woman presents to her physician 6 weeks after suffering a myocardial infarction because of the recent onset of chest pain and dyspnea. Her physical examination is remarkable for a friction rub over the fifth intercostal space in the midclavicular line together with an elevated jugular venous pressure. Which of the following myocardial complications is this individual most likely suffering from?

(A) Cardiac arrhythmia
(B) Dressler's syndrome
(C) Left ventricular failure
(D) Thromboembolism
(E) Ventricular rupture

45. A patient presents for treatment of his severe essential hypertension. He is being treated with numerous medications for high blood pressure, and hydralazine was recently added to his medication regimen. He explains that he has been experiencing unpleasant symptoms since his last visit, when hydralazine therapy was started. Which of the following is an adverse effect of hydralazine?

(A) Angina
(B) Cyanide toxicity
(C) First-dose orthostatic hypotension
(D) Hypertrichosis
(E) Positive Coombs' test

46. A 76-year-old man receives a pacemaker to treat a dangerous form of heart block. This form of heart block is characterized by a constant PR interval with randomly dropped QRS complexes. The patient's ECG prior to treatment is shown here. Which of the following is the abnormality responsible for this type of heart block?

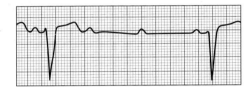

Reproduced, with permission, from USMLERx.com.

(A) Atrioventricular nodal abnormality
(B) Defect in the His-Purkinje system
(C) Independently contracting atria and ventricles
(D) Retrograde conduction
(E) Sinoatrial nodal abnormality

47. A 56-year-old white man is rushed to the emergency department with crushing substernal chest pain. He is morbidly obese, sweating profusely, breathing very rapidly, and clutching at his chest. The patient is stabilized and seems to be doing well when he suddenly goes into cardiac arrest and dies. Which of the following is the most likely cause of death in this patient?

(A) Fatal arrhythmia
(B) Mural thrombosis
(C) Myocardial failure

(D) Myocardial rupture
(E) Ruptured papillary muscle

48. A previously healthy 31-year-old woman is readmitted to the hospital 12 weeks after recovering from severe bacteremia with sudden and complete visual loss in her right eye. She says that she has been feeling feverish for the past couple of weeks. Ophthalmologic examination reveals a gray-white retina with an associated cherry-red spot, two blot hemorrhages, and several segmented vessels with optic edema. Physical examination reveals a new murmur consistent with mitral valve insufficiency. This patient is diagnosed with combined occlusion of the central retinal artery and vein of the right eye. Which of the following is the most likely cause of this patient's central retinal artery occlusion?

(A) Collagen vascular disease
(B) Diabetes mellitus
(C) Endocarditis
(D) Hypertensive crisis
(E) Thromboembolic disease

49. Cardiac output is a function of stroke volume and heart rate. Stroke volume increases when contractility increases, preload increases, or afterload decreases. There are a number of factors that affect each of these components and ultimately cardiac output. Which of the following variations would increase cardiac output?

(A) Aortic stenosis
(B) β-Blocker treatment
(C) Cardiac glycoside treatment
(D) Decreased intracellular calcium concentration
(E) Increased extracellular sodium concentration

50. A 54-year-old woman presents to her physician with swelling in her extremities that pits upon touch. Which of the following conditions is a common cause of this physical finding?

(A) Decreased capillary permeability
(B) Decreased capillary pressure
(C) Increased interstitial fluid colloid osmotic pressure
(D) Increased interstitial fluid pressure
(E) Increased plasma protein levels

1. **The correct answer is E.** The calcium channel blockers verapamil and diltiazem are both effective is slowing the rate and contractility of the heart. Both drugs act via calcium channel blocking of the calcium-dependent conduction in the atrioventricular node. However, verapamil is the more effective agent and is therefore the correct answer.

Answer A is incorrect. Dihydropyridines are the family of drugs to which nifedipine belongs.

Answer B is incorrect. Diltiazem is a calcium channel blocker but is not as effective as verapamil in reducing the rate and contractility of the heart.

Answer C is incorrect. Nifedipine is least effective in reducing the rate and contractility of the heart; conversely, it is most effective in evoking vasodilation.

Answer D is incorrect. Nimodipine is another member of the dihydropyridine family with similar properties, but it is approved only for the management of stroke with subarachnoid hemorrhage.

2. **The correct answer is C.** This individual is likely suffering from polyarteritis nodosa (PAN), which is characterized by necrotizing immune complex inflammation of small or medium-sized arteries. PAN is typically associated with fever, malaise, weight loss, abdominal pain, headache, myalgias, and hypertension. It is also associated with an elevated erythrocyte sedimentation rate, positive perinuclear antineutrophil cytoplasmic autoantibodies, and, in 30% of cases, hepatitis B. Histologically, the intense inflammatory infiltrate in the arterial wall and surrounding connective tissue is associated with fibrinoid necrosis and disruption of the vessel wall.

Answer A is incorrect. Caseating necrosis is associated with tuberculosis infections.

Answer B is incorrect. Eosinophilic infiltrate is a more prominent feature in Churg-Strauss syndrome.

Answer D is incorrect. Granulomatous infiltrate is a more prominent feature in giant cell arteritis.

Answer E is incorrect. Langhans' giant cells are associated with Wegener's granulomatosis.

3. **The correct answer is A.** 3-Hydroxy-3-methylglutaryl coenzyme A reductase (HMGR) is the rate-limiting step in the synthesis of cholesterol. The enzyme converts 3-hydroxy-3-methylglutaryl coenzyme A (HMG-CoA) to mevalonic acid, a cholesterol precursor. Statins competitively inhibit HMGR by obstructing part of the enzyme's active site and preventing sufficient interaction with HMG-CoA to produce mevalonate.

Answer B is incorrect. 3-Hydroxy-3-methylglutaryl coenzyme A (HMG-CoA) synthase is the enzyme that combines acetoacetyl-coenzyme A with acetyl-coenzyme A to form HMG-CoA. It represents a preliminary step in cholesterol synthesis and is not the site of action of the statins.

Answer C is incorrect. Thiolase is another enzyme in the cholesterol synthesis pathway. It is responsible for combining two molecules of acetyl-coenzyme A to form acetoacetyl-coenzyme A. Statins do not affect thiolase activity.

Answer D is incorrect. Citrate synthase is the first enzyme of the Krebs cycle, which combines oxaloacetate with incoming acetyl-coenzyme A to form citrate. It is not involved in cholesterol synthesis and is not affected by statins.

Answer E is incorrect. 3-Hydroxy-3-methylglutaryl coenzyme A (HMG-CoA) lyase is the enzyme that cleaves HMG-CoA into acetoacetate and acetyl-coenzyme A. It proceeds in the reverse order from cholesterol synthesis and is not affected by statins.

4. **The correct answer is D.** The ECG shows peak T waves and widened QRS interval, which are classic changes seen in hyperkalemia. Spironolactone is the most likely medication to affect urinary electrolytes. As an inhibitor of aldosterone receptors in the collecting tubule and an inhibitor of Na^+ channels, spironolactone greatly decreases the excretion of K^+ and mildly increases the excretion of Na^+. Urine volume will be high-normal because the diuretic will increase salt-water wasting.

Answer A is incorrect. Spironolactone decreases K^+ excretion, so there will be decreased levels of K+ in the urine sample.

Answer B is incorrect. Na^+ excretion will be increased with the use of spironolactone; also, diuretics will increase the amount of urine volume excreted.

Answer C is incorrect. Spironolactone will increase Na^+ excretion and decrease K^+ excretion so that K^+ concentrations will be decreased in the urine and Na^+ concentrations will be increased.

Answer E is incorrect. Spironolactone decreases K^+ excretion but increases Na^+ excretion; therefore, Na^+ concentrations will be elevated in the urine.

5. **The correct answer is C.** Tetralogy of Fallot is the most common cause of early cyanosis in infants. The skin becomes bluish because of the malformed right-to-left shunt. The four components of the teratology are (1) ventricular septal defect, (2) overriding aorta, (3) infundibular pulmonary stenosis, and (4) right ventricular hypertrophy.

Answer A is incorrect. Atrial septal defects typically are not clinically apparent until adulthood, when a patient experiences a reversal of blood flow caused by pulmonary hypertension.

Answer B is incorrect. Patent ductus arteriosus typically is not clinically apparent until adulthood, when a patient experiences a rever-

sal of blood flow caused by pulmonary hypertension.

Answer D is incorrect. Transposition of the great vessels is a condition that leads to early cyanosis, but it is not as common as tetralogy of Fallot.

Answer E is incorrect. Ventricular septal defects are the most common cardiac congenital defects, but they do not present with early cyanosis.

6. **The correct answer is C.** Voltage-gated Ca^{2+} channels open slowly in response to the Na^+ upstroke as increasing K^+ conductance during phase 2 gradually depolarizes the cell. The result is a slow conduction velocity that prolongs the transmission from the atria to the ventricles.

Answer A is incorrect. Ion channels in the myocardium are voltage-gated.

Answer B is incorrect. Ion channels in the myocardium are voltage-gated.

Answer D is incorrect. Closing voltage-gated Na^+ channels would hyperpolarize the cell.

Answer E is incorrect. Nodal cells lack the voltage-gated Na^+ channels that are responsible for the upstroke in ventricular cells.

7. **The correct answer is C.** ECG is the gold standard for diagnosing a myocardial infarction within the first 6 hours of the onset of symptoms. ECG changes will include ST-segment elevation (signifying transmural infarct), ST-segment depression (signifying subendocardial infarct), and Q waves (signifying transmural infarct).

Answer A is incorrect. Aspartate aminotransferase is a nonspecific protein that is found in cardiac, liver, and skeletal muscle cells. Levels peak around 2 days post–myocardial infarction (MI) and are negative at 3 days post-MI.

Answer B is incorrect. Creatine kinase-myocardial bound (CK-MB) is the test of choice within the first 24 hours post–myocardial infarction (MI). CK-MB levels peak around 24 hours and are negative at 3 days post-MI.

Answer D is incorrect. Lactate dehydrogenase was once the test of the choice for diagnosing a myocardial infarction (MI); it is elevated from 2–7 days post-MI. Levels peak around 3 days post-MI.

Answer E is incorrect. Troponin I is used within the first 4 hours and for up to 7–10 days post–myocardial infarction (MI). It is more specific than any other protein markers. Troponin I peaks around 24 hours and stays positive for up to 7–10 days post-MI.

8. **The correct answer is A.** Epinephrine is a nonselective agonist at the α- and β-adrenergic receptors. Administering a large dose of epinephrine causes an increase in blood pressure via an increased heart rate and contraction through stimulation of α_1 receptors (the β_2 effect is minimal) and increased systemic vascular resistance through α_1-mediated vasoconstriction. Adding phentolamine blocks the α effects of epinephrine so readministration leaves only the β_1-receptor actions (increased contractility and heart rate) and the β_2-mediated increase in vasodilation, causing a net decrease in blood pressure.

Answer B is incorrect. Isoproterenol is an agonist at the α- and β-adrenergic receptors, although its primary action is at the β receptor. Hence, adding isoproterenol would actually cause a decrease in pressure through β_2-mediated vasodilation. Clonidine is an α agonist at the α_2 receptor leading to decreased sympathetic outflow and possibly causing an additional decrease in pressure. Adding isoproterenol would lead to a further decrease in pressure.

Answer C is incorrect. Norepinephrine is an agonist at the α- and β-adrenergic receptors. It has a more potent β effect than α effect, leading to an increase in vasoconstriction through α_1 stimulation. Propranolol is an α blocker, which would not block the effects of norepinephrine; readministration would cause an increase in pressure.

Answer D is incorrect. Phenylephrine is an α agonist that would cause an increase in pres-

sure through α_1-stimulated vasoconstriction. Metoprolol is a β-blocker, which would not inhibit the effects of phenylephrine. Therefore, readministration of phenylephrine would cause another increase in pressure.

Answer E is incorrect. Phenylephrine is an α agonist, which would result in an increase in pressure through α_1-stimulated vasoconstriction. Phentolamine is a nonselective β-blocker, which would block the increase in pressure caused by phenylephrine and cause no change in pressure.

9. **The correct answer is A.** Coxsackievirus B is the most common cause of viral myocarditis in the United States. It is a member of the Enterovirus group of the Picornaviridae family.

Answer B is incorrect. Hepatitis B is not a frequent cause of viral myocarditis. It has both acute and chronic manifestations that include symptoms such as fever, malaise, headache, anorexia, vomiting, dark urine, and jaundice.

Answer C is incorrect. Poliovirus is not a frequent cause of viral myocarditis. Its infections are mostly asymptomatic; however, poliomyelitis results from viral damage to anterior horn motor neurons.

Answer D is incorrect. Rubella can cross the placenta and is teratogenic. It can cause congenital rubella, leading to patent ductus arteriosus, pulmonary stenosis, cataracts, microcephaly, and deafness.

Answer E is incorrect. Streptococcal infections can lead to rheumatic fever, an immunologic disorder in which antibodies to streptococcal antigens autoreact with human antigens in the heart and other tissues.

10. **The correct answer is D.** The heart has no minimal extraction reserve, which means that it always extracts oxygen at the optimum level. Therefore, the only way to increase oxygen delivery to the heart is to increase coronary blood flow.

Answer A is incorrect. The heart will not decrease coronary blood flow in response to increased oxygen demand. Coronary blood flow will increase.

Answer B is incorrect. The metabolite adenosine is one of the major determinants of coronary blood flow. In response to increased oxygen demand, adenosine production will increase.

Answer C is incorrect. The heart has no minimal extraction reserve; therefore, it does not have the ability to increase or decrease its oxygen extraction.

Answer E is incorrect. The heart has no minimal extraction reserve; therefore, it does not have the ability to increase or decrease its oxygen extraction.

11. **The correct answer is D.** This individual is most likely suffering from Takayasu's arteritis, which is also known as the pulseless disease. It typically affects medium- and large-sized arteries, resulting in thickening of the aortic arch and/or proximal great vessels. Symptoms include fevers, arthritis, night sweats, myalgias, skin nodules, ocular disturbances, and weak pulses in the upper extremities. It is more common in young Asian females and is associated with an elevated erythrocyte sedimentation rate.

Answer A is incorrect. Buerger's disease is associated with smoking and leads to intermittent claudication, cold sensitivity, and, in severe cases, gangrene.

Answer B is incorrect. Giant cell arteritis is also associated with an elevated erythrocyte sedimentation rate, but symptoms include jaw claudication and impaired vision. It typically affects older patients.

Answer C is incorrect. Polyarteritis nodosa is also associated with fevers and myalgias, but typically affects young males. It has an association with hepatitis B infection and perinuclear antineutrophil cytoplasmic autoantibodies.

Answer E is incorrect. Wegener's granulomatosis is associated with pulmonary and renal disease as well as with a focal necrotizing vas-

culitis. It is associated with circulating antineutrophil cytoplasmic autoantibodies.

12. **The correct answer is E.** This patient most likely suffered from a pulmonary embolism (PE). PEs are most often the result of a thromboembolism originating from a deep venous thrombosis (DVT). Individuals are predisposed to DVTs by Virchow's triad: venous stasis, hypercoagulability, and endothelial damage. Postoperative patients are at increased risk for developing DVTs due to immobilization for long periods of time.

Answer A is incorrect. Factor VIII deficiency (hemophilia A) would actually predispose an individual to bleeding. Factor VIII is an integral part of the intrinsic coagulation cascade.

Answer B is incorrect. Hypercoagulability, which is seen in thrombocytosis, factor V Leiden, and disseminated intravascular coagulation, is part of Virchow's triad, not hypocoagulability.

Answer C is incorrect. The endothelial surface needs to be damaged to initiate the coagulation cascade, and therefore an intact endothelial surface would not predispose an individual to a deep venous thrombosis.

Answer D is incorrect. Thrombocytopenia is characterized by a low platelet count, which typically does not predispose an individual to developing deep venous thromboses. Platelets usually are one of the first lines in initiating clot formation.

13. **The correct answer is E.** This patient has suffered rupture of one of the two left ventricular papillary muscles, a complication that may occur 3–10 days after an acute MI, when the infarcted area of myocardium is replaced with granulation tissue and thus is the most weak. Without the anchor of the papillary muscle, there is severe mitral regurgitation, diagnosed by a new holosystolic "blowing murmur" that is loudest at the apex and radiates to the axilla, a severely reduced stroke volume, and evidence of pulmonary edema.

Answer A is incorrect. Aortic stenosis causes a crescendo-decrescendo systolic murmur, not a holosystolic murmur and would not be expected to develop acutely as a complication of an MI.

Answer B is incorrect. Dressler's syndrome is an uncommon form of acute pericarditis that occurs several weeks post-MI and is thought to be a result of autoimmune inflammation. Signs and symptoms of pericarditis include sharp, pleuritic chest pain; fever; and a pericardial friction rub, not a holosystolic murmur.

Answer C is incorrect. Rupture of the interventricular septum may also occur 3–10 days after an acute MI and would also cause a holosystolic murmur. However, the murmur would be loudest over the left sternal border as blood flows from the left to right ventricle during systole. A murmur that is loudest at the apex and radiating to the axilla is characteristic of mitral regurgitation.

Answer D is incorrect. Rupture of the left ventricular (LV) free wall is another complication that can occur 3–10 days post-MI due to weakened myocardium; this development, however, would lead to cardiac tamponade, not to mitral regurgitation. In LV free wall rupture, blood accumulates in the pericardium and the constricted heart cannot pump effectively, causing a severely decreased stroke volume, systemic hypotension with pulsus paradoxus, jugular venous distention, and decreased heart sounds due to the insulating effects of the fluid around the heart. The holosystolic murmur loudest at the apex and radiating to the axilla detected in this patient is characteristic of mitral regurgitation.

Answer F is incorrect. While a ventricular aneurysm is a complication of an acute MI and could lead to a decreased EF, complications of ventricular aneurysm include thrombus formation with resulting emboli and ventricular arrhythmias, not the severe mitral regurgitation seen here.

14. **The correct answer is D.** The ECG shows torsades de pointes. Quinidine is a class IA antiarrhythmic agent used in the treatment of supraventricular arrhythmias. Quinidine slows conduction and can increase the QT interval, leading to torsades de pointes.

Answer A is incorrect. Adenosine is used both to diagnose and to treat supraventricular tachyarrhythmias. However, it is not associated with torsades de pointes.

Answer B is incorrect. Although the class III antiarrhythmics tend to be associated with torsades de pointes, especially sotalol, bretylium is an exception.

Answer C is incorrect. Propranolol is a class II antiarrhythmic but is not associated with torsades de pointes. β-Blockers such as propranolol are used to suppress abnormal pacemakers by decreasing the slope of phase 4 (slow diastolic depolarization in pacemaker cells).

Answer E is incorrect. Bepridil, not verapamil, is a calcium channel blocker and class IV antiarrhythmic associated with torsades de pointes. Verapamil and diltiazem are two calcium channel blockers used in the prevention of nodal arrhythmias (e.g., supraventricular tachycardia).

15. **The correct answer is B.** Aortic stenosis is characterized by a crescendo-decrescendo systolic ejection murmur that radiates to the carotid arteries as well as a weak peripheral pulse termed *pulsus parvus et tardus*. Murmurs of aortic stenosis are commonly the result of a calcified aortic valve, a congenital bicuspid aortic valve, and a valve that is affected by rheumatic heart disease.

Answer A is incorrect. Aortic regurgitation is characterized by a high-pitched blowing diastolic murmur with a widened pulse pressure. It is usually caused by a nondissecting aortic aneurysm, rheumatic heart disease, or syphilitic aortitis.

Answer C is incorrect. Mitral regurgitation is characterized by a holosystolic high-pitched blowing murmur that is at the base of the heart and radiates to the left axilla. It is usually a result of rheumatic heart disease but can also be associated with mitral valve prolapse, infective endocarditis, or damage to papillary muscle post–myocardial infarction.

Answer D is incorrect. Mitral stenosis follows an opening snap with a delayed, rumbling late-diastolic murmur. It is almost always due to rheumatic heart disease.

Answer E is incorrect. Mitral valve prolapse is characterized by a late systolic murmur with a midsystolic click. This is considered the most frequent valvular lesion and is typically caused by myxoid degeneration of the ground substance of the valve. It is associated with a variety of arrhythmias and predisposes an individual to infective endocarditis.

16. **The correct answer is B.** Inferior vena cava (IVC) compression is common in women during the third trimester of pregnancy. The large uterus compresses the IVC, decreasing venous return to the heart. This reduction in preload reduces stroke volume, thus reducing cardiac output. Recall that mean arterial pressure = cardiac output × total peripheral resistance; an acute decrease in either of these parameters will reduce blood pressure.

Answer A is incorrect. Cardiogenic shock can cause hypotension by decreasing the stoke volume and cardiac output, but it would not occur only in the supine position.

Answer C is incorrect. Neurogenic shock can cause hypotension by decreasing both cardiac output and peripheral resistance, but it does not typically occur in pregnant women only when they lie supine.

Answer D is incorrect. When fluid leaves the intravascular space and enters the interstitial space, it is referred to as third spacing. In pregnancy, there is a physiologic amount of third spacing, which causes dependent edema in the hands and feet. Some women may even experience pulmonary edema, which can be dangerous. Third spacing does cause hypertension if the intravascular volume is not replaced, but it would not cause isolated hypotension in the supine position.

Answer E is incorrect. Vasodilation will reduce blood pressure, and pregnant women do

have a constant amount of vasodilation that is greater than that in nonpregnant women. However, there is no reason for all blood vessels to spontaneously vasodilate when changing from an upright to a supine position.

17. **The correct answer is A.** This individual is presenting with signs and symptoms of peripheral vascular disease, also known as intermittent claudication, which can be the presenting sign of atherosclerosis. Atherosclerosis is primarily a disease of elastic arteries (i.e., the aorta) and large and medium-sized muscular arteries that results in the progressive accumulation within the intima of smooth muscle cells, lipids, and connective tissue. Risk factors for atherosclerosis include smoking, hypertension, diabetes mellitus, hyperlipidemia, and a positive family history.

Answer B is incorrect. Arterioles help provide the dynamic regulation of blood flow through the capillary beds and are not affected by atherosclerosis due to the lack of intima, media, and adventitia.

Answer C is incorrect. Capillaries are the smallest form of blood vessel and represent the site of interchange of solutes and cells between the blood and extracellular fluid. They are not typically affected by atherosclerosis but play a major role in the pathophysiology of edema

Answer D is incorrect. Veins are the vessels that return blood back to the heart and are not typically affected by atherosclerosis.

Answer E is incorrect. Venules are the first vessels to collect blood from the capillary beds and are not affected by atherosclerosis.

18. **The correct answer is C.** In tricuspid regurgitation, blood flows back into the atria during ventricular systole. This would affect the C and X waves, replacing them with a large positive deflection. The C wave is thought to be due to pressure on the tricuspid valve during ventricular systole. If the valve allows backflow during ventricular systole, the pressure would drastically increase in the atria. The downward movement of the ventricle causes the X descent during ventricular systole. This would

also be replaced by a positive deflection from blood regurgitating into the atria during ventricular systole.

Answer A is incorrect. These points are not the most likely to be affected in tricuspid regurgitation.

Answer B is incorrect. These points are not the most likely to be affected in tricuspid regurgitation.

Answer D is incorrect. These points are not the most likely to be affected in tricuspid regurgitation.

19. **The correct answer is C.** Constrictive pericarditis interferes with the filling of the ventricles because of granulation tissue formation in the pericardium. It can follow purulent viral infections, trauma, neoplastic diseases, mediastinal irradiation, and other chronic diseases. Pericardial thickening and calcification are sometimes apparent on CT scan and MRI.

Answer A is incorrect. Cardiac tamponade is very similar in presentation to constrictive pericarditis. One defining characteristic of cardiac tamponade is the absence of Kussmaul's sign (failure of cervical venous distention to subside on inspiration).

Answer B is incorrect. Congestive heart failure produces signs and symptoms similar to those of constrictive pericarditis. However, in CHF there would be significant enlargement and hypertrophy of the ventricles.

Answer D is incorrect. Recurrence of breast cancer would not likely present this way unless metastases to the pericardium were present.

Answer E is incorrect. The CT scan and MRI would reveal the hypertrophied ventricular walls that occur in restrictive cardiomyopathies. The absence of Kussmaul's sign also suggests another diagnosis.

20. **The correct answer is C.** The inferior mesenteric artery is located between the renal arteries and the bifurcation of the aorta into the common iliac arteries. This artery is often sacrificed during an infrarenal aortic aneurysm repair. Usually, there is enough collateral flow to the region of the gut supplied by the inferior mesenteric artery that this is not a problem.

Answer A is incorrect. The gastroduodenal artery is a branch of the hepatic artery, which is a branch of the celiac trunk that comes off the aorta superior to the renal arteries.

Answer B is incorrect. The hepatic artery is a branch of the celiac trunk and is found superior to the renal arteries.

Answer D is incorrect. The left gastric artery is a branch of the celiac trunk and is found superior to the renal arteries.

Answer E is incorrect. The splenic artery is a branch of the celiac trunk and is found superior to the renal arteries.

Answer F is incorrect. The superior mesenteric artery is superior to the renal arteries.

21. **The correct answer is D.** This photograph shows the pathognomonic "tree-bark" appearance of syphilitic aortitis. Syphilitic aortitis is characterized by obliterative endarteritis of the vasa vasorum of the media. This disruption of the vasa vasorum can lead to aneurysm, which typically involves the ascending aorta and is a manifestation of tertiary syphilis. Luetic (syphilitic) aneurysms favor the aortic root, where they can be complicated by atherosclerosis. The patient's skin lesions are the gummas of tertiary syphilis.

Answer A is incorrect. Atherosclerosis is most frequently associated with a descending aortic aneurysm, especially one involving the abdominal aorta, and is rarely associated with ascending aortic aneurysms in the absence of underlying pathology, such as that of tertiary syphilis.

Answer B is incorrect. Congenital medial weakness is actually associated with the development of berry aneurysms, which typically occur along the circle of Willis. They are the most frequent cause of subarachnoid hemorrhage and are also associated with adult polycystic kidney disease.

Answer C is incorrect. Cystic medial necrosis (cystic degeneration of the tunica media of the aorta) is the most frequent preexisting histological lesion in aortic dissection, which is not usually associated with aortic dilation. It is also associated with dilation of the ascending aorta, and is commonly seen in connective tissue disorders such as Marfan's syndrome. Although this answer choice is possible, the skin lesions point to tertiary syphilis as the cause of the cardiac pathology.

Answer E is incorrect. Hypertension is often implicated in the etiology of dissecting aneurysms due to a longitudinal intraluminal tear. Dissection is usually not associated with aortic dilation.

22. **The correct answer is A.** A patent ductus arteriosus (PDA) rarely causes cyanosis. PDAs are associated with maternal rubella infection during pregnancy. They are closed with indomethacin, a nonsteroidal anti-inflammatory drug.

    Answer B is incorrect. Tetralogy of Fallot is associated with cyanosis at birth.

    Answer C is incorrect. Transposition of the great vessels is associated with cyanosis at birth.

    Answer D is incorrect. Truncus arteriosus is associated with cyanosis at birth.

    Answer E is incorrect. Ventricular septal defects are the most common congenital cardiac anomaly. They do not cause cyanosis at birth and do not close with nonsteroidal anti-inflammatory drug administration.

23. **The correct answer is A.** Adenosine, a normal component of body chemistry, is extremely useful in abolishing atrioventricular (AV) nodal arrhythmias when given in high-dose intravenous boluses. Adenosine works by hyperpolarizing AV node tissue by increasing the conductance of K^+ (I_{K1}) and by reducing calcium current. As a result, the conduction through the AV node is markedly reduced. In addition to this, adenosine's extremely short duration of action (15 seconds) limits the oc-

currence of its toxicities (i.e., hypotension, flushing, chest pain, and dyspnea).

Answer B is incorrect. Bretylium, a K^+ channel blocker (Class III), is used when other antiarrhythmics fail.

Answer C is incorrect. Encainide is used when ventricular tachycardia progresses to ventricular fibrillation; it is also used in intractable supraventricular tachycardia.

Answer D is incorrect. Lidocaine, a Class Ib antiarrhythmic, is used in the treatment of acute ventricular arrhythmias such as post–myocardial infarction arrhythmias.

Answer E is incorrect. Sotalol, which is both a β-adrenergic-receptor blocker (Class II) and a K^+ channel blocker (Class III), is used when other antiarrhythmics fail.

24. **The correct answer is D.** Norepinephrine, a potent direct-acting α and β agonist, can be useful in cases of septic shock because it stimulates vasoconstriction. It also exerts a mild inotropic effect as a $β_1$ agonist, but this effect may not be clinically relevant.

    Answer A is incorrect. Norepinephrine itself is inotropic and chronotropic, but the potent vasoconstriction that it causes will increase blood pressures to stimulate the baroreceptors, resulting in a reflex bradycardia. However, this is not a direct function of the norepinephrine and is not the reason it would be given to a patient in septic shock.

    Answer B is incorrect. Norepinephrine exerts no $β_2$ effects and thus has no effect on bronchial smooth muscle. If it were a $β_2$ agonist, it would stimulate bronchodilation

    Answer C is incorrect. As a $β_1$ agonist, norepinephrine stimulates a mild increase in cardiac inotropy.

    Answer E is incorrect. Norepinephrine is a vasoconstrictor, not a vasodilator.

25. **The correct answer is F.** The combination of an atrophic heart and lipofuscin accumulation

is referred to as brown atrophy. Lipofuscin is a "wear and tear" pigment that commonly deposits within hepatocytes, splenocytes, and myocardial cells in the elderly. It is comprised of oxidized and polymerized membrane lipids of autophagocytosed organelles accumulated slowly over years.

Answer A is incorrect. Bilirubin can accumulate and stain internal organs, producing yellowish discoloration called jaundice. However, lack of clinical evidence of a hemolytic or obstructive process in this case makes this option highly unlikely.

Answer B is incorrect. Age-related calcification is most often seen on heart valves. It would not appear brown in color, nor would it be associated with generalized cardiac atrophy.

Answer C is incorrect. Cholesterol may accumulate as atheromatous plaques in the arteries; however, its accumulation is not associated with cardiac atrophy nor brown pigmentation.

Answer D is incorrect. Glycogen storage diseases are inherited conditions that appear early in life. Glycogen does not appear pigmented on hematoxylin and eosin stain.

Answer E is incorrect. Iron deposits within the heart could resemble lipofuscin but this would indicate that the patient suffers from hemochromatosis. This is unlikely given the clinical information provided.

26. **The correct answer is E.** This individual is likely suffering from giant cell arteritis (GCA). GCA typically presents in people over the age of 50 and is more common in females. Symptoms include unilateral headache, jaw claudication, and impaired vision. The temporal artery is most often involved.

Answer A is incorrect. The carotid artery is commonly implicated in transient ischemic attacks but not in giant cell arteritis.

Answer B is incorrect. The middle cerebral artery is commonly implicated in cerebrovascular accidents.

Answer C is incorrect. Although this individual is experiencing a loss of vision, ophthalmic artery involvement in giant cell arteritis is typically secondary to temporal artery involvement.

Answer D is incorrect. The subclavian artery is a larger artery that is not typically implicated in giant cell arteritis.

27. **The correct answer is D.** The patient has had a subendocardial infarction, which is caused by ischemic necrosis of less than 50% of the ventricle wall. This area of the myocardium is the last section of the myocardium to be perfused and is the first to undergo necrosis from prolonged ischemia due to diffuse atherosclerosis and a transient thrombosis, followed quickly by clot lysis.

Answer A is incorrect. A complete occlusion of the coronary arteries is a cause of transmural infarcts. On ECG, there is a corresponding ST-segment elevation.

Answer B is incorrect. Coronary artery vasospasm is a condition known as Prinzmetal's variant angina. It is characterized by variant pain at rest and transient ST-segment elevation on ECG.

Answer C is incorrect. Stable angina is characterized by chest pain that arises with physical exertion or stress and passes with rest or decreased stress level. It is often due to greater than 75% occlusion of the coronary arteries by atherosclerosis. Although stable angina may produce slightly elevated cardiac enzymes, this clinical picture is more typical of a bona fide cardiac infarction.

Answer E is incorrect. Ischemic necrosis of greater than 50% of the coronary arteries is a cause of transmural infarcts. On ECG, there is a corresponding ST-segment elevation.

28. **The correct answer is C.** The left anterior descending artery supplies the anterior interventricular septum. It is the artery that is most commonly occluded in coronary artery occlusion. One of two main branches off the left main coronary artery, it descends the left surface of the heart anteriorly and inferiorly in the anterior interventricular groove to the apex of

the heart. Diagonal, septal perforating, and right ventricular branches come off of it, supplying the portions of the anterior aspects of the left atrium, left ventricle, interventricular septum, and right ventricle.

Answer A is incorrect. The acute marginal artery is a branch from the right coronary artery. It runs along the acute margin of the heart and supplies the anterior free wall of the right ventricle.

Answer B is incorrect. The circumflex artery is one of two main branches off the left main coronary artery and it courses along the left atrioventricular groove from the anterior to the posterior surface of the heart. In people who are left-dominant, it will give rise to the posterior descending artery and perfuse the atrioventricular node. Its main branches are the obtuse marginals, which supply blood to the lateral aspect of the left ventricular myocardium. It also has branches that supply blood to the left atrium and, in 40–50% of people, the sinus node.

Answer D is incorrect. The posterior descending artery is a branch of the right coronary artery on the posterior surface of the heart. It courses along the posterior interventricular groove, extending toward the apex of the heart. It has posterior septal perforator branches that run anteriorly in the ventricular septum and supply the posterior one-third of the ventricular septal myocardium.

Answer E is incorrect. The right coronary artery is one of the two main coronary arteries that take off from the aorta, just superior to the aortic valve leaflets. It courses from the aorta anterolaterally to descend in the right atrioventricular groove before curving posteriorly at the acute margin of the right ventricle. It supplies the sinoatrial and atrioventricular nodes, the right atrium, and portions of the right ventricle in addition to providing collaterals to the left anterior descending artery.

29. **The correct answer is C.** This patient is presenting with a classic case of acute bacterial endocarditis (ABE). Endocarditis is often characterized by constitutional symptoms (fever,

malaise, chills), new-onset cardiac murmur, and a combination of other signs and symptoms (e.g., Janeway lesions, Osler nodes, and Roth spots). Acute and subacute endocarditis can be differentiated based on history, as the acute case will have a more severe and sudden onset, as in this patient. *Staphylococcus aureus* is the most common bacteria isolated in cases of infectious endocarditis, and is most often seen in cases of intravenous drug use and indwelling catheters. *S. aureus* is associated with ABE rather than subacute endocarditis, and patients afflicted with ABE often appear much sicker. The murmur described is consistent with tricuspid regurgitation, a sign of right-sided endocarditis that is classic for intravenous drug use or indwelling catheter-related cases. Janeway lesions, Osler nodes, and Roth spots are mostly seen as a complication of left-sided endocarditis, in which septic emboli leave the heart and enter the systemic circulation. In right-sided endocarditis, septic emboli to the lungs leading to bilateral infiltrates are seen more often. This patient is manifesting signs of bilateral infiltrates with signs of hypoxia, decreased breath sounds, and dullness to percussion.

Answer A is incorrect. *Enterococcus faecalis* create a picture of subacute endocarditis. The classic picture is a slow onset of constitutional symptoms with low-grade fever. *Enterococcus* infection is not seen as frequently as viridans streptococci, but it is known to colonize damaged heart valves, especially in patients with a past history of rheumatic fever.

Answer B is incorrect. *Haemophilus aphrophilus* is part of the HACEK group of fastidious gram-negative bacilli that cause 5–10% of cases of bacterial endocarditis that are not related to intravenous drug use. These organisms are difficult to culture, making diagnoses more complex.

Answer D is incorrect. *Streptococcus bovis* also creates a picture of subacute bacterial endocarditis with low-grade fever and insidious onset. It normally inhabits the lower gastrointestinal tract and lesions in the colon, such as those that occur in colon cancer, allow the bacteria access to the bloodstream. It most commonly affects the aortic valve.

Answer E is incorrect. Viridans streptococci are the second most common cause of bacterial endocarditis. This group of bacteria is most often seen in subacute cases In which the onset of symptoms is more chronic and low-grade fevers are more common. Viridans streptococci commonly colonize heart valves previously damaged by rheumatic fever, thus causing left-sided infective endocarditis as opposed to the right-sided version seen more commonly with *Staphylococcus aureus*. One common source of infection is dental procedures during which normal flora can enter the bloodstream.

30. **The correct answer is A.** Cholestyramine and colestipol are bile acid resins that promote binding and excretion of dietary fats that are bile soluble. They decrease serum LDL and total cholesterol.

    Answer B is incorrect. Fibrates such as gemfibrozil decrease peripheral lipolysis, thereby decreasing LDL. They are associated with abdominal cramping and myositis.

    Answer C is incorrect. Niacin acts by increasing lipoprotein lipase activity. Its most significant result is an increase in serum HDL. Adverse effects include flushing.

    Answer D is incorrect. Ezetimibe is a newer lipid-lowering agent that acts by inhibiting cholesterol absorption at the small intestinal brush border. It is frequently given in combination with statins for greater overall LDL reduction.

    Answer E is incorrect. Statins are HMG-CoA reductase inhibitors that inhibit the rate-limiting enzyme in cholesterol synthesis. They cause significant decreases in LDL and modest increases in HDL.

    Answer F is incorrect. There is no available drug that sequesters bile acid resins in hepatocytes.

31. **The correct answer is A.** This patient has von Hippel–Lindau syndrome, an autosomal dominant disorder characterized by abnormal blood vessel growth. The overgrowth of blood vessels leads to angiomas and hemangioblastomas in the retina, brain, and spinal cord, as well as in other regions of the body. Patients also show cystic growths in the kidneys and pancreas, pheochromocytomas, islet cell tumors, and clear cell renal carcinoma. The disease is due to deletion of the *VHL* tumor suppressor gene on the short arm of chromosome 3.

    Answer B is incorrect. In autosomal recessive inheritance, a defective gene from each carrier parent is transmitted to the offspring. Disease is often seen in only one generation. Males and females are equally likely to be affected. Von Hippel–Lindau syndrome is not inherited in this manner.

    Answer C is incorrect. In mitochondrial inheritance, children (male and female) of an affected mother may exhibit the disease. The disease is not transmitted from fathers to any of their children (only maternal transmission). Von Hippel–Lindau syndrome is not inherited in this manner.

    Answer D is incorrect. Spontaneous mutations generally affect only one member of a family and are not seen in multiple generations. Von Hippel–Lindau syndrome is not inherited in this manner.

    Answer E is incorrect. In X-linked recessive inheritance, affected males inherit a defective copy of the X chromosome from heterozygous (asymptomatic) mothers. There is no male-to-male transmission. Von Hippel–Lindau syndrome is not inherited in this manner.

32. **The correct answer is D.** Fat emboli are associated with long bone fractures such as femoral fractures as well as with liposuction. They are caused by particles of bone marrow and other fatty interosseous tissue entering the circulation as a result of severe (often multiple) fractures. They can lodge in the lungs, brain, kidneys, and other organs. They may be asymptomatic or may manifest clinically as a fat embolism syndrome characterized by pulmonary distress, cutaneous petechiae, and various neurologic abnormalities.

Answer A is incorrect. Air emboli result from the introduction of air into the circulation. They can originate from a penetrating chest injury, from a poorly performed abortion, or from decompression sickness that may result in divers who resurface too rapidly.

Answer B is incorrect. Amniotic emboli are caused by the escape of amniotic fluid into the maternal circulation. This can lead to the activation of the coagulation process and may progress to disseminated intravascular coagulation, potentially leading to maternal death.

Answer C is incorrect. Bacterial emboli have an infectious etiology. They typically originate from sources such as bacterial endocarditis.

Answer E is incorrect. Thrombus emboli are caused by fragments of thrombi. They are the most frequent type of embolism and can originate either in the venous system, leading to pulmonary embolisms, or in the arterial system, leading to myocardial infarctions or other end-organ damage.

33. **The correct answer is C.** This individual is presenting with signs typical of congestive heart failure (CHF). In CHF, there is a decrease in effective arterial blood volume due to the inability of the heart to effectively pump blood, which stimulates the renin-angiotensin-aldosterone axis to increase the tubular absorption of Na^+ to help increase intravascular volume.

Answer A is incorrect. Sympathetic outflow would be increased to constrict arteries in order to raise the effective blood volume.

Answer B is incorrect. The venous pressure would actually be increased due to the inability of the heart to effectively pump blood to the arterial system; this would lead to a passive congestion of blood in the venous circulation. This increased venous pressure can result in passive congestion of the liver known as a "nutmeg" liver.

Answer D is incorrect. The effective arterial blood volume would be decreased due to the decreased ability of the heart to pump blood through the arterial circulation.

Answer E is incorrect. Glomerular filtration rate would be decreased because of vasoconstriction of the renal artery due to the release of angiotensin and the increase of sympathetic outflow.

34. **The correct answer is G.** Cardiac troponin I becomes elevated in the first 4 hours after an MI and remains elevated for 7–10 days. CK-MB peaks in the first 24 hours and then falls off. AST is the next to become elevated, as it gradually increases over the first 2 days and then slowly declines; however, it is not specific for damage to the heart. LDH is the last cardiac enzyme to become elevated—by day 2 post-MI—and it remains elevated for up to 7 days post-MI.

Answer A is incorrect. The correct order is troponin, CK-MB, AST, and then LDH.

Answer B is incorrect. The correct order is troponin, CK-MB, AST, and then LDH.

Answer C is incorrect. The correct order is troponin, CK-MB, AST, and then LDH.

Answer D is incorrect. The correct order is troponin, CK-MB, AST, and then LDH.

Answer E is incorrect. The correct order is troponin, CK-MB, AST, and then LDH.

Answer F is incorrect. The correct order is troponin, CK-MB, AST, and then LDH.

35. **The correct answer is C.** Given his age and his history of hypertension and diabetes, this patient is most likely presenting with a stroke. Part of the workup for stroke includes an ultrasound to evaluate the carotid arteries, which in this case showed significant atherosclerosis, the likely cause of the man's stroke. The common carotid arteries, as well as the proximal part of the internal carotids, have their embryologic origins in the third aortic arch. Remember this by noting that "C" is the **third** letter of the alphabet. The aortic arches are responsible for the major arteries in the head and neck regions, while the descending aorta is the origin for the arteries in the rest of the body.

Answer A is incorrect. The first aortic arch gives rise to the maxillary artery, which is not involved in the pathophysiology of stroke.

Answer B is incorrect. The second aortic arch gives rise to the stapedial (**Second = Stapedial**) and hyoid arteries, neither of which is involved in stroke.

Answer D is incorrect. The fourth aortic arch gives rise to the adult arch of the aorta on the left and the proximal part of the right subclavian artery on the right. In theory, it is possible for an embolus from an aortic arch thrombus to travel up the carotid and cause a stroke, but this is not a likely scenario and would not be evaluated by ultrasound. Similarly, a subclavian embolus may travel up the vertebral arteries to cause a posterior stroke, but this would not be evaluated by ultrasound.

Answer E is incorrect. The sixth arch gives rise to the proximal parts of the pulmonary arteries and, on the left, the ductus arteriosus. Note that the fifth aortic arch regresses.

36. **The correct answer is D.** This patient has cardiac tamponade. Pericardiocentesis is required immediately and may be lifesaving. The fluid that has filled the pericardial membrane is removed, thereby restoring the pressure levels that led to the elevated intracardiac pressure, limited ventricular filling, and reduced cardiac output that ultimately caused her symptoms of fatigue and pulsus paradoxus.

Answer A is incorrect. Angioplasty is required for a patient that has greater than 70% blockage of a coronary artery. This diagnosis could not be made by echocardiography.

Answer B is incorrect. Aortic valve replacement would be necessary in situations of valvular failure or rupture. Cardiac tamponade does not affect heart valves.

Answer C is incorrect. Mitral valve replacement would be necessary in situations of valvular failure or rupture. Cardiac tamponade does not affect heart valves.

Answer E is incorrect. Aortic aneurysms do not typically present with pulsus paradoxus or fatigue.

37. **The correct answer is C.** This image shows mitral stenosis, causing a classic "fish-mouth" appearance due to the fusion of the valve leaflets. Mitral stenosis often causes a sharp, high-pitched "opening snap" at the beginning of diastole, due to the opening of the stiffened mitral valve leaflets, followed by a decrescendo-crescendo murmur. The shape of the murmur of mitral stenosis is unique and occurs because the pressure gradient between the left atrium and left ventricle is the greatest when the mitral valve opens and decreases during rapid and slow ventricular filling (decrescendo) and then intensifies slightly during atrial contraction at the end of ventricular diastole (crescendo). The murmur of mitral stenosis is low-pitched and is best heard at the apex of the heart. This woman may have had rheumatic heart disease, which is the most common cause of mitral stenosis.

Answer A is incorrect. A patent ductus arteriosus causes a continuous murmur as blood flows from the higher-pressure aorta to the lower-pressure pulmonary artery during both diastole and systole. The murmur increases during ventricular systole as the pressure in the aorta increases, reaches a maximum at the end of ventricular systole, and decreases throughout diastole, as the pressure in the aorta decreases. This patient, however, has a stenotic mitral valve, not a patent ductus arteriosus.

Answer B is incorrect. Aortic or pulmonic regurgitation, not mitral stenosis, would cause a decrescendo murmur that would be loudest in early diastole, when the pressure gradient between the aorta and the left ventricle is the greatest, and would decrease throughout diastole as the left ventricular pressure increases.

Answer D is incorrect. Aortic stenosis leads to a crescendo-decrescendo murmur best heard at the right sternal border during ventricular systole, as the pressure gradient between the left ventricle and the aorta increases to a maximum during mid-systole and then decreases in late ventricular systole. The characteristic murmur of aortic stenosis may be preceded by a sharp "ejection click" due to the opening of the stiffened aortic valve leaflets. This patient had a stenotic mitral valve, not a stenotic aortic valve.

Answer E is incorrect. Mitral valve prolapse characteristically causes a sharp, high-pitched "click" during mid to late systole followed by the continuous murmur of mitral regurgitation as blood flows from the higher-pressure left ventricle to the lower-pressure left atrium. While the stenotic mitral valve, seen in this patient, could lead to a systolic murmur of mitral regurgitation in addition to the diastolic murmur of mitral stenosis, the murmur of mitral regurgitation due to a stenotic valve would be a holosystolic, continuous murmur. The mid-systolic click followed by a continuous murmur is unique to mitral valve prolapse, which is most commonly caused by enlarged, floppy, and myxomatous mitral valve leaflets.

38. **The correct answer is B.** This is Kawasaki's disease, which typically affects infants and children under 5 years old and is self-limiting. It involves the mouth, skin, and lymph nodes at first, but if left untreated the patient may have arrhythmias due to inflammation of the outer membranes of the heart. The most common histopathologic sign of Kawasaki's disease is acute necrotizing vasculitis of small and medium-sized vessels.

Answer A is incorrect. Buerger's disease is characterized as an idiopathic, segmental thrombosing vasculitis with intermittent claudication, superficial nodular phlebitis, and cold sensitivity. Patients are usually young men (20–40 years old) who are also heavy smokers.

Answer C is incorrect. Polyarteritis nodosa is characterized by cotton-wool spots, microaneurysms, myocarditis, and palpable purpura. This condition most often arises in the fourth or fifth decades of life, and is twice as likely to occur in men. The cardinal histopathologic sign is inflammation throughout the entire arterial wall.

Answer D is incorrect. Takayasu's arteritis is characterized by weak pulses in the upper extremities, fever, arthritis, and night sweats. The condition most often arises in women under the age of 40 years (9:1 female predominance). The classic pulselessness is a result of chronic inflammation and subsequent narrowing of the aorta and its branches, making it a large-vessel vasculitis.

Answer E is incorrect. Wegener's granulomatosis is characterized by necrotizing granulomas in the lung and upper airways together with glomerulonephritis; however, it can occur in any organ. There is a nearly equal gender distribution in incidence, and the condition typically occurs in middle age. Histopathological diagnosis is critical, even though C-ANCA testing is positive in most patients.

39. **The correct answer is F.** This woman is likely suffering from prosthetic valve endocarditis. She may not have taken appropriate prophylactic antibiotics before her root canal procedure, and her susceptible mitral valve has been exposed to transient bacteremia. Her symptoms, including low-grade persistent fever, new-onset murmur, and insidious onset, suggest subacute bacterial endocarditis. This is further supported by her physical examination, which reveals the presence of Roth spots (retinal hemorrhages), Osler's nodes (painful red nodules on digits), and Janeway lesions (dark macules on palms and soles). Given her clinical history and symptoms, the bacterium most likely to have caused this episode is *Streptococcus sanguis*, part of the viridans group. The most appropriate treatment for such an infection is penicillin G.

Answer A is incorrect. Caspofungin is an antifungal used to treat aspergillosis. It would not treat a gram-positive cocci infection.

Answer B is incorrect. Clindamycin, the treatment for several important anaerobic infections, works by blocking peptide bond formation at the 50S ribosomal subunit. This is not an anaerobic infection.

Answer C is incorrect. Mebendazole is an antiparasitic drug used to treat roundworm infections such as pinworm and whipworm.

Answer D is incorrect. Metronidazole is a bactericidal agent used to treat protozoal infections, specifically *Giardia, Entamoeba,* and *Trichomonas* species, as well as anaerobes, specifically *Bacteroides* and *Clostridium* species. Gram-positive cocci are not within metronidazole's spectrum.

Answer E is incorrect. Nafcillin works like penicillin but is used clinically to treat *Staphylococcus aureus,* the cause of acute bacterial endocarditis, among other infections. Nafcillin is used for *S. aureus* because it is penicillinase-resistant due to a bulkier R group. Because of this special property, nafcillin is reserved for suspected *S. aureus* cases, which is not the cause of this patient's condition.

Answer G is incorrect. Pentamidine is an antiparasitic drug used for prophylaxis against *Pneumocystis carinii* pneumonia.

40. **The correct answer is E.** The patient's primary complaints are fatigue and depression that began after she started a new medication. Her physical examination and laboratory studies are within normal limits and reveal no additional side effects of this new medication. Mild sedation and depression are common side effects of β-blockers; disturbance of the sleep cycle, exercise intolerance, and a diminished hypoglycemic response can also occur with the use of β-blockers.

Answer A is incorrect. Enalapril, an angiotensin-converting enzyme inhibitor, has significant side effects such as cough, angioedema, and proteinuria. However, it is not associated with sedation or depression.

Answer B is incorrect. Furosemide is a loop diuretic and thus can cause electrolyte abnormalities such as hypokalemia and metabolic alkalosis. It is not associated with sedation.

Answer C is incorrect. Hydrochlorothiazide, a diuretic, has side effects such as hypokalemia and hyperglycemia. It is not associated with sedation or changes in mood.

Answer D is incorrect. Losartan is an angiotensin receptor blocker; its use can result in hyperkalemia, but it is not associated with sedation.

Answer F is incorrect. Nifedipine is a calcium channel blocker that functions primarily on the vasculature. It can be associated with edema, flushing, and dizziness, but is not usually sedating.

Answer G is incorrect. Prazosin, an α antagonist, can be associated with dizziness, headache, and orthostasis, but is not considered sedating.

41. **The correct answer is E.** The question describes the pathology associated with stable angina. While the exact mechanisms for triggers of stable angina are not known, patients with stable angina do have a dysfunctional endothelium. Atherosclerosis can add to this complication. The most notable sign or symptom associated with stable angina is substernal chest pain lasting 10–15 minutes that is caused by an increased myocardial oxygen demand in times of exercise or emotional stress.

Answer A is incorrect. While arrhythmias can complicate stable angina, they are not a necessary or predominant symptom of the disorder.

Answer B is incorrect. Bradycardia is not associated with stable angina because it does not cause an increase in myocardial oxygen demand.

Answer C is incorrect. Hypertension is associated with, but is not the predominant sign or symptom of, stable angina. Hypertension causes an increase in myocardial oxygen demand because of the increased afterload of the heart, but it does not have to be present in order for a patient to experience stable angina.

Answer D is incorrect. Tachycardia can cause an increase in myocardial oxygen demand due to an increased number of contractions, but it does not have to be present in order for a patient to experience stable angina.

42. **The correct answer is C.** Isovolumetric relaxation (IV in the image) is the period in which

both the aortic and mitral valves are closed, thus keeping ventricular volume constant. Ventricular muscle relaxes from its prior contraction to allow for filling.

Answer A is incorrect. Functions of the atria are not depicted in this diagram.

Answer B is incorrect. Isovolumetric contraction (II in the image) is the period between mitral valve closing and aortic valve opening.

Answer D is incorrect. Ventricular ejection (III in the image) is the period between aortic valve opening and closing.

Answer E is incorrect. Ventricular filling (I in the image) is the period between mitral valve opening and closing.

43. **The correct answer is C.** The carotid sinus baroreceptor sends an afferent signal via the glossopharyngeal nerve to the medulla, which in turn responds with a sympathetic efferent signal that causes vasoconstriction, increased heart rate, increased contractility, and increased blood pressure.

Answer A is incorrect. The baroreceptor located in the aortic arch responds only to an increase in blood pressure.

Answer B is incorrect. The correct efferent response to a decreased baroreceptor afferent firing rate would be increased sympathetic activity and decreased parasympathetic activity.

Answer D is incorrect. The baroreceptor located in the aortic arch responds only to an increase in blood pressure.

Answer E is incorrect. The afferent firing rate would decrease with hypotension.

44. **The correct answer is B.** Dressler's syndrome is an autoimmune phenomenon that results in fibrinous pericarditis. This delayed pericarditis typically develops 2–10 weeks post–myocardial infarction and presents clinically as chest pain and a pericardial friction rub.

Answer A is incorrect. Cardiac arrhythmia is a common cause of post–myocardial infarction (MI) death and typically occurs 2 days post-MI.

Answer C is incorrect. Left ventricular failure occurs in 60% of people who suffer from myocardial infarction and can present as congestive heart failure or cardiogenic shock.

Answer D is incorrect. Thromboemboli are typically systemic emboli that originate from mural thrombi and can lead to cerebrovascular accidents, transient ischemic attacks, and renal artery thrombosis.

Answer E is incorrect. Ventricular rupture is a cause of post–myocardial infarction (MI) death that typically occurs 4–10 days post-MI.

45. **The correct answer is A.** At toxic levels of hydralazine, the body may compensate with severe reflex tachycardia as well as with salt and water retention. Because of these compensations, a patient with cardiac disease may experience angina as a result of increased oxygen demand secondary to increased cardiac output or increased heart rate. With tachycardia, the diastolic time and thus the time available for coronary artery flow is decreased, and angina may result. Furthermore, increased salt and water retention may increase the afterload and oxygen consumption of the heart. Hydralazine is also known to cause a lupuslike syndrome. Hydralazine works by increasing cyclic guanosine monophosphate, which induces smooth muscle relaxation. This smooth muscle relaxation occurs more in the arterioles than in the veins and thus reduces the afterload on the heart.

Answer B is incorrect. Nitroprusside may cause cyanide toxicity due to increased cyanide release.

Answer C is incorrect. Prazosin, an α-blocker, may cause first-dose orthostatic hypotension.

Answer D is incorrect. Minoxidil is known to cause hypertrichosis.

Answer E is incorrect. A positive Coombs' test may be obtained in a patient taking methyldopa.

46. **The correct answer is B.** This is a Mobitz type II second-degree heart block. A defect in the His-Purkinje system is responsible for this type of heart block defect.

     Answer A is incorrect. AV nodal abnormalities lengthen the PR interval and are responsible for first-degree heart block and Mobitz type I second-degree heart block.

     Answer C is incorrect. Independently contracting atria and ventricles occur in the complete absence or ablation of the His-Purkinje system, not simply a defect in the system.

     Answer D is incorrect. Retrograde conductions would result in an increase in the number of P waves and a decrease in the PR interval.

     Answer E is incorrect. SA nodal abnormalities are responsible for problems in automaticity and would not result in randomly dropped QRS complexes.

47. **The correct answer is A.** Fatal arrhythmias following a myocardial infarction, also known as sudden cardiac death, are the most common cause of death in the first few hours following an infarction. Arrhythmias are due to disruption of the conduction system and myocardial irritability following injury.

     Answer B is incorrect. Following myocardial infarction, thrombus formation over the infarcted area of endocardium can lead to a left-sided embolism; however, this is not the most common cause of sudden cardiac death.

     Answer C is incorrect. Myocardial failure can lead to further complications, such as congestive heart failure and cardiogenic shock following an infarction. However, these complications rarely cause immediate death.

     Answer D is incorrect. Myocardial rupture is a complication that most commonly occurs 3–7 days after an infarction, due to the weakened wall strength of the damaged area. The ventricular free wall is the most likely site of rupture; this can lead to bleeding into the pericardial space, causing fatal cardiac tamponade. However, death due to myocardial rupture is unlikely to occur within hours of the ischemic episode.

     Answer E is incorrect. A ruptured papillary muscle is a possible complication of an infarction, but it most commonly occurs 3–7 days after the ischemic event. Thus, papillary muscle rupture would not cause immediate death.

48. **The correct answer is C.** Individuals with central retinal artery occlusion typically present with the acute onset of painless monocular visual loss that is usually the result of thromboembolic phenomena relating to vascular disease. However, since this patient is young and has no consistent prior medical history, one must consider other causes, which in this patient would almost certainly relate to her recent hospitalization for severe bacteremia. In the setting of a new murmur after bacteremia, the most likely cause of this patient's symptoms is a septic embolism that originated in the heart and has lodged in the central retinal artery. Unfortunately, even with treatment, fewer than 25% of patients regain useful vision in the affected eye.

     Answer A is incorrect. Central retinal artery occlusion may result from sequelae of collagen vascular disease, but this is a relatively infrequent cause and is unlikely given the lack of any history consistent with such a diagnosis.

     Answer B is incorrect. Although diabetes is a leading cause of microvascular disease, it is a rare cause of central retinal artery occlusion.

     Answer D is incorrect. Hypertensive crises would be more likely to result in bleeding than thromboembolic phenomena or other causes of central retinal artery occlusion.

     Answer E is incorrect. The overwhelming majority of central retinal artery occlusions are secondary to thromboembolic phenomena. However, given the history and this patient's lack of macrovascular disease, this is a less likely cause of the patient's occlusion.

49. **The correct answer is C.** Cardiac glycosides inhibit the Na$^+$-K$^+$-ATPase transport system to increase intracellular sodium concentration,

which then increases intracellular calcium concentration via the sodium-calcium exchange carrier mechanism. This increased calcium level augments the calcium released to the myofilaments during excitation, resulting in a positive inotropic effect. Increased contractility of the heart directly increases cardiac output.

Answer A is incorrect. Aortic stenosis would increase the afterload necessary to eject blood from the left ventricle. The result would be decreased cardiac output without compensation.

Answer B is incorrect. β-Blockers inhibit cardiac activation by action on catecholamines and would not increase cardiac output.

Answer D is incorrect. A decreased intracellular calcium concentration would decrease the contractility of the heart, resulting in decreased cardiac output.

Answer E is incorrect. Increased extracellular sodium concentration would not increase cardiac output because the sodium-calcium exchange carrier mechanism would not lead to increased calcium concentration intracellularly.

50. The correct answer is C. Net filtration pressure is governed by the equation $P_{net} = [(P_c - P_i) - (\pi_c - \pi_i)]$, where P_c is capillary pressure, P_i is interstitial fluid pressure, π_c is plasma colloid osmotic pressure, and π_i is interstitial fluid colloid osmotic pressure. Increasing P_c, π_i, or the permeability of the capillaries will lead to a net flow of fluid from the capillaries to the interstitium. Likewise, decreasing π_c and P_i will also lead to net outward flow and edema.

Answer A is incorrect. Decreasing capillary permeability would result in fluid being trapped in the vascular space.

Answer B is incorrect. Decreased capillary pressure would decrease the amount of fluid in the interstitial space.

Answer D is incorrect. Increased interstitial fluid pressure would increase fluid flow back into the vascular space.

Answer E is incorrect. Increased plasma protein levels would cause an increase in fluid retention in the vascular space.

CHAPTER 7

Endocrine

1. A 42-year-old woman with a history of pernicious anemia comes to the physician complaining of increased anxiety, heart palpitations, heat intolerance, unexplained weight loss, and multiple daily bowel movements. She has not had a period in 4 months. On physical examination, the patient is found to have a goiter, a thyroid bruit, and mild proptosis. Laboratory studies show elevated triiodothyronine and free thyroxine levels, and an undetectable thyroid-stimulating hormone. Which of the following is the most likely etiology of this patient's disease?

(A) Autoimmune stimulation of thyroid-stimulating hormone receptors
(B) Idiopathic replacement of thyroid tissue with fibrous tissue
(C) Thyroid adenoma
(D) Thyroid hormone–producing ovarian teratoma
(E) Viral infection leading to destruction of thyroid tissue

2. A certain endocrine disorder can lead to an elevated blood pressure, ~~elevated~~ decreased K⁺ levels, Na⁺ and water retention, and decreased renin activity. Which of the following is the most likely diagnosis?

(A) Addison's disease
(B) Hyperthyroidism
(C) Pheochromocytoma
(D) Primary hyperaldosteronism
(E) Secondary hyperaldosteronism

3. A 59-year-old woman with no prior medical history presents to the physician with marked hyperglycemia, diarrhea, and weight loss. A CT scan of the abdomen reveals a pancreatic mass. A trial period on an oral hypoglycemic agent has not helped reduce her glucose levels. Her physical examination is significant for the rash shown in the image. Which of the following is the most likely diagnosis?

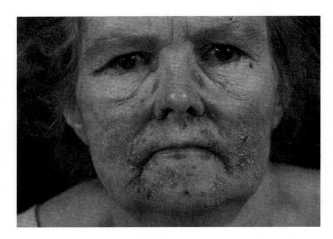

Reproduced, with permission, from Wolff K, Johnson RA, Suurmond D. *Fitzpatrick's Color Atlas & Synopsis of Clinical Dermatolgy,* 5th ed. New York, McGraw-Hill, 2005: Fig. 17-12.

(A) Corticosteroid therapy
(B) Glucagonoma
(C) Insulinoma
(D) Type 1 diabetes mellitus
(E) VIPoma

4. A 5-year-old girl is brought to the pediatrician by her mother because she has noticed a single soft, nontender mass underneath her daughter's tongue. The physician reassures the mother that it is a common congenital ectopic anomaly that does not affect the function of the mass or the hormone it secretes. Hypersecretion of this hormone can cause which of the following conditions?

(A) Amenorrhea
(B) Cold intolerance
(C) Constipation
(D) Hyperlipidemia
(E) Weight gain

5. A 60-year-old patient comes to the physician complaining of polydipsia, polyuria, and polyphagia. A histologic sample of the patient's kidney is shown. Which of the following findings will most likely be apparent on renal biopsy?

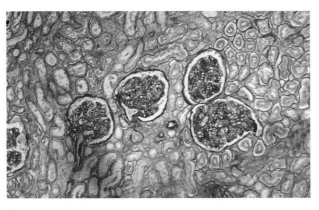

Image courtesy of PEIR Digital Library (http://peir.net).

(A) Amyloid deposits
(B) Crescent formation
(C) Kimmelstiel-Wilson nodules
(D) Segmental sclerosis
(E) Wire loop abnormality

6. A 34-year-old man with moderately severe ulcerative colitis has been on a drug regimen of oral prednisone for 4 months. Which of the following symptoms is the most likely adverse effect of his treatment regimen?

(A) Diabetes insipidus
(B) Diabetes mellitus
(C) Hyperpigmentation of the skin
(D) Hypotension
(E) Muscle hypertrophy
(F) Sodium wasting

7. A 45-year-old man with type 2 diabetes mellitus undergoes a neurologic examination. The patient is unable to sense the vibration produced by a tuning fork placed on his big toe. Which of the following receptors is most likely affected in this patient?

(A) Krause end bulbs
(B) Meissner's corpuscle
(C) Merkel nerve endings
(D) Pacinian corpuscle
(E) Ruffini corpuscle

8. A 53-year-old woman with newly diagnosed type 2 diabetes presents to the emergency department complaining of vomiting, severe headache, dizziness, blurry vision, and difficulty breathing. She says that she had been at a cocktail party when the symptoms began. Her skin is notably flushed on physical examination. Which of the following medications is responsible for this reaction?

(A) Acarbose
(B) Glipizide
(C) Glyburide
(D) Metformin
(E) Tolbutamide
(F) Troglitazone

9. A 25-year-old man comes to the emergency department after experiencing tremors. He appears visibly anxious and relates a recent history of sweats, nausea, vomiting, and lightheadedness. Laboratory studies show a blood glucose level of 50 mg/dL. An abdominal CT scan shows a 1.5-cm mass in the head of the pancreas. Surgical resection of this mass will necessitate ligation of branches from which of the following vascular structures?

(A) The gastroduodenal and inferior mesenteric arteries
(B) The gastroduodenal and superior mesenteric arteries
(C) The left gastric and inferior mesenteric arteries
(D) The left gastric and superior mesenteric arteries
(E) The proper hepatic and inferior mesenteric arteries
(F) The proper hepatic and superior mesenteric arteries

HIGH-YIELD SYSTEMS

Endocrine

10. A 36-year-old woman presents to the physician with amenorrhea. She reports an increase in her ring and shoe sizes over the past year, increased sweating, and increased fatigue. Physical examination is remarkable for a blood pressure of 150/90 mm Hg and coarse facial features with mild macroglossia. Surgery is indicated in her therapy. After surgery, which of the following medications constitutes the most appropriate pharmacotherapy for this patient?

(A) Finasteride
(B) Leuprolide
(C) Octreotide
(D) Recombinant growth hormone
(E) Somatrem

11. A 23-year old man comes to the physician because he has developed intermittent severe headaches, anxiety, and heart palpitations. While he has no significant medical history, he does remember an uncle who had similar symptoms. When probed for a deeper family history, he says that his mother and two cousins have had their thyroids removed. Which of the following most likely accounts for these laboratory findings?

(A) Acromegaly
(B) ACTH-secreting pituitary adenoma
(C) Hyperparathyroidism
(D) Nonfunctioning pituitary adenoma
(E) Pheochromocytoma

12. Growth hormone (GH) is essential to normal human growth and development, and its secretion is tightly regulated via a feedback control system involving the hypothalamus, the pituitary gland, and the peripheral tissues. Which of the following is a stimulus for the secretion of GH?

(A) Hypoglycemia
(B) Obesity
(C) Pregnancy
(D) Somatomedins
(E) Somatostatin

13. The product of the cells shown in this image induces a rise in serum Ca^{2+} levels. Which of the following types of cells are indicated by the arrows in this image?

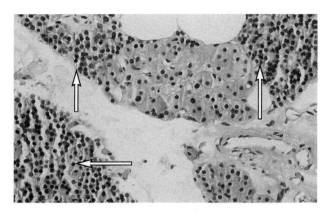

Image courtesy of Armed Forces Institute of Pathology.

(A) Adipocytes
(B) Parathyroid chief cells
(C) Parathyroid oxyphil cells
(D) Thyroid C cells
(E) Thyroid follicle cells

14. A 66-year-old man with history of chronic cough, dyspnea, and a 50-pack-year of cigarette smoking comes to the clinic after noticing some blood in his sputum. He reports that he feels lethargic and has lost 18 kg (40 lb) over the past 3 months with no changes in diet or exercise. Laboratory studies show a serum Na^+ level of 120 mEq/dL. While awaiting a CT scan, the patient suffers a seizure and is rushed to the emergency department of the nearest hospital. Which of the following is most likely to be elevated in this patient?

(A) ACTH
(B) ADH
(C) Parathyroid hormone
(D) Renin
(E) Tumor necrosis factor-α

15. A 65-year-old woman comes to her primary care physician complaining of progressive weakness and fatigue. On further questioning, she notes a recent weight gain and constipation as well as constant subjective chills. Physical examination shows a moderate nontender goiter. A biopsy shows a lymphocytic infiltrate. Which of the following best describes this patient's thyroid-stimulating hormone (TSH) and thyroid hormone levels relative to normal baseline values?

CHOICE	THYROID-STIMULATING HORMONE	TOTAL THYROXINE	FREE THYROXINE
A	↑	↑	↑
B	↑	↓	↑
C	↑	↓	↓
D	↓	↓	↑
E	↓	↓	↓

(A) A
(B) B
(C) C
(D) D
(E) E

16. A 27-year-old woman presents to a new physician with muscle cramping and spasm. On physical examination, the physician notes shortened fourth and fifth metacarpals and metatarsals, short stature, a round face, and abnormal teeth. She has positive Chvostek's and Trousseau's signs. Laboratory studies show a decreased serum Ca^{2+} level and a significantly elevated parathyroid hormone level. There is no evidence of renal disease, thus decreasing the likelihood of renal osteodystrophy. Which of the following is the most common mode of inheritance of this patient's disease?

(A) Autosomal dominant
(B) Autosomal recessive
(C) Mitochondrial
(D) X-linked dominant
(E) X-linked recessive

17. The vascular supply of the hypothalamic-pituitary axis is uniquely designed and functionally resembles the design of the gastrointestinal vasculature in that it includes a portal system. Which of the following is the functional significance of this specialized vascular system?

(A) Delivery of hormones for processing
(B) Delivery of hormones for storage
(C) Delivery of hormones in high concentrations
(D) Delivery of hormones to the hypothalamus
(E) Delivery of preformed trophic hormones systemically

18. A researcher studying type 2 diabetes mellitus is inducing insulin resistance in normal mice. Which of the following types of inhibitors would be effective in producing this effect?

(A) Adenylate cyclase
(B) Guanylate cyclase
(C) Serine kinases
(D) Threonine kinases
(E) Tyrosine kinases

19. A 60-year-old woman with a history of type 2 diabetes mellitus comes to the clinic for a follow-up examination after being placed on a new agent to help her achieve tighter glycemic control. She complains that she has suffered occasional abdominal cramps and diarrhea, adding that she has recently been experiencing increased flatulence, which has become an embarrassing nuisance. Which of the following agents best accounts for this patient's complaints?

(A) Acarbose
(B) Chlorpropamide
(C) Glipizide
(D) Metformin
(E) Troglitazone

20. A 42-year-old man comes to the physician with bitemporal visual field loss and decreased libido. On physical examination, his features appear coarser and larger than in a photograph taken 1 year ago, and he states that his glove size and shoe size have changed over the last year as well. His MRI is shown. Which of the following is the most likely diagnosis for this patient?

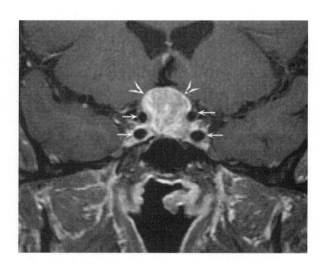

Reproduced, with permission, from Kasper DL, Braunwald E, Fauci AS, Hauser SL, Longo DL, Jameson JL, and Isselbacher KJ, eds. *Harrison's Principles of Internal Medicine*, 16th ed. McGraw-Hill, 2004: Fig. 318-4.

(A) ACTH-secreting pituitary adenoma
(B) Growth hormone–secreting pituitary adenoma
(C) Luteinizing hormone– and follicle-stimulating hormone–secreting pituitary adenoma
(D) Prolactin-secreting pituitary adenoma
(E) Thyroid-stimulating hormone–secreting pituitary adenoma

21. A biopsy of the thyroid gland of a 39-year-old woman is found to contain psammoma bodies and thin projections of epithelium surrounding a fibrovascular core. Which of the following is the most likely diagnosis?

(A) Follicular thyroid carcinoma
(B) Medullary thyroid carcinoma
(C) Papillary thyroid carcinoma

(D) Riedel's thyroiditis
(E) Subacute thyroiditis

22. A patient visits the doctor because she is worried that she is not growing proportionally. The patient claims that her parents are also extremely short. She appears to have a normal head and trunk size but has short arms and legs. Which of the following receptors is defective in achondroplasia?

(A) Antidiuretic hormone receptor
(B) Dihydrotestosterone receptor
(C) Fibroblast growth factor receptor 3
(D) Insulin receptor
(E) LDL receptor

23. Surgery is planned to excise a hyperfunctioning adrenal adenoma from a patient with primary hyperaldosteronism. On CT scan of the abdomen, the adenoma is visible as a 4-cm mass just superior to the right kidney. In order to immediately relieve the patient's hyperaldosteronism, the surgeon must first ligate the primary venous drainage of the tumor. The primary venous drainage flows directly into which of the following structures?

(A) Abdominal aorta
(B) Inferior vena cava
(C) Portal vein
(D) Right gonadal vein
(E) Right renal vein

24. A 54-year-old man with a history of smoking and lung cancer develops hypercalcemia. He is enrolled in a research study to assess the efficacy of a new synthetic agent to treat this condition. After several days of treatment, he reports persistent numbness and tingling around his mouth. Physical examination is significant for positive Chvostek's and Trousseau's signs. An excess of which of the following most likely accounts for this patient's symptoms and signs?

(A) Calcitonin
(B) Parathyroid hormone
(C) Parathyroid hormone–related peptide
(D) Thyroxine
(E) Vitamin D

25. A 34-year-old African-American woman presents to the physician with abdominal cramping that worsens during her menstrual period. The patient also says that her periods often last for more than 7 days. An ultrasound study shows multiple masses on the patient's uterus. Which of the following immunohistochemical stains would be the most appropriate for diagnosing this patient's condition?

    (A) Cytokeratin
    (B) Desmin
    (C) Glial fibrillary acid proteins
    (D) Neurofilament
    (E) Vimentin

26. A 34-year-old woman goes to her primary care physician complaining of a recent feeling that "her heart was racing" and visual changes. During the interview, the physician notices that the patient is clearly anxious. During the review of systems, the patient reveals a recent unintentional 4-kg (8.8-lb) weight loss. On physical examination, the physician notes that the patient is tachycardic and has 2+ nonpitting edema in her lower extremities. Which of the following is the most likely diagnosis?

    (A) Graves' disease
    (B) Hashimoto's thyroiditis
    (C) Iodine deficiency
    (D) Papillary carcinoma of the thyroid gland
    (E) Plummer's disease

27. A 43-year-old woman presents with fatigue, a 4.5-kg (9.9-lb) weight gain over the past 3 months, cold intolerance, hair loss, and concentration problems. Physical examination is significant for dry, coarse skin and bradycardia. She states that she had some slight swelling of her lower neck several months ago, which resolved without treatment. Results of antithyroglobulin antibody and antinuclear antibody tests are negative, but a thyroid peroxidase antibody test is positive. Which of the following statements accurately describes how the antibody that tested positive is contributing to this patient's disease process?

(A) Thyroid peroxidase antibodies bind to and antagonize the thyroid-stimulating hormone receptor of the thyroid gland, causing a decrease in the production and release of thyroid hormone; this results in a state of hypothyroidism

(B) Thyroid peroxidase antibodies bind to and antagonize the thyrotropin-releasing-hormone receptor of the pituitary gland, causing a decrease in the production and release of thyroid-stimulating hormone; this results in a state of hypothyroidism

(C) Thyroid peroxidase antibodies bind to and stimulate the thyroid-stimulating hormone receptor of the thyroid gland, causing an increase in the production and release of thyroid hormone; this results in a state of hyperthyroidism

(D) Thyroid peroxidase antibodies bind to endogenous thyroid peroxidase, thus inhibiting thyroid peroxidase from catalyzing several steps of the thyroid hormone synthesis pathway; this results in a state of hypothyroidism

(E) Thyroid peroxidase antibodies have an agonist effect on the thyroid peroxidase receptor, which leads to downregulation of thyroid hormone synthesis and a state of hypothyroidism

28. A 66-year-old man comes to the emergency department because of weight loss, hypotension, and bronze-colored skin. Laboratory tests show decreased serum levels of sodium, chloride, and cortisol, but increased serum levels of potassium and ACTH. Additionally, the urinary level of 17-OH is decreased. Which of the following most likely explains this patient's symptoms and laboratory values?

    (A) Autoimmune destruction of the adrenal glands
    (B) Cortisol-secreting adrenal adenoma
    (C) Ectopic ACTH production
    (D) Hemochromatosis
    (E) Pituitary corticotropin insufficiency

29. The predominant cells in this photomicrograph from the adrenal medulla secrete which of the following hormones into the bloodstream?

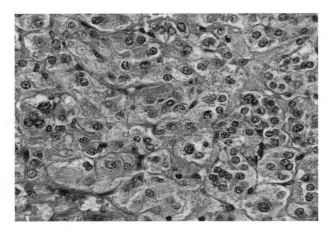

Image courtesy of Armed Forces Institute of Pathology.

(A) Aldosterone
(B) Androgens
(C) Cortisol
(D) Norepinephrine

30. A researcher investigating the action of thyroid hormones wants to develop an assay to analyze the activity of this hormone in various tissues. Which of the following strategies would be most effective in determining the level of activity of these hormones in a tissue sample?

(A) Assessing cAMP levels
(B) Assessing intracellular Ca^{2+} levels
(C) Assessing Na^+/K^+-ATPase mRNA levels
(D) Assessing phospholipase C activity
(E) Assessing phosphorylation of IRS-1

31. A 25-year-old patient presents to a primary care clinic complaining of galactorrhea and loss of libido. Although this tumor is hypersecretory, its presence often causes deficits of other hormones normally produced by the gland in which it resides. Which of the following functions will most likely be preserved in this individual?

(A) Milk synthesis
(B) Ovulation
(C) Parturition
(D) Salt retention
(E) Spermatogenesis

32. A 24-year-old woman who has never been pregnant presents to her physician with galactorrhea. Her past medical history is significant for hypercalcemia and recurrent duodenal ulcers. Maternal family members have been diagnosed with a variety of tumors. Which of the following is the genetic inheritance pattern of this patient's disorder?

(A) Autosomal dominant
(B) Autosomal recessive
(C) Mitochondrial
(D) X-linked dominant
(E) X-linked recessive

33. A 28-year-old man with a history of hypothyroidism comes to the physician because of a 3-day history of abdominal pain, diarrhea, palpitations, and fatigue. Physical examination is remarkable only for tachycardia. Which of the following medications most likely accounts for this patient's presentation?

(A) Dobutamine
(B) Iodide
(C) Leuprolide
(D) Levothyroxine
(E) Propylthiouracil

34. A 22-year-old woman complains of recent-onset polydipsia and polyuria. She has no recent head trauma or known intracranial tumor. A recent blood test reveals that her plasma ADH levels are normal. Her plasma osmolarity is 290 mOsm/L, and her urine flow rate is 10 mL/min. If this patient has nephrogenic diabetes insipidus, which of the following urine osmolarity values most closely reflects her condition?

(A) 100 mOsm/L
(B) 290 mOsm/L
(C) 350 mOsm/L
(D) 425 mOsm/L
(E) 1000 mOsm/L

35. An agitated and confused 44-year-old man is brought to the emergency department after collapsing at his office. The patient has a history of diabetes mellitus and was recently diagnosed with hypertension. He is conscious when the emergency medical team arrives and complains of fatigue and dizziness but denies any chest pain, palpitations, shortness of breath, sweating, fever, or chills. His diabetes has been well controlled with glyburide, but he is unable to recall the name of his antihypertensive drug. Which of the following agents is most likely responsible for this patient's condition?

(A) Enalapril
(B) Hydralazine
(C) Hydrochlorothiazide
(D) Propranolol
(E) Triamterene

36. A 33-year-old woman with diabetes mellitus presents to the physician with loss of vision in both eyes. On physical examination, she is noted to be of tall stature with a lantern jaw, a prominent nose, and supraorbital ridges. She reports excessive sweating and a progressive increase in her ring size. An MRI shows a mass at the base of the patient's brain; a biopsy is performed. Which of the following describes how this biopsied mass would most likely appear on staining?

(A) Acidophilic
(B) Basophilic
(C) Chromophobic
(D) Mixed acidophilic and basophilic
(E) Mixed basophilic and chromophobic

37. A patient undergoes successful radioactive iodine therapy for Graves' disease and returns to a euthyroid state. In a follow-up examination, the patient reports resolution of all prior symptoms except for anxiety and irritability. She also reports frequent muscle spasms. On physical examination, tapping over the facial nerve elicits facial muscle spasm. An ECG shows QT

prolongation. Which of the following most likely describes the current laboratory values of this patient?

Choice	Calcium	Phosphate	Parathyroid Hormone
A	↑	↓	↑
B	↑	↓	↓
C	↓	↑	↑
D	↓	↑	↓
E	Normal	Normal	Normal

(A) A
(B) B
(C) C
(D) D
(E) E

38. A 63-year-old patient using medication to control type 2 diabetes mellitus undergoes an arterial blood gas study that show the following results:

pH: 7.25
P_{O_2}: 90 mm Hg
P_{CO_2}: 28 mm Hg
HCO_3^-: 15 mEq/L
Anion gap: 20 mEq/L

Which of the following agents is the most likely cause of the abnormal blood gas findings?

(A) Acarbose
(B) Glipizide
(C) Metformin
(D) Pioglitazone
(E) Tolbutamide

39. A 65-year-old man comes to the physician because he awakens to urinate several times per night and has developed problems starting and stopping his stream of urine. A biopsy of the prostate shows enlargement and dilation of the prostatic glands but no hyperplasia. Which of the following is the most appropriate pharmacological treatment for this patient?

    (A) Finasteride
    (B) Flutamide
    (C) Ketoconazole
    (D) Spironolactone
    (E) Yohimbine

40. Steroid hormones are unique in that they enter the cell and act directly on the DNA to effect change, rather than acting through intermediary proteins. Which of the following steps in the steroid hormone mechanism is necessary for DNA binding within the nucleus?

    (A) Binding a hormone-specific globulin in plasma
    (B) Binding to DNA enhancer element
    (C) Binding to intracellular receptor
    (D) Exposing the DNA enhancer element
    (E) Transformation of hormone-receptor complex

41. A white, 5-year-old thin boy is brought to the physician complaining of recent weight loss accompanied by excessive hunger, thirst, and urination. His urine is positive for high levels of ketones and glucose. Which of following is the most likely mechanism and associated findings in this disease?

    (A) Autoimmune destruction of the pancreas; association with human leukocyte antigens DR3 and DR4
    (B) Autoimmune inflammation of different locations of the gastrointestinal tract in a skip lesion distribution, usually involving the terminal ileum; association with human leukocyte antigen B27
    (C) Deficiency of a brush border enzyme of the intestinal mucosal cells, causing an inability to break down all of the normally digested carbohydrates

    (D) Increase in the body's resistance to insulin; association with obesity
    (E) Strong genetic predisposition; no association with the human leukocyte antigen system

42. A 56-year-old woman who has type 2 diabetes with recent-onset hypertension comes to the physician because of a rash, changes in taste, and a mild cough. Physical examination shows patchy areas of edema throughout her body. Which of the following medications is the most likely cause of this patient's signs and symptoms?

    (A) Captopril
    (B) Hydrochlorothiazide
    (C) Losartan
    (D) Nifedipine
    (E) Propranolol

43. A 23-year-old nursing student with no significant past medical history comes to the emergency department with light-headedness, nausea, vomiting, and tremors. On physical examination, the patient is tachycardic and diaphoretic. Laboratory studies show a blood glucose level of 30 mg/dL. The patient's symptoms resolve after she drinks a cup of orange juice. Which of the following tests should be ordered to determine whether the student's condition was self-induced?

    (A) Serum B-chain and insulin levels
    (B) Serum C-peptide and insulin levels
    (C) Serum insulin level only
    (D) Serum preproinsulin level
    (E) Serum proinsulin level

44. A 65-year-old man with small cell lung cancer is receiving treatment for ectopic production of ADH. After beginning demeclocycline, he produces large volumes of dilute urine and drinks copious amounts of water. The patient is instructed to not drink any fluid for a 12-hour period. Despite the hold on fluids, the patient continues to produce dilute urine. ADH levels are increased, and serum hyperosmolarity and hypernatremia are noted. Which of the following is the most likely diagnosis?

(A) Nephrogenic diabetes insipidus secondary to demeclocycline treatment

(B) Neurogenic diabetes insipidus secondary to metastatic cancer

(C) Primary hyperaldosteronism

(D) SIADH

(E) Type 2 diabetes mellitus

45. A patient with osteodystrophy of chronic renal disease has abnormal activity of the cell shown in the image. Which of the following hormones plays a key role in stimulating activity of this cell?

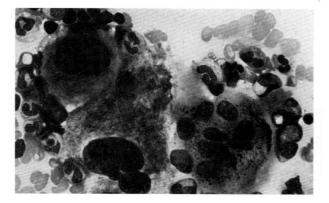

Reproduced, with permission, from Lichtman MA, Beutler E, Kipps TJ, Seligsohn U, Kaushansky K, Prchal JF. *Williams Hematology*, 7th ed. New York, McGraw-Hill, 2006: Plate XV-1.

(A) Angiotensin II

(B) Calcitonin

(C) Parathyroid hormone

(D) Renin

(E) Thyroid hormone

46. Prolactin acts in the negative feedback loop of the hypothalamic-pituitary axis. At which of the following sites does prolactin act?

(A) Inferior hypophyseal artery

(B) Long portal vessels

(C) Neuroendocrine cell nuclei

(D) Superior hypophyseal artery

(E) Trophic hormone–secreting cells of the anterior pituitary

47. A 54-year-old woman presents to the physician with diabetes mellitus, osteoporosis, and hypertension. She has noted a recent weight gain and abdominal striae. Laboratory studies show a decreased ACTH level. A single mass is noted adjacent to the right kidney on abdominal CT scan. Neither low- nor high-dose dexamethasone suppresses the patient's cortisol production. Which of the following is the most likely explanation for these findings?

(A) Adrenal adenoma

(B) Bilateral adrenal hyperplasia

(C) Ectopic ACTH secretion

(D) Exogenous corticosteroid administration

(E) Pituitary adenoma

48. A 60-year-old woman with a 55-pack-year history of smoking presents to the emergency department with nausea and vomiting, headache, malaise, and diffuse aches. A CT scan shows a solitary nodule in the right upper lobe of the lung. Laboratory studies are significant for a serum Ca^{2+} level of 14.2 mg/dL, a serum phosphate level of 1.5 mg/dL, and a serum alkaline phosphatase activity of 81 U/L. The factors that account for this patient's laboratory findings act primarily at which of the following locations?

(A) Adrenal cortex and intestines

(B) Adrenal cortex and renal tubules

(C) Intestines and bones

(D) Renal tubules and bones

(E) Renal tubules and pancreas

49. A 45-year-old man comes to his primary care physician complaining of back pain. On questioning, the patient indicates a recent history of polyuria, polydipsia, hypertension, and weight gain. X-ray film of the spine shows an L4–5 compression fracture. Which of the following is most likely to be elevated in this patient?

(A) Cortisol
(B) Glucagon
(C) Growth hormone
(D) Insulin
(E) Thyroid hormones

50. An 18-year-old woman is referred to a specialist because her periods have stopped. She reports occasional bouts of nausea, vomiting, and generalized weakness. Her blood pressure is 160/99 mm Hg; laboratory studies show a serum K^+ level of 2.2 mEq/L. Her physician remembers that two of the three adrenal hormones are affected in this condition, leaving only one functioning hormone. In which area of the adrenal gland is this one hormone produced?

(A) Capsule
(B) Medulla
(C) Zona fasciculata
(D) Zona glomerulosa
(E) Zona reticularis

1. **The correct answer is A.** This patient presents as a classic case of Graves' disease. The mechanism of Graves' disease centers on thyroid-stimulating IgG antibodies that bind to thyroid-stimulating hormone (TSH) receptors and lead to thyroid hormone production. Similarly, stimulation of the TSH receptor causes glandular hyperplasia and enlargement characteristic of the goiter associated with Graves' disease. Graves' disease is the most common cause of thyrotoxicosis. Patients with this condition may have other autoimmune diseases, such as pernicious anemia or type 1 diabetes mellitus, and frequently present with anxiety, irritability, tremor, heat intolerance with sweaty skin, tachycardia and cardiac palpitations, weight loss, increased appetite, fine hair, diarrhea, and amenorrhea or oligomenorrhea. Other suggestive signs include diffuse goiter, proptosis, periorbital edema, and thickened skin on the lower extremities. Laboratory values are consistent with a hyperthyroid state, with increased thyroid hormone levels and decreased TSH levels.

Answer B is incorrect. Idiopathic replacement of thyroid and surrounding tissue with fibrous tissue is seen in Riedel's thyroiditis; patients can present with dysphagia, stridor, dyspnea, and hypothyroidism, although more than 50% of patients are euthyroid. The disease can mimic thyroid carcinoma, which is high on the list of differential diagnoses for a patient with Riedel's thyroiditis.

Answer C is incorrect. Most thyroid adenomas present as solitary nodules and are usually nonfunctional.

Answer D is incorrect. Thyroid hormone–producing ovarian teratomas are known as struma ovarii, a tumor consisting of thyroid tissue. These tumors can cause hyperthyroidism, but given the patient's history of autoimmune disease, Graves' disease is the better answer choice.

Answer E is incorrect. Viral infections such as mumps or coxsackievirus can lead to destruction of thyroid tissue and granulomatous inflammation, as seen in subacute granulomatous thyroiditis. Patients typically present with flulike symptoms and thyroid tenderness and pain. The disease is typically self-limited and can include a transient hyperthyroid state.

2. **The correct answer is D.** Primary hyperaldosteronism is most commonly caused by an aldosterone-producing adenoma of the adrenal gland. It can also be found in patients with zona glomerulosa hyperplasia. The increased levels of aldosterone lead to hypertension, Na^+ and water retention, and hypokalemia. Increased blood pressure and aldosterone levels can feed back and cause a decreased level of serum renin. Serum renin levels help differentiate between primary hyperaldosteronism, with increased aldosterone and decreased renin levels, and secondary hyperaldosteronism, with increased aldosterone levels and increased renin levels.

Answer A is incorrect. Addison's disease results from adrenal atrophy and causes hypofunction of the adrenal glands. Patients with Addison's disease display signs that are the opposite of those seen in hyperaldosteronism, including hypotension, hyponatremia, and hyperkalemia.

Answer B is incorrect. Patients with hyperthyroidism have heat intolerance, hyperactivity, weight loss, chest pain/palpitations, arrhythmias, diarrhea, hyperreflexia, fine hair, and warm, moist skin.

Answer C is incorrect. Patients with pheochromocytoma have increased levels of epinephrine and norepinephrine, which can lead to elevated blood pressure; however, Na^+, K^+, and renin levels are not affected.

Answer E is incorrect. Lab values in secondary hyperaldosteronism would show hypernatremia and hypokalemia with an increase in renin levels. Secondary hyperaldosteronism occurs in settings in which the kidneys perceive low intravascular volume (renal artery stenosis, chronic renal failure, chronic heart failure, cirrhosis), resulting in an overactive renin-angiotensin system that acts as a stimulus for aldosterone secretion.

3. **The correct answer is B.** This patient has symptoms of a glucagonoma, a rare glucagon-secreting tumor that can cause hyperglycemia, diarrhea, and weight loss. The hyperglycemia seen in these patients will not respond to oral hypoglycemic agents because of the uncontrolled excess glucagon production that continues despite increased insulin levels. Glucagonomas are also associated with necrolytic migratory erythema, a skin rash consisting of painful, pruritic erythematous papules that blister, erode, and crust over.

Answer A is incorrect. Corticosteroid therapy can cause hyperglycemia; however, it is not the best answer choice for this question because it does not satisfactorily explain this patient's pancreatic mass and rash.

Answer C is incorrect. An insulinoma would cause hypoglycemia and not hyperglycemia.

Answer D is incorrect. It is unlikely that a 59-year-old woman would present with type 1 diabetes mellitus. Furthermore, the pancreatic mass and rash cannot be explained by the diagnosis of diabetes mellitus.

Answer E is incorrect. Although VIPomas can cause diarrhea, hyperglycemia, and a pancreatic mass on CT scan, the rash cannot be explained by a diagnosis of VIPoma.

4. **The correct answer is A.** Usually, the thyroid gland develops beneath the tongue, descends along the thyroglossal duct, and eventually resides anterior to the trachea in the neck. Ectopic thyroid tissue may be found anywhere along the course of the duct, including its place of origin—beneath the tongue. This is a common congenital anomaly that does not affect thyroid function, and it should not be removed. Hypersecretion of thyroxine (T_4) from the ectopic gland can result in menstrual abnormalities, including amenorrhea and oligomenorrhea.

Answer B is incorrect. Cold intolerance is characteristic of hypothyroidism, which is a decreased secretion of thyroxine (T_4) from the thyroid gland. Hypersecretion of T_4 would cause heat intolerance, not cold.

Answer C is incorrect. Constipation is characteristic of hypothyroidism, which is a decreased secretion of thyroxine (T_4) from the thyroid gland. Hypersecretion of T_4 is not associated with constipation.

Answer D is incorrect. Hyperlipidemia is characteristic of hypothyroidism, which is a decreased secretion of thyroxine (T_4) from the thyroid gland. Hypersecretion of T_4 is not associated with hyperlipidemia.

Answer E is incorrect. Weight gain is characteristic of hypothyroidism, which is a decreased secretion of thyroxine (T_4) from the thyroid gland. Hypersecretion of T_4 is associated with hypermetabolism and weight loss, not weight gain.

5. **The correct answer is C.** The vignette describes a classic case of type 2 diabetes mellitus: polydipsia, polyuria, and polyphagia in an individual > 40 years old. This condition is due to increased resistance to insulin. The image shows Kimmelstiel-Wilson glomerulosclerosis, which is pathognomonic for diabetes mellitus. These nodules are accumulations of mesangial matrix. Kidneys of diabetic patients also show increased basement membrane thickness and diffuse mesangial matrix proliferation.

Answer A is incorrect. Amyloid deposits are found in renal amyloidosis. The protein is best seen when stained with Congo red. Areas of positive staining are birefringent when viewed with polarized light.

Answer B is incorrect. Crescent formation is an increase in Bowman's capsule epithelial cells. It is classically seen in nephritic syndromes and denotes a poor prognosis.

Answer D is incorrect. Segmental sclerosis is classically seen in focal segmental glomerulosclerosis, a nephrotic syndrome. It is characterized by diffuse infiltration of glomerular capillary tufts with mesangial matrix sclerosis.

Answer E is incorrect. The wire loop abnormality is found in type 4 lupus nephropathy. It is caused by thickening of the glomerular basement membrane in association with accompanying immune complex deposition.

6. **The correct answer is B.** This patient is at risk for prednisone-induced Cushing's syndrome—the most common cause of this disease. Cushing's syndrome is associated with diabetes mellitus, which can be an adverse effect of chronic corticosteroid use owing to decreased glucose tolerance and the counterregulatory action of the hormone.

Answer A is incorrect. Diabetes mellitus, not diabetes insipidus, is an adverse effect of corticosteroids, owing to decreased glucose tolerance and the counterregulatory action of the hormone. Diabetes insipidus can develop due to either pituitary dysfunction (i.e., Sheehan's syndrome) or failure of kidneys to respond to circulating ADH (i.e., renal disease).

Answer C is incorrect. Hyperpigmentation of the skin may develop in a patient with Cushing's disease due to primary pituitary adenoma hypersecretion of ACTH. Elevated ACTH can result in skin hyperpigmentation because of its melanocyte properties. This patient is receiving exogenous corticosteroids; thus, his ACTH levels should be decreased from negative feedback inhibition, and skin hyperpigmentation should not occur.

Answer D is incorrect. Hypertension, not hypotension, is an adverse effect of corticosteroids. This side effect is due to the mineralocorticoid properties of steroids, which lead to increased sodium retention and hence to hypertension.

Answer E is incorrect. Muscle wasting, not muscle hypertrophy, usually develops in Cushing's syndrome due to the catabolic effects of cortisol.

Answer F is incorrect. Sodium retention, not sodium wasting, can be an adverse effect of chronic corticosteroid treatment.

7. **The correct answer is D.** The sensory receptors responsible for transducing the sensation of vibration, pressure, and tension are the large, encapsulated pacinian corpuscles, which are located in the deeper layers of the skin, ligaments, and joint capsules. They can be distinguished histologically by their onionlike appearance on cross section. This patient is presenting with one of the complications of diabetes, neuropathy, and since pacinian corpuscles are responsible for transducing vibratory stimuli, it is these receptors that are involved in this patient's presentation.

Answer A is incorrect. Kraus end bulbs are sensory receptors found in the oropharynx and conjunctiva of the eye.

Answer B is incorrect. Meissner's corpuscles, which are responsible for conveying the sensation of light touch, are small encapsulated sensory receptors found just beneath the dermis of hairless skin, most prominently in the fingertips, soles of the feet, and lips. Meissner's corpuscles are involved in the reception of light discriminatory touch, not vibratory sensation, as is being tested in this case.

Answer C is incorrect. Merkel nerve endings are nonencapsulated and found in all skin types (both hairy and hairless) and, along with Meissner's corpuscles, are believed to be responsible for discriminatory touch.

Answer E is incorrect. Ruffini corpuscles are spindle-shaped, encapsulated mechanoreceptors that are found in the soles of the feet and are responsible for transducing pressure.

8. **The correct answer is E.** This patient had a disulfiramlike reaction after drinking alcohol at a cocktail party. Of the diabetes medications listed, only tolbutamide is associated with causing a disulfiramlike reaction to alcohol consumption.

Answer A is incorrect. Acarbose is an α-glucosidase inhibitor that may cause gastrointestinal disturbances. It does not cause disulfiramlike reactions.

Answer B is incorrect. Glipizide and glyburide are second-generation sulfonylureas that may cause hypoglycemia, but they do not cause disulfiramlike reactions.

Answer C is incorrect. Glyburide and glipizide are second-generation sulfonylureas that may cause hypoglycemia, but they do not cause disulfiramlike reactions.

Answer D is incorrect. Metformin is a hypoglycemic medication used for treatment of type 2 diabetes and can potentially cause lactic acidosis. It does not cause disulfiramlike reactions.

Answer F is incorrect. Troglitazone is a glitazone that may cause weight gain. It does not cause disulfiramlike reactions.

9. **The correct answer is B.** The head of the pancreas and the duodenum share a dual blood supply from the gastroduodenal artery, a branch of the celiac trunk. This artery supplies the anterior and posterior superior pancreaticoduodenal arteries as well as the superior mesenteric artery, which supplies the anterior and posterior inferior pancreaticoduodenal arteries. Therefore, to resect any portion of the duodenum or the head of the pancreas, branches from both the gastroduodenal and superior mesenteric arteries must be ligated.

Answer A is incorrect. While the gastroduodenal artery is an important source of vascular supply to the head of the pancreas, the inferior mesenteric artery does not provide any vascular supply to this structure and thus provides no branches that would need to be ligated to remove the mass described in the question stem.

Answer C is incorrect. Neither the left gastric nor the inferior mesenteric arteries provide any significant arterial supply to the head of the pancreas; thus, no branches from either of these vessels would need to be ligated to complete the resection.

Answer D is incorrect. While the superior mesenteric artery is an important source of vascular supply to the head of the pancreas, the left gastric artery does not provide any vascular supply to this structure and thus provides no branches that would need to be ligated to remove the mass.

Answer E is incorrect. Neither the proper hepatic nor the inferior mesenteric arteries provide any significant arterial supply to the head of the pancreas; thus, no branches from either of these vessels would need to be ligated to complete the resection.

Answer F is incorrect. While the superior mesenteric artery is an important source of vascular supply to the head of the pancreas, the proper hepatic artery does not provide any vascular supply to this structure and therefore provides no branches that would need to be ligated to remove the mass.

10. **The correct answer is C.** This patient presents with acromegaly, the clinical syndrome that is a result of excessive growth hormone (GH) secretion in adults (after closure of the physes). Octreotide is a somatostatin analog that acts at the anterior pituitary to suppress GH secretion, and is used in the treatment of acromegaly. Surgical and radiotherapeutic approaches are also an option, depending on the etiology. Somatostatin is normally secreted by the hypothalamus to help regulate basal GH secretion.

Answer A is incorrect. Finasteride is a 5-α-reductase inhibitor that suppresses the conversion of testosterone to dihydrotestosterone and is used in the treatment of benign prostatic hypertrophy.

Answer B is incorrect. Leuprolide is a gonadotropin-releasing hormone analog that can exhibit both agonist and antagonist actions, depending on the timing of administration. It is used to treat infertility, prostate cancer, and uterine fibroids. Adverse effects include antiandrogen actions (e.g., gynecomastia, decreased libido), nausea, and vomiting.

Answer D is incorrect. Like somatrem, recombinant growth hormone (GH) is useful in the treatment of GH deficiency, but would exacerbate the condition of a patient with acromegaly.

Answer E is incorrect. Somatrem is a somatotropin, or growth hormone (GH) analog, that stimulates the release of somatomedin/insulin-like growth factor-1 from the liver and is useful in the treatment of GH deficiency. It would exacerbate the condition of a patient with acromegaly.

11. **The correct answer is E.** The question stem describes a family of patients that is likely afflicted with one of the multiple endocrine neoplasia (MEN) syndromes. A pheochromocytoma is one of the tumors associated with MEN type 2 and should be considered given his clinical and family history.

Answer A is incorrect. Acromegaly can lead to headaches, however it does not commonly cause palpitations and is not associated with multiple endocrine neoplasia. Clinical signs of acromegaly include coarse facies, enlarged tongue, and increased size of hands and feet.

Answer B is incorrect. An ACTH-secreting pituitary adenoma, which defines Cushing's disease, would cause hypercortisolemia secondary to ACTH stimulation from the anterior pituitary, with elevated serum ACTH levels.

Answer C is incorrect. Up to 80% of patients with hyperparathyroidism are asymptomatic at diagnosis, and their disease is caught by routine blood tests. Some have nonspecific symptoms such as fatigue, mild depression, and anorexia. If severe, metastatic calcification and osteoclastic bone lesions can occur.

Answer D is incorrect. A nonfunctioning pituitary adenoma could account for the undetectable serum ACTH, but such a case would generally be accompanied by hypocortisolemia due to a lack of ACTH stimulation.

12. **The correct answer is A.** In addition to being necessary to normal human growth and development, GH is critical in the stress response to starvation. GH is released in response to hypoglycemia and acts directly to decrease glucose uptake by cells and increase lipolysis, resulting in an increase in blood sugar levels.

Answer B is incorrect. GH secretion is not stimulated by obesity, but rather is reduced by this condition.

Answer C is incorrect. Pregnancy is not a stimulus for GH secretion. Rather, GH secretion actually decreases in pregnancy.

Answer D is incorrect. Somatomedins, or insulin-like growth factors, are secreted by the liver in response to GH and mediate the metabolic changes necessary for growth and development. These intermediaries also act on the hypothalamus and the anterior pituitary via a negative feedback mechanism to reduce GH secretion.

Answer E is incorrect. Somatostatin is not a stimulus for GH secretion but rather is a component of the negative feedback system that regulates GH secretion. Somatostatin is secreted by the hypothalamus in response to stimulation by insulin-like growth factors/somatomedins and acts on the anterior pituitary to reduce GH secretion.

13. **The correct answer is B.** Parathyroid chief cells are small, pale cells with round central nuclei. These cells secrete parathyroid hormone, which raises serum Ca^{2+} levels in three ways: (1) it acts directly on bone to increase osteoclastic resorption; (2) it acts directly on the kidney to increase resorption of calcium and inhibit resorption of phosphate; and (3) it promotes gastrointestinal absorption of calcium via increased levels of activated vitamin D.

Answer A is incorrect. Adipose tissue in the parathyroid gland increases with age but does not secrete hormones related to calcium regulation. The cells contain large vacuoles that appear white on hematoxylin and eosin stain.

Answer C is incorrect. Parathyroid oxyphil cells tend to occur in nodules and have abundant eosinophilic cytoplasm. They are larger than chief cells and do not secrete parathyroid hormone.

Answer D is incorrect. Thyroid C cells secrete calcitonin, which decreases bone resorption of calcium, leading to a decrease in serum calcium levels. C cells are distinguished by their extensive clear cytoplasm. Think "C" for "Clear Cytoplasm."

Answer E is incorrect. Thyroid follicular cells are simple cuboidal cells that line colloid follicles. They are responsible for the synthesis and secretion of triiodothyronine and thyroxine.

14. **The correct answer is B.** This vignette is most consistent with a syndrome of inappropriate secretion of ADH due to a lung neoplasm. ADH is secreted by the posterior pituitary and stimulates the expression of aquaporins in the renal collecting ducts, resulting in transport of water into the renal medulla from the ductal lumen and hence water retention in the kidneys. When levels of this hormone are inappropriately elevated, excessive water retention results in hyponatremia, which can lead to seizures. ADH can be produced ectopically in the setting of malignancy, classically by small cell lung cancer.

Answer A is incorrect. ACTH can be produced ectopically in the setting of malignancy, especially small cell lung cancer. However, excessive levels of ACTH would result in Cushing's syndrome, and the vignette provides no symptoms or signs that would be consistent with this condition.

Answer C is incorrect. Parathyroid hormone (PTH) can be produced ectopically in the setting of malignancy and is associated with a variety of neoplasia, including squamous cell lung cancer, breast cancer, and multiple myeloma. However, excessive levels of PTH would result in hypercalcemia, and the vignette does not provide any indication (circumoral paresthesias, Chvostek's and Trousseau's signs) that would be most consistent with this condition. Note that these symptoms can also occur in the setting of malignancy due to production of PTH-related peptide by tumor cells.

Answer D is incorrect. Hyperreninemia does not typically occur as paraneoplastic syndrome and would generally cause hyperaldosteronism, resulting in hypernatremia and hy-

pokalemia. While seizures can be a consequence of severe hypernatremia, the vignette does not mention any signs or symptoms of hypokalemia (nausea, vomiting, muscle weakness, cardiac dysrhythmias).

Answer E is incorrect. Tumor necrosis factor-α can be produced ectopically in the setting of malignancy and parallels parathyroid hormone both in causing secondary hypercalcemia and in the cancers with which excessive production is associated.

15. **The correct answer is C.** The vignette describes a classic history for hypothyroidism caused by Hashimoto's thyroiditis. This primary hypothyroidism is characterized by reduced secretion of thyroid hormone, resulting in decreased levels of free and total thyroxine (T_4) and increased levels of TSH due to the absence of negative feedback by T_4.

Answer A is incorrect. In the setting of a primary hypothyroidism, both total and free thyroxine levels should be decreased rather than increased.

Answer B is incorrect. Both total and free thyroxine (T_4) levels should be decreased rather than increased in setting of primary hypothyroidism. An elevated T_4 would otherwise result in decreased rather than increased TSH levels due to negative feedback. Furthermore, free and total T_4 levels should vary in the same direction in this setting, as there is no change in the binding capacity of the proteins in the blood.

Answer D is incorrect. Hashimoto's thyroiditis indicates that both total and free T_4 levels should be decreased rather than increased, while TSH levels should be increased rather than decreased. Furthermore, free and total thyroxine levels should vary in the same direction in this setting, as there is no change in the binding capacity of the proteins in the blood.

Answer E is incorrect. In a primary hypothyroidism such as Hashimoto's thyroiditis, the reduction of free and total thyroxine levels in the blood should eliminate feedback inhibition of

TSH secretion, leading to increased rather than decreased TSH levels in the blood.

16. **The correct answer is A.** In all forms of pseudohypoparathyroidism, there is a defect in the peripheral organ response to parathyroid hormone (PTH), leading to increased PTH levels. There are several types of pseudohypoparathyroidism, which vary in clinical presentation. In type I pseudohypoparathyroidism, there is a diminished cAMP response to PTH due to mutations in the stimulatory Gs-α-one protein of the adenylyl cyclase complex (GNAS1). In the majority of cases, type I pseudohypoparathyroidism is inherited in an autosomal dominant manner; the clinical presentation varies depending on whether or not the mutated gene is on the maternally or paternally derived chromosome, due to tissue-specific genetic imprinting. Maternally derived GNAS1 is necessary to get a renal response to PTH, while both maternally and paternally derived GNAS1 seems to be necessary to get negative feedback in the parathyroid gland and to get normal bone response to PTH. This patient has pseudohypoparathyroidism type Ia, which results when the mutated GNAS1 is derived from the maternal chromosome, leading to both the signs and symptoms of hypocalcemia and a pattern of skeletal abnormalities, including round facies, short stature, and short metacarpal and metatarsal bones. In type Ib pseudohypoparathyroidism, the mutated gene is derived from the paternal chromosome and thus the renal response to PTH is intact. These patients often have skeletal abnormalities without hypocalcemia.

Answer B is incorrect. Type I pseudohypoparathyroidism follows an autosomal dominant mode of inheritance.

Answer C is incorrect. Type I pseudohypoparathyroidism follows an autosomal dominant mode of inheritance.

Answer D is incorrect. Type I pseudohypoparathyroidism follows an autosomal dominant mode of inheritance.

Answer E is incorrect. Type I pseudohypoparathyroidism follows an autosomal dominant mode of inheritance.

17. **The correct answer is C.** The hypophyseal portal system allows delivery of trophic hormone-releasing hormones (growth hormone-releasing hormone, corticotropin-releasing hormone, thyrotropin-releasing hormone, and gonadotropin-releasing hormone) from the neuroendocrine cells in the arcuate nucleus of the hypothalamus directly to the trophic hormone-producing cells of the anterior pituitary gland. The portal system keeps these hypothalamic hormones from being diluted in the systemic circulation before reaching their target tissue.

Answer A is incorrect. The cells of the pituitary gland do not carry out any processing of hypothalamic hormones. The posterior pituitary serves as a storage site for ADH and oxytocin, which are synthesized in the hypothalamic supraoptic and paraventricular nuclei and are transported to the posterior pituitary via the supraopticohypophyseal tract.

Answer B is incorrect. The supraopticohypophyseal tract is the conduit through which the ADH and oxytocin, both produced in the hypothalamus, are delivered to the posterior pituitary for storage and later release. Note that this circuit does not involve any vascular structures.

Answer D is incorrect. Hormones are delivered from the anterior pituitary to the hypothalamus via the systemic circulation, just as they are delivered to other tissues. This process does not involve the hypophyseal portal system.

Answer E is incorrect. Trophic hormones of the hypothalamic-pituitary axis (growth hormone, ACTH, thyroid-stimulating hormone, luteinizing hormone, and follicle-stimulating hormone) are synthesized and secreted by the anterior pituitary gland in response to hormonal stimulation by the hypothalamus, but they are not produced in the hypothalamus.

These hormones are secreted from the pituitary into the systemic circulation.

18. **The correct answer is E.** The actions of insulin are mediated at the cellular level by binding of the insulin to its receptor followed by autophosphorylation of tyrosine residues on the insulin receptor; this generates a tyrosine kinase that participates in an intracellular signaling cascade. Inhibition of tyrosine kinase function would preclude downstream signaling and block the physiologic changes associated with insulin action, regardless of the amount of insulin present in the blood.

Answer A is incorrect. Adenylate cyclase and its product, cAMP, are involved in numerous important intracellular signaling systems, including the systems that mediate autonomic sympathetic nervous stimulation, ADH action, renal Ca^{2+} and phosphate transport, and glucagon action. However, adenylate cyclase and cAMP are not involved in the system that mediates insulin action.

Answer B is incorrect. Guanylate cyclase and its product, cGMP, are involved in many intracellular signaling systems, including those that mediate the transduction of visual stimuli into electrical signals in the nervous system and the relaxation of vascular smooth muscle throughout the body. However, guanylate cyclase and cGMP are not involved in the system that mediates insulin action.

Answer C is incorrect. Serine kinases are involved in a number of intracellular signaling cascades, but they are not involved in the signaling cascade that mediates insulin action.

Answer D is incorrect. Threonine kinases are involved in a number of intracellular signaling cascades, but they are not involved in the signaling cascade that mediates insulin action.

19. **The correct answer is A.** Acarbose is an α-glucosidase inhibitor that decreases the hydrolysis and absorption of disaccharides and polysaccharides at the intestinal brush border, thereby reducing postprandial hyperglycemia. This class of agents can be employed as monotherapy or in combination with oral hypoglycemic medications in the management of type 2 diabetes mellitus. These agents commonly cause gastrointestinal adverse effects that include abdominal cramps, diarrhea, and flatulence.

Answer B is incorrect. Chlorpropamide is a sulfonylurea that acts via stimulation of insulin secretion by the pancreas. Hypoglycemia is the most important adverse effect of this drug, but chlorpropamide can also cause disulfiramlike adverse effects. This agent is generally not known to cause significant gastrointestinal disturbances.

Answer C is incorrect. Glipizide is a sulfonylurea that acts via stimulation of insulin secretion by the pancreas. Hypoglycemia is the most important side effect of this drug. Glipizide is generally not known to cause significant gastrointestinal disturbances.

Answer D is incorrect. Metformin inhibits gluconeogenesis, thus reducing blood sugar levels. The most important side effect of this agent is lactic acidosis. Metformin can sometimes cause loose bowel movements but is generally not associated with increased flatulence.

Answer E is incorrect. Troglitazone sensitizes the peripheral tissues to insulin action and is typically associated with weight gain and hepatotoxicity as adverse effects. Gastrointestinal disturbances are not characteristic of this agent or other agents in the same class.

20. **The correct answer is B.** Bitemporal hemianopsia (due to compression of the optic nerves at the chiasm) and diminished libido are common presenting symptoms of pituitary tumors in men. The MRI shows a pituitary adenoma (see *arrowheads*). When these adenomas become large enough, they exert mass effect on the second cranial nerves at the chiasm. Growth hormone (GH)–secreting pituitary adenomas are slow-growing and often go undiagnosed for several years. GH hypersecretion is associated with acromegaly, resulting in bone overgrowth with increased hand and foot size, soft tissue swelling, oily skin, and proximal muscle weakness.

Answer A is incorrect. ACTH-secreting pituitary adenomas account for 70% of cases of Cushing's syndrome. Cortisol excess leads to thin skin, central obesity, hypertension, "moon facies," glucose intolerance, and osteoporosis. ACTH-secreting tumors are typically smaller than 5 mm, and half are undetectable on MRI, rendering the diagnosis a clinical one.

Answer C is incorrect. Gonadotropin-secreting tumors are typically nonfunctioning. These are as common as prolactinomas and are generally diagnosed late because there are few symptoms until mass effect occurs.

Answer D is incorrect. Causes of hyperprolactinemia in men include medications, primary hypothyroidism, and chest wall stimulation (from trauma or herpes zoster reactivation). The diagnosis of idiopathic hyperprolactinemia is made by exclusion of known causes. Forty percent of all pituitary tumors are prolactinomas.

Answer E is incorrect. Thyroid-stimulating hormone–secreting tumors are rare. Patients present with goiter and hyperthyroidism.

21. **The correct answer is C.** Papillary thyroid carcinoma is the most common type of thyroid cancer. It is always distinguished by its fingerlike projections of epithelium surrounding a central fibrovascular core, calcified spheres (psammoma bodies), "Orphan Annie" nuclei, and molding of the nuclei. A prior history of radiation to the neck is often present in the patient. It carries a better prognosis than the other forms of thyroid cancer.

Answer A is incorrect. In follicular thyroid cancer, one would not expect to see a papillary arrangement such as that described in the stem. Instead, one should see uniform follicles containing homogeneous colloid. The presence of psammoma bodies, classically found in papillary thyroid cancer, makes it less likely that this is a follicular carcinoma. This type of cancer carries a worse prognosis than papillary thyroid carcinoma.

Answer B is incorrect. The classic description for medullary thyroid carcinoma is sheets of tu-

mor cells in an amyloid-containing stroma. This type of cancer arises from the C cells of the thyroid, which, due to their calcitonin production, results in hypocalcemia in the patient.

Answer D is incorrect. Although Riedel's thyroiditis can clinically mimic carcinoma, it is not a malignancy. Histologically, the thyroid appears to have been replaced by fibrous tissue.

Answer E is incorrect. Subacute thyroiditis (also known as de Quervain's thyroiditis) is not a malignancy but rather a self-limited inflammation of the thyroid lasting several weeks. It is often accompanied by flulike symptoms, tenderness of the thyroid gland, and a transient hyperthyroidism. Histologically, one would see destruction of thyroid tissue and granulomatous inflammation.

22. **The correct answer is C.** Achondroplasia is due to a defect in the fibroblast growth factor receptor 3. It results in short limbs with a normal-sized head and trunk.

Answer A is incorrect. Diabetes insipidus (DI) can be defined as the inability to concentrate urine due either to lack of antidiuretic hormone (ADH) production (central DI), or to lack of renal response to ADH (nephrogenic DI). In nephrogenic DI, the ADH receptor is ineffective.

Answer B is incorrect. A defective dihydrotestosterone receptor is seen in testicular feminization syndrome (XY-appearing female).

Answer D is incorrect. Type 2 diabetes mellitus is thought to be partially due to insensitivity of the insulin receptor.

Answer E is incorrect. A defective LDL receptor is seen in familial hypercholesterolemia.

23. **The correct answer is B.** The right adrenal gland is drained via the right adrenal vein, which flows directly into the inferior vena cava (IVC). Thus, a right-sided hyperfunctioning adrenal adenoma is drained via the right adrenal vein into the IVC. In contrast, the left

adrenal gland is drained via the left adrenal vein into the left renal vein, which then flows into the IVC.

Answer A is incorrect. The abdominal aorta plays no role in the vascular drainage of any organ but rather provides arterial supply to the abdominal organs, including the kidneys and adrenals glands.

Answer C is incorrect. The portal vein is superior and anterior to the adrenal and renal vasculature and is not involved in the drainage of either of the adrenal glands. Instead, it drains most of the gastrointestinal tract down to the rectum into the liver.

Answer D is incorrect. The right gonadal vein drains the testes or ovaries directly into the inferior vena cava but does not drain the right adrenal gland in either sex.

Answer E is incorrect. Drainage of the right adrenal gland and hence a right-sided adrenal adenoma does not flow through the right renal vein, but instead the adrenal vein flows directly into the inferior vena cava.

24. **The correct answer is A.** This vignette describes a patient with classic symptoms and signs of hypocalcemia. All of these findings can be attributed to the physiologic effects of calcitonin. Calcitonin is normally secreted in response to elevated levels of serum Ca^{2+} and causes decreased bone resorption of Ca^{2+}, resulting in lower serum Ca^{2+} levels.

Answer B is incorrect. Parathyroid hormone (PTH) acts to increase serum Ca^{2+} and phosphate levels by increasing bone resorption and renal reabsorption of Ca^{2+}. Additionally, PTH-related peptide stimulates conversion of inactive 25-OH vitamin D to active 1,25-OH vitamin D, resulting in hypercalcemia rather than hypocalcemia.

Answer C is incorrect. Parathyroid hormone–related peptide (PTHrP) acts like parathyroid hormone (PTH) to increase serum Ca^{2+} and phosphate levels by increasing bone resorption and renal reabsorption of Ca^{2+}. Additionally, PTHrP stimulates conversion of inactive 25-OH vitamin D to active 1,25-OH vitamin D,

resulting in hypercalcemia rather than hypocalcemia. Metastatic small cell lung cancer can plausibly account for a nodule palpable in the neck and is generally associated with paraneoplastic hypercalcemia secondary to elaboration of PTHrP.

Answer D is incorrect. Thyroxine is generally not known to significantly affect serum Ca^{2+} levels. Therefore, excess thyroxine would not be expected to cause hypocalcemia. The functions of thyroxine are summarized by the "**4 B's**": **B**rain maturation, **B**one growth, β-adrenergic effects, and increase **B**asal metabolic rate.

Answer E is incorrect. Vitamin D stimulates Ca^{2+} and phosphate absorption from the intestines and increases bone resorption, resulting in increased serum Ca^{2+} and phosphate levels. Hence, excess vitamin D would result in hypercalcemia rather than hypocalcemia, with nonspecific symptoms of hypercalcemia such as malaise, fatigue, depression, and diffuse aches and pains. Hypercalcemia and hypophosphatemia are evident on laboratory evaluation.

25. **The correct answer is B.** This vignette describes leiomyomas, or fibroids, which are most often seen in African-American women. These tumors are benign and usually present with menstrual pain and menorrhagia (increased bleeding). They are estrogen-sensitive, increasing in size during pregnancy, and decreasing with menopause. As their name suggests, leiomyomas are composed of muscle fibers; thus, the appropriate stain is desmin.

Answer A is incorrect. Cytokeratin staining would be most appropriate for epithelial cells.

Answer C is incorrect. Glial fibrillary acid protein staining would be most appropriate for neuroglia.

Answer D is incorrect. Neurofilament staining would be most appropriate for neurons.

Answer E is incorrect. Vimentin staining would be most appropriate for connective tissue.

26. The correct answer is A. This patient has Graves' disease, an autoimmune disorder resulting from IgG-type autoantibodies to the thyroid-stimulating hormone receptor. The three classic findings associated with Graves' disease are hyperthyroidism, ophthalmopathy, and dermopathy/pretibial myxedema.

Answer B is incorrect. Hashimoto's thyroiditis is an autoimmune disorder characterized by antibodies attacking thyroglobulin or thyroid peroxidase—the two most common autoantibodies in these patients—or antibodies against another part of the thyroid or thyroid hormone synthesis pathway. Although some cases of Hashimoto's thyroiditis may present as a transient hyperthyroidism (with symptoms including palpitations and increased metabolic rate) from an initial disruption of thyroid follicles, the majority of cases present with signs and symptoms of hypothyroidism, such as intolerance to cold weather, weight gain, and mental and physical slowness.

Answer C is incorrect. Iodine deficiency causes hypothyroidism, manifested with signs and symptoms that include intolerance to cold weather, weight gain, and mental and physical slowness.

Answer D is incorrect. Papillary carcinoma of the thyroid, the most common form of thyroid cancer, usually presents as an asymptomatic thyroid nodule with signs of obstruction from the tumor such as hoarseness, cough, dysphagia, or dyspnea or a cervical lymph node mass (as opposed to symptoms of hyper- or hypothyroidism).

Answer E is incorrect. Plummer's disease is characterized by a nodular goiter that has a hyperfunctioning nodule, causing hyperthyroidism. As opposed to Graves' disease, Plummer's disease is not accompanied by ophthalmopathy or dermopathy/pretibial myxedema.

27. The correct answer is D. This patient has Hashimoto's thyroiditis, an autoimmune disorder in which patients have antibodies attacking thyroglobulin, thyroid peroxidase, or another part of the thyroid gland or thyroid hormone synthesis pathway. In this case, antibodies are binding to endogenous thyroid peroxidase, inhibiting thyroid peroxidase from catalyzing several steps of the thyroid hormone synthesis pathway. This results in a state of hypothyroidism, producing the clinical signs and symptoms seen in this patient. The anterior neck swelling that resolved on its own may have represented a goiter from a transient state of hyperthyroidism during the initial disease process, but more clinical information would be needed to make this determination.

Answer A is incorrect. This is not an accurate description of how elevated thyroid peroxidase antibodies lead to Hashimoto's thyroiditis.

Answer B is incorrect. This is not an accurate description of how elevated thyroid peroxidase antibodies lead to Hashimoto's thyroiditis.

Answer C is incorrect. This is not an accurate description of how elevated thyroid peroxidase antibodies lead to Hashimoto's thyroiditis. The mechanism stated in this answer describes the process by which thyroid-stimulating immunoglobulins (NOT thyroid peroxidase antibodies) cause the hyperthyroidism in Graves' disease.

Answer E is incorrect. This is not an accurate description of how elevated thyroid peroxidase antibodies lead to Hashimoto's thyroiditis.

28. The correct answer is A. This patient's laboratory values are consistent with Addison's disease, a primary deficiency of aldosterone and cortisol due to adrenal hypofunction. This condition leads to hypotension and skin hyperpigmentation. Lack of aldosterone production results in the electrolyte imbalance seen in this patient's laboratory values, which then leads to hypotension. ACTH levels increase due to the loss of negative feedback from low cortisol levels. Adrenal atrophy can be due to a number of causes, including autoimmune destruction, infection, and adrenal hemorrhage. Tuberculosis was at one time the most common cause of primary adrenocortical insufficiency.

Answer B is incorrect. An adrenal adenoma producing cortisol would also lead to signs and symptoms consistent with Cushing's syndrome.

Answer C is incorrect. Ectopic ACTH production, as seen in the paraneoplastic syndrome associated with small cell lung cancer, would likely lead to increased, rather than decreased, levels of cortisol production. This would result in signs and symptoms consistent with Cushing's syndrome, including hypertension and weight gain.

Answer D is incorrect. Patients with hemochromatosis can also have changes in skin pigmentation due to deposition of hemosiderin in the skin. Hemochromatosis is associated with a triad of conditions consisting of micronodular pigment cirrhosis, bronze diabetes, and skin pigmentation. Hemochromatosis is not likely to cause the laboratory values seen in this patient. The mnemonic for hemochromatosis is "a tan man with diabetes."

Answer E is incorrect. Pituitary corticotropin insufficiency is an example of secondary adrenocortical insufficiency. Patients with pituitary insufficiency would likely have decreased cortisol and ACTH levels. Secondary insufficiency usually results in less mineralocorticoid malfunction and less, if any, change in skin pigmentation.

29. **The correct answer is D.** Chromaffin cells are neuroendocrine cells derived from the embryonic neural crest. They are found in the medulla of the adrenal gland and in sympathetic nervous system ganglia. Chromaffin cells of the adrenal medulla are innervated by the splanchnic nerve and secrete epinephrine, norepinephrine, and enkephalin into the bloodstream. They derive their name from their ability to be visualized by staining with chromium salts. These cells have large nuclei and are strongly basophilic, in contrast to the more eosinophilic zona reticularis cells. They contain little endoplasmic reticulum and no stored lipid. Norepinephrine-secreting cells are distinguished from epinephrine-secreting cells by virtue of having dense core granules and a more strongly positive chromaffin reaction.

Answer A is incorrect. Aldosterone is secreted by zona glomerulosa cells, which are arranged in irregular ovoid clusters. These cells have round, strongly stained nuclei. The cytoplasm is acidophilic and contains abundant smooth endoplasmic reticulum and mitochondria. Glomerulosa cells contain less lipid and cytoplasm than cells of the zona fasciculata.

Answer B is incorrect. Androgens are secreted by cells in the zona reticularis, the innermost zone of the adrenal cortex. This zone is composed of an irregular network of branching cords and clusters of cells. There are few lipid droplets, and hematoxylin and eosin stains reveal the brown pigment lipofuscin.

Answer C is incorrect. Cortisol is secreted by cells of the zona fasciculata in the adrenal cortex. This zone is the middle and the broadest of the three cortical zones. It is identified histologically by radially arranged cords of single cell width. These cells have abundant, poorly staining cytoplasm and are rich in mitochondria and lipid droplets.

30. **The correct answer is C.** Thyroid hormones act via a nuclear hormone receptor. On binding with its ligand, the receptor translocates from the cytoplasm to the cell nucleus, and the ligand-receptor complex acts as a transcription factor. This results in gene transcription and new protein synthesis. This answer is the only one that involves assessment of gene transcription, and thus represents the only selection that refers to a nuclear hormone receptor mechanism. Furthermore, an important function of thyroid hormones is increasing basal metabolic rate, which is mediated by increasing Na^+/K^+-ATPase expression and activity. Other hormones that act through nuclear steroid hormone receptors include cortisol, aldosterone, vitamin D, testosterone, estrogen, and progesterone.

Answer A is incorrect. Adenylate cyclase and cAMP are critical in the mechanism of a number of different hormones, including glucagon, histamine, epinephrine, dopamine, and vasopressin. However, adenylate cyclase and cAMP are not important in the mechanism of thyroid hormones and other steroid hormones.

Answer B is incorrect. Increases in intracellular Ca^{2+} levels are important in the mechanism of hormones such as norepinephrine, histamine, and vasopressin but are not important in the mechanism of thyroid hormones and other steroid hormones.

Answer D is incorrect. Activation of phospholipase C, resulting in the cleavage of phosphatidylinositol diphosphate into inositol triphosphate and diacylglycerol, is important in the mechanism of several hormones, including histamine and vasopressin, but is not important in the mechanism of thyroid hormones and other steroid hormones.

Answer E is incorrect. Phosphorylation of IRS-1 is important in the mechanism of intracellular insulin action via a tyrosine kinase cascade. Tyrosine kinases are not important in the mechanism of thyroid hormones and other steroid hormones.

31. **The correct answer is C.** ADH and oxytocin are synthesized by the neurons of the supraoptic and paraventricular nuclei, respectively, in the hypothalamus and are transported to the posterior pituitary gland via the supraopticohypophysial tract, where they are stored and eventually released into the capillaries that drain into the hypophysial vein. Oxytocin facilitates milk secretion but not synthesis. It also stimulates uterine contractions during parturition. ADH mediates water absorption in the renal collecting ducts via translocation of aquaporins, thus concentrating the urine. Oxytocin facilitates milk secretion but not synthesis. It also stimulates uterine contractions during parturition.

Answer A is incorrect. Milk synthesis is mediated by prolactin, which is secreted by the anterior pituitary. It would likely be deficient due to impingement of an adenoma on this gland.

Milk synthesis would likely be impaired in such a case.

Answer B is incorrect. Ovulation is stimulated by the surge of luteinizing hormone (LH) just prior to the midpoint of the menstrual cycle. LH is secreted by the anterior pituitary and would likely be deficient due to impingement of an adenoma on the LH-secreting cells of this gland. Ovulation would likely be impaired in such a case.

Answer D is incorrect. Salt retention is a primary action of aldosterone, which acts at the renal distal tubules to increase sodium and chloride reabsorption as well as increase potassium secretion. Aldosterone is produced in a multistep pathway from cholesterol, along with cortisol and the androgens, in response to ACTH stimulation. ACTH is secreted by the anterior pituitary and would likely be deficient due to impingement of an adenoma on this gland.

Answer E is incorrect. Spermatogenesis is stimulated by follicle-stimulating hormone (FSH), which is secreted by the anterior pituitary and would likely be deficient due to impingement of an adenoma on the FSH-secreting cells of this gland. Hence, spermatogenesis would likely be impaired in such a case.

32. **The correct answer is A.** The patient has tumors involving the "3 P's" of multiple endocrine neoplasia (MEN) type 1, also known as Werner's syndrome. Her galactorrhea is likely due to a prolactin-secreting pituitary tumor, and her hypercalcemia is likely due to a parathyroid adenoma. Her recurrent duodenal ulcers are a manifestation of a gastrin-secreting tumor frequently located in the pancreas, as seen in Zollinger-Ellison syndrome. The genetic inheritance of MEN 1 is autosomal dominant, as one would expect if multiple maternal family members are also affected by this disorder.

Answer B is incorrect. Multiple endocrine neoplasia 1 is not inherited in an autosomal recessive pattern.

Answer C is incorrect. Multiple endocrine neoplasia I is not inherited in a mitochondrial pattern.

Answer D is incorrect. Multiple endocrine neoplasia I is not inherited in an X-linked dominant pattern.

Answer E is incorrect. Multiple endocrine neoplasia I is not inherited in an X-linked recessive pattern.

33. **The correct answer is D.** This patient presents with thyrotoxicosis, which can result due to excess endogenous or exogenous thyroid hormone. Levothyroxine is a synthetic form of thyroxine that is used in the treatment of hypothyroidism. Excessively high serum levels of levothyroxine result in symptoms of thyrotoxicosis, including those described in the vignette as well as heat intolerance, unexplained weight loss, agitation, and confusion.

    Answer A is incorrect. Dobutamine is a β-adrenergic agonist that is useful in the acute treatment of congestive heart failure. While the effects of this drug can mimic the symptoms and signs of thyrotoxicosis, this agent cannot account for the gastrointestinal symptoms, the weight loss, and the heat intolerance that are characteristic symptoms of thyrotoxicosis.

    Answer B is incorrect. Pharmacologic doses of iodide are used in the treatment of hyperthyroidism; they inhibit the synthesis of thyroid hormone and the release of preformed thyroid hormone. Iodide is administered orally, and adverse effects include sore mouth and throat, rashes, ulcerations of mucous membranes, and a metallic taste in the mouth, but not thyrotoxicosis.

    Answer C is incorrect. Leuprolide is a gonadotropin-releasing hormone analog that can exhibit both agonist and antagonist actions, depending on the timing of administration. It is used to treat infertility, prostate cancer, and uterine fibroids. Adverse effects include antiandrogen actions (e.g., gynecomastia, decreased libido), nausea, and vomiting.

    Answer E is incorrect. Propylthiouracil, which inhibits the synthesis of thyroxine (T_4) and the peripheral conversion of T_4 to tri-iodothyronine, is used in the treatment of hyperthyroidism. Rare toxicities due to this agent include agranulocytosis, rash, and edema.

34. **The correct answer is A.** Diabetes insipidus is characterized by an inability of the kidney to concentrate urine effectively. Concentration of urine is normally controlled by ADH, which regulates water pores in the renal collecting duct. Central diabetes insipidus results from decreased ADH levels, whereas nephrogenic diabetes insipidus results from a decrease in the kidney's ability to respond to ADH. In either condition, thirst and resulting polydipsia are caused by increased levels of plasma sodium and osmolarity. This change in osmolarity occurs due to loss of free water in the form of hypotonic urine. Since this patient's plasma osmolarity is 290 mOsm/L, only a urine osmolarity less than this value would indicate a hypotonic urine and diabetes insipidus. The correct answer from these choices is therefore 100 mOsm/L.

    Answer B is incorrect. Because this patient's plasma osmolarity is 290 mOsm/L, only a urine osmolarity less than this value would indicate a hypotonic urine and diabetes insipidus.

    Answer C is incorrect. Because this patient's plasma osmolarity is 290 mOsm/L, only a urine osmolarity less than this value would indicate a hypotonic urine and diabetes insipidus.

    Answer D is incorrect. Because this patient's plasma osmolarity is 290 mOsm/L, only a urine osmolarity less than this value would indicate a hypotonic urine and diabetes insipidus.

    Answer E is incorrect. Because this patient's plasma osmolarity is 290 mOsm/L, only a urine osmolarity less than this value would indicate a hypotonic urine and diabetes insipidus.

35. **The correct answer is D.** This patient is most likely hypoglycemic. Normally, hypoglycemia causes an increased sympathetic tone resulting

in tachycardia, diaphoresis, tremor, and anxiety. Diabetic patients who are on β-blockers are unable to produce this sympathetic response, which makes it difficult to recognize the onset of hypoglycemia. Sulfonylureas, such as glyburide and glipizide, are known for causing hypoglycemia—more than other agents, such as metformin.

Answer A is incorrect. Enalapril is an angiotensin-converting enzyme inhibitor that may lead to cough, hypotension, and edema. Adverse events include dizziness and possible syncope, but not agitation or confusion.

Answer B is incorrect. Hydralazine is used to treat severe hypertension and may cause tachycardia and fluid retention.

Answer C is incorrect. Hydrochlorothiazide toxicity includes hyperglycemia, hyperlipidemia, hyperuricemia, and hypercalcemia.

Answer E is incorrect. Triamterene is a potassium-sparing diuretic that may lead to hyperkalemia, which presents with cardiac manifestations.

36. **The correct answer is A.** The patient is showing signs and symptoms of acromegaly. On further testing, the bilateral vision loss is likely to be a bitemporal hemianopsia from the growth hormone (GH)-secreting adenoma compressing the optic chiasm. GH-secreting tumors cause gigantism if the epiphyses have not closed, as in children, and cause acromegaly in adults. Other characteristics of acromegaly include coarse features such as enlarged jaw, face, hands, and feet. Osteoporosis, hyperglycemia, and hypertension may also be associated with excess GH secretion. This second most common pituitary tumor is composed of acidophilic-staining cells.

Answer B is incorrect. Basophilic-staining cells of the pituitary gland can be remembered by the mnemonic "**B-FLAT** Major": Basophilic = FSH, LH, ACTH, TSH, MSH.

Answer C is incorrect. Chromophobic-staining cells of the pituitary gland include prolactin-producing cells.

Answer D is incorrect. A growth hormone–secreting adenoma would not be expected to consist of mixed acidophilic and basophilic components.

Answer E is incorrect. A growth hormone–secreting adenoma would not be expected to consist of mixed basophilic and chromophobic components.

37. **The correct answer is D.** Other causes of hypoparathyroidism include thyroidectomy, metastatic cancer, and DiGeorge's syndrome. Signs and symptoms of hypoparathyroidism include anxiety and irritability, neuromuscular excitability, tetany, intracranial calcifications, dental abnormalities, and cardiac conduction abnormalities. Laboratory values reflect a state of hypocalcemia and hyperphosphatemia with low parathyroid hormone levels.

Answer A is incorrect. These laboratory values are seen in primary hyperparathyroidism.

Answer B is incorrect. The patient would be hypoparathyroid; however, hypoparathyroidism causes hypocalcemia and hyperphosphatemia, not hypercalcemia and hypophosphatemia as indicated in this answer choice.

Answer C is incorrect. These laboratory values are seen in secondary hyperparathyroidism.

Answer E is incorrect. This patient's history of radioactive iodine therapy and signs and symptoms of irritability, neuromuscular excitability, positive Chvostek's sign, and QT prolongation all point to a diagnosis of hypocalcemia secondary to hypoparathyroidism. It is unlikely that his calcium, phosphate, and parathyroid hormone levels are normal.

38. **The correct answer is C.** The mechanism of action of metformin is not entirely understood. It may inhibit gluconeogenesis and increase glycolysis, leading to a decrease in serum glucose levels. Metformin is used as an oral hypoglycemic agent and can be used in patients without islet cell function. Lactic acidosis, one possible cause of an anion-gap metabolic acidosis, is the most serious adverse effect of metformin.

Answer A is incorrect. Acarbose is an intestinal brush border α-glucosidase inhibitor that delays hydrolysis of sugars and absorption of glucose, helping to decrease postprandial hyperglycemia. Because sugars remain in the intestine undigested, patients often experience osmotic diarrhea, an unpleasant side effect that limits the utility of this drug.

Answer B is incorrect. Glipizide is a second generation sulfonylurea that closes K^+ channels in the β-cell membrane, stimulating cell depolarization, an increase in calcium influx, and the release of endogenous insulin in type 2 diabetic patients. This oral hypoglycemic agent requires some residual islet cell function in order to be effective. Common adverse effects include hypoglycemia.

Answer D is incorrect. Pioglitazone can be used as a monotherapy for type 2 diabetes or in combination with other agents. Pioglitazone enhances target cell response to insulin. Weight gain is a side effect of the drug and results from increased responsiveness to insulin, a growth factor.

Answer E is incorrect. Tolbutamide is a first-generation sulfonylurea that works via the same mechanism as glipizide. First-generation sulfonylureas are less likely to cause hypoglycemia than second-generation drugs but are more likely to cause a disulfiram-like effect.

39. **The correct answer is A.** Benign prostatic hypertrophy (BPH) is a common entity in men older than age 50. Pathophysiologically, estradiol levels increase with age and they are thought to sensitize the prostate to the effects of dihydrotestosterone (DHT), causing the prostatic cells to grow. Common symptoms of BPH include increased frequency of urination, nocturia, problems with initiating and stopping urination, and pain on urination. Finasteride is a 5-α-reductase inhibitor that inhibits conversion of testosterone to DHT, therefore preventing further growth of the prostate, as well as promoting hair growth.

Answer B is incorrect. Flutamide is a competitive inhibitor of testosterone and its receptor and is used in the treatment of prostatic carcinoma, not benign prostatic hypertrophy.

Answer C is incorrect. Ketoconazole is a commonly used antifungal that also has antiandrogen effects. In the latter capacity, it is used in the treatment of polycystic ovarian syndrome to prevent hirsutism.

Answer D is incorrect. Spironolactone is a K^+-sparing diuretic that also has antiandrogenic effects. In addition to use in the treatment of hyperaldosteronism, hypokalemia, and congestive heart failure, it can be used in preventing hirsutism in polycystic ovarian syndrome.

Answer E is incorrect. Yohimbine is an α-2-selective inhibitor with questionable usage in the treatment of impotence.

40. **The correct answer is E.** The steroid hormone circulates in the plasma bound to a hormone-specific binding globulin. At the target organ, it enters a cell at the cell membrane due to its lipophilic properties and binds to an intracellular receptor either in the cytoplasm or within the nucleus. The hormone-receptor complex must transform in order to reveal the hormone's DNA binding domain; without this step, it is unable to carry out its action. Once the binding domain is revealed, the hormone binds the DNA enhancer element and generates gene transcription.

Answer A is incorrect. Binding a hormone-specific globulin in the plasma helps the hormone reach its target cell population but does not directly affect its DNA binding capacity.

Answer B is incorrect. Binding to the DNA enhancer element is the desired action of the hormone but does not explain the step necessary to reach this point.

Answer C is incorrect. Binding to the intracellular receptor alone does not enable DNA binding.

Answer D is incorrect. The DNA enhancer element is already exposed.

41. **The correct answer is A.** This patient most likely has diabetes mellitus type 1. The symp-

toms are due to a lack of insulin production by pancreatic β cells, which is believed to be caused by autoimmune/immune-related injury to the pancreas. The genetic predisposition to type 1 diabetes is not as strong as that for type 2 diabetes, but type 1 is associated with human leukocyte antigens (HLA)-DR3 and -DR4. Among whites with type 1 diabetes, 95% have HLA-DR3, HLA-DR4, or both.

Answer B is incorrect. These concepts are used to describe Crohn's disease, a type of inflammatory bowel disease. The term *skip lesions* is used to describe the occurrence of multiple diseased gastrointestinal segments adjacent to normal-appearing uninvolved bowel.

Answer C is incorrect. These concepts are commonly used to describe lactase deficiency, which causes an inability to properly digest the disaccharide lactose into glucose and galactose. The development of some cases is associated with viral or bacterial enteric infections. Note that other brush border enzymes include trehalase, which breaks down the disaccharide trehalose into glucose, and sucrase, which breaks down the disaccharide sucrose into glucose and fructose.

Answer D is incorrect. These are concepts used to describe type 2 diabetes mellitus, which is characterized by erratic insulin secretion (levels may be low, normal, or high) and insulin resistance; the insulin that is secreted from the pancreas does not function properly. About 80% of patients with type 2 diabetes are obese.

Answer E is incorrect. These concepts can be used to describe type 2 diabetes mellitus. There is a 20–40% risk of developing type 2 diabetes mellitus in first-degree relatives of patients, but there is no association with the human leukocyte antigen system.

42. **The correct answer is A.** Captopril is the prototypical angiotensin-converting enzyme (ACE) inhibitor. Common adverse effects are cough, angioedema, taste changes, and rash. Although ACE inhibitors are not indicated as first-line treatment for new-onset hypertension in the general population (think lifestyle modification), those with diabetes should be placed on an ACE inhibitor at the first sign of hypertension.

Answer B is incorrect. Hydrochlorothiazide is used as a first-line pharmacologic treatment for hypertension but is not associated with these adverse effects.

Answer C is incorrect. Losartan is an angiotensin II receptor inhibitor and is indicated for patients who experience the adverse effects of angiotensin-converting enzyme inhibitors.

Answer D is incorrect. Nifedipine is a calcium channel blocker and does not cause these adverse effects.

Answer E is incorrect. β-Blockers such as propranolol can be used for treatment of hypertension but do not cause these adverse effects.

43. **The correct answer is B.** Serum insulin level should be checked to objectively establish hyperinsulinemia. C peptide, which is produced by intracellular cleavage of proinsulin to insulin and released from intracellular vesicles of pancreatic β cells with insulin, will be elevated in patients with hypoglycemia due to endogenous hyperinsulinemia but not in patients with exogenous hyperinsulinemia. Hence, this test can be used to distinguish hypoglycemia due to excessive endogenous insulin secretion, as in an insulinoma, from that due to exogenous insulin administration, as in diabetes and factitious hypoglycemia.

Answer A is incorrect. Insulin is composed of an A chain and a B chain linked by disulfide bonds. The B chain is not found alone in the blood in any appreciable quantity, and it would not allow a distinction between endogenous and exogenous hyperinsulinemia.

Answer C is incorrect. Serum insulin levels will be elevated in both endogenous and exogenous hyperinsulinemia and thus cannot be used to distinguish these two entities.

Answer D is incorrect. Like proinsulin, pre-proinsulin is processed intracellularly. Hence, it is not released into the bloodstream and cannot be detected.

Answer E is incorrect. Proinsulin is produced from preproinsulin and is cleaved intracellularly to produce insulin and C peptide, which are subsequently released into the bloodstream. Hence, proinsulin is not released into the blood and cannot be detected.

44. **The correct answer is A.** Demeclocycline, like lithium, can inhibit the kidneys' response to ADH, resulting in nephrogenic diabetes insipidus. In patients with diabetes insipidus (DI), symptoms include polydipsia, polyuria, hypotonic urine, serum hyperosmolarity, and hypernatremia. In nephrogenic DI, exogenous ADH has no effect because of the inhibition of the kidney's response to the hormone. ADH plasma levels are also elevated.

Answer B is incorrect. In neurogenic DI, unlike nephrogenic DI, exogenous ADH is beneficial because the disease is a result of lack of central ADH production; ADH plasma levels are thus reduced.

Answer C is incorrect. Primary hyperaldosteronism would also cause hypernatremia and hypokalemia. Dilute urine, however, would not be expected.

Answer D is incorrect. ADH levels are frequently elevated in patients with SIADH; however, these patients produce hypertonic urine and have serum hypoosmolarity and hyponatremia.

Answer E is incorrect. Although polydipsia and polyuria are also seen in uncontrolled type 2 diabetes mellitus, hypernatremia would not be expected.

45. **The correct answer is C.** The large cell shown in the image is an osteoclast, which is responsible for bone resorption. Osteoclasts can be identified by their multiple nuclei, ruffled cytoplasmic border adjacent to the surface of bone tissue, and vacuoles and lysosomes within the cytoplasm. Patients with chronic renal disease usually have increased serum phosphorus levels, a tendency toward decreased serum calcium levels, and a compensatory increase in parathyroid hormone (PTH) levels. The increase in PTH levels leads to an increase in osteoclast bone resorption and thus an increase in serum calcium and alkaline phosphatase.

Answer A is incorrect. Angiotensin II, which is converted from angiotensin I in the lung capillaries by ACE, is a product of the renin-angiotensin system and thus can be affected in patients with chronic renal disease; however, angiotensin II does not stimulate activity of osteoclasts.

Answer B is incorrect. Calcitonin inhibits osteoclast activity and thus decreases bone resorption, which would not be the expected physiologic response to hypocalcemia.

Answer D is incorrect. Although renin levels can be affected in patients with chronic renal disease, renin does not stimulate activity of osteoclasts.

Answer E is incorrect. Thyroid hormone does not stimulate activity of osteoclasts.

46. **The correct answer is C.** Prolactin acts on the hypothalamic-pituitary axis to decrease its own secretion by increasing dopamine secretion by the neuroendocrine cell nuclei of the hypothalamus. Dopamine inhibits prolactin secretion by the anterior pituitary, thus producing a negative feedback loop. Bromocriptine is a dopaminergic agonist that acts on this loop to inhibit prolactin secretion.

Answer A is incorrect. The inferior hypophyseal artery provides the arterial supply of the posterior pituitary gland. This vessel plays no role in the prolactin negative feedback loop.

Answer B is incorrect. The long portal vessels of the anterior pituitary carry arterial blood provided via the superior hypophyseal artery, along with dopamine and trophic hormone–releasing hormones secreted by the hypothalamus to the trophic hormone–secreting cells of the anterior pituitary. While these vessels serve as a conduit for the transport of dopamine to the anterior pituitary, they do not represent the site of prolactin negative feedback.

Answer D is incorrect. The superior hypophyseal artery provides the arterial supply to the anterior pituitary gland and feeds into the hypophyseal portal system. This artery is not involved in the negative feedback loop of prolactin.

Answer E is incorrect. The trophic hormone–secreting cells of the anterior pituitary is where dopamine, released in response to prolactin action at the hypothalamus, acts to inhibit prolactin secretion. Hence, these cells are not the site of prolactin negative feedback; rather, these cells are the site of dopaminergic inhibition as a consequence of the action of prolactin action at the hypothalamus.

47. **The correct answer is A.** The patient has signs and symptoms suggestive of hypercortisolism, also known as Cushing's syndrome. Etiologies of hypercortisolism include a cortisol-producing adrenal adenoma, an ACTH-producing pituitary adenoma, paraneoplastic ectopic production of ACTH, and exogenous cortisol or ACTH administration. The dexamethasone suppression test can help distinguish between possible etiologies of hypercorticism. In normal individuals, low doses of dexamethasone suppress cortisol production. In patients with ACTH-producing pituitary adenomas, high doses of dexamethasone are needed to suppress cortisol production. In patients with adrenal adenomas or ectopic sources of ACTH, both low and high doses of dexamethasone fail to suppress cortisol production. Unlike patients with ectopic ACTH production, patients with an adrenal adenoma are expected to have low levels of ACTH due to negative feedback inhibition from the increased cortisol levels, as noted in this patient.

Answer B is incorrect. Bilateral adrenal hyperplasia suggests increased stimulation of the adrenal glands due to increased ACTH production from either a pituitary adenoma or an ectopic ACTH source.

Answer C is incorrect. Ectopic ACTH production is seen in paraneoplastic syndromes associated with bronchogenic cancer, pancreatic cancer, and thymomas. Bilateral adrenal hyperplasia and failed dexamethasone suppression are characteristics of ectopic ACTH production. A single mass noted on abdominal CT scan adjacent to a kidney is more suggestive of an adrenal adenoma than bilateral adrenal hyperplasia.

Answer D is incorrect. Although exogenous corticosteroid administration, like adrenal adenomas, results in decreased levels of ACTH, a mass on abdominal CT scan would be unlikely in a patient with exogenous corticosteroid administration.

Answer E is incorrect. An ACTH-secreting pituitary adenoma would cause bilateral adrenal hyperplasia and elevated ACTH levels, which are usually suppressed with high-dose dexamethasone.

48. **The correct answer is D.** This vignette describes a patient suffering from hypercalcemia secondary to malignancy. The laboratory data show hypercalcemia coupled with hypophosphatemia in the setting of an elevated serum alkaline phosphatase activity. This is consistent with hypercalcemia due to the action of parathyroid hormone–related peptide (PTHrP), which produces physiologic effects that mimic those of parathyroid hormone (PTH): increased bone resorption and increased renal absorption of Ca^{2+} and phosphate, resulting in elevated levels of these electrolytes in the serum.

Answer A is incorrect. Parathyroid hormone (PTH) and PTH-related peptide do not act at the adrenal cortex or the intestines. The adrenal cortex is the primary site of action for ACTH and ACTH-like peptide; the intestines are the primary site of action for 1,25-dihydroxycholecalciferol.

Answer B is incorrect. Parathyroid hormone (PTH) and PTH-related peptide have no action at the adrenal cortex. ACTH and ACTH-like peptide—both of which can be elaborated by neoplastic cells, resulting in Cushing's syndrome—act primarily at the adrenal cortex.

Answer C is incorrect. The intestines and bones are primary sites of action for 1,25 dihydroxycholecalciferol (vitamin D). While parathyroid (PTH) and PTH-related peptide stimulate production of 1,25-dihydroxycholecalciferol, producing secondary effects at the intestines, these hormones do not act primarily on the intestines.

Answer E is incorrect. Parathyroid hormone (PTH) and PTH-releasing peptide act primarily at the renal tubules and bones to increase serum Ca^{2+} levels. These hormones do not influence the pancreas, although pancreatic tumors have been shown to occasionally secrete PTHrP.

49. **The correct answer is A.** This patient's recent history of hyperglycemic symptoms, hypertension, and weight gain are all consistent with a diagnosis of Cushing's syndrome, which is characterized by hypercortisolemia. This leads to exaggeration of the physiologic effects of cortisol, such as hyperglycemia and insulin resistance, immune suppression, and hypertension (a consequence of salt retention due to secondary elevation of aldosterone). One result of this syndrome is osteoporosis, which is caused by increased bone resorption in response to an elevated serum cortisol level. Vertebral compression fractures are common manifestations of osteoporosis.

Answer B is incorrect. Glucagon can account for hyperglycemia via its anti-insulin physiologic effects, but it has no known physiologic effects on bone metabolism.

Answer C is incorrect. Growth hormone (GH) can cause hyperglycemia and insulin resistance but cannot account for increased bone resorption resulting in osteoporosis. Rather, GH stimulates increased bone growth that results in linear growth; it is responsible for the pubertal growth spurt.

Answer D is incorrect. Insulin causes hypoglycemia rather than hyperglycemia and does not exert any physiologic effects on bone metabolism that may be exaggerated and thus manifested as pathology in the setting of insulin excess.

Answer E is incorrect. Thyroid hormones function primarily to increase basal metabolism by increasing the activity of the Na^+/K^+ ATPase but also cause hyperglycemia by stimulating increased glycogenolysis, gluconeogenesis, and lipolysis. However, thyroid hormones do not cause increased bone resorption, but rather stimulate bone growth.

50. **The correct answer is D.** 17-α-Hydroxylase, a form of congenital adrenal hyperplasia, is characterized by deficits in glucocorticoid and sex steroid synthesis. This is coupled with increased mineralocorticoid production due to the increased flow of precursors, such as pregnenolone and progesterone, through mineralocorticoid-yielding pathways. The resultant low serum cortisol and sex steroid levels with elevated mineralocorticoid levels manifest clinically with hypertension, hypokalemia, and a female phenotype with no sexual maturation. Aldosterone is produced in the zona glomerulosa. Aldosterone synthesis requires 21-β-hydroxylase but not 17-α-hydroxylase. Remember the mnemonic "Salt, Sugar, and Sex" for the layers of the adrenal cortex and their respective products.

Answer A is incorrect. The capsule does not produce any hormones.

Answer B is incorrect. The medulla produces catecholamines; neither 17-α-hydroxylase nor 21-β-hydroxylase is required for the synthesis of catecholamines.

Answer C is incorrect. Cortisol is produced in the zona fasciculata of the adrenal cortex. Cortisol synthesis requires 21-β-hydroxylase and 17-α-hydroxylase.

Answer E is incorrect. Sex hormones are produced in the zona reticularis. Synthesis of the sex hormones requires 17-α-hydroxylase but not 21-β-hydroxylase.

CHAPTER 8

Gastrointestinal

1. A 35-year-old woman who is HIV-positive presents to the physician with jaundice and right upper quadrant abdominal pain. The patient reports having had multiple episodes of jaundice over the past 10 years. A hepatitis panel is positive for HBsAg and HBcAb, but negative for HBsAb and HCAb. Which of the following laboratory values would be found in a low level in this patient?

   (A) Albumin
   (B) Alkaline phosphatase
   (C) Bilirubin
   (D) Prothrombin time
   (E) Transaminases

2. A 45-year-old woman who was diagnosed with scleroderma 5 years ago presents to her physician with increasing difficulty swallowing. Which of the following abnormalities of esophageal muscle function is the most likely cause of these symptoms?

   (A) Atrophy of smooth muscle contractions in the lower two-thirds of the esophagus
   (B) Atrophy of smooth muscle contractions in the upper two-thirds of the esophagus
   (C) Atrophy of striated muscle contractions in the lower two-thirds of the esophagus
   (D) Atrophy of striated muscle contractions in the middle one-third of the esophagus
   (E) Atrophy of striated muscle contractions in the upper two-thirds of the esophagus

3. A 35-year-old woman comes to the physician because of painful rectal bleeding for the past month. The pain and bleeding are worse when she defecates. The patient experienced similar symptoms when she was pregnant 5 years ago. Which of the following is the most likely diagnosis?

   (A) Colorectal carcinoma
   (B) External hemorrhoids
   (C) Internal hemorrhoids
   (D) Perianal abscess
   (E) Squamous cell carcinoma

4. A 45-year-old woman presents to her physician with a 2-day history of right upper quadrant pain, nausea, gas, and vomiting. She reports that her symptoms are worse after she eats a fatty meal. Which of the following substances is responsible for this patient's worsening symptoms after fatty meals?

   (A) Cholecystokinin
   (B) Gastrin
   (C) Pepsin
   (D) Secretin
   (E) Somatostatin

5. A 10-year-old girl is brought to the physician because she has had a fever and headache accompanied by abdominal pain and bloody diarrhea. Her stool smear shows leukocytes. A stool culture incubated at 42° C (107.6° F) in a microaerophilic environment shows many comma-shaped organisms. She has no history of recent travel or sick contacts. She has a pet puppy, which the mother says has had diarrhea for the past week. Based on the above information, the physician suspects bacterial gastroenteritis. The organism responsible for this patient's sickness is thought to be associated with the possible development of which of the following symptoms?

   (A) Acute renal failure and thrombocytopenia with hemolytic anemia
   (B) Fever, migratory polyarthritis, and carditis
   (C) Fever, new murmur, small erythematous lesions on the palms, and splinter hemorrhages on the nail bed
   (D) Petechial rash and bilateral hemorrhage into the adrenal gland
   (E) Symmetric ascending muscle weakness beginning in the distal lower extremities

6. A 15-year-old boy presents to the pediatrician with right-sided facial swelling and increased salivation. Which of the following conditions most likely describes the composition of this patient's saliva?

(A) High sodium concentration
(B) Hypotonicity
(C) Low bicarbonate concentration
(D) Low potassium concentration
(E) Small volume

7. This image is from a 30-year-old man with difficulty swallowing. Which of the following actions is most likely absent in this patient?

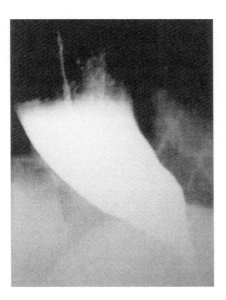

Reproduced, with permission, from Lalwani AK, ed. *Current Diagnosis & Treatment in Otolaryngology—Head & Neck Surgery*. New York. McGraw-Hill, 2004: Fig. 34-3A.

(A) Contraction of the lower esophageal sphincter
(B) Contraction of the upper esophageal sphincter
(C) Initiation of swallowing in the oropharynx
(D) Relaxation of the lower esophageal sphincter
(E) Relaxation of the upper esophageal sphincter

8. A 42-year-old man visits his primary care physician to discuss possible cholesterol-lowering agents. His last blood test showed that he had elevated LDL and triglyceride levels. The physician decides to prescribe gemfibrozil and schedules the man for a follow-up visit in 1 month. Which of the following results are likely to be seen on this patient's next blood test?

(A) A decrease in LDL and a slight increase in triglycerides
(B) A decrease in LDL with little to no effect on HDL or triglycerides
(C) A large decrease in LDL, an increase in HDL, and a slight decrease in triglycerides
(D) A large decrease in triglycerides, a slight decrease in LDL, and a slight increase in HDL
(E) An increase in LDL, a slight decrease in HDL, and a decrease in triglycerides

9. A 50-year-old man presents to his physician because of a 6.8-kg (15-lb) weight loss over the past month, epigastric pain radiating to the back, and jaundice. Laboratory studies show an amylase level of 500 U/L, a lipase level of 300 U/L, and an alkaline phosphatase level of 500 U/L. Levels of CA 19-9 and carcinoembryonic antigen (CEA) are also elevated. Which of the following is most likely responsible for this patient's symptoms?

(A) Acute cholecystitis
(B) Acute pancreatitis
(C) Carcinoid tumor
(D) Colon cancer
(E) Pancreatic adenocarcinoma

10. A 17-year-old girl who is being treated with an extended course of clindamycin for recurrent sinus tract infections presents to the physician with intractable watery diarrhea and cramps. Which of the following organisms is most often associated with this patient's condition?

(A) *Clostridium difficile*
(B) *Clostridium perfringens*
(C) *Escherichia coli*
(D) *Staphylococcus aureus*
(E) *Vibrio cholerae*
(F) *Yersinia enterocolitica*

11. An abdominal CT scan demonstrates a polypoid mass off the gallbladder protruding into the lumen, diffuse thickening of the gallbladder wall, and enlarged lymph nodes. This patient most likely has a history of which of the following?

    (A) *Ascaris lumbricoides*
    (B) Cigarette smoking
    (C) Gallstones
    (D) *Schistosoma haematobium*
    (E) Tuberculosis

12. A 45-year-old man presents with severe anal pain. He is noted to have a fluctuant red and tender mass consistent with a perianal abscess. The patient has had cyclical fevers. He has a temperature of 38.2° C (100.8° F), a heart rate of 89/min, a blood pressure of 129/85 mm Hg, and a respiratory rate of 18/min. The abscess is incised and drained. A specimen of the pus is examined under a microscope and is shown to contain a predominance of neutrophils. Which of the following factors is most abundant in the pus specimen?

    (A) Leukotriene B_4
    (B) Prostaglandin I_2
    (C) Thromboxane A_2
    (D) Vascular endothelial growth factor
    (E) Von Willebrand factor

13. A 46-year-old woman comes to the physician because of voluminous, malodorous, bulky stools. The diarrhea usually abates on fasting. The patient's laboratory values demonstrate an increased stool osmolality. Additional laboratory values include the following:

    Na$^+$: 153 mEq/L
    K$^+$: 3.1 mEq/L
    Cl$^-$: 110 mEq/L
    HCO$_3^-$: 18 mEq/L
    72-hour fecal fat: 32 g/day (normal < 7 g/day)

    Which of the following is the pathologic mechanism most likely responsible for the patient's presentation?

    (A) Exudative diarrhea
    (B) Malabsorption
    (C) Motility derangement

    (D) Osmotic diarrhea
    (E) Secretory diarrhea

14. A 62-year-old woman has had persistent nausea for 5 years with occasional vomiting. On upper gastrointestinal endoscopy, a small area of gastric mucosa is noted in the fundus, which has loss of rugal folds. A biopsy reveals well-differentiated adenocarcinoma confined to the mucosa. Upper gastrointestinal endoscopy performed 5 years previously showed a pattern of gastritis. Microscopy at that time showed chronic inflammation with the presence of *Helicobacter pylori*. Which of the following best characterizes this patient's neoplasm?

    (A) Following resection, a 5-year survival rate of > 90%
    (B) High incidence in the United States
    (C) Linitis plastica
    (D) Metastases limited to regional lymph nodes
    (E) On light microscopy, a signet ring cell pattern

15. A 23-year-old man presents to the physician with abdominal distention and tenderness with no vomiting or diarrhea. Physical examination shows hepatosplenomegaly. Bowel sounds are normal. On questioning, the patient says that he traveled to eastern South America 1 year ago. Several weeks after returning from his trip, he remembers having fever, diarrhea, weight loss, and "funny-looking stools." An ultrasonography shows ascites and hepatic periportal fibrosis. Which of the following conditions is most likely responsible for this patient's present symptoms?

    (A) Appendicitis
    (B) Bowel obstruction
    (C) Enterocolitis
    (D) Portal hypertension
    (E) Ruptured viscus

16. A 62-year-old woman with rheumatoid arthritis and no other past medical history comes to the emergency department complaining of severe epigastric pain, nausea, and vomiting. She says that she vomited blood earlier in the day. A

gross image of the gastric mucosa is shown. Which of the following is the most likely cause of this patient's symptoms?

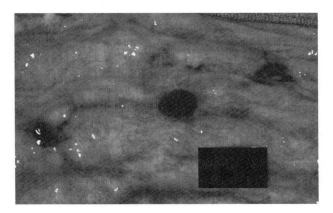

Image courtesy of PEIR Digital Library (http://peir.net).

(A) Amyloidosis
(B) *Helicobacter pylori* infection
(C) Nonsteroidal anti-inflammatory drugs (NSAIDs)
(D) Prednisone
(E) Uremia

17. A 20-year-old man with Crohn's disease refractory to treatment with high-dose methylprednisolone is started on infliximab. Which of the following adverse effects is often associated with infliximab?

(A) Diarrhea
(B) Fever and chills
(C) Headache
(D) Hypertension
(E) Nausea and vomiting

18. A 2-month-old boy is brought to his pediatrician for a regular checkup. His parents report that he has a poor appetite and is very constipated. He has small bowel movements once a week, which his parents believe are very painful. Although he was at the 75th per-

centile for both height and weight at birth, he is currently at the 25th percentile for height and is below the 5th percentile for weight. His abdomen is distended, but his bowel sounds are normal and his abdomen does not appear to be tender. A barium enema shows a narrow rectosigmoid with a dilation of the segment above the narrowing. Which of the following might be missing from this patient on rectosigmoid biopsy?

(A) Enteric neurons
(B) Motor neurons to the external anal sphincter
(C) Pelvic nerves
(D) Sympathetic neurons
(E) Vagus nerve

19. An 8-year-old boy presents to the emergency department with a 2-hour history of vomiting after eating dinner at a seafood buffet. Arterial blood gas analysis reveals a pH of 7.50, an HCO_3^- level of 34 mEq/L, and PCO_2 level of 40 mm Hg. Which of the following best describes the acid-base disturbance occurring in this patient?

(A) Metabolic acidosis
(B) Metabolic alkalosis
(C) Metabolic acidosis/respiratory acidosis
(D) Metabolic acidosis/respiratory alkalosis
(E) Metabolic alkalosis/respiratory acidosis
(F) Metabolic alkalosis/respiratory alkalosis

20. Which of the following conditions is characterized by a fatty liver change, hepatocyte swelling and necrosis, neutrophilic infiltrates, and intracytoplasmic eosinophilic hyaline inclusions derived from cytokeratin intermediate filaments?

(A) Acute viral hepatitis
(B) Alcoholic hepatitis
(C) α-Antitrypsin deficiency
(D) Fatty liver of pregnancy
(E) Neonatal hepatitis

21. A 24-year-old man presents to the physician with diarrhea and abdominal cramps. A fecal occult blood test is positive. On questioning, it is learned that the patient went swimming in a lake during a camping trip 2 days ago. A stool sample is sent for laboratory evaluation. This patient is most likely infected with which of the following parasites?

    (A) *Cryptosporidium*
    (B) *Entamoeba histolytica*
    (C) *Giardia lamblia*
    (D) *Leishmania donovani*
    (E) *Toxoplasma gondii*

22. A 27-year-old man goes to the doctor for an annual physical examination. On rectal examination, masses are palpated. The patient is referred for a colonoscopy, which reveals adenomatous polyps located diffusely throughout the colon. When asked about his family history, the patient states that his father passed away from colon cancer. A diagnosis of familial adenomatous polyposis is suspected, and the patient asks how he got this. Which of the following is the inheritance pattern of this condition?

    (A) Autosomal dominant
    (B) Autosomal recessive
    (C) Autosomal trisomy
    (D) Sex chromosome abnormality
    (E) X-linked recessive

23. A healthy 25-year-old man comes to the physician for a routine examination. His laboratory tests show a serum bilirubin level of 4 mg/dL and a direct bilirubin level of 0.3 mg/dL. The patient's liver function tests are normal. Which of the following steps in bilirubin metabolism is most likely affected in this patient?

    (A) Defects in hepatic excretory function
    (B) Extrahepatic biliary obstruction
    (C) Glucuronosyltransferase deficiency
    (D) Intrahepatic biliary obstruction
    (E) Liver cell damage

24. A 2-year-old girl who has recently been adopted from Singapore is brought to the clinic by her parents. They are concerned because she is having trouble with her vision at night. The vitamin most likely deficient in this child is typically stored in which of the following organs?

    (A) Appendix
    (B) Gallbladder
    (C) Liver
    (D) Pancreas
    (E) Stomach

25. A 46-year-old white woman with rheumatoid arthritis presents with severe pruritus. She denies any history of alcohol or drug use. On physical examination, she is found to have icteric sclera, palpebral xanthomas, and hepatomegaly. She tests positive for antimitochondrial antibody and increased alkaline phosphatase activity. Which of the following mechanisms is most likely responsible for this patient's presentation?

    (A) Destruction of intrahepatic bile ducts
    (B) Hepatic parenchymal destruction
    (C) Obstruction of extrahepatic bile ducts
    (D) Portal vein thrombosis
    (E) Stenosis of extrahepatic and intrahepatic bile ducts

26. A 10-year-old boy presents to the pediatrician with weight loss and multiple purpuric lesions all over his body. The patient has bulky, greasy yellow stools associated with abdominal pain and flatulence that most often occurs after meals. A mucosal biopsy of the small bowel reveals diffuse severe atrophy and blunting of the villi, along with a lymphocytic infiltrate of the lamina propria. Which of the following foods is most likely responsible for this child's presentation?

    (A) Cereals
    (B) Dairy products
    (C) Fish
    (D) Fruits
    (E) Undercooked meat

27. A 26-year-old man with hepatitis C is being medically treated while he awaits liver trans-

plantation. One of the drugs he is taking causes him to have periodic fevers and chills and a sense of depression that he did not have prior to treatment. Which of the following drugs is most likely responsible for this patient's adverse effects?

(A) Intravenous immunoglobulin
(B) Lamivudine
(C) Pegylated interferon
(D) Ribavirin
(E) Tumor necrosis factor-α

28. A 19-year-old woman presents to the emergency department with a new onset of right lower quadrant abdominal pain. On physical examination, the patient has a temperature of 38.5° C (101.3° F) and a WBC count of 13,000/mm^3. Which of the following symptoms is also most likely present in this patient?

(A) Abdominal distention
(B) Hunger
(C) Nausea and vomiting
(D) Profuse watery diarrhea
(E) Vaginal bleeding

29. A 3-year-old child is brought to the pediatrician because of abdominal pain and diarrhea containing mucus and blood. The child has a fever of 39.4° C (103° F). On stool culture, the causative organism is shown to be a non-lactose-fermenting and non–hydrogen sulfide-producing bacterium. Which of the following organisms is most likely responsible for the child's illness?

(A) Enteroinvasive *Escherichia coli*
(B) Enterotoxigenic *Escherichia coli*
(C) *Salmonella* spp.
(D) *Shigella* spp.
(E) *Vibrio cholerae*

30. An unconscious 57-year-old man is brought to the emergency department by ambulance with massive, bright red hemoptysis. On arrival, his blood pressure is 80/40 mm Hg and his heart rate is 124/min. He appears jaundiced with multiple spider angiomas on his chest and arms. He has an enlarged abdomen that is dull to percussion and positive for a fluid wave. He has splenomegaly and muscle wasting in his extremities. Which of the following vessel anastomoses are responsible for the patient's bleeding?

(A) Left gastric artery and left gastric vein
(B) Left gastric vein and azygos vein
(C) Paraumbilical vein and inferior epigastric vein
(D) Portal vein and inferior vena cava
(E) Splenic vein and left renal vein

31. A 76-year-old man with chronic obstructive pulmonary disease presents at his annual clinic visit with complaints of black stools and epigastric pain relieved by meals. He reports a 4.5-kg (10-lb) weight gain over the past 4 months. He has no other medical problems and takes no medications. Physical examination is unremarkable. His plasma Ca^{2+} and phosphate levels are within the normal ranges. Endoscopy reveals mucosal ulceration in the duodenal bulb. Which of the following is the most likely risk factor for this patient's duodenal ulcer?

(A) Alcohol use
(B) Chronic NSAID use
(C) Excessive salt intake
(D) Primary hyperparathyroidism
(E) Tobacco use

32. The alimentary canal is made up of various anatomic layers that function in digestion, absorption, and processing of food particles. An illustration of a longitudinal section through the duodenum is shown. What is the function of the structure to which the arrow is pointing?

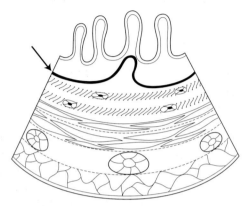

Reproduced, with permission, from USMLERx.com.

(A) Coordinate motility
(B) Inhibit peristalsis
(C) Regulate absorption
(D) Regulate secretions
(E) Smooth muscle contraction

33. A 20-year-old man presents to his physician with a 2-day history of fever, vomiting, and diarrhea. His laboratory studies are unremarkable except for a serum albumin level of 75 g/dL. Which of the following conditions might cause this patient's laboratory abnormality?

(A) Acute infection
(B) Chronic liver disease
(C) Dehydration
(D) Nephrotic syndrome
(E) Poor nutritional status

34. A 33-year-old man with active gastroesophageal reflux disease returns to his physician for the second time in 2 weeks complaining of a worsening sore throat. The patient was previously diagnosed with penicillin-sensitive *Streptococcus pyogenes* on throat culture and, because he is allergic to penicillin, was given ciprofloxacin. Suspicious of an interaction, the physician asks the patient if he has been taking any other medications. Which of the following medications is this patient most likely taking?

(A) Aspirin
(B) Calcium carbonate
(C) Misoprostol
(D) Omeprazole
(E) Ranitidine

35. Which of the following findings is most commonly associated with chronic pancreatitis?

(A) Air-fluid levels in the small intestine on x-ray film of the abdomen
(B) Free air under the right hemidiaphragm on x-ray film of the chest
(C) Pancreatic calcifications on computed tomography
(D) Pancreatic cysts
(E) Pancreatic granuloma formation

36. A 51-year-old man with a long history of medication-dependent reflux esophagitis sees his physician for an annual physical, which reveals a blood gastrin level three times the upper limit of normal. His physician is concerned that the patient might develop atrophic gastritis. Which of the following medications is this patient most likely taking?

(A) Aluminum hydroxide
(B) Bismuth
(C) Cimetidine
(D) Misoprostol
(E) Omeprazole

37. A 22-year-old man presents to the physician with a 1-year history of chronic recurrent right lower quadrant abdominal pain and diarrhea. The patient also has had low-grade fevers and a 6.7-kg (15-lb) weight loss during this period. Endoscopy of his terminal ileum shows multiple erosions. Which of the following is the most likely diagnosis in this patient?

(A) Celiac sprue
(B) Collagenous colitis
(C) Crohn's disease
(D) Irritable bowel syndrome
(E) Ulcerative colitis

38. A 57-year-old woman comes to the physician 3 weeks after returning from a trip to Greece, where she enjoyed one of the local specialties—fresh goat cheese. She has had a fever of 38.8° C (101.8° F) that rises during the day and decreases at night. She says that she feels tired and has lost weight. Her physical exam is notable for hepatosplenomegaly and generalized lymphadenopathy. Which of the following organisms is most likely responsible for this patient's symptoms?

    (A) *Brucella melitensis*
    (B) *Clostridium difficile*
    (C) *Plasmodium malariae*
    (D) *Vibrio cholerae*
    (E) *Yersinia enterocolitica*

39. A 53-year-old man with a history of drinking 1–2 bottles of vodka a day for the past 25 years presents to the emergency department. He has a lengthy history of nausea and vomiting. He experiences a bout of prolonged vomiting, followed by massive hematemesis. At presentation his temperature is 36.7° C (98.1° F), pulse is 110/min, respiratory rate is 23/min, and blood pressure is 80/40 mm Hg. Physical examination reveals a regular rate and rhythm with no murmurs and his lungs are clear to auscultation. There is no abdominal tenderness or distention and bowel sounds are present. His stool is negative for blood. Which of the following is the most likely diagnosis?

    (A) Esophageal laceration (Mallory-Weiss syndrome)
    (B) Esophageal metaplasia (Barrett's esophagus)
    (C) Esophageal squamous cell carcinoma
    (D) Esophageal stricture
    (E) Hiatal hernia

40. A 32-year-old woman presents to the physician with alternating bouts of diarrhea and constipation. She also has chronic abdominal pain relieved by frequent bowel movements. Her symptoms are exacerbated by stress. The patient denies fever or weight loss. She has a negative hemoccult test. Colonoscopy and endoscopy reveal no abnormalities. Which of the following is the most probable diagnosis in this patient?

    (A) Celiac sprue
    (B) Colorectal carcinoma
    (C) Inflammatory bowel disease
    (D) Irritable bowel syndrome
    (E) Pseudomembranous colitis

41. A 34-year-old man is diagnosed with tropical sprue, which causes a decrease in the number of intestinal cells. Which of the following steps in lipid digestion and absorption will this patient most likely have difficulty with?

    (A) Chylomicron formation
    (B) Digestion with lingual lipases
    (C) Emulsification
    (D) Micelle formation
    (E) Mixing

42. A healthy 55-year-old woman presents to the physician with a 1-year history of an unchanging, palpable mass in her left cheek. A parotid gland biopsy reveals groups of well-differentiated epithelial cells in a chondromyxoid stroma surrounded by a fibrous capsule; multiple cell types are visible on light microscopy. The pathologic description of the mass is most consistent with which of the following conditions?

    (A) Adenoid cystic carcinoma
    (B) Mucoepidermoid carcinoma
    (C) Pleomorphic adenoma
    (D) Sialic duct stone
    (E) Warthin's tumor

43. A 7-year-old boy presents to the emergency department with nausea and vomiting. He is diagnosed with a bowel obstruction, and taken to surgery. The appearance of his bowel at surgery is shown in the image. Which of the following conditions is the most likely cause of this patient's symptoms?

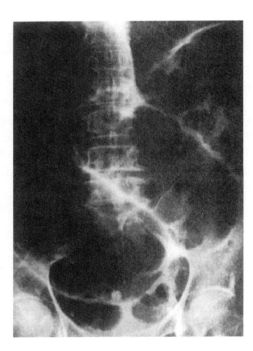

Reproduced, with permission, from Tintinalli JE, Kelen GD, Stapczynski JS, Ma OJ, Cline DM. *Tintinalli's Emergency Medicine: A Comprehensive Study Guide*, 6th ed. New York, McGraw-Hill, 2004: Fig. 79-1.

(A) Bowel infarct
(B) Colorectal carcinoma
(C) Intussusception
(D) Meckel's diverticulum
(E) Volvulus

44. A 34-year-old woman is brought to the emergency department by ambulance due to complaints of dizziness, confusion, and fatigue. She reports that she has had 2–3 similar episodes in the past few months. Physical examination reveals an anxious woman with a heart rate of 120/min and a mild tremor in both hands. Her blood glucose level is 45 mg/dL. The patient reports normal food intake during that day, having had lunch just a few hours prior to the episode. The patient is surprised to hear about the low blood glucose level and says that her husband is the one who has always had "sugar problems" and uses insulin injections daily. The level of which of the following will help differentiate an endogenous cause for the patient's presentation from a factitious cause?

(A) Chloride
(B) C peptide
(C) Insulin
(D) Proinsulin
(E) Sodium

45. A 20-year-old man presents to the clinic after a week-long intravenous heroin binge because of constipation and abdominal fullness. A CT scan shows excess stool present in the colon and rectum. Heroin inhibits bowel motility and causes constipation by which of the following mechanisms?

(A) Inhibition of μ receptors
(B) Inhibition of κ receptors
(C) Partial agonist-antagonist action on μ receptors
(D) Stimulation of κ receptors
(E) Stimulation of μ receptors

46. A woman comes to the physician because of profuse vomiting and watery, nonbloody diarrhea that developed 5 hours after she had eaten tuna salad. She is diagnosed with *Staphylococcus aureus* food poisoning. Which of the following statements is correct?

(A) Microscopic examination will demonstrate gram-positive, catalase-positive, and coagulase-negative bacteria
(B) One would expect to observe a positive quellung reaction
(C) Thayer-Martin media should be used to culture the *Staphylococcus aureus* from this patient's stool
(D) The contaminated canned fish was the source of *Staphylococcus aureus*
(E) The enterotoxin is preformed in food; therefore, there is a short incubation time for the development of the disease

47. A newborn presents to the pediatrician with kernicterus, jaundice, and elevation of serum unconjugated bilirubin; the patient dies soon after her first birthday. This patient most likely had a deficiency in which of the following enzymes?

(A) Aldolase B
(B) Galactose-1-phosphate uridyltransferase
(C) Glucose 6-phosphatase
(D) Uridine diphosphate-glucuronosyltransferase
(E) Uroporphyrinogen decarboxylase

48. Which of the following types of hepatocellular injury is commonly seen following acetaminophen overdose?

(A) Acute hepatitis
(B) Centrilobular necrosis
(C) Fibrosis
(D) Granuloma formation
(E) Microvesicular fatty change

49. A 40-year-old white man presents to the emergency department complaining of burning retrosternal chest pain after meals. His pain is relieved by antacids. The patient's ECG is normal, and his chest x-ray is remarkable for an 8-cm hiatal hernia. This patient is at risk for developing which of the following types of cancer?

(A) Adenocarcinoma of the esophagus
(B) Krukenberg's tumor
(C) Non–small cell adenocarcinoma of the lung
(D) Squamous cell carcinoma of the esophagus
(E) Stomach carcinoma

50. A 43-year-old man with a 20-year history of ulcerative colitis presents to the physician with complaints of worsening bloody diarrhea, progressive fatigue, pruritus, visual disturbances, and arthralgias. On physical examination, he is found to have icteric sclera, finger clubbing, and several small ulcerations with necrotic edges on both legs. Endoscopic retrograde cholangiopancreatography (ERCP) shows alternating strictures and dilations, or "beading," of the bile ducts. Which of the following conditions is consistent with these ERCP findings?

(A) Cholelithiasis
(B) Pancreatic carcinoma
(C) Primary biliary cirrhosis
(D) Primary hemochromatosis
(E) Primary sclerosing cholangitis

1. The correct answer is A. This patient has an acute hepatitis B infection overlying a chronic hepatitis B infection. Hepatitis B typically presents with jaundice and right upper quadrant pain and can be transmitted via parenteral, sexual, and maternal-fetal routes. As this patient has yet to develop antibodies to the hepatitis B surface antigen, she must have an acute hepatitis B infection. A patient with HIV may have a history of risky sexual behavior and would be at risk for hepatitis B infection. This patient's chronic liver disease would lead to a decrease in albumin, as it is typically produced by the liver.

Answer B is incorrect. A patient with chronic liver disease would have an elevation in alkaline phosphatase activity due to decreased function of the biliary tree.

Answer C is incorrect. A patient with chronic liver disease would have an elevation of serum bilirubin, due to difficulty with release into the bile.

Answer D is incorrect. A patient with chronic liver disease would have an increase in prothrombin time, as the liver is the site of production of all major coagulation factors, except factor VIII.

Answer E is incorrect. A patient with chronic liver disease would have an elevation of transaminases, as these indicate hepatocellular damage.

2. The correct answer is A. The upper one-third of the esophagus is made up of striated muscle. The middle one-third of the esophagus is made up of both striated and smooth muscle. The lower one-third of the esophagus is made up of smooth muscle. Patients with scleroderma develop dysphagia secondary to atrophy of smooth muscle contractions in the lower two-thirds of the esophagus and incompetence of the lower esophageal sphincter.

Answer B is incorrect. Patients with scleroderma develop dysphagia secondary to atrophy of smooth muscle contractions in the lower (not upper) two-thirds of the esophagus and incompetence of the lower esophageal sphincter.

Answer C is incorrect. Patients with scleroderma develop dysphagia secondary to atrophy of smooth (not striated) muscle contractions in the lower two-thirds of the esophagus and incompetence of the lower esophageal sphincter.

Answer D is incorrect. Patients with scleroderma develop dysphagia secondary to atrophy of smooth (not striated) muscle contractions in the lower (not middle) two-thirds of the esophagus and incompetence of the lower esophageal sphincter.

Answer E is incorrect. Patients with scleroderma develop dysphagia secondary to atrophy of smooth (not striated) muscle contractions in the lower (not upper) two-thirds of the esophagus and incompetence of the lower esophageal sphincter.

3. The correct answer is B. This patient has external hemorrhoids. External hemorrhoids are thromboses (blood clots) in the veins of the external rectal venous plexus. Since they originate below the pectinate line, external hemorrhoids receive somatic innervation and are therefore painful. Rectal bleeding is also a common symptom seen with hemorrhoids. Some of the predisposing factors for hemorrhoids include, but are not limited to, pregnancy, constipation, heavy weight lifting, or any other cause that results in increased intra-abdominal pressure.

Answer A is incorrect. The peak incidence of colorectal carcinoma is between the ages of 60 and 80. When it is found in a younger person, ulcerative colitis, familial adenomatous polyposis, or another preexisting precancerous syndrome must be suspected. The clinical features of colorectal carcinoma include fatigue, weakness, iron deficiency anemia, constipation, painless rectal bleeding, and abdominal pain. This patient's painful rectal bleeding and lack of other clinical evidence of a malignant lesion make this option unlikely.

Answer C is incorrect. Internal hemorrhoids are prolapses of rectal mucosa containing the normally dilated veins of the internal venous plexus. In contrast to external hemorrhoids, internal hemorrhoids originate above the pectinate line, have an autonomic nerve supply, and usually present with painless rectal bleeding.

Answer D is incorrect. Abscesses are localized collections of purulent inflammatory tissue. Perianal abscess may follow infection of anal fissures or rectal trauma. In this patient, the lack of evidence or history of infection does not support a diagnosis of abscess.

Answer E is incorrect. Squamous cell carcinomas can occur in the lower anal canal and are commonly associated with human papillomavirus infection. They can also present with pain on defecation, bleeding, and obstruction. However, this patient's lack of weight loss, intermittent course, and association of symptoms with pregnancy make this diagnosis highly unlikely.

4. **The correct answer is A.** Gallstones are common in women over 40 years old and often present with right upper quadrant pain, nausea, flatulence, and vomiting. Consumption of fatty foods causes cholecystokinin (CCK) release, leading to worsening pain in a patient with cholelithiasis. CCK is released by the I cells of the duodenum and jejunum and is responsible for gallbladder contraction, pancreatic enzyme secretion, and sphincter of Oddi relaxation.

Answer B is incorrect. Gastrin is released by G cells in the antrum and duodenum and stimulates secretion of gastric acid, intrinsic factor, and pepsinogen.

Answer C is incorrect. Pepsin is secreted by chief cells of the stomach and facilitates protein digestion.

Answer D is incorrect. Secretin is secreted by S cells of the duodenum; it inhibits gastric acid secretion and stimulates HCO_3^- secretion from the pancreas.

Answer E is incorrect. Somatostatin is released by D cells of the pancreas and gastrointestinal mucosa. It inhibits gastric acid, pepsinogen, insulin, glucagon, and pancreatic and small intestine fluid secretion.

5. **The correct answer is E.** Guillain-Barré syndrome is characterized by rapidly progressing ascending paralysis. It is thought to follow a variety of infectious diseases, such as cytomegalovirus, Epstein-Barr virus, HIV, and gastroenteritis caused by *Campylobacter jejuni*. *C. jejuni* gastroenteritis is characterized by bloody diarrhea together with the finding of comma-shaped organisms when incubated at 42° C (107.6° F) in a microaerophilic environment. Domestic animals serve as a source of the bacteria, which are then transmitted to humans via the fecal-oral route.

Answer A is incorrect. Hemolytic-uremic syndrome (HUS) is characterized by acute renal failure and thrombocytopenia with hemolytic anemia. HUS can be a complication of infection caused by *Escherichia coli* O157:H7 and not *Campylobacter jejuni*.

Answer B is incorrect. Rheumatic fever is characterized by fever, migratory polyarthritis, and carditis. It may follow group A streptococcal pharyngitis.

Answer C is incorrect. Fever, a new murmur, Janeway lesions, and nail-bed hemorrhages are all signs of bacterial endocarditis. Acute endocarditis is caused by *Staphylococcus aureus* and subacute infection can be caused by *Streptococcus viridans*.

Answer D is incorrect. Waterhouse-Friderichsen syndrome is characterized by high fever, shock, purpura, and adrenal insufficiency.

6. **The correct answer is B.** This vignette describes a boy with parotiditis. Saliva in patients with this condition is typically hypotonic and copious, with high K^+ and HCO_3^- concentrations, and low Na^+ and Cl^- concentrations.

Saliva also contains α-amylase, kallikrein, and lingual lipase.

Answer A is incorrect. Saliva typically has a low Na^+ concentration.

Answer C is incorrect. Saliva typically has a high HCO_3^- concentration.

Answer D is incorrect. Saliva typically has a high K^+ concentration.

Answer E is incorrect. Since the patient is described as having increased salivation, a small volume of saliva is unlikely in this patient.

7. **The correct answer is D.** The barium swallow study shows esophageal dilatation and a "bird's beak" sign of the distal esophagus, which are characteristic of achalasia. This disease presents with difficulty swallowing, abnormal contractions of esophageal muscles, absence of peristalsis, and absence of relaxation of the lower esophageal sphincter on swallowing.

Answer A is incorrect. In achalasia, the lower esophageal sphincter fails to relax.

Answer B is incorrect. In achalasia, the lower esophageal sphincter is affected, not the upper esophageal sphincter.

Answer C is incorrect. There is no difficulty with initiation of swallowing in achalasia.

Answer E is incorrect. In achalasia, the lower esophageal sphincter is affected, not the upper esophageal sphincter.

8. **The correct answer is D.** Gemfibrozil functions mainly to reduce the circulating level of triglycerides. It is a fibric acid derivative that acts on peroxisome proliferator–activated receptor-γ protein to increase the activity of lipoprotein lipase and facilitate enhanced clearance of triglycerides. There is also a slight reduction in cholesterol synthesis.

Answer A is incorrect. Bile acid resins such as cholestyramine and colestipol bind to bile acids and steroids in the small intestine, preventing their absorption. They cause a reduction in LDL and a slight increase in triglycerides.

Answer B is incorrect. Ezetimibe blocks cholesterol and phytosterol (a plant sterol) absorption in the small intestine, resulting in a decrease in LDL with little to no effect on HDL or triglyceride levels.

Answer C is incorrect. HMG-CoA reductase inhibitors, like the "statins," act to reduce cholesterol biosynthesis in the liver by preventing the formation of the cholesterol precursor mevalonate. They produce a large decrease in LDL, an increase in HDL, and a slight decrease in triglycerides.

Answer E is incorrect. This option describes a drug that would increase LDL levels. This is not caused by any of the cholesterol-lowering drugs.

9. **The correct answer is E.** Patients with pancreatic adenocarcinoma often present with jaundice, epigastric pain radiating to the back, and weight loss. Laboratory studies show an increased amylase, lipase, alkaline phosphatase, CA 19-9, and CEA. Pancreatic cancers are more common in patients with a history of smoking, diabetes mellitus, and chronic pancreatitis. Treatment for pancreatic adenocarcinoma is surgical removal, yet for most patients this is impossible, as the cancer has already metastasized prior to its discovery. If possible, pancreaticoduodenectomy or distal pancreatectomy is preferred to a total pancreatectomy to preserve some of the pancreatic function.

Answer A is incorrect. Patients with acute cholecystitis will present with pain in the right upper quadrant and vomiting. Patients rarely present with jaundice and do not present with weight loss.

Answer B is incorrect. Patients with acute pancreatitis often present with epigastric abdominal pain radiating to the back as well as with nausea and vomiting. Patients do not often present with jaundice or weight loss. Amylase and lipase will also be elevated, but the tumor markers CA 19-9 and CEA will not be elevated in a patient with acute pancreatitis.

Answer C is incorrect. Patients with carcinoid tumor will present with weight loss and symptoms of carcinoid syndrome, including flushing, diarrhea, and valvular heart disease. The laboratory values that are elevated in this patient most likely would not be elevated in a patient with a carcinoid tumor.

Answer D is incorrect. Patients with colon cancer will present with weight loss and may or may not have a change in bowel function, based on the location of the tumor. CEA levels will be elevated in these patients.

10. **The correct answer is A.** Pseudomembranous or antibiotic-associated colitis is an acute colitis characterized by the formation of adherent inflammatory exudates (pseudomembranes) on the injured mucosa. It is usually caused by the two protein exotoxins (A and B) of *Clostridium difficile*, a bacterium normally found in the gut. This disease commonly occurs in patients after a course of broad-spectrum antibiotic therapy (especially clindamycin). Alteration of the normal colonic flora allows these toxin-producing strains to thrive. Patients usually present with severe bouts of watery diarrhea, which can be life threatening. The first step in treating these patients is to immediately discontinue the offending antibiotic.

Answer B is incorrect. *Clostridium perfringens* is not associated with pseudomembranous colitis. Intestinal infection by this organism causes watery diarrhea, with some strains producing a severe necrotizing enterocolitis with perforation.

Answer C is incorrect. *Escherichia coli* is not associated with the development of pseudomembranous colitis. However, clinical features such as fever and diarrhea are common to both *E. coli* and *Clostridium difficile* infections.

Answer D is incorrect. Although *Staphylococcus aureus* has been implicated in pseudomembranous colitis the incidence of *S. aureus* pseudomembranous colitis is rare relative to *Clostridium difficile* colitis.

Answer E is incorrect. *Vibrio cholerae* is not implicated in pseudomembranous colitis. It usually causes massive secretory diarrhea.

Answer F is incorrect. *Yersinia enterocolitica* is not associated with pseudomembranous colitis. However, this organism can also cause fever and diarrhea secondary to intestinal epithelial invasion.

11. **The correct answer is C.** Chronic gallbladder irritation, often as a result of gallstones, is associated with the development of adenocarcinoma of the gallbladder. Gallbladder cancer is a disease of the elderly and is more common in women than men. There is a strong association with cholelithiasis, chronic cholecystitis, and inflammation; 90% of patients with gallbladder cancer have concomitant stones. (Note that cholangiocarcinoma is cancer of the bile duct system, not the gallbladder itself. The risk factors for this tumor include primary sclerosing cholangitis, congenital choledochal cysts, parasitic infections, hepatolithiasis, and toxic exposure. Cholelithiasis, however, has not been associated with cholangiocarcinoma.) In general, the treatment for adenocarcinoma of the gallbladder is surgical excision.

Answer A is incorrect. *Ascaris lumbricoides* is associated with gastrointestinal irritation, cough, and eosinophilia.

Answer B is incorrect. Cigarette smoking is associated with many malignancies, particularly of the lung, pancreas, and esophagus; it has not been linked to adenocarcinoma of the gallbladder.

Answer D is incorrect. *Schistosoma haematobium* infection is associated with the development of squamous cell carcinoma of the bladder.

Answer E is incorrect. Tuberculosis is associated with hemoptysis, cough, and weight loss.

12. **The correct answer is A.** Leukotriene (LT)B$_4$ is a neutrophil chemotactic agent and will be abundant during an acute inflammatory process. LTB$_4$ is produced via the 5-lipoxygenase pathway primarily by neutrophils and macrophages and is one of the most effective chemoattractant mediators known. It is involved in a number of events, including stimulation of leukocyte migration from the blood-

stream, activation of neutrophils, inflammatory pain, host defense against infection, and increased interleukin production and transcription. It is found in elevated concentrations in a number of inflammatory and allergic conditions, such as asthma, psoriasis, rheumatoid arthritis, and inflammatory bowel disease, and has been implicated in the pathogenesis of these diseases.

Answer B is incorrect. Prostaglandin I_2 (PGI_2) is synthesized by vascular endothelium and smooth muscle. Its effects include inhibition of platelet aggregation, relaxation of smooth muscle, reduction of systemic and pulmonary vascular resistance by direct vasodilation, and natriuresis in kidney. It is produced via the cyclooxygenase pathway.

Answer C is incorrect. Thromboxane A_2 (TxA_2) is a potent inducer of platelet aggregation and vasoconstriction. TxA_2 has been thought to play a critical role in the pathogenesis of thrombotic and atherosclerotic disorders.

Answer D is incorrect. Vascular endothelial growth factor (VEGF) is a substance made by cells that stimulates new blood vessel formation, and is a mitogen for vascular endothelial (vessel lining) cells. VEGF is a polypeptide structurally related to platelet-derived growth factor. VEGF initiates the process of new blood vessel growth by binding to endothelial cells that line the blood vessels. VEGF binds to two specific receptor proteins found only on the surface of endothelial cells. The binding of VEGF turns on the receptors, which then generate signals inside the cell, ultimately leading to the growth of new blood vessels.

Answer E is incorrect. Von Willebrand factor (vWF) is made by the cell lining in the walls of blood vessels (veins and arteries). When blood vessels are damaged, platelets clump together at the site of the injury. vWF binds platelet glycoprotein-1b and facilitates platelet adhesion at the site of injury. vWF is also a carrier of factor VIII.

13. The correct answer is B. The patient's symptoms, characterized by voluminous, malodor-

ous bulky stools that improve with fasting combined with increased stool osmolality and 72-hour fecal fat, are suggestive of malabsorption. Malabsorption can result from multiple causes, including defective intraluminal digestion (e.g., pancreatitis), primary mucosal cell abnormalities (e.g., celiac sprue, tropical sprue), reduced small intestinal surface area (e.g., small bowel resection), lymphatic obstruction (e.g., Whipple's disease), and impaired mucosal cell absorption secondary to an infectious agent (e.g., *Giardia lamblia*). One of the easier ways to test for malabsorption is to perform a 72-hour fecal fat collection. This involves putting a patient on a 100-g fat diet for 3 days followed by fecal fat measurement in the stool.

Answer A is incorrect. Exudative diseases are characterized by mucosal destruction that leads to purulent and bloody stools. Exudative diarrhea persists with fasting.

Answer C is incorrect. Motility derangement such as that which occurs with diabetic neuropathy or hyperthyroidism results from failure of gut neuromuscular function. This type of diarrhea would not improve with fasting. Furthermore, stool osmolality would be expected to be normal.

Answer D is incorrect. Osmotic diarrhea is characterized by abundant stool output per day that is relieved with fasting. This type of diarrhea has an osmotic gap ($290 - 2$ [Na_{stool} + K_{stool}] ≥ 50 mOsm) similar to that of malabsorptive diarrhea. However, osmotic diarrhea would not normally increase fecal fat.

Answer E is incorrect. In secretory diarrhea, net intestinal fluid secretion also leads to significantly increased amounts of stool output. Unlike diarrhea secondary to malabsorption, however, secretory diarrhea will be isotonic with respect to plasma and will not abate with fasting.

14. The correct answer is A. This patient has early gastric cancer, defined as adenocarcinoma limited to the gastric mucosa and submucosa regardless of regional lymph node involvement. Prognosis for early gastric carcinoma, compared with other gastric carcinomas, is quite good.

Answer B is incorrect. The incidence of gastric cancer is highest in Japan. Its incidence dropped in the United States with the advent of refrigeration, purportedly due to an increase in the consumption of uncontaminated, fresh foodstuffs.

Answer C is incorrect. Linitis plastica or "leather bottle" stomach is a poor prognostic factor in late-stage gastric carcinoma. It occurs when the neoplasm extends into the muscular layer of the stomach, causing a stiffening and narrowing of the organ.

Answer D is incorrect. Early gastric carcinoma (early because this has occurred at some point in the five years since her last endoscopy/gastric biopsy) does not usually metastasize.

Answer E is incorrect. This would be more indicative of a poorly differentiated, late-stage gastric carcinoma.

15. **The correct answer is D.** Schistosomiasis is a helminthic disease with hepatic involvement. *Schistosoma mansoni* cercaria, which are commonly found in fresh waters of South America, penetrate the host's skin, invade the peripheral vasculature, and eventually settle in the portal or pelvic venous vasculature. Several weeks following infection, patients may develop symptoms similar to the ones described, such as fever, diarrhea, and weight loss; the "funny-looking stools" likely represent *S. cercaria* eggs. Chronic infection may eventually lead to portal hypertension, leading in turn to hepatosplenomegaly, ascites, and eventual cirrhosis.

Answer A is incorrect. Appendicitis commonly presents with right lower quadrant abdominal pain, fever, nausea, vomiting, and leukocytosis. The ascites seen in this patient is not a typical finding with appendicitis.

Answer B is incorrect. Bowel obstruction generally presents with nausea, vomiting, and decreased or absent bowel sounds. This patient has none of these signs or symptoms.

Answer C is incorrect. Enterocolitis would not present with signs and symptoms of ascites. It usually manifests with diarrhea.

Answer E is incorrect. Ruptured viscus may present with signs of peritonitis such as rebound tenderness. It may result from ischemic bowel disease or obstruction. This patient's history, physical examination, and imaging studies are inconsistent with this etiology.

16. **The correct answer is C.** The symptoms of upper gastrointestinal bleeding associated with epigastric pain in a patient with rheumatoid arthritis are most consistent with acute erosive hemorrhagic gastritis. The image shows diffusely hyperemic gastric mucosa, a typical finding in acute gastritis. Given this patient's history of rheumatoid arthritis, the most likely cause of her presentation is NSAID use. As many as 25% of patients who take daily aspirin for rheumatoid arthritis eventually develop acute gastritis.

Answer A is incorrect. Amyloidosis is associated with chronic gastritis, not acute gastritis.

Answer B is incorrect. *Helicobacter pylori* infection is associated with chronic gastritis and not acute erosive hemorrhagic gastritis. *H. pylori* infection can be associated with a mild acute gastritis, but the patient's history of rheumatoid arthritis should prompt the consideration of NSAID use.

Answer D is incorrect. Steroid treatment is not a known risk factor for acute gastritis.

Answer E is incorrect. Although uremia is a risk factor for developing acute gastritis, this patient has no evidence of kidney failure or symptoms to suggest uremia.

17. **The correct answer is B.** Recent studies have demonstrated the benefit of infliximab for the treatment of Crohn's disease that is refractory to steroid treatment. Infliximab is a monoclonal antibody that blocks the effects of TNF-α and thereby decreases the body's inflammatory response. Adverse effects of infliximab include fever and chills, as well as anaphylactoid reactions.

Answer A is incorrect. Diarrhea is not often associated with infliximab.

Answer C is incorrect. Headache is not often associated with infliximab.

Answer D is incorrect. Hypotension, not hypertension, is often associated with infliximab.

Answer E is incorrect. Nausea and vomiting are not often associated with infliximab.

18. **The correct answer is A.** This patient suffers from Hirschsprung's disease. This disease develops when neural crest cells fail to migrate to the distal colon. Enteric neurons do not form in a segment of the rectosigmoid; these neurons are normally responsible for relaxation of the rectum to allow defecation. These patients present in infancy with abdominal distention, prolonged passage of meconium, absent or infrequent bowel movements, and poor nutrition/weight gain. The barium enema also suggests Hirschsprung's disease, as these patients typically have a narrow segment in the rectosigmoid with a massively dilated segment above this narrowing. A full-thickness biopsy showing absence of enteric neurons in the rectum and possibly sigmoid colon would provide a definitive diagnosis.

Answer B is incorrect. Motor function to the external anal sphincter is provided via the pudendal nerve. Defects in this nerve would lead to involuntary defecation with a full rectum.

Answer C is incorrect. The pelvic nerve regulates the defecation reflex, in which a full rectum brings about relaxation of the internal anal sphincter and constriction of the external anal sphincter, leading to the urge to defecate.

Answer D is incorrect. Sympathetic nerves stop colonic movements. Thus, absent sympathetic innervation would actually increase colonic movement.

Answer E is incorrect. The vagus nerve causes contractions in the proximal colon. The absence of the vagus effect on the colon would decrease defecation but would not lead to increased stool in the sigmoid colon.

19. **The correct answer is B.** Vomiting typically induces a metabolic alkalosis due to a loss of hydrogen ions from the stomach, leading to

an increase in pH. This leaves an increased HCO_3^- concentration in the bloodstream. In this case, the P_{CO_2} is still normal; thus, no respiratory compensation has occurred, and the patient has uncompensated metabolic alkalosis.

Answer A is incorrect. This patient is presenting with a metabolic alkalosis, not an acidosis.

Answer C is incorrect. The metabolic alkalosis in this patient is uncomplicated.

Answer D is incorrect. The metabolic alkalosis in this patient is uncomplicated.

Answer E is incorrect. The metabolic alkalosis in this patient is uncomplicated.

Answer F is incorrect. The metabolic alkalosis in this patient is uncomplicated.

20. **The correct answer is B.** The histopathologic changes described are consistent with hepatitis seen in severe exposure to alcohol. Intracytoplasmic hyaline inclusions derived from cytokeratin intermediate filaments are called Mallory bodies, which are also seen in primary biliary cirrhosis, Wilson's disease, chronic cholestatic syndromes, and hepatocellular tumors. Prolonged alcohol abuse may result in alcoholic cirrhosis, an irreversible condition characterized by nodular fibrosis of the liver parenchyma.

Answer A is incorrect. In acute viral hepatitis, hepatocyte injury takes the form of diffuse swelling (ballooning degeneration). Fatty change is unusual, with the exception of hepatitis C virus. In contrast to alcoholic hepatitis, Mallory bodies are not seen.

Answer C is incorrect. α-Antitrypsin deficiency is an autosomal recessive disorder that may result in both liver failure and emphysema. Histologically, this condition is characterized by the presence of cytoplasmic globular inclusions in hepatocytes. These inclusions are strongly periodic acid-Schiff (PAS) positive, a specific feature for this disease.

Answer D is incorrect. Fatty liver of pregnancy is an acute hepatic failure during the third trimester of pregnancy associated with microvesicular liver change. Pathologically, this condition is not characterized by Mallory body formation and neutrophilic infiltrates.

Answer E is incorrect. Neonatal hepatitis commonly results in jaundice during the first few weeks of life. Liver biopsy in neonatal hepatitis may reveal panlobular multinucleated giant cells among other morphologic manifestations. Mallory bodies and neutrophilic infiltrates are not typically seen in this condition.

21. **The correct answer is B.** *Entamoeba histolytica* infection presents with bloody diarrhea (dysentery), abdominal cramps with tenesmus, and pus in the stool. It can also cause right upper quadrant pain and liver abscesses. *E. histolytica* is transmitted via cysts in water (fecal-oral transmission). On microscopy, one observes amebas with ingested RBCs. Treatment for *E. histolytica* infection includes metronidazole and iodoquinol.

Answer A is incorrect. *Cryptosporidium* species infection presents with severe diarrhea in HIV-positive patients and with mild watery diarrhea in HIV-negative patients. *Cryptosporidium* is transmitted via cysts in water (fecal-oral transmission). Microscopically, acid-fast staining cysts are found. Unfortunately, there is no treatment available for *Cryptosporidium* species infection. In healthy patients, however, cryptosporidiosis is self-resolving.

Answer C is incorrect. *Giardia lamblia* infection presents with bloating, flatulence, foul-smelling diarrhea, and light-colored fatty stools. *G. lamblia* is transmitted via cysts in water (fecal-oral transmission). On microscopy, one observes teardrop-shaped trophozoites with a ventral sucking disc or cysts. Metronidazole is used to treat *G. lamblia* infection.

Answer D is incorrect. *Leishmania donovani* presents with hepatomegaly and splenomegaly, malaise, anemia, and weight loss. *L. donovani* is transmitted via the sandfly. Microscopically, macrophages containing amastigotes are observed. Sodium stibogluconate is used to treat *L. donovani* infection.

Answer E is incorrect. *Toxoplasma gondii* infection presents with brain abscesses in HIV-positive patients and with birth defects if infection occurs during pregnancy (toxoplasmosis is one of the TORCHeS organisms). *Toxoplasma gondii* is transmitted via cysts in raw meat or cat feces. The definitive stage (sexual stage) occurs in cats. Microscopically, acid-fast staining cysts are found. Sulfadiazine and pyrimethamine are used to treat toxoplasmosis.

22. **The correct answer is A.** Familial adenomatous polyposis is an autosomal dominant condition characterized by a deletion on chromosome 5.

Answer B is incorrect. Examples of autosomal recessive conditions include cystic fibrosis, sickle cell anemia, and hemochromatosis.

Answer C is incorrect. Examples of autosomal trisomy conditions include Down's syndrome (trisomy 21), Edwards' syndrome (trisomy 18), and Patau's syndrome (trisomy 13).

Answer D is incorrect. Examples of conditions related to sex chromosome abnormalities include Klinefelter's syndrome (XXY), Turner's syndrome (XO), and double-Y males (XYY).

Answer E is incorrect. Examples of X-linked recessive conditions include fragile X syndrome, hemophilia A and B, glucose-6-phosphate dehydrogenase deficiency, and Lesch-Nyhan syndrome

23. **The correct answer is C.** This patient has an indirect bilirubinemia with a high total serum bilirubin but a normal direct bilirubin. In a healthy 25-year-old individual, this is most likely due to a deficiency in functional glucuronosyltransferase, otherwise known as Gilbert's disease. Glucuronosyltransferase deficiency causes an indirect hyperbilirubinemia only, while the other answer choices cause an elevation in both direct and indirect bilirubin levels.

Answer A is incorrect. Defects in hepatic excretion are due to either intrahepatic obstruction or extrahepatic obstruction and result in an increase in both indirect and direct bilirubin.

Answer B is incorrect. Extrahepatic biliary obstruction due to a tumor, stone, or stricture causes an elevation of both indirect and direct bilirubin levels.

Answer D is incorrect. Intrahepatic biliary obstruction causes a defect in excretion and results in an increase in both direct and indirect bilirubin levels.

Answer E is incorrect. Liver cell damage such as that seen in chronic hepatitis causes an elevation of both direct and indirect bilirubin due to an impairment of uptake, conjugation, and excretion of bilirubin.

24. **The correct answer is C.** This patient has vitamin A deficiency (characterized by early symptoms of night blindness, dry conjunctivae, and gray plaques, as well as late symptoms of corneal ulceration and necrosis leading to perforation and blindness), which is commonly seen in children and pregnant women whose diets are deficient in vitamin A, especially those from Southeast Asia. Vitamin A deficiency can also result from malabsorption following intestinal surgery, storage abnormalities secondary to liver disease, and excessive secretion due to proteinuria. Vitamin A is typically stored in the liver as retinyl esters.

Answer A is incorrect. Vitamin A is not typically stored in the appendix.

Answer B is incorrect. Vitamin A is not typically stored in the gallbladder.

Answer D is incorrect. Vitamin A is not typically stored in the pancreas.

Answer E is incorrect. Vitamin A is not typically stored in the stomach.

25. **The correct answer is A.** The triad of jaundice (icteric sclera), hypercholesterolemia (palpebral xanthomas), and pruritus with positive antimitochondrial antibody titers and elevated alkaline phosphatase activity is classic for primary biliary cirrhosis. Primary biliary cirrhosis is a cholestatic disease with chronic, progressive,

and often fatal liver injury characterized by the destruction of medium-sized intrahepatic bile ducts with eventual liver failure. Liver transplantation is the definitive treatment.

Answer B is incorrect. Hepatic parenchymal destruction occurs only as a late sequela of primary biliary cirrhosis secondary to intrahepatic bile duct compromise. This patient's acute presentation suggests early disease.

Answer C is incorrect. Obstruction of extrahepatic bile ducts is seen with secondary biliary cirrhosis resulting from obstructive conditions such as cholelithiasis, neoplasms, surgical procedures, biliary atresia, and cystic fibrosis. Primary biliary cirrhosis is not characterized by extrahepatic bile duct obstruction.

Answer D is incorrect. Portal vein thrombosis is not a mechanism responsible for this patient's presentation. Portal vein thrombosis has multiple etiologies, including hypercoagulable states, inflammatory diseases (e.g., ulcerative colitis), iatrogenic causes, infections, and liver disease. Unlike primary biliary cirrhosis, it commonly presents with variceal hemorrhage and/or melena.

Answer E is incorrect. Stenosis of extrahepatic and intrahepatic bile ducts is seen with primary sclerosing cholangitis and not with primary biliary cirrhosis.

26. **The correct answer is A.** This patient's history and biopsy results are consistent with celiac disease. The physical examination would most likely reveal an anorexic-appearing child with temporal wasting and multiple nonblanching purpuric lesions located on the upper and lower extremities. Celiac disease (gluten-sensitive enteropathy) is characterized by small intestine mucosal damage and the malabsorption of most nutrients, resulting in the symptoms and physical examination findings presented in this case. The gliadin fraction in wheat is responsible for disease activation. Thus, cereals are responsible for this patient's presentation. Discontinuation of gliadin-containing foods such as cereals usually results in complete remission.

Answer B is incorrect. Dairy products are not associated with celiac disease but can be associated with lactose intolerance, which usually appears benign on mucosal biopsy.

Answer C is incorrect. Fish is not associated with celiac disease.

Answer D is incorrect. Fruits and vegetables are not associated with celiac disease.

Answer E is incorrect. Undercooked meat is commonly associated with infectious enteropathies and not celiac disease. There are variable appearances on mucosal biopsy.

27. **The correct answer is C.** Pegylated interferon is a cytokine derivative that improves the body's antiviral response. It is used in the treatment of hepatitis B and C. Adverse effects of interferon therapy include a flulike reaction that manifests as episodic fevers and chills, as well as occasional profound depression. As a result, interferon is contraindicated in severely depressed or suicidal patients. Although interferon is not a cure for hepatitis, it is recommended to slow the progression of cirrhotic liver disease in some patients. Pegylated interferon is a longer-acting form of interferon.

Answer A is incorrect. Intravenous immunoglobulin is an engineered antibody that is used to clear the serum of protein products. It is often used in treatment of autoimmune diseases such as Guillain-Barré syndrome. Adverse effects include flulike reaction and anaphylactoid reaction.

Answer B is incorrect. Lamivudine is a nucleotide reverse transcriptase inhibitor used in the treatment of HIV and hepatitis B. Its principal adverse effect is hepatotoxicity.

Answer D is incorrect. Ribavirin is an antiviral drug used in the treatment of hepatitis C, respiratory syncytial virus, and, occasionally, other viral illnesses. It is not associated with depression or a flulike reaction.

Answer E is incorrect. Tumor necrosis factor-α is a cytokine involved in the antiviral and antitumor response. It is not currently used as a treatment for hepatitis C.

28. **The correct answer is C.** New onset of right lower quadrant abdominal pain in a young patient with a fever and an elevated WBC count is suggestive of appendicitis. Patients with appendicitis typically present with periumbilical or right lower quadrant abdominal pain. Fifty to sixty percent will also present with nausea and vomiting.

Answer A is incorrect. Distention is rare in a patient with appendicitis unless diffuse peritonitis has developed.

Answer B is incorrect. Patients with appendicitis typically present with anorexia. Hunger in a patient with appendicitis should make one reconsider the diagnosis.

Answer D is incorrect. While diarrhea can occur in a patient with appendicitis, profuse watery diarrhea is more suggestive of acute gastroenteritis than appendicitis.

Answer E is incorrect. Vaginal bleeding does not typically occur in appendicitis but would be suggestive of rupture of a corpus luteum cyst, rupture of a graafian follicle, or a ruptured tubal pregnancy.

29. **The correct answer is D.** *Shigella* species produce gastroenteritis characterized by abdominal pain and bloody diarrhea. Additionally, since *Shigella* species invade intestinal epithelial cells, the illness is accompanied by fever. *Shigella* is a nonlactose fermenter, and it does not produce gas or hydrogen sulfide.

Answer A is incorrect. *Escherichia coli* can also cause a bloody diarrhea, and the enteroinvasive species can cause fever. Unlike *Shigella*, however, *E. coli* is a lactose fermenter.

Answer B is incorrect. Enterotoxigenic *Escherichia coli* infection causes gastroenteritis characterized by watery diarrhea. *E. coli* is a lactose fermenter.

Answer C is incorrect. Although *Salmonella* species cause bloody diarrhea, it does not invade intestinal epithelial cells and therefore does not cause fever. It is a nonlactose fermenter but, unlike *Shigella*, produces gas and hydrogen sulfide.

Answer E is incorrect. *Vibrio cholerae* produces a gastroenteritis characterized by high-volume, watery diarrhea.

30. **The correct answer is B.** The patient's presentation is consistent with ruptured esophageal varices. Portal systemic shunting of blood occurs when the liver becomes so scarred and fibrotic that there is an increase in resistance in blood flow from the portal vein and portal hypertension develops. When the pressure in the portal system is greater than the venous pressure in the systemic system, blood will find alternate routes to return to the heart. One of those alternate routes is from the left gastric vein into the azygos vein. The veins around the esophagus and upper stomach that carry this blood may become enlarged and rupture, as in this case. Mortality from ruptured esophageal varices approaches 50%, so it is important to look for symptoms of liver disease and portal hypertension in anyone with massive hemoptysis. It is also important to screen cirrhotic patients with serial endoscopies to look for varices that can be treated before they rupture.

Answer A is incorrect. The portal system is a system of veins that drain the gastrointestinal tract and deliver the blood to the liver. The left gastric artery is upstream of the portal system, and an anastomosis between the left gastric artery and vein would bypass the portal system altogether and would not contribute to the formation of esophageal varices.

Answer C is incorrect. Anastomoses between these two vessels leads to the formation of caput medusae, the spokes-of-a-wheel veins radiating from the umbilicus in patients with portal hypertension.

Answer D is incorrect. There is no route for blood to flow from the portal vein to the inferior vena cava. If there were, however, this would relieve the pressure in the portal system and would reduce the risk of bleeding from varices. In fact, creating a portacaval shunt (TIPS, or transjugular intrahepatic portosystemic shunt) is a current treatment for portal hypertension with massive ascites.

Answer E is incorrect. Anastomoses between the splenic vein and the left renal vein are retroperitoneal vessels that are not near the esophagus.

31. **The correct answer is E.** Given this patient's history of chronic obstructive pulmonary disease, the most likely factor contributing to the development of his duodenal ulcer is tobacco use. The incidence of peptic ulcers in smokers is twice as great as in nonsmokers.

Answer A is incorrect. Unlike acute gastritis, alcohol use is not a known risk factor for peptic ulcer development.

Answer B is incorrect. Chronic use of NSAIDs is a known risk factor for peptic ulcer disease. However, in this patient, there is no reason to suspect long-term use of these medications.

Answer C is incorrect. Excessive salt intake is not a risk factor for peptic ulcer disease.

Answer D is incorrect. Primary hyperparathyroidism is associated with peptic ulcer disease. This condition is a possibility in this patient given his increased risk for bronchogenic squamous cell carcinoma; however, his recent weight gain and normal Ca^{2+} and phosphate plasma levels argue against primary hyperparathyroidism.

32. **The correct answer is A.** This illustration depicts the muscularis externa, which is composed of an inner circular layer, cut transversely (seen in the upper left half of the field), and an outer longitudinal layer, sectioned longitudinally (seen at the lower right). The arrows are pointing to one of the components of the enteric nervous system (cells with large nuclei and darkly stained nucleoli consistent with neurons) called Auerbach's myenteric plexus, situated between the two muscle layers. The myenteric plexus functions mainly in coordinating motility along the entire gut wall.

Answer B is incorrect. Inhibition of peristalsis is mediated via sympathetic innervation derived from the splanchnic nerves. In general, the sympathetic nervous system, not the myenteric, inhibits peristalsis and activates sphincter muscles.

Answer C is incorrect. Meissner's plexus, not the myenteric plexus, regulates absorption.

Answer D is incorrect. Meissner's submucosal plexus regulates secretions. This component of the enteric nervous system is located between the mucosa and the inner layer of smooth muscle in the gastrointestinal tract wall. The image shows the myenteric plexus, which does not function in regulating secretion.

Answer E is incorrect. Smooth muscle contraction in the gastrointestinal tract is mediated primarily by parasympathetic stimulation via the vagus nerve. The myenteric plexus, however, does not perform that function.

33. **The correct answer is C.** Hyperalbuminemia is only significant when it may indicate dehydration. A patient with a 2-day history of vomiting and diarrhea is most likely dehydrated due to loss of volume.

Answer A is incorrect. Acute infection typically causes hypoalbuminemia due to decreased protein synthesis.

Answer B is incorrect. Chronic liver disease causes hypoalbuminemia as albumin is typically produced in the liver.

Answer D is incorrect. Nephrotic syndrome causes hypoalbuminemia due to excessive protein loss.

Answer E is incorrect. Poor nutritional status causes hypoalbuminemia due to poor protein intake.

34. **The correct answer is B.** The ciprofloxacin has been rendered ineffective due to chelation with calcium in antacids.

Answer A is incorrect. Aspirin is associated with gastric ulcers and Reye's syndrome.

Answer C is incorrect. Misoprostol is a prostaglandin E_1 analog that can be used to prevent NSAID-induced peptic ulcers. It is also used as a medical abortifacient in many countries and is therefore strictly contraindicated in pregnant women

Answer D is incorrect. Omeprazole is a proton pump inhibitor and is associated with atrophic gastritis due to hypergastrinemia and carcinoid tumors.

Answer E is incorrect. Although cimetidine, another H_2 antagonist, is associated with inhibition of the cytochrome P450 system, ranitidine is relatively free of this adverse effect.

35. **The correct answer is C.** Chronic pancreatitis is a disease characterized by recurrent episodes of pancreatic inflammation with associated loss of pancreatic parenchyma. It is commonly associated with alcoholism. Chronic pancreatitis is a disabling disease. Chronic malabsorption may develop secondary to exocrine insufficiency. Diabetes mellitus is also a common manifestation of chronic pancreatitis. A relatively specific finding in chronic pancreatitis is visualization of pancreatic calcifications on CT scan.

Answer A is incorrect. An abdominal x-ray finding of air-fluid levels in the small intestine is suggestive of bowel obstruction. This feature is not common with chronic pancreatitis.

Answer B is incorrect. Free air under the right hemidiaphragm on chest x-ray suggests a ruptured abdominal viscus. This feature is not common with chronic pancreatitis.

Answer D is incorrect. Pancreatic cysts contain serous fluid enclosed by ductlike cuboidal epithelium. They can occur with pancreatic neoplasms, polycystic disease, von Hippel–Lindau disease, or congenitally. In contrast, chronic pancreatitis may be characterized by pseudocysts and not cystic lesions. Pseudocysts are collections of fluid, usually pancreatic secretions that form after inflammation of the pancreas. Unlike pancreatic cysts, they lack true epithelial lining.

Answer E is incorrect. Pancreatic granuloma formation is not commonly seen in chronic pancreatitis. Pancreatic granuloma is a rare condition that may be seen with extrapulmonary tuberculosis and, uncommonly, with sarcoidosis. It is not commonly associated with chronic pancreatitis.

36. **The correct answer is E.** Omeprazole is a proton pump inhibitor and is associated with atrophic gastritis due to hypergastrinemia. It may also be associated with carcinoid tumors.

    Answer A is incorrect. Aluminum hydroxide is an antacid and is associated with constipation and hypophosphatemia.

    Answer B is incorrect. Bismuth binds to ulcers, allowing a physical protective barrier, and has no known significant adverse effects.

    Answer C is incorrect. Cimetidine is an H_2 antagonist and is associated with inhibition of the cytochrome P450 system.

    Answer D is incorrect. Misoprostol is a prostaglandin E_1 analog that can be used to prevent NSAID-induced peptic ulcers. It is also used as a medical abortifacient in many countries and is therefore strictly contraindicated in pregnant women.

37. **The correct answer is C.** A history of recurrent right lower quadrant abdominal pain with diarrhea, fevers, and weight loss is indicative of a chronic gastrointestinal inflammatory process. One of the most common inflammatory bowel diseases is Crohn's disease. The signs and symptoms of this disease are sequelae of chronic transmural inflammation of the bowel, which usually starts in the terminal ileum. Patients typically present in their 20s with complaints similar to those described in the vignette.

    Answer A is incorrect. Celiac sprue is a disorder of malabsorption secondary to gluten sensitivity. However, it would not present with fevers and mucosal erosions. Instead, colonoscopy would show villous flattening.

    Answer B is incorrect. Patients with collagenous colitis usually have normal endoscopic findings.

    Answer D is incorrect. Irritable bowel syndrome is a functional disorder and would not present with abnormalities on colonoscopy.

    Answer E is incorrect. This patient's clinical presentation and mucosal erosions in the terminal ileum are suggestive of Crohn's disease. Ulcerative colitis can share many features with Crohn's disease. However, it is usually limited to the colon.

38. **The correct answer is A.** *Brucella melitensis* enters the body after the ingestion of contaminated milk products or direct contact with contaminated livestock. It is an intracellular bacterium that causes undulating fever, weakness, and loss of appetite.

    Answer B is incorrect. *Clostridium difficile* causes severe nonbloody diarrhea associated with pseudomembranes. It is associated with previous antibiotic treatment.

    Answer C is incorrect. *Plasmodium malariae* is a protozoan that causes malaria. This disease is characterized by episodes of fever and chills every 72 hours. It is spread through the bite of the *Anopheles* mosquito. While splenomegaly is often present, lymphadenopathy is not.

    Answer D is incorrect. *Vibrio cholerae* causes food poisoning that is characterized by watery diarrhea (rice-water stool). This patient reports no such symptoms.

    Answer E is incorrect. *Yersinia enterocolitica* is also transmitted to humans through the consumption of unpasteurized milk. It causes enterocolitis with symptoms that can be indistinguishable from enterocolitis caused by *Salmonella* or *Shigella* species. Hepatosplenomegaly and lymphadenopathy are typically absent, however.

39. **The correct answer is A.** This patient has Mallory-Weiss syndrome. Repeated bouts of prolonged vomiting can cause longitudinal lacerations in the distal esophagus, with extension to submucosal arteries that can bleed massively. Untreated, this bleeding can be fatal. Bleeding from esophageal varices should also be suspected in a patient with a history like this.

    Answer B is incorrect. Metaplasia of esophageal mucosa is associated with reflux causing inflammation, sometimes leading to ulceration. This can cause bleeding, but it is usually not massive. Barrett's esophagus is of concern primarily because of its association with adenocarcinoma.

Answer C is incorrect. Esophageal squamous cell carcinoma would cause ulceration of the esophageal mucosa, but massive bleeding is uncommon.

Answer D is incorrect. Esophageal stricture are typically caused by scaring, from reflux, toxic ingestions, or scleroderma. It is a chronic problem most commonly manifesting as dysphagia, not hematemesis.

Answer E is incorrect. Hiatal hernia is usually an incidental finding, most commonly causing nausea and substernal pain. Bleeding is very uncommon and is rarely massive.

40. **The correct answer is D.** Irritable bowel syndrome is a functional gastrointestinal disorder characterized by abdominal pain and altered bowel habits in the absence of demonstrable organic pathology. It is a diagnosis of exclusion based on clinical features such as the ones presented. Most commonly, patients have alternating diarrhea and constipation, chronic abdominal pain that improves with stools, a change in stool frequency and consistency, and onset after emotional and/or stressful life events. These symptoms occur in the absence of fevers, lower gastrointestinal bleeding, leukocytosis, and weight loss.

Answer A is incorrect. Celiac sprue is a disease of malabsorption characterized by bulky, fatty stools following meals. Endoscopic findings reveal villous flattening in the small intestine.

Answer B is incorrect. Colorectal carcinoma is unlikely given the patient's young age, absence of weight loss, negative hemoccult test, and benign colonoscopy findings.

Answer C is incorrect. Inflammatory bowel disease has a highly variable presentation; however, mucosal lesions are readily evident on colonoscopy and/or endoscopy.

Answer E is incorrect. Pseudomembranous colitis usually follows broad-spectrum antibiotic therapy and is characterized by bloody diarrhea, fever, and leukocytosis. Absence of these manifestations in the patient argues against this diagnosis.

41. **The correct answer is A.** Micelles contact the intestinal cell membrane so that hydrophobic products can be absorbed. In intestinal cells, digestive products are reesterified and chylomicrons are formed. Chylomicrons are exocytosed from intestinal cells and transported through the lymph to the bloodstream.

Answer B is not correct. Lingual lipases digest triglycerides to monoglycerides and fatty acids in the stomach.

Answer C is not correct. Emulsification with bile acids occurs in the small intestine. This process also increases surface area for digestion.

Answer D is not correct. Micelle formation occurs in the small intestine to solubilize hydrophobic products so that they can be transported across the intestinal cell membrane.

Answer E is not correct. Mixing breaks lipids into smaller droplets in the stomach. This increases the surface area for enzyme digestion.

42. **The correct answer is C.** The most common tumor of the parotid gland is the pleomorphic adenoma. The pleomorphic adenoma is a benign, well-differentiated, well-circumscribed mass that grows slowly over the course of months to years. On histopathology, it is characterized by the presence of multiple cell types, classically epithelial cells in a chondromyxoid stroma.

Answer A is incorrect. Adenoid cystic carcinoma is an invasive, poorly differentiated cancer characterized by gland-forming tissue and a cystic, fluid-filled cavity. It tends to infiltrate perineurial spaces and cause pain.

Answer B is incorrect. Mucoepidermoid carcinoma is an invasive, poorly differentiated cancer composed of mucosal and epidermal cell types.

Answer D is incorrect. A sialic duct stone is an inorganic precipitate mechanically obstructing the opening of the sialic duct, resulting in an erythematous and inflamed oral mass.

Answer E is incorrect. Warthin's tumor is a benign mass of lymphoid cells. A well-circumscribed mass of lymphoid cells in a salivary gland is virtually pathognomonic for a Warthin's tumor.

43. **The correct answer is E.** This is an example of volvulus, a twisting of the bowel that is more prevalent in adults than in children. In adults, volvulus occurs with equal frequency in both the small and large intestine. In children, volvulus almost always occurs in the small intestine and is often the result of intestinal malrotation that occurred during development of the embryonic gut. Volvulus is associated with bowel obstruction in both young and old patients.

Answer A is incorrect. A gross image of infarcted bowel would appear dark red or purple as a result of accumulated luminal hemorrhage. Bowel infarction can result from various causes including acute arterial thrombosis or venous occlusion.

Answer B is incorrect. Colorectal carcinoma may be papillary or polypoid. A gross image would commonly demonstrate proximal bowel dilation.

Answer C is incorrect. Intussusception occurs when one segment of the small intestine telescopes into the immediately distal segment of the bowel. Although intussusception can cause vomiting in children, the gross image shows volvulus and not intussusception.

Answer D is incorrect. Meckel's diverticulum is a remnant of vitelline duct that appears as an outpouching of the small intestine. The image demonstrates no such anomaly.

44. **The correct answer is B.** The patient's condition is likely secondary to excess insulin. This

could be caused by an endogenous source of insulin as seen in insulinomas or due to exogenously administered insulin. One way to rule out a factitious cause of high insulin levels is to check the C-peptide level. C peptide is formed from the cleavage of endogenously produced insulin but is not present in manufactured pharmaceutical insulin, and therefore would be high only if the source of insulin were endogenous.

Answer A is incorrect. Chloride levels will be unaffected by the source of insulin.

Answer C is incorrect. Insulin levels will be high in both exogenous and endogenous causes of hyperinsulinemia.

Answer D is incorrect. Proinsulin levels will be high in both exogenous and endogenous causes of hyperinsulinemia.

Answer E is incorrect. Sodium levels will be unaffected by the source of insulin.

45. **The correct answer is E.** Heroin and other opiates function primarily by stimulation of μ receptors in the brain and gastrointestinal tract. μ-Receptor stimulation is responsible not only for the pleasure sensation derived from opiates but also for the decreased bowel motility and constipation with which opiates are associated. Narcotic pain medications have similar adverse effects because they are opiate-derived drugs. It is important to minimize opiate use in patients with suspected small bowel obstruction, ileus, or infectious diarrhea because these patients poorly tolerate constipation and slowed gastrointestinal motility.

Answer A is incorrect. Naloxone and naltrexone inhibit μ receptors and serve to block the effects of opiates. They are used for opiate overdose.

Answer B is incorrect. μ Receptors are not the primary receptors involved in the heroin response. Naloxone has an inhibitory effect on κ receptors.

Answer C is incorrect. Buprenorphine is a partial agonist-antagonist at μ receptors. It is being used in drug treatment programs to attempt to wean heroin addicts off of opiate drugs.

Answer D is incorrect. κ Receptors are not the primary receptors involved in the heroin response. Instead, they are activated by butorphanol.

46. **The correct answer is E.** *Staphylococcus aureus* food poisoning is characterized by more vomiting than diarrhea. Since the enterotoxin is preformed in food, the incubation time is short (1–8 hours). Contaminated mayonnaise has been shown to be a frequent source of S. *aureus* food poisoning.

Answer A is incorrect. *Staphylococcus aureus* is a gram-positive, catalase-positive, and coagulase-positive bacterium.

Answer B is incorrect. A positive quellung reaction is seen with encapsulated bacteria only. *Staphylococcus aureus* is not an encapsulated bacterium.

Answer C is incorrect. *Neisseria gonorrhoeae* is cultured on Thayer-Martin media.

Answer D is incorrect. Contaminated seafood is a common source of *Vibrio parahaemolyticus* and *V. vulnificus*. *Staphylococcus aureus* is commonly found in the mayonnaise portion of the tuna salad.

47. **The correct answer is D.** This constellation of symptoms is suggestive of Crigler-Najjar syndrome type I, a hereditary hyperbilirubinemia that is fatal within 18 months of life secondary to kernicterus (bilirubin deposition in brain tissue). Multiple genetic defects in the allele for the bilirubin uridine diphosphate-glucuronosyltransferase (UGT1) may give rise to this disorder. This enzyme is responsible for conjugating bilirubin with one or two molecules of glucuronic acid. The liver is morphologically normal by light and electron microscopy.

Answer A is incorrect. Aldolase B is responsible for conversion of fructose-1-phosphate to dihydroxyacetone phosphate and glyceraldehyde. The deficiency of this enzyme leads to jaundice, cirrhosis, and hypoglycemia, not ker-

nicterus, as seen in Crigler-Najjar syndrome type I.

Answer B is incorrect. Deficiency in galactose-1-phosphate uridyltransferase (responsible for synthesis of glucose-1-phosphate from galctose-1-phosphate) causes cataracts, hepatosplenomegaly, and mental retardation and not the presentation seen in Crigler-Najjar syndrome type I.

Answer C is incorrect. Glucose-6-phosphatase is an enzyme that catalyzes the dephosphorylation of glucose-6-phosphate to glucose. Its deficiency results in severe fasting hypoglycemia and increased glycogen deposition in the liver (von Gierke's disease). Presentation of this disease is drastically different from Crigler-Najjar syndrome type I.

Answer E is incorrect. A deficiency of uroporphyrinogen decarboxylase (involved in heme synthesis) leads to porphyria cutanea tarda, the most commonly diagnosed porphyria. In some instances this disorder can result in secondary hemochromatosis, but not in the presentation of Crigler-Najjar syndrome type I.

48. **The correct answer is B.** Acetaminophen is known to cause centrilobular necrosis. This type of necrosis occurs immediately around the terminal hepatic vein. In addition to acetaminophen, centrilobular necrosis can be caused by carbon tetrachloride, bromobenzene, halothane, and rifampin. Diffuse hepatic necrosis has also been reported with acetaminophen toxicity.

Answer A is incorrect. Drugs causing acute hepatitis include methyldopa, isoniazid, nitrofurantoin, and phenytoin. Acetaminophen is not associated with acute hepatitis.

Answer C is incorrect. Hepatic fibrosis is commonly associated with drugs that cause chronic hepatitis and/or hepatocellular injury. Some of the culprits include ethanol, methotrexate, and amiodarone. Acetaminophen is not associated with fibrotic liver changes.

Answer D is incorrect. Granuloma formation does not occur with acetaminophen overdose.

HIGH-YIELD SYSTEMS

Gastrointestinal

Some of the drugs associated with granuloma formation include sulfonamides, methyldopa, quinidine, hydralazine, and allopurinol.

Answer E is incorrect. Microvesicular fatty change does not occur with acetaminophen overdose. It is usually seen with tetracycline, salicylates, and ethanol use.

49. **The correct answer is A.** The quality and location of this patient's pain, combined with alleviation with medication and the radiographic findings, are suggestive of gastroesophageal reflux disease (GERD). This disorder increases the risk of developing esophageal mucosal metaplasia, called Barrett's esophagus. In turn, patients with Barrett's esophagus are at increased risk for developing adenocarcinoma of the esophagus.

Answer B is incorrect. Krukenberg's tumor is bilateral involvement of the ovaries by metastatic carcinoma of the stomach. This neoplasm bears no relation to gastroesophageal reflux disease.

Answer C is incorrect. Non–small cell adenocarcinoma of the lung is commonly caused by cigarette smoking but is not associated with gastroesophageal reflux disease.

Answer D is incorrect. Squamous cell carcinoma is not known to correlate with gastroesophageal reflux disease. Squamous cell carcinoma is thought to be associated with tobacco and alcohol use.

Answer E is incorrect. Stomach cell carcinoma is not associated with gastroesophageal reflux disease. Risk factors for stomach adenocarcinoma include *Helicobacter pylori* infection, nitrosamine exposure, excessive salt intake, and low intake of fresh fruit and vegetables. This type of carcinoma is predisposed by achlorhydria and chronic gastritis.

50. **The correct answer is E.** This patient presents with a number of classic extraintestinal manifestations of ulcerative colitis (UC). Progressive fatigue, pruritus, and icteric sclera are clinical manifestations of primary sclerosing cholangitis, an irreversible condition characterized by inflammation, obliterative fibrosis, and segmental constriction of intrahepatic and extrahepatic bile ducts seen in patients with UC. On endoscopic retrograde cholangiopancreatography (a radiographic visualization of the pancreatic duct and biliary tree), these bile duct changes are visualized as alternating strictures and dilations, or "beading."

Answer A is incorrect. Cholelithiasis, also known as gallstones, is not associated with ulcerative colitis. Endoscopic retrograde cholangiopancreatography may be used to visualize a ductal stone but is not a modality of choice for gallstone detection.

Answer B is incorrect. Pancreatic carcinoma is not associated with ulcerative colitis. On endoscopic retrograde cholangiopancreatography, it is characterized by a double-duct sign that results from tumor obstruction of both the common bile duct and the main pancreatic duct, not beading

Answer C is incorrect. Primary biliary cirrhosis is a nonsuppurative, granulomatous destruction of medium-sized intrahepatic bile ducts. It is not associated with ulcerative colitis. Endoscopic retrograde cholangiopancreatography findings in this condition are nonspecific.

Answer D is incorrect. Primary hemochromatosis is a familial defect in control of iron absorption with massive accumulation of hemosiderin in hepatic and pancreatic parenchymal cells. This condition is not associated with ulcerative colitis and has no specific endoscopic retrograde cholangiopancreatography findings.

CHAPTER 9

Hematology and Oncology

HIGH-YIELD SYSTEMS

Hematology and Oncology

1. A 23-year-old woman presents to her physician with a nevus on her arm that is asymmetrical with irregular borders. She has noticed a change in the color of this nevus in recent weeks. The nevus is removed and sent to the pathologist. On examination of the specimen, the pathologist determines that it is a melanoma. Which of the following features of this lesion may be a prognostic factor for the patient?

(A) Average size of neoplastic cells
(B) Degree of angiogenesis
(C) Degree of atypia
(D) Depth within the dermis
(E) Lateral spread within the epidermis

2. Which of the following is expected when the hemoglobin dissociation curve shown in this image switches from A to B?

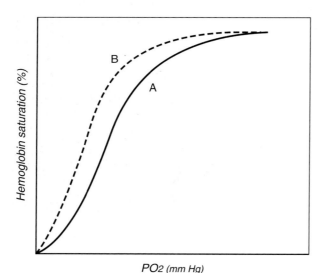

PO2 (mm Hg)

Reproduced, with permission, from USMLERx.com.

(A) A decrease in H⁺ bound to hemoglobin
(B) A decrease in oxygen-binding capacity
(C) A decrease in the affinity of oxygen for hemoglobin
(D) An increase in hemoglobin molecules in the taut state
(E) An increase in off-loading to peripheral tissues

3. A 43-year-old man comes to the physician because of increasing epigastric pain, heartburn, and weight loss over the past 4 months. When asked about bowel habits, the patient recalls a few occasions on which he had black, tarry stools. On physical examination, the physician notes that the patient is thin and pale and has diffuse tenderness over the epigastric area. Serum levels of which of the following substances are likely to be elevated in this patient?

(A) Cholecystokinin
(B) Gastrin
(C) Intrinsic factor
(D) Secretin
(E) Somatostatin

4. A 65-year-old man presents with a 2-month history of a cough. He also complains of a droopy right eyelid and dry facial skin. On a head and neck examination, the physician finds anisocoria, with the right eye more constricted than the left. A CT scan reveals a 3-cm nodule in one lung. Based on these symptoms, which of the following is the most likely location of the tumor found on CT scan?

(A) Apex of left upper lobe
(B) Apex of right upper lobe
(C) Hilum
(D) Right lower lobe
(E) Right middle lobe

5. A 58-year-old woman presented to her physician after discovering a lump in her left breast. The physician examines the lump and finds it to be hard, nontender, and moveable. Which of the following increases this woman's risk of breast cancer?

(A) Drinking 4 cups of coffee every day
(B) Having a history of a cyst that drained straw-colored fluid
(C) Having a history of fibroadenoma of the left breast
(D) Having gone through menopause 2 years ago
(E) Taking St. John's wort every day

6. Low-molecular-weight heparins are distinct from heparin is several ways, including their predominant action on which of the following?

(A) Antithrombin III
(B) Factors II, VII, IX, and X
(C) Factor IIa
(D) Factor VII
(E) Factor Xa

7. A 4-year-old girl is brought to the emergency department with an 8-hour history of projectile vomiting and headache. Her parents say that the patient was well until 2 months ago, when they noted that she was becoming increasingly clumsy. Physical examination shows nystagmus in all directions of gaze, as well as truncal ataxia. Laboratory studies of blood show a WBC count of 7200/mm^3, a hemoglobin level of 12.3 g/dL, and a platelet count of 225,000/mm^3. A CT scan shows a lesion in the cerebellar vermis with associated dilation of the third and lateral ventricles. Which of the following is most likely to be evident on histopathologic examination of the lesion?

(A) Deeply staining nuclei with scant cytoplasm arranged in pseudorosettes
(B) Pleomorphic anaplastic cells with foci of necrosis in a palisading pattern
(C) Regular round cells aligned smoothly with spherical nuclei surrounded by clear cytoplasm and finely granular chromatin associated with calcifications
(D) Stratified squamous epithelial cells embedded in spongy reticular stroma with prominent peripheral gliosis
(E) Whorls of meningothelial cells with oval-shaped nuclei with indistinct cytoplasm and psammoma bodies

8. A 17-year-old boy presents to the emergency department with severe abdominal pain. Laboratory tests show a deficit in uroporphyrinogen I synthetase and excess δ-aminolevulinate and porphobilinogen in the urine. Which of the following symptoms might also be present in this patient?

(A) Chest pain
(B) Hypotension
(C) Neuropsychiatric disturbances
(D) Polyphagia
(E) Stiff neck

9. A 35-year-old woman makes an appointment with her primary care physician after feeling a hard lump in her neck. Her physician notes that she has a single hard, nontender nodule in the left lobe of her thyroid that moves when she swallows. There is no cervical lymphadenopathy. The patient denies any changes in her recent health, no tremor, no restlessness, no heat intolerance, and no increased level of anxiety. Blood tests show normal thyroid hormone and calcitonin levels. A scintiscan shows a cold nodule in the left lobe of her thyroid, so a fine needle aspiration is done. The pathology is shown in the image. This patient most likely has which of the following?

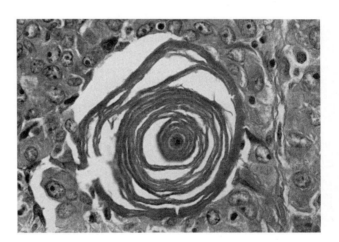

Image courtesy of Armed Forces Institute of Pathology.

(A) Follicular carcinoma
(B) Papillary carcinoma
(C) Medullary carcinoma
(D) Multinodular goiter
(E) Thyroglossal duct cyst

10. An individual with hemophilia A is unable to solidify the platelet plug formed following endothelial damage; this leads to abnormal bleeding. This condition is caused by a defect in the coagulation cascade. Which of the following elements of the coagulation cascade is defective in people with hemophilia A?

(A) Factors II, VII, IX, and X
(B) Factor VIII
(C) Factor IX
(D) Lack of protein C
(E) Mutations in antithrombin III

11. A 16-year-old boy is brought to the emergency department because of the acute onset of fever, chills, and a productive cough. Samples taken of the sputum show α-hemolytic gram-positive cocci in chains that show a positive quellung reaction. The patient says that he has had similar infections over the past year. A peripheral blood smear is done, and results show several sickle-shaped RBCs. Which of the following explains why this patient is susceptible to this particular type of infection?

(A) Bone marrow infiltration resulting in neutropenia and compromised immune function
(B) Large vessel occlusions in the cerebral vasculature resulting in neurologic events and aspiration pneumonia
(C) Microvascular infarcts resulting in pulmonary failure
(D) Microvascular infarcts resulting in splenic dysfunction
(E) Vaso-occlusion in the renal medulla resulting in renal failure and uremia

12. A 55-year-old man presents to the physician with easy bruising, splenomegaly, and fatigue. A peripheral blood smear is shown. Which of the following is the most likely diagnosis?

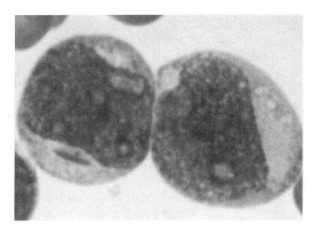

Reproduced, with permission, from Lichtman MA, Beutler E, Kipps TJ, Seligsohn U, Kaushansky K, Prchal JF. *Williams Hematology*, 7th ed. New York, McGraw-Hill, 2006: Color Plate XVI-2.

(A) Acute myeloid leukemia
(B) Chronic idiopathic myelofibrosis
(C) Chronic lymphocytic leukemia
(D) Chronic myelogenous leukemia
(E) Hairy cell leukemia

13. During autopsy of a 65-year-old woman, the liver is examined, revealing multiple tumors of various sizes throughout both lobes. This pattern, along with the fact that most tumors found in the liver are metastases, leads the pathologist to suspect that a primary tumor exists in another organ. Which of the following is the most likely location of the primary tumor?

(A) Breast
(B) Colon
(C) Kidney
(D) Lung
(E) Thyroid

14. Lead poisoning causes anemia because it does which of the following?

    (A) Binds to hemoglobin with high affinity, preventing oxygen from binding
    (B) Causes increased iron absorption from the gut, disrupting heme synthesis
    (C) Disrupts DNA synthesis, causing megaloblastic changes in RBCs
    (D) Inhibits ferrochelatase, disrupting heme synthesis
    (E) Increases the action of aminolevulinate dehydratase, disrupting heme synthesis

15. A 20-year-old man comes to the physician for a physical examination before beginning college. He states that he has been in good health except for a complaint of bloody stools that he attributes to occasional constipation. On further questioning, the physician discovers that the patient's mother died of colorectal cancer at the age of 42 years. The physician sends the patient for a colonoscopy; results show hundreds of polyps throughout the large intestine. This disorder results from an abnormality of which of the following chromosomes?

    (A) 1
    (B) 5
    (C) 11
    (D) 21
    (E) 22

16. A 60-year-old woman presents to her physician with findings of decreased proprioception in her lower extremities and gait instability consistent with subacute combined degeneration secondary to cobalamin deficiency. However, blood tests show normal hematocrit and near-normal mean cell volume. The physician orders additional tests. Which of the following laboratory results would support a diagnosis of cobalamin deficiency?

    (A) Decreased level of lactate dehydrogenase
    (B) Elevated methylmalonic acid
    (C) Elevated WBC count
    (D) Increased cobalamin level
    (E) Microcytosis
    (F) Negative anti-intrinsic factor antibody
    (G) Negative Schilling test

17. A 22-year-old man is diagnosed with medullary thyroid carcinoma, and his blood tests are significant for hypercalcemia and increased plasma catecholamine levels. He reports that his mother also had medullary thyroid carcinoma in her 20s and that she recently had surgery to remove her parathyroid glands. These findings suggest a possible mutation in which of the following genes?

    (A) *erb-B2*
    (B) *MEN I*
    (C) *ras*
    (D) *Rb*
    (E) *ret*

18. Breast cancer is the leading cause of cancer in women in the United States and the second leading cause of cancer deaths in women. Age, a family history of breast cancer, and mutations in the *BRCA1* and *BRCA2* genes are important risk factors for the development of breast cancer. Which of the following drugs are used as prophylactic treatment in women at high risk for developing breast cancer?

    (A) Abciximab and aspirin
    (B) Flutamide and leuprolide
    (C) Tamoxifen and raloxifene
    (D) Testosterone and prednisone
    (E) Vincristine and vinblastine

19. A 47-year-old woman from the Middle East presents with general malaise and weight loss. On physical examination, the woman is found to have hepatomegaly and splenomegaly. Blood samples are taken and show moderate anemia. Macrophages containing amastigotes are seen on histologic analysis. Which of the following parasites does the woman most likely harbor?

    (A) *Babesia* spp.
    (B) *Giardia lamblia*
    (C) *Leishmania donovani*
    (D) *Plasmodium ovale*
    (E) *Trichomonas vaginalis*

20. A type of lymphoma is characterized by onset in middle age and by neoplastic cells that resemble normal germinal center B lymphocytes. Additionally, it is the most common type of non-Hodgkin's lymphoma in the United States. What is the characteristic chromosomal translocation and protein that is produced by this translocation?

(A) t(8;14), c-myc
(B) t(9;22), bcr-abl
(C) t(11;22), EWS-FL-1
(D) t(14;18), bcl-2
(E) t(15;17), PML-RAR-α

21. A 52-year-old heart transplant patient on chronic immunosuppressive therapy that includes cyclosporine develops bacterial sinusitis. The patient's physician decides to start him on antibiotic therapy but is having difficulty choosing between amoxicillin and erythromycin to treat the infection. Concurrent use of erythromycin and cyclosporine would most likely lead to which of the following serum drug levels?

(A) Decreased cyclosporine serum concentrations
(B) First decreased, then increased serum cyclosporine concentrations
(C) First increased, then decreased serum cyclosporine concentrations
(D) Increased cyclosporine serum concentrations
(E) Unchanged cyclosporine serum concentrations

22. A 56-year-old man is diagnosed with transitional cell carcinoma and treated with excision and chemotherapy. Which of the following risk factors most likely lead to this patient's cancer?

(A) Alcohol use
(B) Exposure to asbestos
(C) Exposure to phenacetin
(D) Hypertension
(E) Previous pyelonephritis

23. A 70-year-old man with no prior surgical history presents with numbness/tingling of the extremities, weakness, and glossitis (sore, smooth, enlarged tongue). Preliminary laboratory studies are negative for antinuclear antibodies and antimitochondrial antibodies, but positive for antibodies against intrinsic factor. What is the function of the protein that is deficient and/or affected in this disease process?

(A) Binding free vitamin B_{12} in ileal cells for transport through the bloodstream
(B) Binding free vitamin B_{12} in the small intestine and then to ileal receptors
(C) Binding free vitamin B_{12} in the stomach
(D) Splitting R-protein/vitamin B_{12} complexes in the duodenum
(E) Splitting vitamin B_{12} from its exogenous ingested protein-bound form

24. A 2-year-old boy is brought to a clinic because his mother noticed a large, unilateral, painless abdominal mass while she was bathing him. While performing an ultrasound-guided biopsy (histologic image shown), the technician notes that the kidney calyces are highly distorted by the mass. Which of the following is most likely the origin of this lesion?

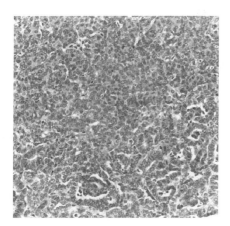

Reproduced, with permission, from Tanagho EA, McAninch. *Smith's General Urology*, 16th ed. New York, McGraw-Hill, 2004: Fig. 21-10.

(A) An autosomal dominant gene that also leads to cystic masses in the liver
(B) Embryonic renal cells from the embryonic kidney

(C) Malignant transformation of renal tubular cells

(D) Malignant transformation of uroepethilial cells

(E) Primitive neural crest cells

25. An 8-year-old boy is brought to the pediatrician after his parents noticed very dark urine in the toilet earlier that morning. Initial laboratory studies show intravascular hemolysis; further testing shows that his RBCs are susceptible to complement-mediated lysis. This patient most likely has which of the following conditions?

(A) Autoimmune hemolytic anemia
(B) Common bile duct stricture
(C) Hereditary spherocytosis
(D) Paroxysmal nocturnal hemoglobinuria
(E) Thrombotic thrombocytopenic purpura

26. Which of the following chemotherapeutic agents should be avoided in a patient with impaired renal function?

(A) Bleomycin
(B) Cisplatin
(C) Cytarabine
(D) Doxorubicin
(E) Tamoxifen

27. A 3-year-old girl was in her usual state of good health 1 month ago when she developed an acute viral upper respiratory infection. She now presents to the emergency department with nonblanching purple skin lesions. The rest of her physical examination is unremarkable. The complete blood count demonstrates a low platelet count, while the peripheral blood smear is notable only for large platelets. Which of the following laboratory findings might be present in this patient?

(A) Antiplatelet antibodies
(B) Decreased megakaryocytes on bone marrow biopsy
(C) IgA deficiency
(D) Increased fibrin split products
(E) Vitamin K deficiency

28. A 57-year-old woman is diagnosed with small-cell lung carcinoma. She has gained weight, and she says that her face has recently "ballooned." Which of the following symptoms is this patient likely to be experiencing in addition to the ones mentioned?

(A) Cold intolerance and hair loss
(B) Galactorrhea and amenorrhea
(C) Insatiable thirst and polyuria
(D) Poor wound healing and hirsutism
(E) Restlessness and tremor

29. A 45-year-old woman arrives in the emergency department complaining of intense pain in her upper abdomen for the past 4 hours. She had a similar episode in the past, but it went away within an hour. Her history is significant for a recent flulike infection and a prolonged feeling of fatigue and general exhaustion. Physical examination reveals that her sclerae are icteric, her palate is abnormally pigmented, and her skin has a yellow hue. Ultrasound shows radiopaque gallstones. A Coombs' test is negative. A peripheral blood smear shows small RBCs, several of which have no central pallor. Which of the following is the most likely cause of this patient's condition?

(A) A mutation in the gene encoding ankyrin
(B) A mutation in the glucose-6-phosphate dehydrogenase gene
(C) Circulating antibodies targeted against erythrocytes
(D) Iron deficiency anemia
(E) RBC hemolysis because of a mechanical heart valve

30. A recent study in a small community of 6000 people in central Africa showed that 0.5% are homozygotes for hemoglobin S and therefore have sickle cell disease. Ten percent of the community is heterozygotes for the mutant allele. Last year, six new infants were diagnosed with sickle cell disease. Which of the following is the current prevalence of homozygous sickle cell disease among this population?

(A) 0.001
(B) 3
(C) 6
(D) 30
(E) 600

31. A 65-year-old man comes to a local clinic complaining of back pain. After ruling out the most common causes of back pain, the treating physician becomes suspicious of a malignant process. He sends the patient for a bone marrow biopsy, with the results shown in the image. What is the most likely diagnosis for this patient?

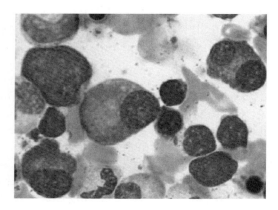

Reproduced, with permission, from Lichtman MA, Beutler E, Kipps TJ, Seligsohn U, Kaushansky K, Prchal JF. *Williams Hematology*, 7th ed. New York, McGraw-Hill, 2006: Color Plate XXI-2.

(A) Bone marrow suppression
(B) Lymphoma
(C) Metastatic prostate cancer
(D) Multiple myeloma
(E) Normal bone marrow

32. A 23-year-old woman presents to the emergency department following a motor vehicle crash. Her injuries are minor, and she states that she feels a bit dizzy and tired but has felt this way recently anyway. The physician notices that her laboratory results are consistent with megaloblastic anemia. Upon further questioning, she reports that she has been taking antibiotics off and on over the last several months for frequent urinary tract infections. Which of the following medications is this patient most likely taking?

(A) Chloramphenicol
(B) Clindamycin
(C) Erythromycin
(D) Gatifloxacin
(E) Trimethoprim

33. A 60-year-old woman presents to the physician with painless reddish-brown blood in her stool. Initial laboratory tests show the following results:

Hematocrit: 33%
Hemoglobin: 11 g/dL
Mean corpuscular volume: 73 μm^3
WBC count: 8000/mm^3
Platelet count: 200,000/mm^3

Which of the following is the most important next step in the management of this patient?

(A) Abdominal plain films
(B) Colonoscopy
(C) CT scan of the abdomen
(D) Esophagoduodenoscopy
(E) Pelvic ultrasound

34. A patient with relapsing Hodgkin's disease presents with weight gain, foot ulcers, vision problems, elevated blood sugar, oral candidiasis, and new onset of wildly swinging mood changes. What is the most likely etiology of this patient's psychiatric symptoms?

(A) Adverse effects of bleomycin
(B) Adverse effects of prednisone
(C) Adverse effects of vincristine
(D) Normal psychiatric response to having cancer
(E) Progression of disease

35. A 41-year-old pregnant woman sees her obstetrician because of new-onset vaginal bleeding. Although she is only 4 months pregnant, her doctor notes that her uterus is the size usually seen at 6 months of gestation. Maternal blood works shows a β-human chorionic gonadotropin (β-hCG) level > 5 times the upper limit of normal. Which of the following should concern the doctor the most?

(A) The fetus may have a neural tube defect
(B) The patient has a hydatidiform mole
(C) The patient has a tubal pregnancy
(D) The patient has preeclampsia
(E) The patient is having triplets

36. An 8-year-old boy comes to the physician with his mother, who wants to discuss respiratory problems that have arisen since an upper respiratory infection 4 months ago. The mother says that the patient has attacks characterized by wheezing and shortness of breath that usually resolve after an hour. On one occasion an attack required a visit to the emergency department, and the mother remembers the emergency department physician saying something about an abnormally high level of eosinophils in the patient's blood. Which of the following is the most likely diagnosis for this patient?

(A) Asbestosis
(B) Asthma
(C) Coronavirus infection
(D) Croup
(E) Cystic fibrosis

37. A 56-year-old man who is a health care worker presents to his physician with vague abdominal discomfort. A physical examination reveals a tender liver, palpable to 6 cm below the costal margin and scleral icterus. His laboratory studies are significant for an aspartate aminotransferase activity of 200 U/L and an alanine aminotransferase activity of 450 U/L. A CT scan of the abdomen shows a dominant solid nodule in the liver. The marker most likely to be elevated in this patient is also a good indicator of which of the following malignancies?

(A) Choriocarcinoma
(B) Colorectal carcinoma
(C) Melanoma
(D) Neuroblastoma
(E) Prostatic carcinoma
(F) Yolk sac carcinoma

38. The marker for prostatic carcinoma is prostate-specific antigen. The presence of a hepatoma has no effect on this marker. Which of the following types of neoplastic cell is most common in non-Hodgkin's lymphoma?

(A) B lymphocyte
(B) Myeloblast
(C) Plasma cell
(D) Reed-Sternberg cell
(E) T lymphocyte

39. A 29-year-old man presents to his primary care physician with a painless testicular mass. Laboratory studies show an elevated serum human chorionic gonadotropin level, suggesting a germ cell tumor. Which of the following is the most likely site of nodal metastasis in this tumor?

(A) Deep inguinal lymph nodes
(B) External iliac lymph nodes
(C) Gluteal lymph nodes
(D) Retroperitoneal lymph nodes
(E) Superficial inguinal lymph nodes

40. Heme synthesis occurs in the bone marrow and liver. Which of the following catalyzes the committed step in heme synthesis?

(A) δ-Aminolevulinic acid dehydratase
(B) δ-Aminolevulinic acid synthase
(C) Ferrochelatase
(D) Heme oxygenase
(E) Uroporphyrinogen I synthase

41. A 74-year-old man comes to the physician because of bone pain in his left femur. An x-ray shows lytic lesions, and a diagnosis of multiple myeloma is made. The patient is placed on a regimen of melphalan, vincristine, doxorubicin, and ifosfamide. What is the mechanism of action of vincristine?

(A) Alkylating agent
(B) Intercalation between DNA strands
(C) Microtubule disassembly inhibitor
(D) Microtubule formation inhibitor
(E) Topoisomerase II inhibitor

42. A 35-year-old man comes to the emergency department with meningeal symptoms. He says he was taken to a trauma center in rural Ecuador 2 years ago after experiencing blunt abdominal trauma. He does not remember exactly what was done, but he believes they took drastic measures to control intra-abdominal bleeding. Before leaving the trauma center, he was counseled about a new susceptibility to encapsulated organisms. Laboratory tests show an increased platelet count. Which of the following findings would be seen in a peripheral blood smear from this patient?

(A) Heinz bodies, target cells, perhaps more platelets than usual
(B) Megaloblastic anemia
(C) Schistocytes
(D) Sickle cells
(E) Spherocytes

43. A 20-year-old African-American woman develops anemia after being treated for a urinary tract infection. A peripheral blood smear shows RBC lysis and precipitates of hemoglobin within the RBCs. Which of the following drug classes most likely caused her hemolytic anemia?

(A) Aminoglycosides
(B) Fluoroquinolones
(C) Macrolides
(D) Sulfonamides
(E) Tetracyclines

44. Several drugs are used to prevent myocardial infarction in patients with acute coronary syndrome. One class of drugs binds to the glycoprotein receptor IIb/IIIa on activated platelets, thereby interfering with platelet aggregation. This prevents renewed formation of clots that could block the lumen of the cardiac vessels. Which of the following is an example of this class of drug?

(A) Abciximab
(B) Clopidogrel
(C) Leuprolide
(D) Selegiline
(E) Ticlopidine

45. A 49-year-old man presents to the emergency department complaining that "my skin has turned yellow." Physical examination reveals the man is significantly jaundiced. He has no abdominal pain and has a negative Murphy's sign. The physician is concerned that he can feel the patient's gallbladder and orders a CT scan. What is the most likely cause of this patient's jaundice?

(A) Acute hepatitis
(B) Choledocholithiasis
(C) Cholelithiasis
(D) Hemolytic anemia
(E) Pancreatic cancer

46. A 34-year-old man comes to the emergency department complaining of the sudden onset of vomiting and epigastric abdominal pain radiating to the back. On physical examination, the patient is afebrile and has abdominal tenderness; decreased bowel sounds are noted, as is diffuse bruising that he describes as having appeared suddenly. He also reports continuous epistaxis. Laboratory tests show a slightly elevated WBC count, thrombocytopenia, increased amylase and lipase activity, increased prothrombin time (PT) and partial thromboplastin time (PTT), and the presence of fibrin split products. An abdominal ultrasound performed at the bedside shows a dilated common bile duct. Which of the following is the most likely etiology of this patient's abnormal coagulation profile?

(A) Abdominal aortic aneurysm
(B) Acute pancreatitis
(C) Appendicitis
(D) Gastric ulcer
(E) Gram-negative sepsis

47. A 70-year-old man comes to his physician for a routine physical examination. Although he is asymptomatic, a blood test shows an abnormal level of immunoglobulin. After further testing, he is diagnosed with monoclonal gammopathy of undetermined significance. Which of the following is the current treatment for monoclonal gammopathy of undetermined significance?

(A) Anticoagulation
(B) High-dose steroids
(C) No treatment
(D) Restrictive diet
(E) Vinca alkaloids

48. An 8-year-old boy has a chronic history of severe hemolytic anemia, hepatosplenomegaly, and maxillary overgrowth. He has received blood transfusions since early infancy but has not received a transfusion in over 4 months. A hemoglobin electrophoresis shows marked elevation of HbF, increased HbA_2, and absence of HbA_1. Which of the following diagnoses is most consistent with this patient's electrophoresis?

(A) α-Thalassemia minor
(B) β-Thalassemia major
(C) β-Thalassemia minor
(D) Glucose-6-phosphate dehydrogenase deficiency
(E) HbH disease
(F) RBCs containing hemoglobin Barts

49. A 69-year-old male has a tumor removed from the cerebellopontine angle because a CT scan shows a 2-cm sharply circumscribed mass adjacent to the right pons that extends into the right cerebellar hemisphere. He reports a 3-month history of dizziness and a 4-year history of progressive hearing loss. Grossly, the tumor specimen appears as a single irregular fragment of tan-pink soft tissue that measures slightly less than 2 cm. A microscopic pathology report indicates that the specimen consist Which of the following types of tumors would most likely result in these findings?

(A) Medulloblastoma
(B) Meningioma
(C) Neurofibroma
(D) Oligodendroglioma
(E) Schwannoma

50. A 73-year-old woman is brought to the emergency department after passing out on the subway. The patient has a 3-month history of burning epigastric pain that is worse after eating, along with dark stool. Physical examination shows a blood pressure of 95/52 mm Hg, a pulse of 97/min, epigastric tenderness, and guaiac-positive stool. Laboratory tests show a hemoglobin level of 9.5 g/dL, a hematocrit of 28%, and a mean corpuscular volume of 75 μm^3. Which of the following is the most likely diagnosis?

(A) Anemia of chronic disease secondary to peptic ulcer disease
(B) Iron deficiency anemia secondary to blood loss
(C) Iron deficiency anemia secondary to pernicious anemia
(D) Megaloblastic anemia secondary to blood loss
(E) Megaloblastic anemia secondary to pernicious anemia

1. **The correct answer is D.** The vertical growth phase of melanoma describes the extent of neoplastic cells into the dermis. During this time, the melanoma is very likely to metastasize. The depth of invasion into the dermis is an established prognostic factor for the patient, since most melanoma patients die due to complications of metastatic melanoma involvement of other organs (lung or brain).

Answer A is incorrect. Size of neoplastic cells is not a factor in determining prognosis.

Answer B is incorrect. Melanoma growth is associated with increased tumor angiogenesis, but it is not an established clinical prognostic factor.

Answer C is incorrect. Degree of atypia is not as important as depth, since highly atypical cells may be confined to the epidermis.

Answer E is incorrect. Lateral spread within the epidermis is not as important as depth in determining metastatic potential.

2. **The correct answer is A.** A shift in the hemoglobin dissociation curve from A to B will lead to a shift in the P50 (50% hemoglobin saturation) to the left or, equivalently, to an increase in the affinity of oxygen for hemoglobin. Since at any given PO_2 hemoglobin will have higher affinity for oxygen, there will be less deoxyhemoglobin. Because deoxyhemoglobin is a better buffer for H^+ than oxyhemoglobin, there will be less H^+ bound to hemoglobin. Conversely, the Bohr effect states that increasing H^+ causes decreased oxygen affinity for hemoglobin, thus promoting off-loading in peripheral tissues. Therefore, increasing H^+ promotes the deoxyhemoglobin state, which can act as a carrier for H^+, providing negative feedback regulation

Answer B is incorrect. Oxygen-binding capacity will be unaffected; with high PO_2, hemoglobin saturation would be near 100% in both states A and B.

Answer C is incorrect. Hemoglobin will have greater affinity for oxygen in state B.

Answer D is incorrect. A shift leftward suggests an increase in the number of hemoglobin molecules in the relaxed state (which has higher affinity for oxygen) rather than in the taut state (which has a lower affinity for oxygen).

Answer E is incorrect. Less off-loading to peripheral tissues would be expected with more relaxed hemoglobin.

3. **The correct answer is B.** The question stem describes a case of a pancreatic gastrinoma leading to Zollinger-Ellison syndrome. This syndrome results from hypergastrinemia. Gastrin is normally produced by the G cells of the antrum and duodenum. For example, ectopic and unregulated production of gastrin by malignant pancreatic islet cells stimulates excess secretion of acid by parietal cells of the stomach. Gastrin also promotes hypertrophy of the stomach. Increased stomach acid leads to symptoms of gastroesophageal reflux disease and to ulceration and gastric bleeding, as evidenced by the patient's pallor and melena. Elevated serum gastrin would be diagnostic of gastrinoma.

Answer A is incorrect. Cholecystokinin (CCK) is produced by the I cells of the duodenum and jejunum. CCK stimulates gallbladder contraction and pancreatic enzyme secretion. CCK inhibits gastric acid secretion.

Answer C is incorrect. Intrinsic factor is also released by the parietal cells of the stomach; its function is to bind vitamin B_{12} to enable its absorption. High intrinsic factor levels would be unlikely to produce the symptoms of elevated gastrin secretion in this case.

Answer D is incorrect. Secretin is produced normally by the S cells of the duodenum and promotes pancreatic bicarbonate secretion while inhibiting gastric acid secretion.

Answer E is incorrect. Somatostatin is produced by the pancreatic islets and gastrointestinal mucosa. Unlike gastrin, somatostatin inhibits gastric acid and pepsinogen secretion in addition to counteracting the actions of CCK and secretin. Somatostatin also inhibits the release of insulin and glucagons.

4. **The correct answer is B.** The question stem describes a case of Pancoast's tumor, in which a lung neoplasm of any type located in the apex impinges on the cervical sympathetic plexus. This impingement results in Horner's syndrome of ptosis, miosis, and anhidrosis, as described in this patient. The symptoms are ipsilateral to the damaged plexus, so the tumor must be located in the apex of the right upper lobe.

Answer A is incorrect. The symptoms are ipsilateral to the injured plexus, so a tumor in the left apex would have presented with Horner's syndrome on the left side, not the right.

Answer C is incorrect. Squamous cell carcinoma of the lung usually appears at the hilum, but such a tumor mass would not cause Horner's syndrome.

Answer D is incorrect. A tumor in the right lower lobe would not manifest in these symptoms.

Answer E is incorrect. A tumor located in the right middle lobe could not result in these symptoms because it would not be located near the cervical sympathetic plexus.

5. **The correct answer is D.** Late menopause (> 50 years old) is associated with an increased risk of breast cancer. Other risk factors include being female, older age, early first menarche (< 12 years old), delayed first pregnancy (> 30 years old), and family history of a first-degree relative with breast cancer at a young age.

Answer A is incorrect. Breast cancer risk is not increased by caffeine intake.

Answer B is incorrect. Breast cancer risk is not increased by nonhyperplastic cysts. Had the cyst drained bloody fluid, it would have been more worrisome for a malignant process.

Answer C is incorrect. Breast cancer risk is not increased by fibroadenoma.

Answer E is incorrect. Breast cancer risk is not increased by use of St. John's wort.

6. **The correct answer is E.** Low-molecular-weight heparins act predominantly on Xa, whereas heparin targets both antithrombin III and Xa.

Answer A is incorrect. Heparin targets both antithrombin III and Xa.

Answer B is incorrect. Warfarin blocks the activation of vitamin K–dependent factors II, VII, IX, and X.

Answer C is incorrect. Factor IIa, or thrombin, is the enzyme that catalyzes the final step of the clotting cascade, the formation of fibrin. Thrombin is a vitamin K–dependent factor that is not influenced by low-molecular-weight heparin.

Answer D is incorrect. Factor VII is part of the extrinsic pathway and is one of the vitamin K–dependent factors.

7. **The correct answer is A.** The diagnosis is medulloblastoma, which occurs predominantly in children and is found exclusively in the cerebellum, accounting for 20% of brain tumors in children. On microscopic examination, the tumor is very cellular with sheets of anaplastic cells. Each tumor cell is small with little cytoplasm and crescent-shaped, deeply staining nuclei arranged in pseudorosettes. These tumors are frequently radiosensitive.

Answer B is incorrect. This micropathologic description is characteristic of glioblastoma multiforme, which is the most common primary brain tumor of adults and occurs in the cerebral hemispheres. It carries a particularly grave prognosis, with a survival rate at 5 years of almost zero. Most patients live less than 1 year after diagnosis. This is seldom a tumor of childhood.

Answer C is incorrect. This description is consistent with a diagnosis of oligodendroglioma, which is a relatively rare, slow-growing, benign tumor that is most often found in the frontal lobes. The micropathologic appearance is classically described as consisting of "fried egg" cells that have round nuclei with clear cytoplasm and are often calcified.

Answer D is incorrect. This histopathology describes a craniopharyngioma, the most common supratentorial tumor in children, which is embryologically derived from remnants of Rathke's pouch. It has a bimodal distribution of affected ages, with a second peak in the fifth decade.

Answer E is incorrect. This is a description of a nonmalignant tumor known as a meningioma, which is a common primary intracranial neoplasm arising from arachnoid granulations. These tumors are slow-growing and expand locally rather than by infiltration.

8. **The correct answer is C.** This patient suffers from acute intermittent porphyria, an autosomal dominant disorder caused by a lack of uroporphyrinogen I synthetase. The buildup of toxic levels of α-aminolevulinate (ALA) and porphobilinogen lead to the associated symptoms of abdominal pain (more than 90% of cases), neuropathy, high sympathetic tone, and neuropsychiatric disturbances, including anxiety, depression, seizures, and paranoia.

Answer A is incorrect. The differential diagnosis for chest pain is long and includes cardiac, pulmonary, gastrointestinal, and musculoskeletal etiologies. However, attacks of acute intermittent porphyria are not associated with chest pain.

Answer B is incorrect. Due to the high sympathetic tone caused by the pain of the crisis, hypertension may be associated with acute intermittent porphyria, but not hypotension.

Answer D is incorrect. Polyphagia, or greatly increased hunger, is one of the cardinal symptoms associated with diabetes mellitus, not acute intermittent porphyria.

Answer E is incorrect. A stiff neck may be associated with meningeal irritation and can be

found in meningitis or with musculoskeletal problems, but it is not found in acute intermittent porphyria.

9. **The correct answer is B.** This patient has papillary carcinoma, the most common form of thyroid cancer. Patients are frequently in their 20s–40s and many have a history of exposure to ionizing radiation. On histology papillary carcinomas show branching papillae with a fibrovascular stalk. These papillae are lined by epithelial cells with empty-looking, ground-glass nuclei often called "Orphan Annie eye nuclei." Also characteristic of papillary carcinoma is the concentrically calcified psammoma bodies shown in the image above. Psammoma bodies are almost never seen in follicular or medullary carcinomas. The prognosis of papillary carcinoma is excellent. The overall 10-year survival rate is about 98%, especially in patients without lymph node metastases.

Answer A is incorrect. Follicular carcinoma is the second most common form of thyroid cancer and generally presents in women in their 40s and 50s. Follicular carcinomas may present as well-circumscribed nodules or infiltrative lesions. Like papillary carcinomas, they show up as cold lesions on scintigrams; however, their histology is different. Microscopically, follicular carcinomas present as uniform cells surrounding colloid-filled follicles with Hurthle cells (cells with abundant granular eosinophilic cytoplasm). There are no psammoma bodies seen in follicular carcinoma. The prognosis is excellent, with 10-year survival rates > 92%.

Answer C is incorrect. Medullary carcinoma is a neoplasm of the parafollicular or C cells of the thyroid. These cells secrete calcitonin, which causes increased serum calcitonin levels. Medullary carcinoma can be sporadic, in which it tends to be unilateral or may be associated with multiple endocrine neoplasia types IIA and IIB, in which case it tends to affect both the right and left lobe of the thyroid. On histology, sheets of spindle-shaped cells are seen in amyloid stroma.

Answer D is incorrect. Multinodular goiters are asymmetrically enlarged thyroid glands that may by toxic or nontoxic—that is, they may or may not overproduce thyroid hormone. Because the gland can get very large in this disorder, symptoms may include dysphagia because of compression of the esophagus or compression of the large vessels in the neck. The presentation of multinodular goiter does not correlate with the clinical picture presented in this case.

Answer E is incorrect. A thyroglossal cyst is a congenital abnormality caused by the persistence of the diverticulum formed during the migration of the thyroid gland from the foramen cecum to the tracheal cartilage. These lesions are found in the midline and do not localize to one lobe.

10. **The correct answer is B.** Hemophilia A is an X-linked disorder caused by factor VIII deficiency. Bleeding frequently occurs in joints and the retroperitoneal space. Laboratory tests would reveal an increased partial thromboplastin time due to an isolated problem with the intrinsic coagulation cascade. Platelet count would be normal in patients with this condition.

Answer A is incorrect. Factors II, VII, IX, and X are all vitamin K–dependent clotting factors. None of them is deficient in patients with hemophilia A.

Answer C is incorrect. Factor IX deficiency is the cause of hemophilia B, another X-linked disorder. Clinically, this condition is similar to hemophilia A. The partial thromboplastin time would be elevated.

Answer D is incorrect. Protein C or S deficiency is another uncommon inherited cause of hypercoagulability.

Answer E is incorrect. Mutations leading to antithrombin III deficiency result in a rare cause of inherited hypercoagulability.

11. **The correct answer is D.** This patient has sickle cell disease, as evidenced by the erythrocyte sickling in the peripheral blood smear. Pa-

tients with this disease are prone to microvascular infarcts in several vascular beds in the body. Over time, multiple micro-infarcts in the spleen result in functional asplenia, making patients particularly susceptible to infections with encapsulated organisms. This patient presents with pneumonia caused by *Streptococcus pneumoniae*. This is an encapsulated bacterium, which is confirmed by the positive quellung reaction.

Answer A is incorrect. Sickle cell patients are at risk of having an aplastic crisis, often associated with parvovirus B19 infection, during which time bone marrow activity is suppressed. Some patients may subsequently develop bone marrow necrosis. Although these patients are at risk of developing a host of infections, this particular complication is not specifically associated with susceptibility to infections with encapsulated organisms.

Answer B is incorrect. Sickle cell patients are at risk of having an aplastic crisis, often associated with parvovirus B19 infection, during which time bone marrow activity is suppressed. Some patients may subsequently develop bone marrow necrosis. Although these patients are at risk of developing a host of infections, this particular complication is not specifically associated with susceptibility to infections with encapsulated organisms.

Answer C is incorrect. Microvascular infarcts resulting in pulmonary failure

Answer E is incorrect. The renal medulla is particularly prone to vaso-occlusive complications in sickle cell patients; renal failure and uremia could be possible complications. However, this is not related to infection susceptibility.

12. **The correct answer is A.** The cytoplasmic inclusions seen in the myelocytic precursors on this peripheral blood smear are fused lysosomal granules known as Auer rods. Release of these fused granules may cause acute disseminated intravascular coagulation and fatal hemorrhage. Auer rods define a cell as being of myelocytic lineage as opposed to lymphocytic

and are seen in acute myeloid leukemia (AML), especially in the subgroup of acute promyelocytic leukemia. AML is the most common form of leukemia in adults and constitutes approximately one-fifth of acute leukemia cases in children. The prognosis for patients with AML is poor; many patients die within a few years of diagnosis.

Answer B is incorrect. Chronic idiopathic myelofibrosis also can present with splenomegaly and fatigue; however, peripheral blood smear would show teardrop-shaped RBCs, nucleated red cell precursors, and granulocytic precursor cells without the presence of Auer rods.

Answer C is incorrect. Chronic lymphocytic leukemia is more common in patients greater than 60 years of age. The disease has an insidious onset, with patients presenting early on with fatigue and weight loss and later with lymphadenopathy and hepatosplenomegaly. The peripheral blood smear reflects a marked lymphocytosis, with a typically normocytic normochromic anemia. As the disease progresses, platelet count may drop. Auer rods are not a feature of lymphocytic lymphomas or leukemias.

Answer D is incorrect. Characteristics of chronic myelogenous leukemia include lymphadenopathy, splenomegaly, marked leukocytosis, mature myeloid precursor cells, and minimal blasts and promyelocytes.

Answer E is incorrect. Although hairy cell leukemia affects middle-aged men who tend to present with massive splenomegaly and fatigue, Auer rods are not present in leukemic cells of this disease. Hairy cell leukemia derives its name from the hairlike filamentous projections characteristic of affected leukemic cells.

13. **The correct answer is B.** Remember that the liver and lung are the most common sites of metastasis (after lymph nodes) due to the high blood flow through these organs. Therefore, primary tumors in any of the locations listed may metastasize to the liver. However, given that the blood vessels from the gastrointestinal tract drain into the hepatic circulation, the most likely primary tumor that metastasizes to the liver would be from a gastrointestinal source such as the colon.

Answer A is incorrect. Breast tumors may also metastasize to the liver, but with less frequency than gastrointestinal cancers. Breast metastases are more often found in brain and bone.

Answer C is incorrect. Tumors of the kidney, such as renal cell carcinoma, metastasize to the brain and bone, and less so to the liver.

Answer D is incorrect. Lung tumors often metastasize to brain and bone, and less often to the liver.

Answer E is incorrect. Thyroid cancer often leads to bone metastases.

14. **The correct answer is D.** Lead inhibits α-aminolevulinate (ALA) dehydratase and ferrochelatase, preventing both porphobilinogen formation and the incorporation of iron into protoporphyrin IX, the final step in heme synthesis. Inhibition of both of these steps results in ineffective heme synthesis and subsequent microcytic (hemoglobin-poor) anemia.

Answer A is incorrect. Lead does not have a high affinity for hemoglobin. This type of pathology is seen in carbon monoxide (CO) poisoning. CO binds to hemoglobin with much higher affinity than oxygen, resulting in decreased oxygen-carrying capacity.

Answer B is incorrect. Hemochromatosis is a disorder of excess iron levels in the body due to increased iron absorption from the gut. This leads to pathology because humans have no good pathway to rid the body of excess iron without active hemorrhage. Lead poisoning does not affect iron absorption from the gut.

Answer C is incorrect. Folate and B_{12} deficiency disrupt DNA synthesis, specifically thiamine synthesis, resulting in megaloblastic changes in RBCs.

Answer E is incorrect. Lead inhibits α-aminolevulinate (ALA) dehydratase, preventing porphyrin synthesis beyond the formation of ALA; it does not increase its actions. This causes ALA to accumulate in the urine.

15. **The correct answer is B.** This patient has familial adenomatous polyposis (FAP), which is an autosomal dominant disease caused by a mutation of chromosome 5. FAP classically presents with rectal bleeding in a 20- to 40-year-old people with a family history of colon polyps and/or colorectal cancer. On colonoscopy, a patient with FAP will have hundreds of polyps present, in contrast to hereditary nonpolyposis colorectal cancer, in which tens of polyps are present. Nearly 100% of patients with FAP will go on to develop colorectal cancer; treatment is complete resection of the affected bowel.

Answer A is incorrect. Chromosome 1 is affected in retinoblastoma and osteosarcoma.

Answer C is incorrect. Chromosome 11 is affected in Wilms' tumor.

Answer D is incorrect. Chromosome 21 is affected in Down's syndrome.

Answer E is incorrect. Chromosome 22 is affected in neurofibromatosis type 2.

16. **The correct answer is B.** In a minority of patients with cobalamin (B_{12}) deficiency, hematocrit and mean corpuscular volume can be normal. In these cases, laboratory testing for elevated homocysteine and methylmalonic acid can be used to make the diagnosis.

Answer A is incorrect. LDH would be increased in B_{12} deficiency due to failed hematopoiesis.

Answer C is incorrect. Neutropenia with hypersegmented neutrophils is typically seen in B_{12} deficiency.

Answer D is incorrect. Decreased cobalamin levels would support a diagnosis of B_{12} deficiency.

Answer E is incorrect. B_{12} deficiency presents as a macrocytic anemia. Peripheral blood smear typically shows macro-ovalocytosis of RBCs.

Answer F is incorrect. A positive anti-intrinsic factor antibody would suggest autoimmune destruction of parietal cells in the stomach leading to decreased intrinsic factor and B_{12} absorption.

Answer G is incorrect. In the Schilling test, radioactive cobalamin is given orally with a nonradioactive parenteral load. Radioactivity measured in the urine can be used to estimate oral cobalamin absorption. A positive Schilling test would suggest a defect in absorption.

17. **The correct answer is E.** The characteristics described in the question are found in patients with the most common hyperplasias/tumors associated with multiple endocrine neoplasia (MEN) type 2A, also known as Sipple's syndrome. MEN 2A is associated with parathyroid hyperplasia or tumor leading to hypercalcemia, medullary carcinoma of the thyroid, and pheochromocytoma, which commonly causes elevated plasma catecholamine levels. The MEN syndromes follow an autosomal dominant pattern of inheritance and both MEN 2A and MEN 2B (MEN 3) are linked to distinct mutations in the ret oncogene.

Answer A is incorrect. The *erb-B2* oncogene is associated with breast, ovarian, and gastric carcinomas.

Answer B is incorrect. Mutations in the *MEN 1* gene are found in patients with multiple endocrine neoplasia 1, also known as Werner's syndrome, which is characterized by hyperplasia or tumor of the "**3 P's**": **P**ituitary, **P**arathyroid, and **P**ancreas.

Answer C is incorrect. The *ras* oncogene mutation is associated with carcinoma of the colon.

Answer D is incorrect. The *Rb* gene is a tumor suppressor gene located on chromosome 13q. Mutation of the gene is associated with retinoblastoma and osteosarcoma.

18. **The correct answer is C.** Use of tamoxifen and raloxifene as prophylaxis in women at high risk for breast cancer has been shown to reduce the incidence of breast cancer by

50–80% in this population. It is thought that selective estrogen receptor modulators have a selective benefit in reducing the incidence of estrogen receptor–positive cancers for *BRCA2*-positive women.

Answer A is incorrect. Abciximab is an antiplatelet drug used in the treatment of acute coronary syndromes. Aspirin is an irreversible inhibitor of cyclooxygenase.

Answer B is incorrect. Flutamide is a nonsteroidal antiandrogen that competitively inhibits androgens at the testosterone receptor. Gonadotropin-releasing hormone analogs such as leuprolide are used in continuous dosing regimens in the treatment of prostate cancer.

Answer D is incorrect. Testosterone is an androgen that is approved by the Food and Drug Administration for palliation therapy in metastatic breast cancer. Adverse effects of testosterone treatment include virilization, edema, and jaundice. Prednisone is a systemic corticosteroid that is used in various anticancer treatment regimens. The combination of testosterone and prednisone is not used as prophylaxis treatment for women at high risk for breast cancer.

Answer E is incorrect. Vincristine and vinblastine are microtubule inhibitors used to treat testicular carcinoma as well as Hodgkin's and non-Hodgkin's lymphomas.

19. **The correct answer is C.** *Leishmania donovani* infection presents with hepatomegaly and splenomegaly, malaise, anemia, and weight loss. *L. donovani* is transmitted via the sandfly. Microscopically, macrophages containing amastigotes are observed. Sodium stibogluconate is used to treat *L. donovani* infection.

Answer A is incorrect. *Babesia* species infection presents with a malaria-like syndrome. Babesiosis is transmitted by the *Ixodes* tick. On microscopic examination, one observes no red blood cell pigment and the Maltese cross–appearing parasite. Quinine is used to treat babesiosis.

Answer B is incorrect. *Giardia lamblia* infection presents with bloating, flatulence, foul-smelling diarrhea, and light-colored fatty stools. *G. lamblia* is transmitted via cysts in water (fecal-oral transmission). On microscopy, one observes teardrop-shaped trophozoites with a ventral sucking disc or cysts. Metronidazole is used to treat *G. lamblia* infection.

Answer D is incorrect. *Plasmodium ovale* infection has a 48-hour cyclic fever. A unique feature of both the *P. ovale* and *P. vivax* organisms is that they can form hypnozoites that can remain dormant in the liver for long periods of time, only to resurface later.

Answer E is incorrect. *Trichomonas vaginalis* is the cause of vaginitis. Symptoms of vaginitis include a foul-smelling greenish discharge, itching, and burning. *T. vaginalis* is transmitted sexually. On microscopic wet mount, one finds trophozoites. Metronidazole is used to treat *T. vaginalis* infection.

20. **The correct answer is D.** The question stem describes follicular lymphoma, the most common type of non-Hodgkin's lymphoma in the United States. The characteristic chromosomal translocation is t(14;18), which juxtaposes the IgH locus on chromosome 14 next to the BCL2 locus on chromosome 18. This causes overproduction of the bcl-2 protein, an anti-apoptotic factor, facilitating the survival of the cancer. An important simplifying fact to help remember the different chromosomal translocations is that those involving the immunoglobulin loci on chromosome 14 tend to be cells that normally produce antibodies (e.g., B lymphocytes). Thus, these translocations are common in B-lymphocyte lymphomas.

Answer A is incorrect. The t(8;14) rearrangement is most commonly found in Burkitt's lymphoma as well as in some cases of acute lymphocytic leukemia. Translocation of the c-myc gene next to the immunoglobulin heavy chain locus results in constitutive overproduction of the c-myc oncogene, promoting neoplastic proliferation.

Answer B is incorrect. The t(9;22) translocation results in the Philadelphia chromosome, which is most commonly found in chronic myelogenous leukemia as well as in other chronic myeloproliferative disorders and acute lymphocytic leukemia, where it confers a poor prognosis. The translocation results in a bcr-abl fusion protein that functions as a constitutively active tyrosine kinase to promote leukemia growth.

Answer C is incorrect. The t(11;22) chromosomal translocation is associated with Ewing's sarcoma. (Note that it does not involve the immunoglobulin locus.) It overproduces a chimeric transcription factor that activates the c-myc promoter and produces excessive amounts of the EWS-FL-1 protein. Ewing's sarcoma is a small round cell tumor of the bone usually found in the long bones of teenagers. X-ray will show a lytic tumor with reactive bone deposited around it in an onion-skin fashion.

Answer E is incorrect. The t(15;17) translocation denotes the acute promyelocytic leukemia (APL) subtype of acute myelogenous leukemia. The characteristic fusion of the promyelocytic leukemia (PML) gene with the retinoic acid receptor-α (RAR-α) gene blocks differentiation of immature myeloid blasts, most likely by blocking activity of other retinoic acid receptors. Treatment with all-trans retinoic acid (termed **differentiation therapy**) overwhelms the blockade of the other retinoic acid receptors, restores differentiation, and can induce temporary remission. Combination differentiation treatment together with conventional chemotherapy can result in long-term survival rates of 70–80%, unique among the acute leukemias. APL patients also typically present with dysfunctional coagulopathies, predisposing them to excess bleeding, a major source of mortality.

21. **The correct answer is D.** Cyclosporine is an immunosuppressant that binds to cyclophilins, thereby blocking the differentiation and activation of T lymphocytes by inhibiting the production of interleukin-2 (IL-2). Erythromycin is a macrolide antibiotic that binds to the 50S ribosomal subunit and inhibits protein synthesis. Amoxicillin is a β-lactam antibiotic that inhibits bacterial cell wall synthesis. Studies have shown similar results with amoxicillin and erythromycin in the treatment of bacterial sinusi-

tis. Concurrent use of erythromycin and cyclosporine could lead to elevated cyclosporine serum concentrations because erythromycin inhibits the cytochrome P450 enzyme system in the liver. The cytochrome P450 enzyme superfamily is a major site of drug metabolism and is responsible for the oxidation, reduction, and hydrolysis of drug compounds, including cyclosporine.

Answer A is incorrect. Erythromycin will increase, not decrease, cyclosporine concentrations.

Answer B is incorrect. Erythromycin will increase cyclosporine concentrations both initially and over time.

Answer C is incorrect. Erythromycin will increase cyclosporine concentrations both initially and over time.

Answer E is incorrect. Erythromycin will increase cyclosporine concentration

22. **The correct answer is C.** Transitional cell carcinoma (TCC) is a malignant tumor that arises from the transitional epithelium of the renal pelvis. It can spread to adjacent tissues and often recurs after removal. It is the most common tumor of the urinary tract system. While it can occur in renal calyces, the renal pelvis, and the ureters, the most common site for TCC is in the bladder. There is significant association of TCC with phenacetin (a common painkiller), smoking, aniline dyes, and cyclophosphamide (a chemotherapeutic drug); remember the mnemonic "Associated problems in your **Pee SAC.**" Hematuria is the most common presenting sign of TCC. The presence of otherwise unexplained hematuria denotes cancer in the urinary tract in individuals over the age of 40 years until proven otherwise. Commonly, TCC is treated surgically. Other treatment modalities include radiation and chemotherapy as either adjuvant or primary treatment, depending on the case.

Answer A is incorrect. Alcohol use is not a risk factor associated with transitional cell carcinoma.

Answer B is incorrect. Exposure to asbestos is not a risk factor associated with transitional cell carcinoma.

Answer D is incorrect. Hypertension is not a risk factor associated with transitional cell carcinoma.

Answer E is incorrect. Previous pyelonephritis is not a risk factor associated with transitional cell carcinoma.

23. **The correct answer is B.** The above clinical and laboratory findings are consistent with pernicious anemia, a chronic progressive anemia that is caused by a failure to absorb vitamin B_{12} because of a lack of availability of intrinsic factor. It is believed to be caused by immune-mediated destruction of gastric mucosa, leading to a loss of parietal cells (parietal cells produce intrinsic factor, which is essential for vitamin B_{12} absorption). Several studies have also suggested that autoantibodies may play a role by blocking the binding of vitamin B_{12} to intrinsic factor, preventing the binding of intrinsic factor or intrinsic factor/vitamin B_{12} complex to receptors in the ileum of the intestine, or attacking the gastric proton pumps of parietal cells. The normal physiologic function of intrinsic factor is to bind free vitamin B_{12} in the small intestine and bind the resulting complex to receptors on cells on the ileum of the intestine.

Answer A is incorrect. Transcobalamin II, a plasma protein, binds free vitamin B_{12} in ileal cells for transport through the bloodstream.

Answer C is incorrect. R proteins are vitamin B_{12}–binding proteins produced by the salivary gland that bind vitamin B_{12} once it has been split from its exogenous protein-bound form by pepsin in the stomach.

Answer D is incorrect. Pancreatic proteases are secreted into the duodenum, which split the R-protein/vitamin B_{12} complexes, producing vitamin B_{12} that is free to bind intrinsic factor to form intrinsic factor/vitamin B_{12} complexes.

Answer E is incorrect. Pepsin, which is active in creating the acidic pH of the stomach, splits vitamin B_{12} from its exogenous protein-bound form, leaving it free to bind R proteins produced by the salivary gland.

24. **The correct answer is B.** Wilms' tumor arises from neoplastic embryonal renal cells of the metanephros. Wilms' tumor is the most common solid tumor of childhood (most commonly occurring between the ages of 2 and 4 years) and is rarely seen in adults. It commonly presents with a huge palpable flank mass and is seen with hemihypertrophy (abnormal enlargement of one side of the body). It is associated with the deletion of tumor suppressor gene WT1 on chromosome 11. Since it arises from the kidney parenchyma, it distorts the kidney calyces as it grows.

Answer A is incorrect. Adult polycystic disease is an autosomal dominant genetic disorder that presents with bilateral cystic enlargement of the kidneys. Individuals with this disorder also suffer from cystic enlargement of the liver, berry aneurysms, and mitral valve prolapse.

Answer C is incorrect. Clear cell carcinoma of the kidney is a malignancy derived from the renal tubular cells. It is common for patients to present with an abdominal mass, but patients with clear cell carcinoma are commonly male adults between the ages of 50 and 70 years, with an increased incidence found in smokers. Patients with renal cell carcinoma present with a range of symptoms, such as hematuria, a palpable mass, polycythemia, flank pain, and fever.

Answer D is incorrect. Transitional cell carcinoma (TCC) is a malignant tumor that arises from the uroepithelial cells of the urinary tract. TCC is the most common tumor of the urinary tract (as it can occur in the renal calyx, renal pelvis, ureters, and bladder). Painless hematuria and urinary outflow obstruction are the most common presenting signs of TCC.

Answer E is incorrect. Malignancy that is derived from the primitive neural crest cells as an abdominal mass in a young child is neuroblastoma. The tumor does not arise in the kidney;

instead, it forms from the adrenal medulla and paraspinal sympathetic ganglia. Therefore, it does not distort the kidney architecture.

25. **The correct answer is D.** This patient suffers from paroxysmal nocturnal hemoglobinuria, an acquired disease caused by RBC susceptibility to complement-mediated cell lysis. This is due to insufficient synthesis of GPI anchors, which anchor proteins that protect RBCs from this process. Clinical manifestations include intravascular hemolysis with hemoglobin release into the blood and subsequent hemoglobinuria, thrombotic complications (such as Budd-Chiari syndrome), and anaplastic anemia.

Answer A is incorrect. Autoimmune hemolytic anemia (AIHA) is caused by IgG antibodies that are targeted against RBC antigens. This patient's symptoms are all due to acute intravascular hemolysis. However, in AIHA, the hemolysis is antibody-mediated and is not due to susceptibility for complement-mediated lysis.

Answer B is incorrect. Although common bile duct (CBD) stricture may cause darker urine due to elevated bilirubin in the blood, it would not cause intravascular hemolysis or complement-mediated lysis. CBD strictures caused by carcinomas of the pancreatic head are the most common causes of painless jaundice.

Answer C is incorrect. Hereditary spherocytosis is caused by mutations that result in an unstable erythrocyte cytoskeleton. When those erythrocytes pass through the spleen, the reticuloendothelial cells remove pieces of the membrane, causing spherocyte formation. This results in extravascular hemolysis and is not due to complement-mediated lysis.

Answer E is incorrect. The normal von Willebrand factor (vWF) protease is absent in patients with thrombotic thrombocytopenic purpura (TTP), resulting in high levels of large vWF multimers and causing excessive platelet adhesion and clearance. Because of diffuse thrombus formation in the microvasculature,

evidence of intravascular hemolysis is found due to microangiopathy. The classic pentad of TTP consists of fever, thrombocytopenia, microangiopathic hemolysis, neurologic symptoms, and renal insufficiency. RBC lysis is caused by shear trauma in the vessels and is not secondary to complement-mediated lysis.

26. **The correct answer is B.** Cisplatin has been shown to cause nephrotoxicity and acoustic nerve damage. Use of cisplatin requires that the patient be vigorously hydrated in order to prevent kidney damage. In patients with documented kidney dysfunction, cisplatin should be avoided altogether due to these patients' greater susceptibility to dose-related nephrotoxicity.

Answer A is incorrect. Bleomycin toxicity includes pulmonary fibrosis, hypertrophic skin changes, and minimal myelosuppression. It is not associated with nephrotoxicity.

Answer C is incorrect. Cytarabine causes leukopenia, thrombocytopenia, and megaloblastic anemia. It is not associated with nephrotoxicity.

Answer D is incorrect. Toxic effects of doxorubicin include cardiotoxicity, myelosuppression, and alopecia. It is not associated with nephrotoxicity.

Answer E is incorrect. Tamoxifen has been noted to cause hot flashes, nausea/vomiting, skin rash, and vaginal bleeding. It is not associated with nephrotoxicity.

27. **The correct answer is A.** This patient presents with clinical features of idiopathic thrombocytopenic purpura (ITP), the most common cause of thrombocytopenia in childhood. ITP is an autoimmune disease and is most commonly instigated by a viral illness. Bleeding disorders due to platelet defects or deficiencies will present with microhemorrhage of the mucous membranes and of the skin, like the non-blanching purple skin lesions (purpura) seen in this patient. ITP is a diagnosis of exclusion but classically presents with thrombocytopenia, antiplatelet antibodies, as well as signs of a

compensatory increase in platelet production, including large platelets on peripheral blood smear and increased megakaryocytes on bone marrow biopsy. As ITP only affects platelets, patients will have normal prothrombin time and normal partial thromboplastin time.

Answer B is incorrect. Decreased megakaryocytes on bone marrow biopsy suggest a defect in platelet production which can result from malignancy, infection, or drug reactions.

Answer C is incorrect. Patients with IgA deficiency present with frequent respiratory, urinary, and gastrointestinal infections and would not present with isolated thrombocytopenia.

Answer D is incorrect. Increased fibrin split products are a sign of activation of the coagulation cascade and may be associated with thrombocytopenia in the case of disseminated intravascular coagulation (DIC). DIC is caused by a systemic activation of the clotting cascade leading to global depletion of clotting factors in addition to depletion of platelets. DIC leads to complications from both the systemic microthrombi and the increased risk of bleeding from clotting factor and platelet depletion. While patients with DIC will present with thrombocytopenia, they will also have an increased prothrombin time and partial thromboplastic time and schistocytes on their peripheral blood smears. In addition to the microhemorrhage of the skin and mucous membranes due to the platelet deficiency, patients with DIC can also develop macrohemorrhage in joints and internal organs as a result of the clotting factor deficiencies

Answer E is incorrect. Vitamin K deficiency leads to a deficiency in the Vitamin K–dependent clotting factors, II, VII, IX, and X, causing an elevated prothrombin time and increasing the risk of macrohemorrhage. Vitamin K deficiency, however, should not lead to thrombocytopenia seen in this patient.

28. **The correct answer is D.** Although her symptoms may be somewhat nonspecific, the fact that this patient has small-cell lung carcinoma (SCLC) should be a clue that her symptoms may be part of a paraneoplastic syndrome.

SCLC is notorious for production of ACTH and ADH. In this case, excessive ACTH production has lead to increased glucocorticoids. Weight gain and redistribution of body fat (in contrast to the cachexia typical of cancers alone) and moon facies are classic signs of Cushing's syndrome. Poor wound healing (due to inhibition of collagen synthesis by glucocorticoids) and hirsutism (stimulation of androgen production by ACTH) are also part of Cushing's syndrome.

Answer A is incorrect. Cold intolerance and hair loss are symptoms of hypothyroidism.

Answer B is incorrect. Galactorrhea and amenorrhea are symptoms of hyperprolactinemia, as may occur in cases of anterior pituitary tumors.

Answer C is incorrect. Insatiable thirst and polyuria are symptoms of antidiuretic hormone deficiency or diabetes insipidus.

Answer E is incorrect. Restlessness and tremor are symptoms of hyperthyroidism.

29. **The correct answer is A.** This woman suffers from hereditary spherocytosis (HS), typically caused by mutations in the genes that code for either ankyrin or spectrin. Both of these proteins contribute to the erythrocyte cytoskeleton. When the erythrocytes with abnormal membranes pass through the spleen, the reticuloendothelial cells remove pieces of the membrane, causing a decreased membrane-to-cytoplasm ratio. This results in spherocyte formation. HS is often associated with hemolytic crisis resulting in jaundice and pigmented gallstones.

Answer B is incorrect. Glucose-6-phosphate dehydrogenase (G6PD) deficiency is due to an X-linked mutation and therefore typically occurs only in males. Although hemolysis in the setting of G6PD could be secondary to infection, Heinz bodies and bite cells will be found in the peripheral blood smear, not spherocytes.

Answer C is incorrect. Autoimmune hemolytic anemia is due to antibodies against erythrocytes. This will cause a positive Coombs' test and therefore is unlikely in this setting.

Answer D is incorrect. Iron deficiency anemia causes a microcytic anemia. This does not fit the hemolytic picture and is not associated with spherocytes.

Answer E is incorrect. Hemolysis because of a mechanical valve is caused by mechanical trauma as the erythrocytes flow across the foreign surface. This results in schistocytes in a peripheral blood smear. This diagnosis is unlikely given the absence of a unique heart sound on examination and an absence of schistocytes in the smear.

30. **The correct answer is D.** Prevalence is the total number of cases in a population at a given time. Since the study was done recently, we can assume that the current prevalence of the disease can be deciphered from the results of that study (0.5% of the population is 30). Therefore, the prevalence of sickle cell disease in this community is 30 individuals. Prevalence is commonly confused with incidence, which is the number of new cases in a population per unit of time. In this example, the incidence is 6/year. Prevalence exceeds incidence for chronic diseases.

    Answer A is incorrect. This number is the result of dividing the number of new cases last year by the total number of people in the community. This does not give the prevalence.

    Answer B is incorrect. This is not a relevant number and is perhaps the result of incorrect calculations.

    Answer C is incorrect. The incidence is the number of new cases in a population per unit of time. Six is the incidence of the disease last year.

    Answer E is incorrect. This answer is the prevalence of people with heterozygotes, not the prevalence of those with sickle cell disease.

31. **The correct answer is D.** This bone marrow biopsy is consistent with multiple myeloma. Plasma cells can be clearly seen throughout this slide, recognized by their off-center nuclei and clock-face chromatin distribution. Also commonly seen on a bone marrow biopsy of multiple myeloma are stacked RBCs, in what's known as a rouleaux formation.

    Answer A is incorrect. Bone marrow suppression appears as a paucity of cells on histology. This image has too many plasma cells to represent bone marrow suppression.

    Answer B is incorrect. Lymphoma is a neoplastic disorder of the lymphoid tissue. There are many different types of lymphoma, two of the most distinctive histologic types being Burkitt's lymphoma and Hodgkin's lymphoma. Burkitt's lymphoma shows a "starry sky" pattern on histology. This pattern is created by macrophage ingestion of tumor cells. Hodgkin's lymphoma is distinguished by its Reed-Sternberg cells. The Reed-Sternberg cells are binucleate and display prominent nucleoli.

    Answer C is incorrect. Prostate cancer is typically adenocarcinoma. It commonly metastasizes to the axial skeleton and can cause back pain and spinal cord compression. It causes osteoblastic lesions in bone.

    Answer E is incorrect. This image shows too many plasma cells to represent normal bone marrow.

32. **The correct answer is E.** Trimethoprim is associated with megaloblastic anemia, leukopenia, and granulocytopenia. These effects may be reduced with a folic acid supplement.

    Answer A is incorrect. Chloramphenicol is a broad-spectrum antibiotic that is particularly effective against bacterial meningitis and is associated with aplastic anemia and gray baby syndrome.

    Answer B is incorrect. Clindamycin is associated with pseudomembranous colitis due to *Clostridium difficile* overgrowth.

    Answer C is incorrect. Erythromycin is a macrolide and is associated with cholestatic hepatitis.

    Answer D is incorrect. Gatifloxacin is a fluoroquinolone and is associated with tendinitis.

33. The correct answer is B. Rectal bleeding or anemia in anyone age 50 years or older is considered colorectal cancer until proven otherwise. The gold standard for diagnosis of colorectal cancer is colonoscopy with possible tissue biopsy of suspicious lesions. Current cancer screening recommendations suggest colonoscopy or double-contrast barium enema every 10 years, sigmoidoscopy every 5 years, and/or fecal occult blood testing in people age 50 and above.

Answer A is incorrect. Abdominal plain films are best used to visualize radiopaque renal lithiasis, free air, or fluid.

Answer C is incorrect. Abdominal CT scans can visualize many abdominal pathologies; however, colonoscopy is a more sensitive test for colorectal cancer screening.

Answer D is incorrect. Esophagoduodenoscopy is best used to evaluate for lesions of the upper gastrointestinal tract.

Answer E is incorrect. Pelvic ultrasound is best used to evaluate abnormalities of the ovaries, uterus, and vagina.

34. The correct answer is B. In addition to the physical signs of Cushing's syndrome (weight gain, moon face, thin skin, muscle weakness, and brittle bones) along with cataracts, hypertension, increased appetite, elevated blood sugar, indigestion, insomnia, nervousness, restlessness, and immunosuppression, prednisone is known to produce profound mood changes known as glucocorticoid psychosis.

Answer A is incorrect. The typical adverse effects of bleomycin are pulmonary fibrosis, skin changes, and myelosuppression. Bleomycin is part of the **ABVD** cancer chemotherapy regimen against Hodgkin's: **A**driamycin (doxorubicin), **B**leomycin, **V**inblastine, and **D**acarbazine.

Answer C is incorrect. Common adverse effects of vincristine are areflexia and peripheral neuritis. Vincristine is part of the **MOPP** cancer chemotherapy regimen used against Hodgkin's disease: **M**echlorethamine, vincristine (**O**ncovin), **P**rocarbazine, and **P**rednisone.

Answer D is incorrect. Wildly swinging mood is suggestive of cyclothymic disorders, which are common in patients with chronic medical illness. However, given that this disorder requires 2 years for diagnosis, the most likely cause is glucocorticoid psychosis.

Answer E is incorrect. The progression of Hodgkin's disease typically does not involve profound psychiatric symptoms.

35. The correct answer is B. Hydatidiform moles are cystic swellings of the chorionic villi. They usually present in the fourth and fifth months of pregnancy with vaginal bleeding. On exam the uterus is larger than expected for gestational age and the serum β-hCG level is much higher than normal. Moles can be either partial or complete and are caused by either fertilization of an egg that has lost its chromosomes or fertilization of a normal egg with two sperm. Partial moles may contain some fetal tissue but no viable fetus, and a complete mole contains no fetal tissue. Hydatidiform moles must be surgically removed because the chorionic villi may embolize to distant sites and because moles may lead to choriocarcinoma, an aggressive neoplasm that metastasizes early but is very responsive to chemotherapy.

Answer A is incorrect. Neural tube defects are usually detected in utero by increased α-fetoprotein levels in amniotic fluid and maternal serum; β-hCG levels are normal in these patients.

Answer C is incorrect. The fallopian tubes are the most common site for ectopic pregnancies. If undetected, tubal pregnancies may rupture, causing unilateral lower quadrant pain and uterine bleeding. Because the patient may exsanguinate, ruptured ectopic pregnancy is a surgical emergency. This patient does not have the symptoms of a tubal pregnancy. Also, because of the small size of the fallopian tubes, tubal pregnancies present long before 4 months of gestation.

Answer D is incorrect. While all obstetricians are concerned about and should monitor their patients for signs of preeclampsia, that is not the main cause of concern for this patient. Preeclampsia is the triad of hypertension, proteinuria, and edema. Eclampsia occurs when seizures are added to the list of symptoms. This patient does not have any of these symptoms.

Answer E is incorrect. A woman carrying more than one fetus tends to have a larger uterus and higher levels of β-hCG than a woman with a single pregnancy at the same point in gestation. However, the β-hCG level in multiple pregnancy is never as abnormally high as in a hydatidiform mole. While a multiple pregnancy is something the physician should investigate, a β-hCG level this high indicates hydatidiform mole.

36. **The correct answer is B.** This boy suffers from asthma, which is characterized by airway hyperresponsiveness and airflow obstruction. This condition can be precipitated by several factors, including allergens, upper respiratory infections, drugs, and stress. Clinically, asthmatics experience episodes of wheezing, coughing, and dyspnea. Sputum samples may demonstrate Curschmann's spirals and Charcot-Leyden crystals. Blood tests will typically reveal eosinophilia. Other causes of eosinophilia include neoplasms, parasites, collagen vascular diseases, and allergic processes.

Answer A is incorrect. Asbestosis is characterized by diffuse interstitial fibrosis and an increased risk of mesothelioma and bronchogenic carcinoma. Intermittent obstructive episodes are not associated with asbestosis. Ferruginous bodies in the lungs are necessary for this diagnosis.

Answer C is incorrect. Asbestosis is characterized by diffuse interstitial fibrosis and an increased risk of mesothelioma and bronchogenic carcinoma. Intermittent obstructive episodes are not associated with asbestosis. Ferruginous bodies in the lungs are necessary for this diagnosis.

Answer D is incorrect. Croup is laryngotracheobronchitis due to infection with the RNA virus parainfluenza. Croup is characterized by a seal-like barking cough, not intermittent obstructive episodes.

Answer E is incorrect. Cystic fibrosis is an autosomal recessive disease resulting from ineffective chloride transport due to a defective *CFTR* gene. This condition is characterized by pulmonary infections, chronic bronchitis, and pancreatic insufficiency. High concentrations of chloride in a sweat test would confirm this diagnosis, not high levels of eosinophils.

37. **The correct answer is F.** This vignette suggests a malignancy of the liver. Hepatomas are highly associated with chronic hepatitis B and C infections, which are often found in health care workers due to needle stick injuries. Other risk factors for hepatomas include Wilson's disease, hemochromatosis, alcoholic cirrhosis, α_1-antitrypsin deficiency, and carcinogens. α-Fetoprotein is a marker for hepatomas but can also be elevated in patients with germ cell tumors, such as yolk sac tumors. Tumor markers should not be used for primary diagnoses, but for confirmation and to monitor therapy.

Answer A is incorrect. This vignette suggests a malignancy of the liver. Hepatomas are highly associated with chronic hepatitis B and C infections, which are often found in health care workers due to needle stick injuries. Other risk factors for hepatomas include Wilson's disease, hemochromatosis, alcoholic cirrhosis, α_1-antitrypsin deficiency, and carcinogens. α-Fetoprotein is a marker for hepatomas but can also be elevated in patients with germ cell tumors, such as yolk sac tumors. Tumor markers should not be used for primary diagnoses, but for confirmation and to monitor therapy.

Answer B is incorrect. The marker for colorectal carcinoma is carcinoembryonic antigen. This marker is nonspecific and is also produced by pancreatic, gastric, and breast carcinomas. The presence of a hepatoma has no effect on this marker.

Answer C is incorrect. The marker for melanoma is S-100. This marker also is elevated with neural tumors and astrocytomas.

The presence of a hepatoma has no effect on this marker.

Answer D is incorrect. The marker for neuroblastoma is bombesin. This marker also is elevated with lung and gastric cancers. The presence of a hepatoma has no effect on this marker.

Answer E is incorrect. The marker for prostatic carcinoma is prostate-specific antigen. The presence of a hepatoma has no effect on this marker.

38. **The correct answer is A.** Neoplastic B lymphocytes are the cells of origin in most non-Hodgkin's lymphomas (90% of cases), with the notable exception of lymphoblastic lymphoma, which is typically dominated by T lymphocytes.

    Answer B is incorrect. Myeloblasts are the neoplastic cells in acute myelogenous leukemia.

    Answer C is incorrect. Plasma cells are the neoplastic cells in multiple myeloma. Multiple myeloma also affects patients in their 50s and 60s. However, at presentation patients with multiple myeloma usually have pathologic fracture caused by lytic lesions, hypercalcemia because of bone resorption, and repeated infection because of decreased production of normal immunoglobulins. Urine analysis in patients with multiple myeloma shows Bence Jones proteinuria with a monoclonal spike on electrophoresis.

    Answer D is incorrect. Reed-Sternberg cells are the neoplastic cells in Hodgkin's disease. Under light microscopy, Reed-Sternberg cells appear as large binucleate cells with abundant cytoplasm and large "owl-eye" nucleoli.

    Answer E is incorrect. T-lymphocyte lymphomas are less common and include lymphoblastic lymphomas and a minority of diffuse large cell lymphomas.

39. **The correct answer is D.** The testes begin life high in the abdomen and descend to their final resting place in the scrotum. The lymphatic drainage from the testes, therefore, is to the nodes around the aorta in the lumbar region just inferior to the renal arteries.

    Answer A is incorrect. The deep inguinal nodes drain the vessels in the spongy urethra and may become enlarged in some sexually transmitted diseases or other causes of urethritis.

    Answer B is incorrect. External iliac nodes drain the bladder.

    Answer C is incorrect. Gluteal lymph nodes drain the deep tissue of the buttocks.

    Answer E is incorrect. Tumors of the scrotum itself, but not of the testes, may spread to the superficial inguinal lymph nodes. The scrotum is an outpouching of abdominal skin, and drainage of this skin is to the superficial inguinal nodes. The testes, however, which lie inside the scrotum, begin life in the abdomen, and lymph drainage follows embryologic origins, not final locations.

40. **The correct answer is B.** δ-Aminolevulinic acid synthase catalyzes the first reaction, glycine + succinyl-CoA → δ-aminolevulinic acid. This is the rate-limiting and committed step in heme synthesis.

    Answer A is incorrect. δ-Aminolevulinic acid dehydratase catalyzes the second step in heme synthesis, 2δ-aminolevulinic acid → porphobilinogen.

    Answer C is incorrect. Ferrochelatase catalyzes the final reaction in heme synthesis, which is insertion of an iron atom into the protoporphyrin IX ring structure, forming heme.

    Answer D is incorrect. Heme oxygenase catalyzes the first step in heme metabolism in which heme is oxidized, producing biliverdin, ferric iron, and carbon monoxide.

    Answer E is incorrect. Uroporphyrinogen I synthase condenses four molecules of porphobilinogen together to form hydroxymethylbilane; this is the third step in heme synthesis. Uroporphyrinogen I synthase can also be called porphobilinogen deaminase.

41. The correct answer is D. Vincristine is a vinca alkaloid antineoplastic agent that inhibits microtubule formation. It is used in the treatment of leukemias, Hodgkin's and non-Hodgkin's lymphoma, Wilms' tumor, neuroblastoma, rhabdomyosarcoma, and multiple myeloma.

Answer A is incorrect. Melphalan and ifosfamide are two among many alkylating agents. Melphalan is an alkylating agent that inhibits DNA and RNA synthesis through the formation of carbonium ions. It is used in the treatment of multiple myeloma, ovarian carcinoma, neuroblastoma, rhabdomyosarcoma, and breast cancer. Ifosfamide is an alkylating agent, also known as nitrogen mustard, used in the treatment of lung cancer, Hodgkin's and non-Hodgkin's lymphoma, breast cancer, lymphocytic leukemias, ovarian cancer, and multiple myeloma.

Answer B is incorrect. Chemotherapeutic drugs such as doxorubicin act by noncovalently intercalating between DNA strands, creating breaks in the strands to decrease replication and generate free radicals. Doxorubicin is used in the treatment of Hodgkin's lymphoma, myelomas, sarcomas, and solid tumors of the breast, ovary, and lung.

Answer C is incorrect. Chemotherapeutic agents such as paclitaxel act by binding to tubulin and hyperstabilizing polymerized microtubules, preventing the mitotic spindle from breaking down. It is used in the treatment of ovarian and breast cancers.

Answer E is incorrect. Chemotherapeutic drugs such as etoposide act by inhibiting topoisomerase II and increasing DNA degradation. Etoposide is used to treat oat cell carcinoma of the lung and prostate and testicular cancer.

42. The correct answer is A. This man likely underwent a splenectomy to control bleeding. Splenic injury is the most common injury following blunt trauma. After splenectomy, individuals are highly susceptible to encapsulated organisms, including *Neisseria meningitides*, *Streptococcus pneumoniae*, *Haemophilus influenzae*, and *Klebsiella pneumoniae*. In fact, those who undergo splenectomy should receive vaccinations for the first three organisms in this list within 2 weeks of the procedure. This man likely did not receive these vaccinations before leaving the hospital. Due to the loss of splenic processing of immature and irregular erythrocytes, Heinz bodies and target cells could be expected in the peripheral blood smear. Because many platelets are sequestered in the spleen, splenectomy will cause a rise in platelet count, typically transiently.

Answer B is incorrect. A peripheral blood smear containing large RBCs, hypersegmented polymorphonuclear leukocytes, and anisocytosis/poikilocytosis suggests megaloblastic anemia secondary to either B_{12} or folate deficiency. Splenectomy will not result in the picture of megaloblastic anemia.

Answer C is incorrect. Schistocytes are typically due to disseminated intravascular coagulation or traumatic hemolysis. One form of traumatic hemolysis is microangiopathic hemolytic anemia found in thrombotic thrombocytopenic purpura. Schistocytes would not be expected following splenectomy.

Answer D is incorrect. Sickle cells in the peripheral blood smear are evidence of sickle cell anemia, a condition that this patient shows no evidence of having. Although autosplenectomy is a possibility with sickle cell anemia, the patient clearly received his splenectomy due to trauma, not repeated vaso-occlusive crises.

Answer E is incorrect. Spherocytes are evidence of hereditary spherocytosis (HS), a condition caused by mutations in either the ankyrin or the spectrin gene, both of which contribute to the erythrocyte cytoskeleton. In HS, when erythrocytes with abnormal membranes pass through the spleen, the reticuloendothelial cells remove pieces of the membrane causing spherocyte formation, not Heinz bodies or target cells.

43. The correct answer is D. This patient has glucose-6-phosphate dehydrogenase deficiency, which is common in African-Americans, and demonstrates characteristic Heinz bodies (precipitates of hemoglobin) within RBCs. Hemolysis can be precipitated by certain drugs, such as sulfonamides, isoniazid, aspirin, ibuprofen, primaquine, and nitrofurantoin.

Answer A is incorrect. Aminoglycosides are commonly associated with nephro- and ototoxicity.

Answer B is incorrect. Fluoroquinolones may cause some gastrointestinal upset, damage to cartilage in children, and tendonitis and tendon rupture in adults.

Answer C is incorrect. Macrolide toxicity includes gastrointestinal discomfort, acute cholestatic hepatitis, eosinophilia, and skin rashes.

Answer E is incorrect. Tetracycline toxicity includes gastrointestinal distress, tooth discoloration and inhibition of bone growth in children, and photosensitivity reactions.

44. **The correct answer is A.** Abciximab functions by binding to the glycoprotein receptor IIb/IIIa on activated platelets, preventing fibrinogen from binding and interfering with platelet aggregation. It is used in acute coronary syndrome and angioplasty.

Answer B is incorrect. Both clopidogrel and ticlopidine function by inhibiting the ADP pathway involved in the binding of fibrinogen to platelets during platelet aggregation.

Answer C is incorrect. Leuprolide is a gonadotropin-releasing hormone analog that acts as an agonist when administered in a pulsatile fashion and as an antagonist when administered in a continuous fashion. It is used to treat infertility (when administered as an agonist), prostate cancer (when administered as an antagonist), and uterine fibroids.

Answer D is incorrect. Selegiline is a selective monoamine oxidase B inhibitor that causes an increase in the availability of dopamine. It is used with levodopa in the treatment of Parkinson's disease.

Answer E is incorrect. Both clopidogrel and ticlopidine function by inhibiting the ADP pathway involved in the binding of fibrinogen to platelets during platelet aggregation.

45. **The correct answer is E.** This patient's physical exam demonstrates Courvoisier's sign—jaundice and a palpable, enlarged, nontender gallbladder. This sign is often found in patients with cancer in the head of the pancreas, which is obstructing the gallbladder from emptying.

Answer A is incorrect. Acute hepatitis is associated with tenderness in the right upper quadrant, and it should not produce an enlarged gallbladder.

Answer B is incorrect. Choledocholithiasis is the presence of a stone in the common bile duct. It is a common cause of cholecystitis, which is associated with tenderness in the right upper quadrant.

Answer C is incorrect. Cholelithiasis simply refers to stones within the gallbladder. It is generally painless, and does not cause jaundice or an enlarged gallbladder.

Answer D is incorrect. Hemolytic anemia is a cause of painless jaundice, however, it is not associated with an enlarged gallbladder.

46. **The correct answer is B.** This patient is in disseminated intravascular coagulation (DIC) secondary to an acute case of pancreatitis. Common causes of DIC are gram-negative sepsis, malignancy, acute pancreatitis, trauma, transfusion reactions, and obstetric complications. During DIC, there is a massive activation of the coagulation cascade that results in thrombus formation throughout the microvasculature. Rapid consumption of both platelets and coagulation factors follows. Concurrent with this consumptive coagulopathy is activation of the fibrinolytic system. In this patient, thrombocytopenia, elevated prothrombin time/partial thromboplastin time, and the presence of fibrin split products all suggest DIC. Pancreatitis as the cause is supported by the clinical presentation, the increased amylase and lipase activity, and the presence of a dilated common bile duct, suggesting gallstones as a possible cause of the pancreatitis episode.

Answer A is incorrect. Abdominal aortic aneurysms (AAAs) are characterized by tearing hypogastric pain that may radiate to the back and by the detection of a pulsatile abdominal mass. The development of an AAA that does not rupture will not result in DIC or cause pancreatitis.

Answer C is incorrect. Appendicitis may present initially with diffuse abdominal tenderness, typically in the periumbilical region, and with an elevated white blood cell count. However, pain radiating to the back and increased amylase and lipase activity suggest pancreatitis. Additionally, appendicitis is not a typical cause of disseminated intravascular coagulation.

Answer D is incorrect. Gastric ulcers may present clinically as epigastric pain radiating to the back and may be associated with increased amylase activity, especially if perforation has occurred. However, ulcers are not typical causes of disseminated intravascular coagulation and will not cause increased amylase and lipase activity.

Answer E is incorrect. Gram-negative sepsis is a common cause of disseminated intravascular coagulation. There is no evidence in this case to suggest that the patient is suffering from sepsis, including a fever, a very high white blood cell count, or a previous infection. All physical and laboratory evidence supports pancreatitis.

47. **The correct answer is C.** Monoclonal gammopathy of undetermined significance (MGUS) is characterized as a plasma cell dyscrasia, defined by the presence of a monoclonal immunoglobulin, also called an M protein, in the serum or urine of persons without evidence of multiple myeloma, Waldenström's macroglobulinemia, amyloidosis, or other lymphoproliferative disorders. MGUS is a preneoplastic condition. There is no accepted treatment for this disorder because one cannot predict which patients will progress to develop multiple myeloma.

Answer A is incorrect. Anticoagulation is not the recommended treatment for MGUS

Answer B is incorrect. High-dose steroids are not a current treatment modality for MGUS.

Answer D is incorrect. A restrictive diet is not a current treatment modality for MGUS.

Answer E is incorrect. Vinca alkaloids such as vincristine and vinblastine are microtubule inhibitors used in the treatment of some cancers. However, vinca alkaloids are not currently the recommended treatment for MGUS.

48. **The correct answer is B.** The correct answer is β-thalassemia major. The thalassemias can be divided into genetic diseases involving decreased synthesis/absence of either the α-globin chain (leading to α-thalassemia) or the β-globin chain (leading to β-thalassemia). These genes are responsible for encoding protein chains found in the hemoglobin molecule. This patient has classic symptoms of thalassemia: hemolytic anemia, hepatosplenomegaly, and "chipmunk facies." The requirement for blood transfusions since birth should raise the suspicion for β-thalassemia major in this patient, but the hemoglobin electrophoresis results alone can be used to arrive at this conclusion. This patient shows increased HbF (α-2 γ-2) and HbA$_2$ (α-2 β-2); thus, synthesis of the α chain is intact. Absence of HbA$_1$ (α-2 β-2) supports an absence of β-chain synthesis and, therefore, a diagnosis of β-thalassemia major.

Answer A is incorrect. α-Thalassemia minor is associated with a two-gene deletion of α globin (two gene regions are intact). Deletion of only a single α gene results in an asymptomatic carrier with no hematologic manifestations.

Answer C is incorrect. β-Thalassemia minor (the heterozygous defect) would show decreased but not absent HbA$_1$.

Answer D is incorrect. Glucose-6-phosphate dehydrogenase deficiency would not present with abnormal hemoglobin electrophoresis.

Answer E is incorrect. HbH is less severe than Hb Barts and is associated with three-gene deletion of α globin. The abnormal hemoglobin molecule contains four β chains.

Answer F is incorrect. Because there are two separate α-globin loci and therefore four distinct α-globin alleles, there are four genotypes possible in α-thalassemia. Hb Barts is the most severe of these genotypes; it is associated with complete absence of all α-globin chains. This results in the absence of all fetal hemoglobins that require this chain, and in the formation of tetramers of the γ chain (normally a component of HbF). This condition leads to hydrops fetalis and intrauterine fetal death.

49. The correct answer is E. This patient had an acoustic schwannoma removed from the cerebellopontine angle. Schwann cell tumors are the third most common primary brain tumor; they are often localized to cranial nerve VIII. Most are benign, slow-growing tumors that can be resected. Histologically, two patterns are found: (1) Antoni A, or spindle cells palisading and forming whorls; and (2) Antoni B, or loosely arranged tissue after degeneration in the tumor. The histopathologic description of this patient's tumor is consistent with Antoni A.

Answer A is incorrect. Medulloblastomas are highly malignant radiosensitive tumors that are typically found in the posterior fossa. These tumors are of neuroectodermal origin, and histopathologic examination shows a rosette or perivascular pseudorosette pattern. Peak incidence occurs in childhood.

Answer B is incorrect. Meningiomas are slow-growing tumors that most often occur in the hemispheric convexities and parasagittal regions. Although meningiomas are rare, they can appear in the cerebellopontine angle. However, the histology would classically show psammoma bodies, or areas of calcification.

Answer C is incorrect. Neurofibromas are tumors of peripheral origin. This patient's tumor is intra-axial, as shown on the CT scan. Histologically, these cells appear as loosely arranged spindle cells with intervening collagen.

Answer D is incorrect. Oligodendrogliomas are relatively uncommon, slow-growing tumors that occur most often in the frontal lobes. The

tumor comprises homogeneous sheets of cells with uniformly rounded nuclei and an associated network of finely branching blood vessels.

50. The correct answer is B. This patient is suffering from iron deficiency anemia secondary to blood loss from the gastrointestinal tract. Since the body possesses a limited ability to absorb iron from the gut, occult blood loss can quickly lead to a depletion of existing iron stores and hence to an iron deficiency anemia. The burning epigastric pain that worsens after eating is consistent with a gastric ulcer. The black stool is melena, which occurs with blood loss in the upper gastrointestinal tract (bleeding in the lower gastrointestinal tract causes visibly bloody red stools). Iron deficiency anemia is shown by the low hematocrit level and mean corpuscular volume. The most common cause of iron deficiency anemia in postmenopausal women is occult blood loss, often from a gastrointestinal source.

Answer A is incorrect. Anemia of chronic disease is typically a normocytic anemia due to a chronic inflammatory, infectious, malignant, or autoimmune disease. This patient's anemia is microcytic and is likely due to a condition involving blood loss.

Answer C is incorrect. Although this patient's lab values are consistent with iron deficiency anemia, pernicious anemia results instead in megaloblastic anemia.

Answer D is incorrect. The low mean corpuscular volume is not consistent with megaloblastic anemia, which is normally caused by a deficiency of folate or vitamin B_{12}, not blood loss.

Answer E is incorrect. Although pernicious anemia is a common cause of B_{12} deficiency, the low mean corpuscular volume is not consistent with megaloblastic anemia.

CHAPTER 10

Musculoskeletal and Connective Tissue

1. A 33-year-old woman develops an erythematous, finely punctate, blanchable rash. The rash first develops on her trunk and neck. Within a day, it progresses to her extremities but spares the face. The rash is worse in the creases of her axillae and groin. On physical examination, the physician notes a strawberry-colored tongue, a beefy-red oropharynx, and paleness around the mouth. Which of the following is the most likely diagnosis?

    (A) Bacterial meningitis
    (B) Rubella
    (C) Scarlet fever
    (D) Streptococcal pharyngitis
    (E) Toxic shock syndrome

2. A 19-year-old woman presents to the emergency department with malaise and a diffuse red rash over most of her body except the palms of her hands and the soles of her feet. Physical examination is remarkable for fever, tachycardia, elevated respiratory rate, and orthostatic hypotension. No obvious signs of infection are found. The patient reports that this is the second day of her menstrual cycle. She denies alcohol use, drug use, or recent exposure to febrile individuals. The patient is immediately started on intravenous antibiotics and gradually improves. Which of the following is the most likely causative agent in this patient's condition?

    (A) *Clostridium perfringens* enterotoxin
    (B) Disseminated *Staphylococcus aureus* infection
    (C) *Rickettsia rickettsii*
    (D) *Staphylococcus aureus* exotoxin
    (E) *Treponema pallidum*

3. A 76-year-old man is scheduled to undergo repair of an abdominal hernia that is easily reduced by pushing the abdominal contents back through the external ring. During repair, the surgeon sees that the hernial sac protrudes from the abdominal wall superior to the inguinal ligament and medial to the inferior epi-

gastric vessels. Which of the following types of hernia does this patient have?

    (A) Diaphragmatic hernia
    (B) Direct inguinal hernia
    (C) Femoral hernia
    (D) Hiatal hernia
    (E) Indirect inguinal hernia

4. A 22-year-old college student presents to the school health service complaining of worsening weakness in his arms and legs. He says that over the past day he has also begun to feel weakness in his chest and back. He mentions that he thinks he had food poisoning earlier in the week, which caused stomach pain and bloody diarrhea. Physical examination reveals that the deep tendon reflexes in his lower extremities are absent. His physician sends his stool to be cultured. The results show infection with *Campylobacter jejuni*. Which one of the following statements is most consistent with the disease process connecting the patient's gastrointestinal infection and his neurological symptoms?

    (A) An excessive immune response to a gastrointestinal *Campylobacter jejuni* infection led to an autoimmune inflammation of peripheral nerves
    (B) Dissemination of *Campylobacter jejuni* gastrointestinal infection led to infiltration of peripheral muscle cells with *Campylobacter jejuni*
    (C) Dissemination of *Campylobacter jejuni* gastrointestinal infection led to infiltration of peripheral nerves with *Campylobacter jejuni*
    (D) Toxins secreted by *Campylobacter jejuni* infiltrated into peripheral muscle cells
    (E) Toxins secreted by *Campylobacter jejuni* infiltrated into peripheral nerves, causing destruction

5. An 81-year-old man complains of back pain that is dull and constant, regardless of his activity level. Laboratory tests reveal an elevated

serum alkaline phosphatase level. Results of a vertebral biopsy are shown. What is the most likely cause of this patient's pain?

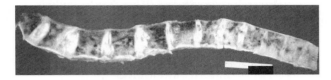

Image courtesy of PEIR Digital Library (http://peir.net).

(A) Chondrosarcoma
(B) Ewing's sarcoma
(C) Metastatic carcinoma
(D) Osteosarcoma
(E) Paget's disease of bone

6. An otherwise healthy infant boy born via vaginal delivery has an abnormal appearance of his right upper limb. His arm hangs by his side, pronated and medially rotated. Which of the following muscles is still functioning in this patient?

(A) Biceps
(B) Deltoid
(C) Infraspinatus
(D) Supraspinatus
(E) Triceps

7. A 19-year-old woman comes to the physician after returning from a vacation in Tennessee with a fever of 39.5° C (103.1° F). She also has a severe headache and red conjunctivae. A couple of hours after the onset of these symptoms, a rash appears on her palms and soles. The physician diagnosis her with Rocky Mountain spotted fever. Which of the following statements is correct?

(A) Cold antibody agglutination is a classic finding for rickettsial infections
(B) *Rickettsia rickettsii* is a facultative intracellular parasite
(C) *Rickettsia rickettsii* is the largest bacterium known

(D) She should promptly be treated with doxycycline
(E) The bacterium is spread by the tsetse fly

8. A 16-year-old gymnast presents to the emergency department after landing awkwardly on her ankle. She is diagnosed with a sprained ankle. Which of the following ligaments is most commonly injured in an ankle sprains?

(A) Anterior talofibular ligament
(B) Calcaneofibular ligament
(C) Talonavicular ligament
(D) Tibiocalcaneal ligament
(E) Tibiotalar ligament

9. A 16-year-old boy with sickle cell disease presents to his primary care physician complaining of pain in his chest and left thigh for the past week. He has recently had fevers spiking to 39.4° C (103° F) and chills. The physician has known the patient for many years and while the chest pain has been chronic, the pain in his left thigh is of recent onset. With a review of the patient's records, the physician discovers that the pain started soon after he was last admitted for a sickle cell crisis. On physical examination, the patient has a fever of 39.0° C (102.3° F), and his left thigh is warm, erythematous, and edematous. It is also very tender to palpation. The physician is very concerned and wants the patient to be admitted to the hospital. He orders an x-ray and MRI of the left thigh and draws blood for culturing before he begins antibiotic treatment. What pathogen is most likely responsible for the infection in this patient?

(A) *Mycobacterium tuberculosis*
(B) *Neisseria gonorrhoeae*
(C) *Pseudomonas aeruginosa*
(D) *Salmonella typhi*
(E) *Staphylococcus aureus*

10. A 13-month-old boy is admitted to the hospital with a broken tibia. This is the fourth broken bone the patient has sustained. On physical examination, the patient is found to have multiple poorly healing superficial wounds on his arms and legs; he also has a blue tint to his sclerae. The patient is subsequently diagnosed with the most common form of this disease. Which of the following sets of tissues would most likely be affected in this patient?

(A) Blood vessels, skin, uterus
(B) Bone, interstitial tissue, cartilage
(C) Bone, tendons, skin
(D) Cartilage, blood vessels, vitreous humor
(E) Skin, cellular basement membrane, blood vessels

11. A 17-year-old girl comes to the physician complaining of a painful, swollen left elbow and fever. She notes that in the previous few days her right knee was also swollen and slightly painful. Upon physical examination, the physician notices an edematous and tender left elbow. He also notices that the patient's cheeks are slightly red but do not appear tender to the touch. Laboratory tests are negative for anti–double-stranded DNA antibodies but positive for antibodies against Smith nuclear antigen and antinuclear antibodies. Also, results of Venereal Disease Research Laboratory testing are positive. The patient is shocked when informed of her positive result for syphilis, stating that she has no past sexual history. Which of the following is the most likely diagnosis?

(A) Polyarteritis nodosa
(B) Rheumatoid arthritis
(C) Secondary syphilis
(D) Systemic lupus erythematosus
(E) Tertiary syphilis

12. A 14-year-old boy presents to his family physician with complaints of muscle weakness affecting his ability to play on his soccer team. Physical examination reveals pseudohypertrophy of his calf muscles. The boy's family history is positive for similar symptoms in a maternal uncle, whose condition progressed to a wheelchair-bound state by the age of 30 years. After further diagnostic tests, including muscle biopsy and genetic analysis, it is determined that the patient has Becker's muscular dystrophy. Which of the following is the etiology of this disorder?

(A) Autosomal dominant
(B) Autosomal recessive
(C) Mitochondrial inheritance
(D) Somatic mutation
(E) X-linked dominant
(F) X-linked recessive

13. A biopsy of one of several red, tender, subcutaneous nodules from the anterior lower legs of a 27-year-old man is obtained by a dermatologist. On histopathology, she sees a panniculitis (inflammation of subcutaneous fat) with widening of tissue septa from edema, increased neutrophils, and fibrin exudation. Which of the following diseases is often present in someone with these nodules?

(A) Acne vulgaris
(B) Crohn's disease
(C) Eczema
(D) Pancreatitis
(E) Psoriasis

14. A 23-year-old man comes to the clinic complaining of a severe headache that started 2 hours ago. He describes the headache as being "the worst in his life." His blood pressure is 138/95 mm Hg, and his heart rate is 56/min. On examination, the physician notes flexible joints and decreased skin elasticity. The examination is otherwise unremarkable. The patient states that he has not had any medical problems in the past. A CT scan of the head reveals blood in the sulci indicative of a subarachnoid hemorrhage. What is the most likely defect associated with this patient's disease?

(A) Arteriovenous malformation
(B) Atrial fibrillation
(C) Defect in type IV collagen synthesis
(D) Hydroxylation of propyl and lysyl residues
(E) Hypertension

15. An 8-year-old boy is brought to his pediatrician by his parents with complaints of swelling and pain over his right femur for the past 2–3 weeks. The child and parents deny any history of trauma to the region. The patient reports that the pain is often worse at night, and his mother states that he has been having low-grade fevers of 37.8°–38.1° C (100.0°–100.6° F). On physical examination there is no erythema of the region, but a firm immobile tender mass is palpable. Fine needle aspiration cytology of the region reveals anaplastic small blue cells. Genetic evaluation of this patient is most likely to reveal which of the following?

(A) t(9;22) chromosomal translocation
(B) t(11;22) chromosomal translocation
(C) Trisomy 18
(D) Trisomy 21
(E) XXY

16. A 31-year-old man comes to the clinic complaining of red and itchy eyes for the past 8 hours. The patient has had pain on urination and diffuse joint pain for 1 month, but tested negative for gonorrhea and chlamydia on a previous visit 3 weeks ago. He has also tested negative for rheumatoid factor, and his human leukocyte antigen (HLA) status is HLA-B27. When asked about any recent illnesses, all the patient can recall is going to the emergency department 2 months ago for a bad case of diarrhea. Which of the following is the most likely diagnosis?

(A) Lyme arthritis
(B) Psoriatic arthritis
(C) Reiter's syndrome
(D) Rheumatoid arthritis
(E) Systemic lupus erythematosus

17. A 50-year-old slightly obese man comes to the emergency department with his wife at 3 A.M. complaining of severe pain in his left great toe. He said the pain began 5 hours ago while he was walking home after dinner, which consisted of steak and a few beers. His serum studies are unremarkable except for negative blood cultures and an elevated uric acid level. When asked about allergies, the patient states that he

is allergic to nonsteroidal anti-inflammatory drugs (NSAIDs). An aspiration of the toe reveals negatively birefringent crystals. Which of the following is the best acute treatment for this condition?

(A) Allopurinol
(B) Ceftriaxone
(C) Colchicine
(D) Hydrochlorothiazide
(E) Ibuprofen
(F) Indomethacin
(G) Naproxen

18. A 20-year-old woman presents to the emergency department with several deep lacerations on the medial side of her wrist after a suicide attempt. She receives prompt psychiatric evaluation. The function of which of the following muscles might be affected by these wounds?

(A) Abductor pollicis brevis
(B) Adductor pollicis
(C) Flexor pollicis brevis
(D) Lumbricals (1 and 2)
(E) Opponens pollicis

19. A 50-year-old man presents to the emergency department because of severe pain with even slight abduction of his arm following a skiing accident. He is diagnosed with a rotator cuff tear. Which of the following is most commonly injured in a rotator cuff tear?

(A) Infraspinatus tendon
(B) Subacromial bursa
(C) Subscapularis tendon
(D) Supraspinatus tendon
(E) Teres minor tendon

20. A 58-year-old man is prescribed a medication by his physician. After 4 months on this medication, the patient develops arthralgias in his hands and knees, mild fever, and hepatomegaly. On examination, there is no rash or neurologic findings, and laboratory studies show no hematologic abnormalities or renal disease. The patient is positive for antinuclear antibody and negative for anti-DNA antibodies. The medication is discontinued, and the patient's symptoms resolve. Which of the following medications did this patient most likely receive?

(A) Bleomycin
(B) Enalapril
(C) Haloperidol
(D) Hydralazine
(E) Rifampin

21. A 34-year-old man injures his lateral pterygoid muscle. Which of the following activities will be adversely affected by this injury?

(A) Drinking liquids
(B) Forming a fist
(C) Kicking a soccer ball
(D) Moving eyelids
(E) Opening doors

22. A recent immigrant from Central America presents to the dermatologist with the cutaneous hypopigmented lesions shown in the image. The lesions are concentrated in the extremities and buttocks. The patient reports recent loss of facial hair and eyebrows along with several episodes of epistaxis. Past medical history is significant for childhood asthma and atopic dermatitis. Suspecting a case of lepromatous leprosy, the dermatologist performs both a sensory neurologic examination and a biopsy of the cutaneous nodules. Which of the following cytokines, when administered locally, would most likely improve this patient's condition?

(A) Interferon-γ
(B) Interleukin-4
(C) Interleukin-5
(D) Interleukin-10
(E) Transforming growth factor-β

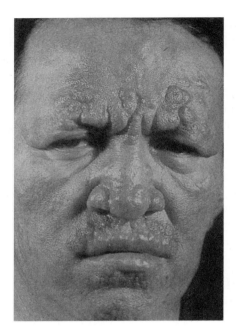

Reproduced, with permission, from Kasper DL, Braunwald E, Fauci AS, Hauser SL, Longo DL, Jameson JL, and Isselbacher KJ, eds. *Harrison's Principles of Internal Medicine*, 16th ed. McGraw-Hill, 2004: Fig. 151-1.

23. A 21-year-old man home from college for spring break decides to cook dinner for his family. While he is chopping carrots, the knife slips and he gets a large cut across his palm. His parents rush him to the emergency department, where the bleeding is controlled. On further examination, the physician finds that the patient is unable to bring his thumb and fifth finger together. Which of the following intrinsic hand muscles contributes to this motion of the thumb and the fifth finger?

(A) Abductor digiti minimi
(B) Abductor pollicis brevis
(C) Adductor pollicis
(D) Interosseous muscles
(E) Lumbrical

24. The skeletal system develops via a process known as ossification, in which bones are created from preexisting mesoderm. Which of the following is the name of the mechanism by which long bones of the limbs ossify, and how can this mechanism be described?

(A) Endochondral ossification—bones form directly from mesoderm

(B) Endochondral ossification—bones form on a hyaline cartilage mold

(C) Intramembranous ossification—bones form directly from mesoderm

(D) Intramembranous ossification—bones form on a hyaline cartilage mold

(E) Intrathoracic ossification—bones form in the thorax and migrate to the limbs

25. A 14-year-old girl presents with difficulty walking after injuring her ankle during a soccer match. She is diagnosed with a Pott's fracture, with fractures of the medial malleolus and fibula. Which of the following types of forceful movement causes this injury?

(A) Avulsion
(B) Dorsiflexion
(C) Eversion
(D) Inversion
(E) Plantar flexion

26. Late one evening, a 57-year-old man has sudden-onset, severe pain in his left great toe. He presents to his primary care physician the next day, and reports no history of trauma. On physical examination there is edema with erythema and pain on movement of the left first metatarsophalangeal joint, but there is no overlying skin ulceration. A joint aspirate is performed and microscopy reveals numerous neutrophils. Over the next 4 weeks, he has two similar episodes. On physical examination between these attacks, there is minimal loss of joint mobility. Which of the following laboratory findings is most characteristic for his underlying disease process?

(A) Hypercalcemia
(B) Hyperglycemia
(C) Negatively birefringent crystals in joint aspirate
(D) Positively birefringent crystals in joint aspirate
(E) Positive rheumatoid factor

27. A 42-year-old woman comes to the clinic complaining of blurry vision. She states that for the past 3 weeks her eyes have been very dry and itchy, and she is unable to make tears. She also states that she has had a very dry mouth despite drinking adequate fluids. Physical exami-

nation reveals bilateral dry, ulcerated corneas and fissures on the sides of her lips. In addition, both of her knees are erythematous and swollen. When asked about her knees, she says, "Yes, my knees and wrists tend to be swollen and stiff in the morning, but my mom had arthritis." You run a test for several autoantibodies, which reveals that she is rheumatoid factor–positive and antibody-SS-B (La)–positive. Which of the following is the most likely diagnosis?

(A) CREST syndrome
(B) Cystic fibrosis
(C) Sicca syndrome
(D) Sjögren-Larsson syndrome
(E) Sjögren's syndrome

28. A 14-year-old football player is side tackled during a high school football game. When he tries to stand up, his right leg buckles. He is taken to the emergency department, where physical examination reveals that the patient's tibia is easily moved anterior in relation to the femur. An MRI of the patient's knee is shown. Which injured structure is responsible for the findings in the patient's physical examination?

(A) Anterior cruciate ligament
(B) Lateral collateral ligament
(C) Medial collateral ligament
(D) Posterior cruciate ligament
(E) Ulnar collateral ligament

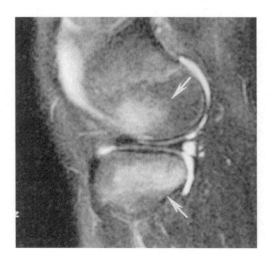

Reproduced, with permission, from Chen MYM, Pope TL, Ott DJ. *Basic Radiology*. New York, McGraw-Hill, 2004: Fig. 7-21.

29. A 25-year-old man comes to the emergency department because of rapidly spreading cellulitis on his right hand. He tells the physician that he was bitten by a cat the previous day. Which of the following organisms is most likely responsible for this patient's infection?

(A) *Pasteurella multocida*
(B) Rabies virus
(C) *Sporothrix schenckii*
(D) *Staphylococcus aureus*
(E) *Trypanosoma brucei gambiense*

30. The association between autoimmune diseases and the expression of certain cytokines has prompted several advances in pharmacotherapy. Which of the following is an accurate statement regarding the drug therapy of autoimmune disease?

(A) Adalimumab, a synthetic TNF-α analog, is indicated for mild rheumatoid arthritis, a disease associated with an overexpression of TNF-α
(B) Anakinra, a monoclonal antibody against the interleukin-1 receptor, is indicated for rheumatoid arthritis, a disease associated with an overexpression of endogenous interleukin-1-receptor antagonist
(C) Etanercept, a fusion protein of a TNF-α receptor and IgG$_1$, is indicated for rheumatoid arthritis, a disease associated with an overexpression of TNF-α
(D) Infliximab, a monoclonal antibody against TNF-α, is indicated for systemic lupus erythematosus, a disease associated with an underexpression of TNF-α
(E) Infliximab, a synthetic TNF-α analog, is indicated for rheumatoid arthritis, a disease associated with an overexpression of TNF-α

31. A 21-year-old man presents to the emergency department following an injury to his shoulder that he sustained while playing football. His shoulder appears flattened, and he is not able to abduct his arm. He is found to have a fracture at the surgical neck of his humerus. Which of the following muscles is most likely to be affected by this injury?

(A) Biceps
(B) Brachialis
(C) Deltoid
(D) Infraspinatus
(E) Supraspinatus

32. A 42-year-old woman has had increasing pain and swelling of the joints of her hands and feet for several months. It is becoming very difficult for her to perform common household tasks. A microscopic image of the synovium of a proximal interphalangeal joint in her hand is shown. Which of the following laboratory serologic findings would most likely be positive in this patient?

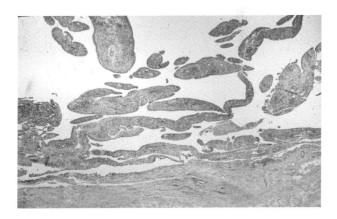

Image courtesy of PEIR Digital Library (http://peir.net).

(A) Anticentromere antibody
(B) Antinuclear antibody
(C) *Borrelia burgdorferi* antibody
(D) HLA-B27
(E) Rheumatoid factor

33. A 60-year-old man presents to the physician with a limp that he has had since childhood. His left hip falls whenever he lifts his right leg. He reports one major illness as a child, after which he developed this limp. Which of the following muscles is most likely affected in this patient?

(A) Gluteus maximus
(B) Gluteus medius
(C) Obturator internus

(D) Piriformis
(E) Quadratus femoris

34. A 45-year-old computer programmer notices atrophy and weakness of his opponens pollicis, abductor pollicis brevis, and flexor pollicis brevis muscles. Laboratory tests reveal an increased erythrocyte sedimentation rate and leukocyte count. Sensation to which of the following cutaneous areas is most likely to be decreased?

(A) Dorsal aspect of pinky finger
(B) Dorsal aspect of ring finger
(C) Palmar aspect of index finger
(D) Volar aspect of lateral wrist
(E) Volar aspect of medial wrist

35. A 50-year-old man who recently returned from a trip to Southeast Asia comes to the physician with exquisitely tender and enlarged lymph nodes. He also complains of fever, chills, and general weakness. On physical examination, the physician notes eschars and purpura on his right arm over the area where, according to the patient, a flea had bitten him 5 days ago. Which of the following organisms is most likely responsible for this patient's symptoms?

(A) *Babesia microti*
(B) *Bacillus anthracis*
(C) *Leishmania donovani*
(D) *Trichinella spiralis*
(E) *Yersinia pestis*

36. A 22-year-old woman who is a professional tennis player presents to the physician with pain on the lateral aspect of her elbow radiating down her forearm. Repetitive use of which of the following muscles most likely lead to this patient's condition?

(A) Biceps
(B) Extensor carpi radialis
(C) Extensor carpi ulnaris
(D) Flexor carpi ulnaris
(E) Pronator teres

37. A 61-year-old man presents to the physician with frequent headaches and increasing deafness. The patient notes that his winter hat fits more snugly than usual. Laboratory values show a marked increase in alkaline phosphatase activity. A diagnosis of Paget's disease is made. Dysfunction of the cell type shown by the arrow in the image is associated with Paget's disease. Which of the following is the embryologic origin of this dysfunctional cell?

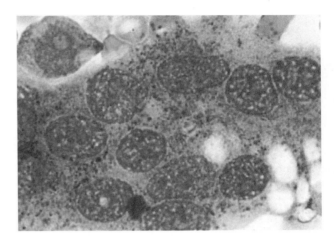

Reproduced, with permission, from Lichtman MA, Beutler E, Kipps TJ, Seligsohn U, Kaushansky K, Prchal JF. *Williams Hematology*, 7th ed. New York, McGraw-Hill, 2006: Color Plate VI-2.

(A) Endoderm
(B) Neural crest cells
(C) Neuroectoderm
(D) Mesoderm
(E) Surface ectoderm

38. A 64-year-old man with no prior medical history has had increasing back pain and right hip pain for the past decade. The pain is worse at the end of the day. On physical examination, he has bony enlargement of the distal interphalangeal joints. A CT scan of the spine reveals the presence of prominent osteophytes involving the vertebral bodies. X-ray of the pelvis shows sclerosis with narrowing of the joint space at the right acetabulum. Which of the following diseases is most likely the cause of this patient's symptoms?

(A) Gout
(B) Osteoarthritis
(C) Osteomyelitis
(D) Pseudogout
(E) Rheumatoid arthritis

39. A 38-year-old man comes to the clinic with a swollen, sausagelike left middle finger along with diffuse joint swelling of his left hand and right foot over the past 3 days. The patient also has scaly, silvery red plaques with well-defined borders along the skin just distal to both elbows. His uric acid level is within normal limits. Which of the following is the most likely diagnosis?

(A) Gouty arthritis
(B) Ichthyosis
(C) Psoriatic arthritis
(D) Reiter's syndrome
(E) Seborrheic keratosis

40. A 20-year-old man presents to the physician with a nontender indurated mass over his mandible. He has had this mass for 4 months and decided to come to the physician because the mass started to ooze a thick yellow exudate. Yellow granules are seen on microscopic examination of the discharge. Which of the following organisms is responsible for this man's lesion?

(A) *Actinomyces israelii*
(B) *Nocardia asteroides*
(C) *Prevotella melaninogenica*
(D) *Staphylococcus aureus*
(E) *Trichinella spiralis*

41. A 29-year-old man develops a flulike illness 10 days after a trip to upstate New York. On physical examination, he has lymphadenopathy and a red, flat, round rash over his left arm. One red spot is particularly big and has a clear area in the center. Which of the following statements is correct?

(A) A diagnosis of Lyme disease must be made based on clinical presentation
(B) Erythema multiforme is the characteristic rash of Lyme disease
(C) Lyme disease is best treated with a fluoroquinolone
(D) The late stage of Lyme disease is characterized by encephalopathy
(E) The reservoir of *Borrelia burgdorferi* is the white-tailed deer

42. The histologic section shows a cross-section of normal human skin. Pemphigus vulgaris patients suffer from production of autoantibodies against which of the following labeled layers in this image?

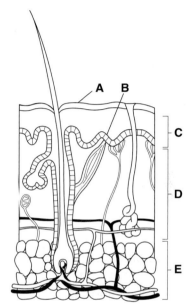

Reproduced, with permission, from USMLERx.com.

(A) A
(B) B
(C) C
(D) D
(E) E

43. A 25-year-old man develops acute onset of fever, malaise, muscle pain, hypertension, abdominal pain, bloody stool, and prerenal failure 6 months after recovering from an acute hepatitis B infection. Which of the following disease processes is most likely responsible for the patient's findings?

(A) Buerger's disease
(B) Giant cell (temporal) arteritis
(C) Kawasaki's syndrome
(D) Polyarteritis nodosa
(E) Takayasu's arteritis

44. A 56-year-old man undergoes surgery to remove a thyroid tumor. The next day, his wife notices that his voice has become much hoarser than it was previously. The doctor concludes that a particular nerve must have been accidentally injured during surgery. What is the embryologic origin of the muscles supplied by this nerve?

(A) First branchial cleft
(B) First branchial pouch
(C) Fourth branchial pouch
(D) Sixth branchial arch
(E) Third branchial arch
(F) Third branchial cleft

45. A 10-year-old boy is brought to the pediatrician by his mother because he has been complaining of difficulty using his right hand. On examination, he is found to have a right wrist drop. The loss of which of the following muscles contributes to this patient's condition?

(A) Extensor carpi radialis longus
(B) Flexor carpi radialis
(C) Palmaris longus
(D) Pronator quadratus
(E) Pronator teres

46. Rheumatoid arthritis is classified as a type II hypersensitivity disease. Approximately what percentage of rheumatoid arthritis patients are rheumatoid factor–positive, and rheumatoid factor is usually of what antibody isotype?

(A) 0%, IgG
(B) 25%, IgM
(C) 50%, IgM
(D) 80%, IgM
(E) 95%, IgG

47. A 27-year-old man comes to the physician's office with a 6-month history of low back pain and stiffness that wakes him up during the night and is worst in the morning. The patient was diagnosed with bilateral sacroiliitis 4 months ago because of his tenderness to percussion of the sacroiliac joints and pain on springing the pelvis up. He has severe limitation of motion of his lumbar spine. Laboratory test results are negative for antinuclear antibody and rheumatoid factor, and show the pa-

tient's human leukocyte antigen status is B27-positive. Which of the following is the most likely diagnosis?

(A) Ankylosing spondylitis
(B) Osteoarthritis
(C) Psoriatic arthritis
(D) Reiter's syndrome
(E) Rheumatoid arthritis
(F) Vertebral compression fracture

48. A 15-year-old boy is brought to the emergency department because he has pain in his hand following a fist fight. The physician tells the patient that he has broken his hand. Which of the following is the most likely site of this patient's fracture?

(A) Distal radius
(B) Hamate
(C) Metacarpals
(D) Phalanges
(E) Scaphoid

49. A 5-year-old boy comes to the emergency department with fever, malaise, nausea, decreased urine output (despite normal fluid intake), and smoky brown urine that began 10 days after he had recovered from a sore throat. What would be the most likely pathologic findings on biopsy of one of this patient's kidneys?

(A) Enlarged hypercellular glomeruli on light microscopy; dense humps found on the epithelial side of the glomerular basement membrane on electron microscopy
(B) Linear deposition of antibodies against glomerular basement membrane found on immunofluorescence
(C) Mesangial proliferation on light microscopy; mesangial deposition of IgA on immunofluorescence
(D) Normal-appearing glomeruli on light microscopy; effacement of the foot processes of the visceral epithelial cells on electron microscopy
(E) Widespread and pronounced thickening and splitting of the glomerular basement membrane on electron microscopy

50. A 2-year-old boy presents to the pediatrician with multiple fractures and no history of trauma. The boy's father and paternal grand-mother also suffered from bones breaking very easily. Physical examination is significant for blue sclera, loose joints, and low muscle tone. This patient most likely has a defect in which of the following types of collagen?

(A) Type I collagen
(B) Type II collagen
(C) Type III collagen
(D) Type IV collagen
(E) Type X collagen

1. **The correct answer is C.** Scarlet fever is caused by *Streptococcus pyogenes* and is characterized by a typical sandpaper rash, strawberry tongue, beefy-red pharynx, and circumoral pallor. As the rash heals, the skin peels off in fine scales.

Answer A is incorrect. The signs of meningitis are fever, headache, photophobia, nuchal rigidity, and possibly seizures. This patient does not have these symptoms.

Answer B is incorrect. Rubella presents with a prodrome of malaise and suboccipital lymphadenopathy. A maculopapular rash develops first on the face and then generalizes and resolves in 3–5 days. The patient's rash is not consistent with a diagnosis of rubella.

Answer D is incorrect. Inflammation, exudates, fever, and tender cervical lymph nodes characterize pharyngitis. While scarlet fever may sometimes complicate cases of primary *Streptococcus pyogenes* pharyngitis, pharyngitis does not appear to be a prominent feature of this particular presentation.

Answer E is incorrect. *Staphylococcus aureus* and *Streptococcus pyogenes* toxic shock syndromes are characterized by abrupt onset of local or diffuse pain, fever, confusion, and signs of soft tissue infection. The former is sometimes (but not exclusively) associated with women using hyperabsorbable tampons during menses. A diffuse erythema that subsequently desquamates as the patient recovers may be present in 10% of patients. It does not involve the symptoms described in the question.

2. **The correct answer is D.** Bacterial/viral superantigens are proteins that bind to the major histocompatibility complex (MHC) class II molecule outside of the peptide-binding groove. They also bind to the V-β domain of certain T-cell receptor (TCR) subsets, thus leading to the "nonspecific" activation of certain T-lymphocyte subsets. Depending on the superantigen, anywhere from 2–20% of all T lymphocytes can be activated. *Staphylococcus*

aureus toxic shock syndrome toxin 1 (TSST-1) is one of these superantigens, and it can additionally cross-link class II molecules, leading to dendritic cell and macrophage activation independent of the MHC-TCR cross-linking. The massive T-lymphocyte activation leads to supraphysiologic production of cytokines, including interleukin (IL)-1, tumor necrosis factor-(, IL-6, IL-12, and interferon-γ. It is these cytokines that are most responsible for the clinical symptoms of toxic shock syndrome. Thus, the most likely cause of the menstruating female's symptoms is a toxin released from *S. aureus* TSST-1 and not the bacterium itself.

Answer A is incorrect. While *Clostridium perfringens* enterotoxin is also a superantigen, physical examination revealed no signs of cutaneous infections, and thus this pathogen is less likely to be the causative agent. Additionally, the patient's symptoms improved following *Staphylococcus aureus* antibiotic treatment.

Answer B is incorrect. The clinical vignette is most likely indicative of toxic shock syndrome, a result of a circulating staphylococcal toxin and not the bacterium itself. In fact, blood cultures are most often negative. In this patient's case, vaginal cultures may be positive for *S. aureus* and may have been taken.

Answer C is incorrect. In Rocky Mountain spotted fever, the rash is often a presenting symptom, but this rash often includes the palms and soles.

Answer E is incorrect. In syphilis, the rash is often a presenting symptom, but this rash often includes the palms and soles.

3. **The correct answer is B.** Direct inguinal hernias protrude directly through the abdominal wall in Hesselbach's triangle, which is bordered by the inguinal ligament, rectus abdominis muscle, and inferior epigastric vessels. Remember that the issue of direct versus indirect has nothing to do with whether or not the hernia enters the scrotum through the external ring, as both direct and indirect hernias can do

this. Direct versus indirect distinguishes where the hernia enters the inguinal canal—either through the internal ring (indirect) or straight through the abdominal wall (for direct hernias, think **directly** through the wall). In this case, the abdominal contents pierced through the abdominal wall and through the external inguinal ring. Direct hernias are often discovered in older patients, as the hernia is a result of pressure and tension exerted over time that eventually leads the abdominal wall to give way. Direct hernias are less common and have less risk of strangulation than indirect hernias.

Answer A is incorrect. Diaphragmatic hernias are serious birth defects that are lethal unless repaired soon after birth. A defective development of the diaphragm leads to herniation of abdominal contents into the thorax, displacing the lung. Even after repair of such lesions, children may have poor pulmonary function due to poor lung development in utero.

Answer C is incorrect. Femoral hernias protrude inferior to the inguinal ligament and do not go through the external inguinal ring.

Answer D is incorrect. Hiatal hernias are hernias of the stomach protruding superiorly through the diaphragm.

Answer E is incorrect. Indirect inguinal hernias occur when abdominal contents enter the internal inguinal ring through a patent processus vaginalis, exit the inguinal canal through the external ring, and, often, enter the scrotum of male patients. The examiner's finger would go through the external ring and would pass posterior to the epigastric vessels and through the internal ring. These hernias are the most common type found in both men and women, and the recommendation is that they be repaired when they are discovered to avoid the complication of strangulation and bowel infarction.

4. **The correct answer is A.** This patient has Guillain-Barré as a result of his gastroenteritis. The important message here is that Guillain-Barré syndrome is thought to be primarily an autoimmune disorder against peripheral nerves and the cells that myelinate them (Schwann cells). Thus, it makes sense that an excessive immune response to an infection (such as from a pathogen like *Campylobacter jejuni*) can lead to an autoimmune process. Histologically, this disease is characterized by perivenular and endoneurial infiltration with lymphocytes, macrophages, and plasma cells.

Answer B is incorrect. Guillain-Barré syndrome is a disease that primarily attacks peripheral nerves and Schwann cells. The ascending paralysis and muscle weakness that occur as a consequence are secondary to the neuropathy.

Answer C is incorrect. The mechanism suggested in this answer choice is not thought to be the primary disease process in Guillain-Barré syndrome.

Answer D is incorrect. Guillain-Barré syndrome is a disease that primarily attacks peripheral nerves and Schwann cells. The ascending paralysis and muscle weakness that occur as a consequence are secondary to the neuropathy.

Answer E is incorrect. While *Campylobacter jejuni* can penetrate through the intestinal mucosa to cause septicemia, the mechanism described in this answer choice is not the major hypothesized pathogenesis of Guillain-Barré syndrome.

5. **The correct answer is C.** This image shows several nodular, tan lesions, indicative of metastases. Metastatic neoplasia should be strongly considered in older adults with elevated alkaline phosphatase levels, particularly older men with back pain, often a sign of bone lesions due to prostate cancer. Metastases to bone are far more common than primary bone tumors. The most common cancers that metastasize to bone are breast, lung, thyroid, testes, kidney, and prostate.

Answer A is incorrect. Chondrosarcoma is a malignant cartilaginous tumor. It is most common in men 30–60 years old. Chondrosarcoma is rarely seen in the spine, but it would not cause an elevated alkaline phosphatase.

Answer B is incorrect. Ewing's sarcoma is an anaplastic blue cell malignant tumor most common in boys under 15 years of age. It is typically aggressive but highly responsive to chemotherapy.

Answer D is incorrect. Osteosarcoma is the most common malignant tumor of bone, with a peak incidence in teenage males (10–20 years old). It is most commonly found in the metaphysis of long bones, most commonly in the lower extremities. It commonly presents with systemic symptoms and a palpable soft tissue mass.

Answer E is incorrect. Paget's disease of bone is characterized by accelerated bone turnover leading to increased bone formation and resorption, resulting in its characteristic "mosaic" pattern. It presents most commonly with pain, skeletal deformities, and fractures. It is associated with secondary osteosarcoma and fibrosarcoma. It does not cause nodular lesions like those shown here.

6. **The correct answer is E.** This infant has Erb-Duchenne palsy, a condition seen following trauma during delivery, due to traction/tear of the C5–6 roots in the brachial plexus (superior trunk). This condition results in paralysis of abductors, lateral rotators, and biceps. Of the muscles listed above, only the triceps is not involved in these actions; it functions to extend the elbow and adduct the arm. It is innervated by the radial nerve, which is supplied by C6–8.

Answer A is incorrect. The biceps muscle functions to supinate and flex the arm. It is innervated by the musculocutaneous nerve, which comes from the superior trunk of the brachial plexus.

Answer B is incorrect. The deltoid is supplied by the axillary nerve, which comes from the superior trunk of the brachial plexus. It functions to abduct the arm.

Answer C is incorrect. The infraspinatus muscle helps laterally rotate the arm and is supplied by the suprascapular nerve from the superior trunk of the brachial plexus.

Answer D is incorrect. The supraspinatus muscle helps abduct the arm and is supplied by the suprascapular nerve from the superior trunk of the brachial plexus.

7. **The correct answer is D.** Rocky Mountain spotted fever should promptly be treated—even before confirmatory laboratory test are in—with a tetracycline (such as doxycycline) or chloramphenicol, as delay in antibiotic therapy can lead to death.

Answer A is incorrect. Cold antibody agglutination is used to detect *Mycoplasma* infection. The Weil-Felix reaction can detect a rickettsial infection due to cross-reacting antigens from *Proteus vulgaris*.

Answer B is incorrect. *Rickettsia rickettsii* is an obligate intracellular parasite that replicates freely in the cytoplasm.

Answer C is incorrect. *Rickettsia rickettsii* is a small, rod- to coccoid-shaped, gram-negative bacterium the size of a large virus.

Answer E is incorrect. *Rickettsia rickettsii* has two arthropod vectors, the tick *Dermacentor andersoni* and *D. variabilis*. The tsetse fly spreads African sleeping sickness.

8. **The correct answer is A.** The lateral ligaments are more commonly injured than the medial ligaments, since they are weaker. The anterior talofibular ligament is the most common of the lateral ligaments to be injured.

Answer B is incorrect. The calcaneofibular ligament is a lateral ligaments that is injured frequently, but less frequently than the anterior talofibular ligament.

Answer C is incorrect. The lateral ligaments are more commonly injured than the medial ligaments, since they are weaker. The talonavicular ligament is a medial ligament so it is much less likely to be injured.

Answer D is incorrect. The lateral ligaments are more commonly injured than the medial ligaments, since they are weaker. The tibiocalcaneal ligament is a medial ligament so it is much less likely to be injured.

Answer E is incorrect. The lateral ligaments are more commonly injured than the medial ligaments, since they are weaker. The tibiotalar ligament is a medial ligament so it is much less likely to be injured.

9. **The correct answer is D.** This patient is presenting with osteomyelitis of his left femur. Classic signs include fever (often exceeding 38.9° C [102° F]), erythema, and edema. Pain is also a classic finding. Most often, there is some form of external injury that allows bacteria to colonize the bone, such as an ulcer or puncture from an intravenous needle. However, in patients with sickle cell disease, osteomyelitis often occurs secondary to bone infarction and can follow a sickle crisis. The bacteria are hematogenously spread from elsewhere in the body, colonizing the dead bone. While the majority of osteomyelitis cases are caused by *Staphylococcus aureus*, in patients with sickle cell disease the most common pathogen is *Salmonella typhi*.

Answer A is incorrect. *Mycobacterium tuberculosis* is a rare cause of osteomyelitis. As an extrapulmonary manifestation of the disease, tuberculosis may be observed in the vertebral column of immunosuppressed patients.

Answer B is incorrect. *Neisseria gonorrhoeae* is a rare cause of osteomyelitis. It is seen most often as a sexually transmitted disease (STD). In complicated cases it can lead to septic arthritis. In even rarer cases, the septic arthritis can be complicated by osteomyelitis. In a sexually active patient with a history of STDs, it is an important pathogen to consider when the presentation is consistent with osteomyelitis.

Answer C is incorrect. *Pseudomonas aeruginosa* is a common cause of osteomyelitis in patients with diabetes mellitus. It is most often seen in diabetic foot ulcers and infections.

Answer E is incorrect. *Staphylococcus aureus* is the most common cause of osteomyelitis in the general population and is seen at even higher rates in intravenous drug users. However, in patients with sickle cell disease, *Salmonella typhi* is more often identified as the causative agent.

10. **The correct answer is C.** The most likely diagnosis for this patient is osteogenesis imperfecta (OI). OI is characterized by multiple spontaneous bone fractures, retarded wound healing, and characteristically blue sclerae. This disease is caused by a variety of gene defects leading to abnormal collagen synthesis. The most common form of OI is an autosomal dominant defect in type I collagen synthesis. Type I collagen has high tensile strength and is found in skin, bone, tendons, eyes, ears, and teeth. Other symptoms of type I OI include hearing impairment and joint laxity.

Answer A is incorrect. Type III cartilage is characterized by thin, pliable fibrils found in blood vessels, skin, and the uterus. This collagen is not abnormal in type I osteogenesis imperfecta.

Answer B is incorrect. Interstitial tissue is composed of types V and VI collagen. Cartilage contains type II and IX collagen. Of these tissues only bone contains type I cartilage, the type of cartilage affected by osteogenesis imperfecta.

Answer D is incorrect. Type II collagen is primarily found in cartilage and vitreous humor. Blood vessels contain collagen types III and V, Thus, none of these tissues are affected in type I osteogenesis imperfecta.

Answer E is incorrect. Skin contains type I collagen and type VII collagen at the dermal-epidermal junction. Cellular basement membrane is composed of type IV collagen. Blood vessels contain types III and V cartilage. Of these three structures, only skin contains the collagen affected most commonly in osteogenesis imperfecta.

11. **The correct answer is D.** This patient has systemic lupus erythematosus (SLE), which is diagnosed by the presence of four of the following 11 findings designated by the American Rheumatism Association, and summarized by the mnemonic **"BRAIN SOAP, MD"**: **B**lood dyscrasias (such as hemolytic anemia or thrombocytopenia), **R**enal disorder, **A**rthritis (in two or more peripheral joints), **I**mmunologic disor-

der (such as anti-DNA antibody and anti-Smith antibody), **N**eurologic disorder, **S**erositis (such as pleuritis or pericarditis), **O**ral ulcers, **A**ntinuclear antibody (elevated titers in the absence of drugs associated with drug-induced lupus syndrome), **P**hotosensitivity, **M**alar rash, and **D**iscoid rash. Many patients with SLE have antiphospholipid antibodies, which are actually believed to be antibodies against proteins that complex to phospholipids. Since these antibodies also bind to the cardiolipin antigen used in syphilis serology, patients with SLE may test false positive for syphilis.

Answer A is incorrect. Polyarteritis nodosa, a necrotizing immune complex vasculitis that usually affects small or medium-sized muscular arteries, commonly presents with fever, malaise, myalgias, and hypertension. Findings may include pericarditis, myocarditis, palpable purpura, and cotton-wool spots (white opacities in the retina).

Answer B is incorrect. The American Rheumatism Association diagnostic criteria for rheumatoid arthritis requires four out of the following seven findings: (1) Morning stiffness for more than 6 weeks; (2) Arthritis of hand joints for more than 6 weeks; (3) Arthritis involving three or more joint areas for more than 6 weeks; (4) Symmetric arthritis for more than 6 weeks; (5) Rheumatoid nodules (small lumps of tissue most commonly found over bony prominences, that are histologically characterized by a center of fibrinoid necrosis surrounded by histiocytes, numerous lymphocytes, and plasma cells); (6) Positive serum rheumatoid factor; and (7) Radiologic changes (such as bony erosion in or near the area of symptomatic joints).

Answer C is incorrect. Secondary syphilis often develops 6 weeks after an untreated primary chancre of syphilis has healed and is characterized by fever, lymphadenopathy, skin rashes (widespread small, flat lesions that particularly involve the palms, soles, and oral mucosa), and condylomata lata (painless wartlike lesions that present in the vulva, the scrotum, or other warm, moist areas of the body).

Answer E is incorrect. Tertiary syphilis may develop 6–40 years after primary syphilis and may present with gummas (noninfectious granulomatous lesions, often found in skin and bone), tabes dorsalis (inflammatory damage to the posterior columns and dorsal roots of the spinal cord), aneurysm of the ascending aorta or aortic arch, and Argyll-Robertson pupils (pupils that constrict during accommodation but do not react to light).

12. **The correct answer is F.** X-linked recessive inheritance shows affected male individuals inheriting a defective copy of the X chromosome from heterozygous (asymptomatic) mothers. There is no male-to-male transmission. Heterozygous females may be affected, but usually not as severely as males. Becker's muscular dystrophy is a milder, slower-developing form of dystrophinopathy with manifestations similar to those of Duchenne's muscular dystrophy.

Answer A is incorrect. Autosomal dominant inheritance shows disease in many generations, with both males and females affected. It is possible for a male or a female to transmit the defective gene to their offspring. Becker's muscular dystrophy is not inherited in this manner.

Answer B is incorrect. In autosomal recessive inheritance, a defective gene from each carrier parent is transmitted to the offspring. Disease is often seen in only one generation. Males and females are equally likely to be affected. Becker's muscular dystrophy is not inherited in this manner.

Answer C is incorrect. In mitochondrial inheritance, all children (male and female) of an affected mother exhibit the disease. The disease is not transmitted from fathers to any of their children (only maternal transmission). Becker's muscular dystrophy is not inherited in this manner.

Answer D is incorrect. Somatic mutations occur in the somatic (nongerm) tissues; they are unable to be transmitted to offspring and often occur in isolated individuals within a family.

Males and females are equally susceptible to somatic mutations. Becker's muscular dystrophy is not inherited in this manner.

Answer E is incorrect. X-linked dominant inheritance shows disease in any offspring who inherit the affected X chromosome. It is transmitted from fathers to all their daughters but none of their sons, and from mothers to sons or daughters. Becker's muscular dystrophy is not inherited in this manner.

13. **The correct answer is B.** This patient has erythema nodosum, an inflammation of subcutaneous fat that is often accompanied by fever and malaise that is described clinically and pathologically in the question stem. The exact mechanism is unknown, but it often occurs together with inflammatory bowel disease (Crohn's disease or ulcerative colitis), sarcoidosis, certain drugs (such as oral contraceptives and sulfonamides), certain malignant neoplasms, and certain infections (such as tuberculosis, β-hemolytic streptococci, coccidioidomycosis, histoplasmosis, and leprosy).

Answer A is incorrect. Acne vulgaris is a disorder of the epidermis that has both inflammatory and noninflammatory variants. It is associated with the bacterium *Propionibacterium acnes.*

Answer C is incorrect. Eczema is an inflammatory skin disorder that is associated with contact allergies, asthma, ultraviolet light exposure, repeated physical skin rubbing, and certain drugs. It is not associated with erythema nodosum.

Answer D is incorrect. Pancreatitis, which is associated with many cases of biliary tract disease and alcoholism, is not associated with erythema nodosum.

Answer E is incorrect. Psoriasis is a nonpruritic inflammatory skin disorder associated with arthritis, enteropathy, spondylitic disease, and certain human leukocyte antigen (HLA) types, including HLA-B27, HLA-13, and HLA-17.

14. **The correct answer is C.** The patient's presentation is consistent with that of Ehlers-Danlos syndrome. Patients with this condition have decreased skin elasticity and hypermobile joints. Ehlers-Danlos syndrome is a heritable disorder of connective tissues (specifically type IV collagen synthesis) that leads to a decrease in tensile strength and in the integrity of skin, joints, blood vessels, and other tissues. The disease is associated with intracranial aneurysms resulting from the decreased tensile strength of the vessel walls. These aneurysms can rupture, leading to subarachnoid hemorrhage.

Answer A is incorrect. Arteriovenous malformations (AVMs) are a common cause of subarachnoid hemorrhages. However, the examination findings of hypermobile joints and decreased skin elasticity would not be explained by an AVM.

Answer B is incorrect. In up to 10% of cases, atrial fibrillation may result in mural thrombi that embolize to the brain, producing an ischemic stroke. However, this diagnosis is less likely given the patient's age and the absence of a prior history of heart problems. In addition, the CT scan is more consistent with a subarachnoid hemorrhage than with an ischemic stroke.

Answer D is incorrect. Vitamin C deficiency results in an inability to hydroxylate the propyl and lysyl residues between tropocollagen molecules necessary for the production of collagen. This deficiency may lead to scurvy, a disease that is characterized by hypertrophic, bleeding gums and poor wound healing.

Answer E is incorrect. Hypertension is a cause of hemorrhagic stroke. However, most patients with hemorrhagic stroke are typically much older. This patient's increased blood pressure and low heart rate are due to increased intracranial pressure (Cushing's reflex).

15. **The correct answer is B.** The patient's presentation and histology is most consistent with Ewing's sarcoma and is associated with t(11;22) translocations.

Answer A is incorrect. Chronic myelogenous leukemia is associated with t(9;22) translocation (the Philadelphia chromosome) and is not associated with blue cell histology.

Answer C is incorrect. Trisomy 18 is Edward's syndrome, which is associated with severe mental retardation, rocker bottom feet, micrognathia, and death within the first year of life.

Answer D is incorrect. Trisomy 21 is diagnostic of Down's syndrome a genetic disease associated with mental retardation and characteristic facial features. While individuals with Down's syndrome are at a higher risk of acute lymphocytic leukemia, they are not at an increased risk for bone masses or blue cell tumors.

Answer E is incorrect. XXY is Klinefelter's syndrome, a genetic disturbance of the sex chromosomes associated with testicular atrophy, eunuchoid body shape, long extremities, and gynecomastia.

16. **The correct answer is C.** The correct answer is Reiter's syndrome, which is diagnosed by conjunctivitis in a patient who has had both urethritis (or cervicitis) and arthritis for at least 1 month. Most patients are in their 20s or 30s, and 80% are positive for HLA-B27. It is thought to be caused by an autoimmune reaction within several weeks of a gastrointestinal or genitourinary infection.

Answer A is incorrect. Lyme arthritis, usually caused by a bite from a tick harboring the spirochete *Borrelia burgdorferi*, presents as an initial local skin infection followed by monarticular/polyarticular arthritis. Its late sequelae include myocardial, pericardial, and neurologic changes.

Answer B is incorrect. Patients with psoriatic arthritis can have joint pain, conjunctivitis, and human leukocyte antigen-B27, but the diagnosis requires the presence of psoriasis, which is characterized by nonpruritic scaly/silvery erythematous plaques with well-defined borders.

Answer D is incorrect. While rheumatoid factor is not necessary to diagnose rheumatoid arthritis, the patient's human leukocyte anti-

gen status, urethritis, and conjunctivitis make it a less likely diagnosis.

Answer E is incorrect. Systemic lupus erythematosus is diagnosed by the presence of four of the 11 symptoms summarized by the mnemonic **"BRAIN SOAP, MD"**: **B**lood dyscrasias (such as hemolytic anemia or thrombocytopenia), **Re**nal disorder, **A**rthritis, **I**mmunologic disorder (such as anti-DNA antibody and anti-Smith antibody), **N**eurologic disorder, **S**erositis (such as pleuritis or pericarditis), **O**ral ulcers, **A**ntinuclear antibody (elevated titers in the absence of drugs associated with drug-induced lupus syndrome), **P**hotosensitivity, **M**alar rash, and **D**iscoid rash.

17. **The correct answer is C.** Gout is characterized by a raised blood uric acid level that leads to uric acid deposition in tissues, particularly the joints. In some patients, gout is precipitated by eating foods rich in purine, such as meats (especially organ meats, like kidneys). The first-line therapy in the treatment of gout consists of nonsteroidal anti-inflammatory drugs (NSAIDs) such as ibuprofen, naproxen, and indomethacin. However, since the patient is allergic to NSAIDs, colchicine is the next best therapy for an acute gouty attack. (It is considered an alternate drug because side effects include diarrhea, gastrointestinal upset, and, in patients with renal or hepatic insufficiency, bone marrow suppression, myopathy, and neuropathy.)

Answer A is incorrect. Allopurinol is used in the chronic treatment of gout but has no beneficial effect in an acute gouty attack; in fact, it may initially precipitate an attack or make an existing attack worse.

Answer B is incorrect. Ceftriaxone would be given for gonococcal arthritis, which most frequently involves the knee. Early stages yield positive blood cultures for gonococci and later stages may yield positive joint cultures and/or purulent synovial fluid.

Answer D is incorrect. Hydrochlorothiazide is a diuretic and is not indicated for gout. In fact, people who take hydrochlorothiazide may develop gout because it increases the renal tubular reabsorption of uric acid.

Answer E is incorrect. The patient is allergic to NSAIDs, so ibuprofen is not a good choice.

Answer F is incorrect. The patient is allergic to NSAIDs, so indomethacin is not a good choice.

Answer G is incorrect. The patient is allergic to NSAIDs, so naproxen is not a good choice.

18. **The correct answer is B.** Wrist slashing on the medial aspect of the arm may injure the ulnar artery and ulnar nerve. The adductor pollicis is innervated by a branch of the ulnar nerve and adducts the thumb. Other muscles innervated by the ulnar nerve include the hypothenar muscles, lumbricals (3 and 4), dorsal interossei, and palmar interossei.

Answer A is incorrect. The abductor pollicis brevis is innervated by a branch of the median nerve and functions in abduction and opposition of the thumb.

Answer C is incorrect. The flexor pollicis brevis is innervated by a branch of the median nerve and flexes the thumb.

Answer D is incorrect. The first and second lumbricals are innervated by the median nerve.

Answer E is incorrect. The opponens pollicis is innervated by a branch of the median nerve and functions in opposition of the thumb.

19. **The correct answer is D.** The supraspinatus tendon is most commonly injured in a rotator cuff tear. This muscle aids the deltoid in abduction of the arm, especially in the first 15 degrees. Rotator cuff tear is very uncommon in the young but often occur in older individuals when an abducted arm receives an indirect force.

Answer A is incorrect. The infraspinatus muscle is less commonly injured in rotator cuff tears. It functions to laterally rotate the arm.

Answer B is incorrect. The subacromial bursa separates the supraspinatus tendon from the coracoacromial ligament, acromion, and deltoid. Injury to this bursa causes severe pain with abduction from 50 to 130 degrees, not slight abduction.

Answer C is incorrect. The subscapularis muscle is less commonly injured in rotator cuff tears. It functions to medially rotate and adduct the arm.

Answer E is incorrect. The teres minor muscle is less commonly injured in rotator cuff tears. It functions to medially rotate and adduct the arm.

20. **The correct answer is D.** This is the clinical picture of drug-induced lupus. This type of lupus is different from systemic lupus erythematosus in that the male:female ratio is about equal, renal and central nervous system features are absent, hypocomplementemia and anti-DNA antibodies are absent, and the symptoms resolve when the drug is discontinued. Hydralazine is the only drug among those listed that is associated with this syndrome. Other drugs known to cause lupus are procainamide, isoniazid, chlorpromazine, penicillamine, sulfasalazine, methyldopa, and quinidine.

Answer A is incorrect. Bleomycin is most commonly associated with pulmonary fibrosis.

Answer B is incorrect. Enalapril, an angiotensin-converting enzyme inhibitor, is most often associated with a dry cough.

Answer C is incorrect. Haloperidol can lead to hepatomegaly but would not cause this clinical picture.

Answer E is incorrect. Isoniazid, not rifampin, is associated with drug-induced lupus.

21. **The correct answer is A.** The muscles involved in jaw movement are fourfold: lateral pterygoid, masseter, temporalis, and medial pterygoid. The lateral pterygoid opens the jaw while the other three close the jaw. All four are innervated by the trigeminal nerve (V3). One can remember this with the mnemonic "**M**'s Munch" and "**L**ateral **L**owers." Clearly, drink-

ing liquids would be impaired with a lateral pterygoid injury.

Answer B is incorrect. The lateral pterygoid has no role in finger movement; it is located in the head.

Answer C is incorrect. The lateral pterygoid has no role in leg or foot movement; it is located in the head.

Answer D is incorrect. The lateral pterygoid has no role in eyelid movement.

Answer E is incorrect. The lateral pterygoid has no role in arm or hand movement; it is located in the head.

22. **The correct answer is A.** This patient's condition is a clinical example that demonstrates the importance of CD4+ T-helper (TH)–cell differentiation into a TH_1 or TH_2 phenotype. TH_1 cells drive a cell-mediated immune response that includes activation of macrophages and cytotoxic T lymphocytes. TH_2 cells orchestrate an antibody-mediated response. As an intracellular pathogen that infects macrophages, *Mycobacterium leprae* is most effectively controlled by TH_1 cells. The patient described here presents with severe lepromatous disease, which results when the CD4 TH cells differentiate into TH_2 instead of TH_1 effectors. Indeed, the biopsy would most likely show widespread acid-fast bacilli inside of macrophages. Individuals that mount a TH_1 response to the mycobacteria can better control the disease (their clinical condition is named tuberculous leprosy), and their macrophages can contain the bacilli within granulomas. Interferon-γ is secreted by TH_1 cells, and one important role of this cytokine is to activate macrophage. Therefore, local administration of this cytokine will alleviate the cutaneous lesions.

Answer B is incorrect. Interleukin-4 is a TH_2 cytokine important in antibody class switching.

Answer C is incorrect. Interleukin-5 is a TH_2 cytokine important in antibody class switching.

Answer D is incorrect. Interleukin-10 is also a TH_2 cytokine.

Answer E is incorrect. Transforming growth factor-β has immunosuppressive effects.

23. **The correct answer is B.** Although opposition of the thumb and fifth digit involves adducting both fingers toward the midline, the abductor pollicis brevis is involved. It abducts the thumb and contributes to the medial rotation of the thumb in the beginning of the opposition motion. This muscle is innervated by the median nerve, which can be damaged by deep cuts.

Answer A is incorrect. The abductor digiti minimi abducts the little finger, pulling it away from the other fingers, and is essentially the opposite motion needed for opposition.

Answer C is incorrect. The adductor pollicis adducts the thumb toward the palm; this is a different motion than opposition. This muscle makes a person's grip stronger but does not contribute to the opposition motion.

Answer D is incorrect. The interossei are responsible for adduction and abduction of the fingers; the dorsal interossei abduct the fingers and the palmar interossei adduct the fingers.

Answer E is incorrect. The lumbricals are intrinsic hand muscles that flex the metacarpophalangeal joints and extend the interphalangeal joints. Opposition of the thumb and fifth digit involves adducting both fingers to the midline and medially rotating them.

24. **The correct answer is B.** The long bones of the limbs form via endochondral ossification. In this process, mesoderm is first converted to a cartilaginous model. Bone then forms at the primary ossification center at the diaphysis. Besides the long bones, other bones that form via endochondral ossification include the sphenoid, ethmoid, incus, stapes, malleus, limb girdles, vertebrae, sternum, and ribs.

Answer A is incorrect. While long bones do form via endochondral ossification, this is not the correct description of this process. In endochondral ossification, bones form from a cartilaginous mold that is derived from mesoderm; the bones do not form directly from mesoderm.

Answer C is incorrect. In the process of intramembranous ossification, bone forms directly from mesoderm without an intermediate cartilaginous mold. The long bones do not undergo this process, but rather form via endochondral ossification with a cartilaginous intermediate. Bones that form via intramembranous ossification include the frontal, parietal, maxilla, zygomatic, palatine, and mandible.

Answer D is incorrect. Although long bones do form from mesoderm by means of ossification of a hyaline cartilage mold, this is termed *endochondral ossification*, not intramembranous ossification.

Answer E is incorrect. The process of intrathoracic ossification does not exist.

25. **The correct answer is C.** A Pott's fracture typically occurs following forceful eversion of the foot. The medial malleolus is immediately injured, and the talus then fractures the lateral malleolus and fibula.

    Answer A is incorrect. Avulsion injuries typically cause a fracture of the malleolus, but these are not known as a Pott's fracture.

    Answer B is incorrect. Dorsiflexion injuries are rare at the ankle joint.

    Answer D is incorrect. Inversion injuries typically cause an ankle sprain.

    Answer E is incorrect. Plantar flexion injuries are rare at the ankle joint.

26. **The correct answer is C.** This man is suffering from gout. Gout causes painful swelling of joints, most commonly the metatarsophalangeal joint, caused by precipitation of monosodium urate crystals. It can be caused by hyperuricemia, thiazide diuretics, and Lesch-Nyhan syndrome. It is diagnosed by viewing the crystals in the joint's synovial fluid, which are negatively birefringent.

    Answer A is incorrect. Hypercalcemia can be caused by hyperparathyroidism, which can cause bone lesions, but does not typically affect joints, nor does it cause swelling or redness.

Answer B is incorrect. Hyperglycemia is a feature of diabetes mellitus, a systemic endocrine disorder. Through nonenzymatic glycosylation it causes peripheral vascular disease, increasing the risk of foot ulcerations and osteomyelitis.

Answer D is incorrect. Pseudogout causes symptoms that mimic those of gout, but is caused by the precipitation of calcium pyrophosphate crystals within the joint space. These crystals are positively birefringent. This disease classically affects large joints, most commonly the knee, in men over 50 years old.

Answer E is incorrect. Positive rheumatoid factor is present in 80% of patients with rheumatoid arthritis. This pain is typically persistent for weeks to months and is associated, eventually, with significant joint deformity.

27. **The correct answer is E.** This patient has Sjögren's syndrome. The vast majority of patients with this syndrome are women between the ages of 35 and 45 years, and the disease is characterized by dry eyes (keratoconjunctivitis sicca), dry mouth (xerostomia), and one other connective tissue or autoimmune disease (such as rheumatoid arthritis). The eye and mouth dryness is from autoimmune destruction of the lacrimal and salivary glands.

    Answer A is incorrect. CREST syndrome is a variant of scleroderma (progressive systemic sclerosis), which is a disease characterized by extensive fibrosis throughout the body (most notably of the skin). **CREST** stands for **C**alcinosis, **R**aynaud's phenomenon, **E**sophageal dysfunction, **S**clerodactyly, and **T**elangiectasia.

    Answer B is incorrect. Cystic fibrosis also causes dysfunction of the exocrine glands (such as the lacrimal and salivary glands), but it is due to a mutation in the cystic fibrosis transmembrane conductance regulator gene on chromosome 7. Individuals with cystic fibrosis also tend to have pulmonary and pancreatic dysfunction.

    Answer C is incorrect. When only the first two criteria are present—dry eyes and dry mouth—it is called sicca syndrome.

Answer D is incorrect. Sjögren-Larsson syndrome is an autosomal recessive syndrome that is characterized by congenital ichthyosis (dry and scaly fishlike skin) and associated with mental retardation and spastic paraplegia; it is caused by a mutation in the fatty aldehyde dehydrogenase gene on chromosome 17p.

28. **The correct answer is A.** The anterior cruciate ligament (ACL) is one of four major ligaments of the knee and bridges the femur and tibia. Part of the "unhappy triad" (ACL, medial collateral ligament, and medial meniscus) of structures involved in common knee injuries, it limits anterior movement of the tibia in relation to the femur. The arrows in the image point to the classic "kissing contusions" of the lateral femoral condyle and the lateral tibial plateau. To test the integrity of the ACL, one can check for the so-called anterior drawer sign. With the patient's knees in a flexed position, stand in front of the patient and place your hands behind the calf muscles. The sign is positive if, as you pull toward yourself, there is significant anterior dislocation.

Answer B is incorrect. The lateral collateral ligament is one of four major ligaments of the knee and bridges the femur and the fibula. It prevents excessive lateral movement of the knee.

Answer C is incorrect. The medial collateral ligament is one of four major ligaments of the knee and bridges the femur and the tibia. Part of the "unhappy triad" (anterior cruciate ligament, medial collateral ligament, and medial meniscus) of structures involved in common knee injuries, it prevents excessive medial movement of the knee.

Answer D is incorrect. The posterior cruciate ligament is one of four major ligaments of the knee and bridges the femur and tibia. It acts to limit posterior dislocation of the tibia on the femur.

Answer E is incorrect. The ulnar collateral ligament is in the upper extremity at the elbow. It forms connections between the ulna and the humerus.

29. **The correct answer is A.** *Pasteurella multocida* is associated with cat and dog bites. Cellulitis appears around the bite site and can sometimes lead to osteomyelitis.

Answer B is incorrect. Rabies virus causes rabies. The signs of this disease include a prodrome of fever and anorexia followed by confusion, lethargy, and increased salivation.

Answer C is incorrect. *Sporothrix schenckii* is a fungus that typically causes necrotizing, granulomatous lymphocutaneous skin infections in the distribution of draining lymph nodes following trauma by tainted vegetation. Its association with recent outdoor activity, particularly gardening, accounts for its nickname, "rose gardener's disease."

Answer D is incorrect. *Staphylococcus aureus* is one of the major causes of cellulitis but is not particularly associated with an animal bite.

Answer E is incorrect. *Trypanosoma brucei gambiense* is transmitted by the bite of a tsetse fly and causes African sleeping sickness.

30. **The correct answer is C.** All of the facts in this statement are correct. Tumor necrosis factor-α (TNF-α) is a potent inflammatory cytokine found in increased amounts in the serum and synovial fluid of people with rheumatoid arthritis. TNF-α also promotes the release of other pro-inflammatory cytokines. Furthermore, it makes logical sense that one would treat rheumatoid arthritis with etanercept, a drug that can bind the excess TNF-α and remove it via an IgG-mediated immune response.

Answer A is incorrect. Adalimumab binds and inhibits tumor necrosis factor-α (TNF-α); it is sometimes prescribed for moderate to severe cases of rheumatoid arthritis. It is not a synthetic TNF-α analog.

Answer B is incorrect. Anakinra is a synthetic interleukin-1-receptor antagonist, not a monoclonal antibody. Rheumatoid arthritis is associated with an underexpression of endogenous interleukin-1-receptor antagonist (i.e., it causes an excess of available interleukin-1 receptors), and thus some cases can be treated with anakinra, a synthetic interleukin-1-receptor antagonist.

Answer D is incorrect. Systemic lupus erythematosus is associated with an underexpression of tumor necrosis factor-α (TNF-α), but this answer choice can be ruled out by (1) knowing that infliximab is a monoclonal antibody against TNF-α, and (2) realizing that one would not treat an underexpression of TNF-α with an antibody against TNF-α.

Answer E is incorrect. Infliximab is a monoclonal antibody against tumor necrosis factor-α (TNF-α), not a synthetic TNF-α analog. But infliximab is indicated for the treatment of rheumatoid arthritis, since it is a monoclonal antibody against TNF-α, which is overexpressed in rheumatoid arthritis.

31. **The correct answer is C.** The axillary nerve courses around the surgical neck of the humerus and is often injured in fractures at this region. The deltoid muscle will atrophy following axillary nerve damage. This leads to a flattening of the shoulder and inability to abduct the arm.

    Answer A is incorrect. The biceps muscle functions to supinate and flex the forearm. It is innervated by the musculocutaneous nerve, which comes from the lateral cord of the brachial plexus.

    Answer B is incorrect. The brachialis muscle functions to flex the forearm. It is innervated by the musculocutaneous nerve, which comes from the lateral cord of the brachial plexus.

    Answer D is incorrect. The infraspinatus muscle helps laterally rotate the arm and is supplied by the suprascapular nerve from the superior trunk of the brachial plexus.

    Answer E is incorrect. The supraspinatus muscle helps abduct the arm and is supplied by the suprascapular nerve from the superior trunk of the brachial plexus.

32. **The correct answer is E.** Rheumatoid factor would most likely be positive in this woman,

who is suffering from rheumatoid arthritis. Eighty percent of patients with rheumatoid arthritis have positive rheumatoid factor (anti-IgG antibody). This autoimmune condition causes a marked influx of inflammatory cells into the joint synovium, as seen here, resulting in destructive change, pannus formation, and eventually joint deformity. The disease is more common in women, and classically symmetrically affects the proximal interphalangeal joints, as described here.

Answer A is incorrect. Anticentromere antibody is associated with the **CREST** variant of scleroderma (progressive systemic sclerosis). In this disease patients suffer from **C**alcinosis, **R**aynaud's phenomenon, **E**sophageal dysmotility, **S**clerodactyly, and **T**elangiectasia. Arthritis is not associated with this syndrome.

Answer B is incorrect. Antinuclear antibody is associated with systemic lupus erythematosus, an autoimmune disease with a wide variety of symptoms including fever, rash, joint pain, and photosensitivity. The joint pain in lupus is typically transient, asymmetrical, and nondeforming.

Answer C is incorrect. *Borrelia burgdorferi* is the cause of Lyme disease. The third stage of Lyme disease can manifest as migratory polyarthritis, but this patient has none of the other signs and symptoms associated with this disease.

Answer D is incorrect. HLA-B27 is strongly associated with arthritides without rheumatoid factor, such as ankylosing spondylitis. This condition most commonly affects men and causes severe stiffening of the spine and sacroiliac joints, as well as uveitis. The hands are not typically involved.

33. **The correct answer is B.** As a child this patient had polio. Patients who develop polio experience injury to the nerve roots that supply the superior gluteal nerve, which innervates the gluteus medius and minimus. These muscles typically abduct and medially rotate the thigh and keep the pelvis level. When these muscles do not function properly, the patient

is unable to keep the pelvis level and develops a characteristic limp.

Answer A is incorrect. The gluteus maximus is innervated by the inferior gluteal nerve and functions to extend and laterally rotate the thigh. It also assists in standing from a sitting position. Individuals with injury to this muscle would have difficulty rising to a standing position.

Answer C is incorrect. The obturator internus is innervated by branches of L5 and S1 and functions to laterally rotate when the leg is extended and to abduct when the thigh is flexed.

Answer D is incorrect. The piriformis muscle is innervated by branches of S1–2 and functions to laterally rotate when the leg is extended and to abduct when the thigh is flexed.

Answer E is incorrect. The quadratus femoris muscle is innervated by branches of L5 and S1 and functions to laterally rotate the thigh.

34. **The correct answer is C.** The syndrome described here is carpal tunnel syndrome, which is compression of the median nerve. This compression is often caused by synovitis, which can manifest in an increased erythrocyte sedimentation rate and WBC count. The median nerve has motor and sensory functions. It supplies the three thenar muscles as well as the following cutaneous regions: the palmar aspect of the lateral hand up to the lateral half of the ring finger, and the areas distal to the (proximal) interphalangeal joints of the thumb, index, and middle finger and the radial half of the ring finger. The mnemonic for the three thenar muscles is **Oaf: O**ppose (**O**pponens pollicis), abduct (**A**bductor pollicis brevis), and flex (**F**lexor pollicis brevis). The "a" and "f" are lowercase because those muscles are "brevis."

Answer A is incorrect. This area is innervated by the branches of the ulnar nerve, which is unaffected in carpal tunnel syndrome.

Answer B is incorrect. This area is innervated by the branches of the ulnar nerve, which is unaffected in carpal tunnel syndrome.

Answer D is incorrect. This area is innervated by the lateral cutaneous nerve of the forearm, a branch of the musculocutaneous nerve.

Answer E is incorrect. This area is innervated by the medial cutaneous nerve of the forearm.

35. **The correct answer is E.** *Yersinia pestis* is the organism responsible for the plague, also known as the Black Death. The bacterium can be spread by fleas. The disease develops after 2–8 days of incubation and is characterized by the presence of exquisitely tender lymph nodes called buboes.

Answer A is incorrect. *Babesia microti* is transmitted to humans through the bite of a tick. It causes a sickness similar to malaria with symptoms of fever and anemia.

Answer B is incorrect. *Bacillus anthracis* can cause cutaneous anthrax, which is characterized by a painless ulcer with a black scab.

Answer C is incorrect. *Leishmania donovani* is transmitted through the bite of a sandfly and causes visceral leishmaniasis. This disease is characterized by abdominal pain and distention, anorexia, weight loss, and fever.

Answer D is incorrect. A person infected with *Trichinella spiralis* presents with fever, periorbital and facial edema, myalgia, and eosinophilia.

36. **The correct answer is B.** This patient suffers from lateral epicondylitis, better known as tennis elbow. This condition stems from overuse of the superficial extensor muscles of the forearm and wrist, including the extensor carpi radialis muscle. This muscle also inserts at the lateral epicondyle.

Answer A is incorrect. The biceps muscle functions to supinate and flex the forearm.

Answer C is incorrect. The extensor carpi ulnaris muscle functions to extend and adduct the hand at the wrist but does not extend the forearm.

Answer D is incorrect. The flexor carpi ulnaris muscle functions to flex and abduct the hand at the wrist.

Answer E is incorrect. The pronator teres muscle functions to pronate and flex the forearm.

37. **The correct answer is D.** Paget's disease is abnormal bone remodeling associated with dysfunction of both osteoblasts and osteoclasts. In the early resorptive period of the disease, excessive osteoclast resorption occurs. The cell pictured in the image is an osteoclast, a large multinucleated cell with a ruffled cytoplasmic border frequently found adjacent to bone surfaces undergoing resorption. Osteoclasts are derived from blood or marrow monocytes and are thus of mesodermal origin.

    Answer A is incorrect. Endoderm forms gut tube epithelium and derivatives. Osteoclasts are not derived from endoderm.

    Answer B is incorrect. Neural crest cells form the autonomic nervous system, melanocytes, dorsal root ganglia, chromaffin cells of the adrenal medulla, enterochromaffin cells, pia, celiac ganglion, Schwann cells, odontoblasts, parafollicular cells of the thyroid, laryngeal cartilage, and aorticopulmonary septum. Osteoclasts are not derived from neural crest cells.

    Answer C is incorrect. Neuroectoderm forms the neurohypophysis, central nervous system neurons, oligodendrocytes, astrocytes, and pineal gland. Osteoclasts are not derived from neuroectoderm.

    Answer E is incorrect. Surface ectoderm forms the adenohypophysis, the lens of the eye, the epithelial linings, and the epidermis, with the exception of melanocytes. Osteoclasts are not derived from surface ectoderm.

38. **The correct answer is B.** Osteoarthritis is a disease of wear and tear leading to destruction of articular cartilage, subchondral bone formation, osteophytes, sclerosis, and other degenerative changes. It is common and progressive, and becomes more so with age. It classically presents in weight-bearing joints as pain after use, improving with rest. It commonly affects the distal interphalangeal joints as well.

Answer A is incorrect. Gout is a painful swelling of a joint, most commonly the metatarsophalangeal joint, caused by precipitation of monosodium urate crystals. It is diagnosed by viewing the crystals in the joint's synovial fluid, which are negatively birefringent. It is not associated with osteophytes or sclerosis with narrowing.

Answer C is incorrect. Osteomyelitis is an infection in the bone. It presents most commonly with tenderness, warmth, swelling, and more acute pain, rather than joint narrowing. The pain typically is present with and without movement.

Answer D is incorrect. Pseudogout causes symptoms that mimic those of gout, but is caused by the precipitation of calcium pyrophosphate crystals within the joint space. These crystals are positively birefringent. This disease classically affects large joints, most commonly the knee, in men over 50 years old. It is not associated with osteophytes or sclerosis with narrowing.

Answer E is incorrect. Rheumatoid arthritis is an autoimmune arthritis caused by inflammatory destruction of synovial joints. It is associated with pain that is worst in the morning, improving with use, and classically affects the proximal interphalangeal joints. It is not associated with osteophytes or sclerosis with narrowing.

39. **The correct answer is C.** This patient has psoriatic arthritis, which presents with psoriasis (nonpruritic scaly or silvery erythematous plaques with well-defined borders) and joint symptoms that are of acute onset in one-third of patients. More than 50% of patients have an asymmetric distribution of joint swelling in the distal interphalangeal joints of the hands and feet. Some patients may develop a sausagelike finger from inflammation of the digital tendon sheaths.

    Answer A is incorrect. Gout is characterized by a raised blood uric acid level that leads to uric acid deposition in tissues, particularly the joints. The presence of arthritic symptoms and the absence of elevated uric acid make the diagnosis of gouty arthritis unlikely.

Answer B is incorrect. While the term *scaly* may also be used to describe ichthyosis, the scaly skin of ichthyosis appears fishlike and is usually due to an inherited or acquired disorder leading to an accumulation of excessive keratin at the skin surface. It is not associated with joint inflammation.

Answer D is incorrect. While this patient does have arthritis, Reiter's syndrome is diagnosed by conjunctivitis in a patient who has had both urethritis (or cervicitis) and arthritis for at least 1 month. It is thought to be caused by an autoimmune reaction within several weeks of a gastrointestinal or genitourinary infection.

Answer E is incorrect. Seborrheic keratosis is characterized by benign, raised papules that appear as if they were stuck or pasted onto the body. If the keratoses occur in large numbers and with sudden onset, it is called a Leser-Trélat sign, which is associated with internal malignancy. Seborrheic keratosis is not associated with joint inflammation.

40. **The correct answer is A.** The infection caused by *Actinomyces israelii* typically presents as a chronic, slowly progressing mass that eventually evolves into a draining sinus tract. Characteristic sulfur granules are seen in the thick yellow exudate.

Answer B is incorrect. Nocardiosis is caused by *Nocardia asteroides*. This disease begins as a respiratory infection followed by abscess and sinus tract formation. The organism does not produce sulfur granules but is often acid-fast.

Answer C is incorrect. *Prevotella melaninogenica* is part of the normal oral flora and is most commonly responsible for abscess formation in the mouth, pharynx, brain, and lung. It does not produce sulfur granules.

Answer D is incorrect. *Staphylococcus aureus* can also cause abscesses in various body locations but is not associated with the presence of sulfur granules.

Answer E is incorrect. A person infected with *Trichinella spiralis* presents with fever, periorbital and facial edema, myalgia, and eosinophilia.

41. **The correct answer is E.** The white-footed mouse and the white-tailed deer are the reservoirs of *Borrelia burgdorferi*. The bacterium is spread to humans by the Ixodes tick. Lyme disease has three characteristic stages: stage 1 is characterized by erythema chronicum migrans (ECM); stage 2 is marked by the appearance of multiple small ECM rashes and by neurologic, cardiac, and brief arthritic symptoms; and stage 3 involves chronic arthritis and encephalopathy.

Answer A is incorrect. Early, localized Lyme is more reliably diagnosed clinically—i.e., on the basis of a tick exposure and rash—due to the delay in the development of antibodies. Serologic tests for Lyme are, however, particularly helpful in evaluating patients for the later stages of Lyme disease.

Answer B is incorrect. Erythema chronicum migrans is the characteristic rash of Lyme disease. It is a round, flat rash with a clear center that spreads out over time.

Answer C is incorrect. Lyme disease can be treated with doxycycline or any antibiotic from the penicillin family.

Answer D is incorrect. The late stage (stage 3) of Lyme disease is characterized by encephalopathy and chronic arthritis.

42. **The correct answer is C.** C is the epidermis. Pemphigus vulgaris is an autoimmune disorder in which pathogenic antibodies are directed against a cell-cell adhesion protein, desmoglein-3, which is expressed by the keratinocytes of the epidermis. The destruction of desmoglein leads to intraepidermal acantholysis with sparing of the basal layer. Physical exam typically shows flaccid epidermal bullae that easily slough off leaving large denuded areas of skin (Nikolsky's sign), subject to secondary infection. Treatment is usually steroids.

Answer A is incorrect. A is the stratum corneum, which is composed of enucleated, keratinized, flat keratinocytes. The autoantibodies that mediate pemphigus vulgaris are directed against desmoglein-3, a protein involved in cell-cell adhesion within the other layers of the epidermis, not within the stratum corneum.

Answer B is incorrect. B is the dermoepidermal junction. The autoantibodies that mediate this disease are directed against a protein expressed in the epidermis.

Answer D is incorrect. D is the dermis. The autoantibodies that mediate this disease are directed against a protein expressed in the epidermis.

Answer E is incorrect. E is the hypodermis. The autoantibodies that mediate this disease are directed against a protein expressed in the epidermis.

43. **The correct answer is D.** Polyarteritis nodosa is a vasculitis (i.e., inflammation of a blood vessel) characterized by inflammation affecting small to medium-sized arteries, particularly the renal, cardiac, and gastrointestinal tract vessels (usually not the pulmonary vasculature). As many as 30% of patients have been reported to have a history of a prior hepatitis B infection.

Answer A is incorrect. Buerger's disease, also known as thromboangiitis obliterans, is a vasculitis that mostly affects arteries and veins of the extremities. As such, patients often have intermittent claudication and Raynaud's phenomenon. The majority of patients are men who are heavy smokers and show hypersensitivity to tobacco injected into the skin.

Answer B is incorrect. Giant cell (temporal) arteritis is a type of vasculitis that affects the arteries of the head, especially, of course, the temporal arteries. The highlights of this disease can be remembered by the mnemonic **JOE:** patients get **J**aw pain and **O**cular disturbances from ischemia to the arteries supplying them. Patients also often have markedly elevated **E**rythrocyte sedimentation rates. The disease is often associated with the presence of polymyalgia rheumatica.

Answer C is incorrect. Kawasaki's disease is a self-limited vasculitis that normally occurs in in-

fants and children and is characterized by conjunctival and oral erythema, fever, erythema and edema of the palms and soles, generalized rash, and cervical lymph node swelling. About 20% of patients may go on to develop coronary artery inflammation and/or aneurysm.

Answer E is incorrect. Takayasu's arteritis is a vasculitis characterized by fibrotic thickening of the aortic arch (it also affects the pulmonary arteries, the branches of the aortic arch, and the rest of the aorta in up to one-third of patients). Clinically, patients often have lower blood pressure and weaker pulses in the upper extremities than in the lower extremities; some patients have ocular disturbances as well.

44. **The correct answer is D.** The left and right recurrent laryngeal nerves (branches of cranial nerve X) supply all the intrinsic muscles of the larynx except the cricothyroid. Paralysis of the intrinsic laryngeal muscles results in hoarseness. Because the recurrent laryngeal nerves rest on the anterior surface of the thyroid, they are easily injured during thyroid surgery. The intrinsic laryngeal muscles (except the cricothyroid) are derivatives of the sixth branchial (pharyngeal) arch. The branchial arches are composed of mesoderm and neural crest cells. Branchial arch mesoderm becomes arterial and muscle tissue, while the branchial arch neural crest cells become skeletal components and connective tissue.

Answer A is incorrect. The first branchial cleft becomes the external auditory meatus.

Answer B is incorrect. The first branchial pouch develops into the middle ear cavity, the Eustachian tubes, and the mastoid air cells.

Answer C is incorrect. The branchial pouches are pouches of the foregut endodermal lining, and therefore form endodermal structures. The fourth branchial pouch develops into the superior parathyroid glands.

Answer E is incorrect. The greater horn of the hyoid and the stylopharyngeus muscle are derived from the third branchial arch. Cranial nerve IX supplies the third branchial arch derivatives.

Answer F is incorrect. In contrast to the branchial arches, which are mesodermal and form anatomical structures, the branchial clefts are pockets of ectoderm and form modified holes in the embryo. The second, third, and fourth pharyngeal clefts form temporary cervical sinuses, which are normally obliterated during development. Abnormal persistence of one of these sinuses results in a branchial cyst in the neck.

45. **The correct answer is A.** Wrist drop is due to injury to the radial nerve, leading to loss of the extensor muscles of the wrist, including the extensor carpi radialis longus. The wrist appears flexed due to the unopposed action of the flexor muscles.

    Answer B is incorrect. The flexor carpi radialis muscle flexes and abducts the hand at the wrist. It is innervated by the median nerve.

    Answer C is incorrect. The palmaris longus muscle flexes the hand at the wrist and is innervated by the median nerve.

    Answer D is incorrect. The pronator quadratus muscle pronates the forearm and binds the radius and ulna together. It is innervated by the anterior interosseous nerve, which stems from the median nerve.

    Answer E is incorrect. The pronator teres muscle pronates and flexes the forearm at the elbow and is innervated by the median nerve.

46. **The correct answer is D.** Rheumatoid factor (RF) is an autoantibody that is usually of the IgM isotype. It is directed against the Fc (constant) region of the patient's (self) IgG. Interestingly, while RF has been implicated in the pathogenesis of some extra-articular manifestations of rheumatoid arthritis (RA) (such as subcutaneous rheumatoid nodules), only 80% of RA patients are RF-positive, and thus it is believed not to contribute to the main pathogenesis of RA. It is also interesting to note that many patients suffering from Sjögren's syndrome are RF-positive but do not suffer from the symptoms of RA.

Answer A is incorrect. This percentage is too low, and the most common rheumatoid factor is IgM.

Answer B is incorrect. This percentage is too low.

Answer C is incorrect. This percentage is too low.

Answer E is incorrect. This percentage is too high, and the most common rheumatoid factor is IgM.

47. **The correct answer is A.** This patient has ankylosing spondylitis, a chronic inflammatory disease of the spine and sacroiliac joints that often leads to the stiffening or consolidation of the bones that make up the joints. Common findings are low back pain, stiffness for over 3 months, pain and stiffness in the thoracic region, limited movement in the lumbar area, and limited chest expansion. Around 90% of patients are human leukocyte antigen-B27–positive, and common complications include uveitis and aortic regurgitation.

Answer B is incorrect. Osteoarthritis is joint inflammation and destruction secondary to wear and tear. Unlike the symptomatology seen in the above patient, osteoarthritis presents with pain that is worse after use of the joints (i.e., at the end of the day) and tends to present in individuals older than age 50.

Answer C is incorrect. Patients with psoriatic arthritis can have joint pain and be human leukocyte antigen-B27–positive, but the diagnosis requires the presence of psoriasis, which is characterized by nonpruritic scaly or silvery erythematous plaques with well-defined borders.

Answer D is incorrect. While this patient does have sacroiliitis and is human leukocyte antigen-B27–positive, Reiter's syndrome is diagnosed by conjunctivitis in a patient who has had both urethritis (or cervicitis) and arthritis for at least 1 month. It is thought to be caused by an autoimmune reaction within several weeks after a gastrointestinal or genitourinary infection.

HIGH-YIELD SYSTEMS

Musculoskeletal

Answer E is incorrect. Rheumatoid arthritis is an autoimmune disorder of synovial joints and often presents with morning joint stiffness, subcutaneous joint nodules (particularly in the proximal interphalangeal joints), and symmetric joint involvement. Eighty percent of patients have positive rheumatoid factor in their serum, and the disease may include systemic symptoms (such as fever, pleuritis, and pericarditis).

Answer F is incorrect. Vertebral compression fractures are a complication of osteoporosis and present with acute back pain, loss of height, and kyphosis.

48. **The correct answer is C.** This patient most likely suffers from a "boxer's fracture," which occurs when individuals strike a blow with a closed fist. The most commonly injured sites for experienced boxers are the first and second metacarpals, whereas for inexperienced boxers the fifth metacarpal is the most common site of injury. The metacarpals have a good blood supply and thus heal rapidly.

Answer A is incorrect. A complete transverse fracture of the distal radius is commonly called a Colles' fracture. This occurs most commonly in the elderly following forced dorsiflexion.

Answer B is incorrect. Fracture of the hamate is not common but can be complicated, as the ulnar nerve can often be injured. There are healing difficulties associated with this type of fracture.

Answer D is incorrect. Fracture of the phalanges is a common injury and is often due to crushing or hyperextension injuries.

Answer E is incorrect. Fracture of the scaphoid commonly occurs when individuals fall onto an abducted hand.

49. **The correct answer is A.** Nephritic syndrome is characterized by hematuria, hypertension, oliguria, and azotemia. The patient is exhibiting pathologic findings consistent with poststreptococcal glomerulonephritis. This disease is classically found in children who present 1–2 weeks after recovering from a sore throat with fever, malaise, oliguria (a pathologically small amount of urine relative to fluid intake), nausea, and hematuria.

Answer B is incorrect. This answer describes the pathologic findings of Goodpasture's syndrome, a type II hypersensitivity against collagen type IV, which is found in the lungs and the kidneys. The disease commonly presents with concurrent hemoptysis and hematuria. Exposure to hydrocarbon solvents such as those found in the dry-cleaning industry as well as cigarette smoking have been associated with an increased risk of developing Goodpasture's syndrome.

Answer C is incorrect. This answer describes the pathologic findings of IgA nephropathy (also known as Berger's nephropathy), one of the most common causes of recurrent gross or microscopic hematuria from glomerulonephritis worldwide.

Answer D is incorrect. This answer describes the pathologic findings of minimal change disease, the most common cause of nephrotic syndrome in children. It tends to respond very well to corticosteroid therapy. Remember, you have to **LEAP** to nephrotic syndrome, as it is characterized by **L**ipiduria/hyper**L**ipidemia, **E**dema (generalized), hypo**A**lbuminemia, and **P**roteinuria.

Answer E is incorrect. This answer describes the pathologic findings of Alport's syndrome, which usually presents between the ages of 5 and 20 years with nerve deafness and ophthalmopathy, accompanied with signs and symptoms of nephritis (such as gross or microscopic hematuria).

50. **The correct answer is A.** This child has osteogenesis imperfecta, a group of inherited disorders that mainly affect the bones. It results from a type I collagen mutation that affects bone, skin, and tendon. Patients present with fragile bones and frequent bone fractures. Some types are associated with brittle teeth, hearing loss, a blue tint to the sclera, scoliosis, and loose joints. The most frequent mode of inheritance is autosomal dominant.

Answer B is incorrect. Type II collagen is found mostly in hyaline-type cartilage, vitreous body, and nucleus pulposus. One condition associated with a mutation in type II collagen is Stickler syndrome, which involves a characteristic facial appearance, eye abnormalities, hearing loss, and joint problems.

Answer C is incorrect. Type III collagen is found in skin, blood vessels, uterus, fetal tissue, and granulation tissue. A mutation in this type of collagen is often seen in Ehlers-Danlos syndrome. Patients present with hypermobility that often results in dislocation and early-onset arthritis. Patients with Ehlers-Danlos syndrome also have characteristic soft, highly elastic, and fragile skin. When the vasculature is involved,

patients can present with potentially life-threatening complications such as blood vessel and organ rupture.

Answer D is incorrect. Type IV collagen is found in the basement membrane in the kidneys and ears. A mutation in this collagen results in Alport's syndrome, an X-linked disease that leads to the development of glomerulonephritis and hearing loss and that often presents in patients before the age of 30.

Answer E is incorrect. Type X collagen is found in the epiphyseal plate. A mutation in this collagen has been associated with Schmid metaphyseal chondrodysplasia. This presents clinically with short stature and a waddling gait.

CHAPTER 11

Neurology and Psychiatry

1. A couple presents to the emergency department (ED) with their 5-month-old son. The parents report that their son has never been fussy. However, last night he began to cry incessantly and neither changing his diapers nor feeding was able to calm him. This morning he had become very lethargic and warm, and his temperature reached 39.4° C (103° F). The physician examines the baby and notices some rigidity in his nuchal region. The ED physician becomes extremely concerned and orders a lumbar puncture which reveals an elevated opening pressure, elevated protein level, decreased glucose level, and numerous polymorphonuclear cells. What is the most likely cause of this patient's symptoms?

(A) *Cryptococcus neoformans*
(B) Cytomegalovirus
(C) Enterovirus
(D) *Escherichia coli*
(E) *Haemophilus influenzae*
(F) *Neisseria meningitides*

2. A 35-year-old woman who was hospitalized for mania 2 weeks ago shows substantial improvement. Her mania has resolved; she is now sleeping through the night. She no longer has delusions of grandiosity, and her speech is not pressured and does not show flight of ideas. She is ready for discharge. Which of the following drugs could be prescribed as maintenance therapy for this patient?

(A) Bupropion
(B) Carbamazepine
(C) Fluoxetine
(D) Olanzapine
(E) Reserpine

3. A 27-year-old man presents to his primary care physician for a pre-employment physical examination. The patient states that he has been healthy and has no complaints except that he has been drinking a lot of water for what feels like an unquenchable thirst for the past couple of weeks. He reports that he has also been urinating excessively and is unable to sleep through the night due to his thirst and frequent urination. Urine analysis is significant only for a specific gravity of 1.002. Serum analysis is significant for a osmolality of 320 mOsm/L and a serum glucose level of 120 mg/dL. The patient is admitted to the hospital, where subcutaneous vasopressin is administered. Subsequent urine analysis revealed a specific gravity of 1.009 and serum analysis reveals an osmolality of 300 mOsm/L and a serum glucose level of 124 mg/dL. The patient is most likely to benefit from treatment with which of the following?

(A) Desmopressin
(B) Fluid restriction
(C) Hydrochlorothiaz
(D) Insulin
(E) Metformin

4. A 70-year-old man is referred to a specialist for evaluation because of progressive memory loss and cognitive decline. His wife reports that he is always getting lost in their neighborhood and that she now pays the bills because he has become unreliable. She adds that her husband has lost interest in his stained glass creations, which he had enjoyed for nearly 20 years. She also states that the patient's appetite has remained normal and that his weight has not changed. His sleeping patterns and energy level are largely unchanged as well. Although the neurologic examination is normal, he scores only a 19/30 on the Mini-Mental State Examination, with errors in figure drawing, recall, language, and concentration. Laboratory studies are unremarkable. Which of the following symptoms is most likely to develop in this patient over the next 3 months?

(A) Depression
(B) Gait disturbances
(C) Hyperorality
(D) Stereotyped perseveration
(E) Symmetric muscular weakness

5. A medical student anteriorly dislocates her shoulder while playing softball. With the help of her fellow students, she is able to reduce the dislocation without going to the emergency department, but for the next 10 days she experiences numbness in her arm. Which of the following is the most likely location of the numbness and the nerve responsible?

(A) Lateral dorsal surface of the hand, radial nerve
(B) Lateral palm, thumb and radial 2.5 fingers, median nerve
(C) Lateral upper arm over deltoid muscle, axillary nerve
(D) Medial anterior and posterior surfaces of the forearm, medial cutaneous nerve
(E) Medial palm and ulnar 1.5 fingers, ulnar nerve

6. A 45-year-old man presents to the physician with a history of back pain that is aggravated by bending or straining and relieved by resting on the unaffected side. Physical examination shows pain and sensory loss over the back of the thigh, lateral calf, and foot, with associated motor deficit of the gastrocnemius muscle (4/5 strength on the affected side). Given the most likely nerve root affected, which of the following reflexes might be abnormal on physical examination?

(A) Achilles
(B) Biceps
(C) Patella
(D) Supinator
(E) Triceps

7. A 67-year-old woman presents to the physician with right-sided Horner's syndrome, dysarthria, diplopia, numbness, and ataxia with contralateral impairment of pain and temperature sensation. No other motor or hearing deficits are evident. Which of the following groups of structures is supplied by the artery involved in this condition?

(A) Caudal lateral pontine tegmentum, including cranial nerve VII, the spinal tegmental tract of cranial nerve V, and the inferior surface of the cerebellum
(B) Cochlea and vestibular apparatus
(C) Dorsolateral quadrant of the medulla, including the nucleus ambiguus and the inferior surface of the cerebellum
(D) Internal capsule, caudate nucleus, putamen, and globus pallidus
(E) Lateral geniculate body, globus pallidus, and posterior limb of the internal capsule

8. A 40-year-old man was admitted to the neurology service for evaluation of persistent numbness over his left jaw and lower face. MRI reveals a schwannoma, which is compressing a cranial nerve (CN) as the nerve exits the skull. The CN involved in this case exits the skull through which of the following foramina?

(A) Foramen ovale
(B) Foramen rotundum
(C) Foramen spinosum
(D) Jugular foramen
(E) Superior orbital fissure

9. A 47-year-old man presents with dysarthria and progressive muscle weakness of the bilateral upper and lower extremities in the absence of any history of neurologic disease or recent illness, weight loss, or trauma. Physical examination is notable for muscle atrophy and weakness in all extremities. Deep tendon reflexes are absent in the upper extremities but are 3+ in the lower extremities; some fasciculations are present. Babinski's sign is upgoing bilaterally, and cranial nerves are intact. Laboratory and imaging studies are all within normal limits. Which of the following would be expected on microscopic examination of the central nervous system?

(A) Demyelination of axons in the dorsal columns and spinocerebellar tracts in the spinal cord
(B) Demyelination of axons in the posterior limb of the internal capsule in the cerebrum
(C) Neuronal loss in the region of the anterior horn cells and corticospinal tracts in the spinal cord
(D) Neuronal loss in the region of the anterior horn cells and posterior columns in the spinal cord
(E) Neuronal loss only in the region of the anterior horn cells in the spinal cord

10. A 3-week-old neonate is noted to have enlargement of the head on a routine physical examination. His birth history is remarkable for an episode of group B streptococcal meningitis that resolved after a course of intravenous antibiotics. Which of the following mechanisms is most likely responsible for this patient's symptoms?

(A) Accumulation of blood in the subarachnoid space
(B) Decreased absorption of cerebrospinal fluid by the arachnoid villi
(C) Increased cerebrospinal fluid reabsorption
(D) Increased choroid plexus production
(E) Ventricle blockage

11. A 19-year-old college student presents to the emergency department with severe vomiting after taking an unknown pill on a night out with her friends. Which of the following labeled areas of the brain is most likely involved in this patient's vomiting?

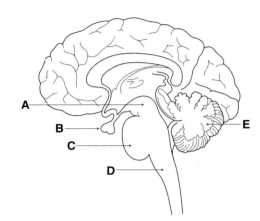

Reproduced, with permission, from USMLERx.com.

(A) A
(B) B
(C) C
(D) D
(E) E

12. A 76-year-old woman dies at home from sudden cardiac arrest after the onset of ventricular fibrillation. The family consents to an autopsy that reveals several small infarcts throughout the basal ganglia. Assuming that the defects arise from a single vessel within the central nervous system, pathology from which artery would be most consistent with this finding?

(A) Anterior cerebral artery
(B) Anterior communicating artery
(C) Lateral striate artery
(D) Posterior cerebral artery
(E) Vertebral cerebral artery

13. A 63-year-old homeless woman is brought to the emergency department (ED) by the police, who noted her to be disoriented and confused.

On questioning, the patient appears to be having problem with her short-term memory, frequently forgetting what question she had been asked. She provides plausible details of the events prior to her coming to the hospital, but the police report to be untrue. On physical examination she is emaciated and has nystagmus and an unsteady gait. Examination of the ED records reveals that she has presented multiple times in the past for alcohol withdrawal. The lesion accounting for the patient's symptoms is located in which part of the brain?

(A) Basal ganglia
(B) Broca's area
(C) Cerebellar vermis
(D) Mamillary bodies
(E) Wernicke's area

14. A 72-year-old woman presents to her physician with worsening low back pain that radiates over her anterior thighs. The pain has affected her for nearly 3 years; it occurs during walking and prolonged standing and is relieved by rest and sitting. The patient also says that she has begun to experience a decreased urinary stream. Physical examination is notable for reduced mobility over the lumbar spine; there is no pain elicited with leg raising in the supine position. Posterior tibial and dorsalis pedis pulses are 2+. Ankle reflexes are 1+ bilaterally. Which of the following represents the most likely process responsible this patient's back pain?

(A) Conus medullaris syndrome
(B) Lumbar spinal stenosis
(C) Lumbosacral disc herniation
(D) Peripheral vascular disease
(E) Polymyalgia rheumatica

15. An 82-year-old woman suffers an ischemic stroke with numerous sequelae, including uvular deviation to the right side. Assuming the defect is in the lower motor neuron, damage to which of the following cranial nerves is consistent with this abnormality?

(A) Left IX
(B) Left X

(C) Left XII
(D) Right IX
(E) Right X
(F) Right XII

16. A 45-year-old man who has received long-term treatment for schizophrenia has recently been noted to display involuntary movements that include lateral deviations of the jaw and "fly-catching" motions with his tongue. Which of the following agents is the most likely cause of his involuntary movements?

(A) Clozapine
(B) Fluphenazine
(C) Lithium
(D) Risperidone
(E) Selegiline

17. A 26-year-old woman presents to her primary care physician with a 2-month history of difficulty reading, pain in her right eye, and paresthesias in her hands and legs. The patient describes a similar episode that occurred 1 year ago; she assumed that it was a viral illness because it was self-limited. During the physical examination, the patient is noted to have hyperemia and edema of her right optic disc and mild hyperreflexia. The patient undergoes an MRI, which confirms the diagnosis. Histopathology of the lesions would demonstrate which of the following?

(A) Duplication and fragmentation of the internal elastic lamina
(B) Granulomatous inflammatory infiltrate of the adventitial and medial layers with fragmentation of the internal elastic lamina
(C) Inflammation of white matter associated with multinucleate giant cells and aggregates of mononuclear cells
(D) Lymphocyte and macrophage infiltration associated with areas of demyelination
(E) Spongiform degeneration without inflammatory changes

18. A 2-month-old boy is brought to his pediatrician for a regular checkup. His parents report that he has a poor appetite and is very constipated. He has small bowel movements once a week, which his parents believe are very painful. Although he was at the 75th percentile for both height and weight at birth, he is currently at the 25th percentile for height and is below the 5th percentile for weight. His abdomen is distended, but his bowel sounds are normal and his abdomen does not appear to be tender. A barium enema shows a narrow rectosigmoid with a dilation of the segment above the narrowing. Which of the following might be missing from this patient on rectosigmoid biopsy?

(A) Enteric neurons
(B) Motor neurons to the external anal sphincter
(C) Pelvic nerves
(D) Sympathetic neurons
(E) Vagus nerve

19. During the autopsy of a patient who complained of the "worst headache of her life" shortly before dying, the pathologist removes the calvarium with the dura attached. On the surface of the brain, there is frank blood on visual inspection that the pathologist is unable to remove by rubbing or scraping the surface. Which of the following types of hemorrhages most likely caused this finding?

(A) Epidural hemorrhage
(B) Intradural hemorrhage
(C) Parenchymal hemorrhage
(D) Subarachnoid hemorrhage
(E) Subdural hemorrhage

20. A psychologist whose first child is now 4 years old is determined to use behavioral treatment techniques to raise her child. For instance, if the child throws a temper tantrum in a store because she will not buy him candy, she just picks up the child and leaves the store; however, if the child behaves in the store, she takes him to the zoo. This is an example of which of the following kinds of behavior modification?

(A) Aversive conditioning
(B) Classical conditioning
(C) Learned helplessness
(D) Operant conditioning
(E) Stimulus generalization

21. A 33-year-old woman presents to the emergency department complaining of right facial weakness and pain behind her right ear since that morning. Neurological examination confirms complete paralysis of the right side of her face, decreased taste sensation on the right side of her tongue, and increased sensitivity to loud sounds in her right ear. The rest of her neurological examination is normal. The patient is given a short course of steroids and her facial weakness improved gradually over the next few weeks. In addition to the symptoms described above, this patient may also develop:

(A) Decreased sensation over her left cheek
(B) Decreased sensation over her right cheek
(C) Deviation of the uvula and soft palate to the left when the patient is asked to say "Ahh"
(D) Deviation of the uvula and soft palate to the right when the patient is asked to say "Ahh"
(E) Dryness in her left eye
(F) Dryness in her right eye

22. During a right temporal craniotomy, the neuronal radiations projecting to the inferior bank of the calcarine sulcus are injured. Which of the following is the most likely visual disturbance to occur in this patient?

(A) Left upper quadrantanopia
(B) Left hemianopia with macular sparing
(C) Left lower quadrantanopia
(D) Right upper quadrantanopia
(E) Right hemianopia with macular sparing
(F) Right lower quadrantanopia

23. A 19-year-old inpatient on a psychiatry ward has a contentious relationship with his attending psychiatrist. The patient has been diagnosed with major depression and questionable borderline personality disorder. His reactions

to the psychiatrist have been aggressive and have included such behavior as spitting in the psychiatrist's face. In morning conference, which of the following is a mature defense mechanism that the psychiatrist might use when talking with other staff members about the patient?

(A) Dissociation
(B) Humor
(C) Identification
(D) Projection
(E) Reaction formation

24. The high-power micrograph shown here demonstrates a key histologic finding obtained from the brain of a 75-year-old patient at autopsy. The patient had a neurologic illness that was primarily characterized by motor symptoms without evidence of dementia. Which of the following findings might this patient have exhibited?

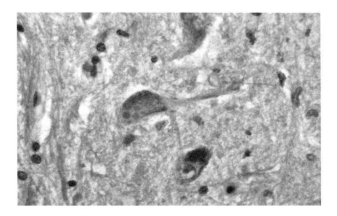

Image courtesy of PEIR Digital Library (http://peir.net).

(A) Bradykinesia
(B) Grand mal seizures
(C) Myoclonic fasciculations
(D) Symmetrical proximal muscle weakness
(E) Tongue fasciculations

25. A 40-year-old woman comes to the physician because of hoarseness following surgery for removal of a thyroid nodule. Which of the following nerves was most likely injured during her surgery?

(A) Accessory nerve
(B) External laryngeal nerve
(C) Glossopharyngeal nerve
(D) Internal laryngeal nerve
(E) Recurrent laryngeal nerve

26. As part of the neurologic examination of an infant, reflexes are tested. One of the reflexes is tested by firmly stroking the bottom of the foot with a tool such as the metal end of a reflex hammer. At what age does this tested reflex usually disappear?

(A) 1 month
(B) 6 months
(C) 12 months
(D) 24 months
(E) 48 months

27. After a brain tumor resection, a right-handed patient presents to the physician with his wife, who reports that the patient can no longer balance his checkbook or count his money. Recently, he has also had difficulty identifying individual fingers when she points to them and will confuse his left and right sides. Additionally, she reports that although he can read without effort, he has extreme difficulty with writing. The damage can be localized to which of the following areas of the brain?

(A) Left angular gyrus
(B) Left posterior inferior frontal lobe
(C) Left posterior superior temporal gyrus
(D) Left sylvian region
(E) Left temporoparieto-occipital junction

28. A 26-year-old African-American woman presents to her primary care physician because of fatigue and insomnia for the past 7 months. She also complains of difficulty concentrating and irritability as well as feeling continually worried. She states that nothing seems to make her feel better or worse; she is still able to perform all of her work duties as a public relations officer and in fact was recently promoted. Her past medical history is unremarkable. Physical examination shows no focal findings, but the woman appears markedly agitated. Which of the following is this patient's most likely diagnosis?

(A) Attention-deficit/hyperactivity disorder
(B) Avoidant personality disorder
(C) Generalized anxiety disorder
(D) Obsessive-compulsive disorder
(E) Social phobia disorder

29. A 38-year-old woman comes to the physician with a 4-month history of episodic nausea and a sensation of abnormal motion that lasts for 4–5 minutes. Her symptoms have intensified over the past week, and the episodes now last more than an hour. A particularly severe episode this morning resulted in vomiting and buzzing in her right ear. On physical examination, the patient appears healthy with normal vital signs, mild sensorineural hearing loss in the right ear, and no nystagmus. The patient's laboratory tests are unremarkable. Audiologic testing demonstrates unilateral hearing loss on the right side, most pronounced in the low-frequency range. Which of the following locations is the most likely origin of the abnormality responsible for this patient's symptoms?

(A) Cochlea
(B) Endolymphatic sac
(C) Semicircular canals
(D) Utricle and saccule
(E) Vestibulocochlear nerve

30. The ability of language requires many intricate movements of the tongue and lips and involves multiple cranial nerves. Glottal sounds (kah) require different muscles and nerves than lingual (lah) sounds. A defect in which of the following muscles, innervated by which nerve, can affect lingual sounds?

(A) Genioglossus, hypoglossal nerve
(B) Genioglossus, vagus nerve
(C) Palatoglossus, hypoglossal nerve
(D) Palatoglossus, vagus nerve
(E) Styloglossus, glossopharyngeal nerve

31. A 42-year-old woman presents to the emergency department with bilateral leg weakness and paresthesias involving the toes. On physical examination the patient has diminished ankle-jerk and knee-jerk reflexes bilaterally and abnormal sweating, but has normal sensation despite the paresthesias. Past medical history is notable for diarrheal illness 3 weeks prior to admission. Over the course of the next 24 hours, the weakness progresses, involving the upper limbs and the face. Diagnostic studies confirm the presence of an antibody-mediated autoimmune disease. Which of the following is the function of the cells targeted by antibodies in this condition?

(A) Conduction of nerve impulses from central nervous system neurons to peripheral muscle
(B) Conduction of nerve impulses from the cerebral cortex to spinal motor neurons
(C) Contraction in response to changes in membrane potential
(D) Myelination of central nervous system axons
(E) Myelination of peripheral nervous system axons

32. A 43-year-old man presents to emergency department complaining of vision problems for the past 2 days. He informs the physicians that he has AIDS and that his last CD4 count 3 months ago was 24 cells/μL. He stopped taking antiretroviral therapy 2 years ago. Neurologic examination reveals problems with speech, memory, and coordination. He is admitted to the hospital but his symptoms rapidly worsen, and 3 weeks after admission the patient dies. What is the most likely cause of death in this patient?

(A) *Cryptococcus neoformans*
(B) Herpes simplex virus
(C) JC virus
(D) *Pneumocystis jiroveci*
(E) *Toxoplasmosa gondii*

33. A 32-year-old woman presents to the physician with worsening anesthesia, weakness of both upper extremities, and headaches. The patient has no prior significant medical history and cannot recall any recent episodes of trauma. Physical examination is notable for the absence of motor deficits in both upper extremities, but positive for the absence of pain and temperature sensation and reflexes in both upper extremities. Position and vibration sense are intact in the upper extremities and there are no lower extremity abnormalities. An MRI of the spinal column shows dilation within the cervical spinal cord. Which of the following diagnoses is consistent with this patient's findings?

(A) Arnold-Chiari I malformation
(B) Arnold-Chiari II malformation
(C) Communicating hydrocephalus
(D) Congenital aqueductal stenosis
(E) Dandy-Walker syndrome

34. A 5-year-old boy is brought to the emergency department by his mother after she found him having convulsions on the kitchen floor. On the way to the hospital, he experienced another seizure. On admission, the patient appears weak and disoriented and has no recollection of the event. He is given a dose of phenytoin for seizure prophylaxis. One hour after the drug is administered, his plasma concentration is 50 µg/mL; 2 hours after drug administration, it is 30 µg/mL. Assuming that phenytoin undergoes zero-order elimination, what will be the plasma concentration 3 hours after the drug's administration?

(A) 5 µg/mL
(B) 10 µg/mL
(C) 15 µg/mL
(D) 20 µg/mL
(E) 25 µg/mL

35. A 35-year-old man with depression presents to the emergency department with flushing, diarrhea, sweating, and muscle rigidity. During the physical examination, he says that he began seeing a new psychiatrist because his sertraline was not working for him. His new doctor gave him a different medication, but he decided to use both medicines to "get rid of the depression." Which of the following medications did the new doctor most likely prescribe for this patient?

(A) Citalopram
(B) Lithium
(C) Nortriptyline
(D) Tranylcypromine
(E) Trazodone

36. A 7-year-old boy is brought to the emergency department after falling from a tree; an x-ray film shows that he has a midshaft fracture of the humerus. Which of the following structures could be injured with this type of fracture?

(A) Anterior circumflex humeral artery
(B) Axillary nerve
(C) Median nerve
(D) Radial nerve
(E) Ulnar nerve

37. A 35-year-old woman presents to the emergency department with trembling hands and a facial tic. According to her mother, she has been seeing a psychiatrist for the past year. She has no other significant medical history. Which of the following medications has this patient most likely been taking?

(A) Chlorpromazine
(B) Imipramine
(C) Lithium
(D) Sertraline
(E) Trazodone

38. A 65-year-old man is being evaluated because his speech has been noted to lack appropriate fluency. Throughout the evaluation, the patient has trouble finding certain words but seems to understand everything asked of him. His ability to repeat is poor, but it is preserved more than his ability to generate spontaneous responses to posed questions. When he responds to questions, he frequently uses the wrong word. These clinical findings are most consistent with which of the following types of aphasia?

(A) Broca's
(B) Conduction
(C) Global
(D) Thalamic
(E) Transcortical motor
(F) Transcortical sensory
(G) Wernicke's

39. While on a rotation in the hospital, a resident physician observes an attending physician giving a patient a dose of physostigmine. For which of the following drug overdoses is physostigmine indicated?

(A) Atropine
(B) Bethanechol
(C) Echothiophate
(D) Neostigmine
(E) Pralidoxime

40. A 32-year-old man comes to the physician because of headaches that occur at night and without warning. They begin in his left eye and then generalize to the left side of his face. Alcohol can precipitate the attacks, which last for less than 1 hour. The patient rates the pain as a 10/10, and multiple over-the-counter analgesics have resulted in minimal benefit. He is given a prescription for sumatriptan. Which of the following is the most likely diagnosis?

(A) Cluster headache
(B) Medication-overuse headache
(C) Migraine headache
(D) Temporomandibular joint dysfunction syndrome
(E) Tension headache

41. A 42-year-old African-American woman is brought to a psychiatric crisis center by police after exhibiting bizarre and aggressive behavior in a public square. On initial examination, she is mute and exhibits poor eye contact; she is also unkempt and bizarrely dressed. The patient is admitted to the inpatient psychiatric floor and started on antipsychotic medication. In subsequent days, the patient is able to interact more appropriately with other patients on the unit, although she still exhibits poor eye contact. Her delusions are incomplete and bizarre. She frequently giggles during her daily interviews and smiles broadly when talking about her delusions. The nurses report that the patient's behavior is childlike, and she has a tendency to expose herself to the other patients. Assuming the patient has schizophrenia, which of the following subtypes would best describe this patient?

(A) Catatonic
(B) Disorganized
(C) Paranoid
(D) Residual
(E) Undifferentiated

42. Perineal pain from childbirth can be alleviated by numbing which of the following nerves?

(A) Inferior gluteal
(B) Obturator
(C) Pudendal
(D) Sciatic
(E) Superior gluteal

43. A medical student is performing experiments on an anesthetized animal for her pharmacology class. An arterial line is inserted to monitor blood pressure, and the animal is given an intravenous dose of epinephrine, which produces the expected increase in blood pressure. The student then injects an unknown drug, followed 15 minutes later by readministration of epinephrine. The second administration of epinephrine now produces a decrease in blood pressure. To which of the following classes does the unknown drug belong?

(A) Acetylcholinesterase inhibitor
(B) Nicotinic ganglionic blocker
(C) Nonselective α-receptor agonist
(D) Nonselective α-receptor antagonist
(E) Nonselective β-receptor antagonist

44. A 40-year-old woman presents to a psychiatrist after a referral from her family physician. She states that she feels anxious all of the time. Her family physician diagnosed her with generalized anxiety disorder and prescribed buspirone; however, the patient does not report feeling any better. She works from home as a transcriptionist and has no close friends. She views herself as stupid and unappealing. She still lives at home with her mother and says that she is afraid to live by herself. Which of the following personality disorders best describes this patient?

(A) Avoidant
(B) Dependent
(C) Histrionic
(D) Narcissistic
(E) Schizoid
(F) Schizotypal

45. A 2-year-old boy is brought to the pediatrician because his mother discovered a large abdominal mass while bathing him. Examination shows that the child has marked hypertension and dark circles around his eyes. Urine catecholamine levels are elevated. A biopsy of the mass reveals small round cells with hyperchromatic nuclei, often forming a pseudorosette pattern around central primitive nerve fibers. Amplification of which of the following oncogenes is associated with this tumor?

(A) bcl-2
(B) c-myc
(C) erb-B2
(D) n-myc
(E) ras

46. A 7-year-old boy is brought to his pediatrician by his mother after a troubling parent-teacher conference. The teacher informed the mother

that the child is disruptive in class and generally does not finish his homework assignments. The mother reports that the child's room is always messy and that he has difficulty completing chores in a timely fashion. In the office, the child is restless and interrupts his mother often. He does not exhibit pressured speech, although he does speak in a very loud voice. He has always cried easily—mainly due to frustration—but the mother does not believe that they have a difficult relationship. Which of the following is the most likely diagnosis?

(A) Antisocial personality disorder
(B) Attention-deficit/hyperactivity disorder
(C) Childhood bipolar disorder
(D) Conduct disorder
(E) Oppositional defiant disorder

47. A 2-week-old baby girl is brought to the pediatrician for her first doctor's appointment. On examination, the baby is found to have a tuft of hair on her lower back, but no lesion is found. Ultrasound shows no herniation of any kind. Which of the following conditions does this baby have?

(A) Anencephaly
(B) Meningocele
(C) Meningomyelocele
(D) Spina bifida cystica
(E) Spina bifida occulta

48. A 43-year-old woman presents to her primary care physician for a regular checkup. A neurologic examination shows that when the patient looks to the left, the right eye stops at the midline and the left eye shows monocular horizontal nystagmus. When the patient looks to the right, both eyes seem to move appropriately. Convergence is normal. What is the most likely cause of this patient's findings?

(A) Internuclear ophthalmoplegia
(B) Medial rectus damage
(C) Pupillary light-near dissociation
(D) Relative afferent pupillary defect
(E) Sixth-nerve palsy

49. Neurofibromatosis type 1, also known as von Recklinghausen's disease, has certain associated physical findings. Which of the following is a physical finding in a patient with neurofibromatosis type 1?

    (A) Brushfield spots
    (B) Lisch's nodules
    (C) Macro-orchidism
    (D) Mitral valve prolapse
    (E) Tendon xanthomas

50. A 42-year-old woman presents to her primary care physician with a chief complaint of paresthesias that started in her fingers and toes about 1 week ago. Since then, her symptoms have progressed to include paresthesias and muscle weakness in her lower legs. A nerve conduction study is performed and shows slowed nerve conduction velocities. The patient is diagnosed with Guillain-Barré syndrome. As her disease progresses, which of the following acid-base disorders would she be expected to develop?

    (A) Metabolic acidosis (anion-gap)
    (B) Metabolic acidosis (non–anion-gap)
    (C) Metabolic alkalosis
    (D) Respiratory acidosis
    (E) Respiratory alkalosis

1. **The correct answer is D.** The concern for this patient is meningitis, which can be caused by bacteria, viruses, or fungi. The classic triad is fever, headache, and nuchal rigidity. Other symptoms such as rash and photophobia are also commonly present. In neonates, though, it may be difficult to identify these symptoms. Inference from the history, such as severe crying in a normally quiet baby, may indicate headache or muscle stiffness. A lumbar puncture and cerebrospinal fluid (CSF) analysis is essential in determining the cause. Classic CSF findings for bacterial meningitis are elevated opening pressure, elevated levels of polymorphonuclear leukocytes, elevated protein levels, and decreased glucose levels, as seen in this patient. In newborns from 0 to 6 months old, the three most common causes of meningitis are all bacterial and include group B streptococci, *Escherichia coli*, and *Listeria*. Culture and microbiology analysis will be able to differentiate between these species. However, the mortality rate for meningitis is high if untreated, and patients can quickly deteriorate. Therefore, empiric treatment should be initiated prior to obtaining the results of CSF analysis.

Answer A is incorrect. *Cryptococcus* mostly causes meningitis in patients with HIV/AIDS. Cerebrospinal fluid findings for fungal meningitis are most often an elevated opening pressure, elevated lymphocytes, elevated protein level, and decreased glucose level. The number of polymorphonuclear leukocytes is normal, differentiating it from bacterial etiologies.

Answer B is incorrect. Cytomegalovirus is another pathogen that causes meningitis in patients with HIV/AIDS and immunosuppressed patients. Findings on cerebrospinal fluid analysis are typical for viral meningitis (normal or slightly elevated opening pressure, elevated lymphocytes, normal protein level, and normal glucose level).

Answer C is incorrect. Enterovirus commonly causes viral meningitis in patients 6 months to 60 years old. Clinically, the specific virus causing viral meningitis is not always determined, but the family of enterovirus is most commonly seen. Cerebrospinal fluid analysis in viral meningitis reveals normal or slightly elevated opening pressure, elevated lymphocytes, normal protein level, and normal glucose level.

Answer E is incorrect. *Haemophilus influenzae* type B used to be a very common cause of bacterial meningitis in children between the ages of 6 months and 6 years. However, the incidence has dramatically decreased in the past 15 years with the introduction of *H. influenzae* vaccines.

Answer F is incorrect. *Neisseria meningitides* is the most common cause of meningitis in patients 6–60 years old. It is also seen less frequently in patients age 6 months to 6 years. It is rarely seen in newborns. Findings of cerebrospinal fluid analysis would be consistent with bacterial meningitis.

2. **The correct answer is B.** Carbamazepine is an anticonvulsant that is also prescribed for mood stabilization in patients with mania, poor anger management, and lack of impulse control. Valproic acid is another anticonvulsant medication that is used for mood stabilization. Valproic acid and carbamazepine have a wider therapeutic range than lithium, although lithium is typically the first-line maintenance therapy in bipolar disorder.

Answer A is incorrect. Bupropion is an atypical antidepressant. More typical antidepressants, such as selective serotonin reuptake inhibitors, have a place in the treatment of bipolar disorder, but the effect on a patient's mood must be carefully monitored for a cycling into a manic state.

Answer C is incorrect. Fluoxetine is a selective serotonin reuptake inhibitor that can elevate mood. Antidepressants have a place in the treatment of bipolar disorder, but the effect on a patient's mood must be carefully monitored for a cycling into a manic state.

Answer D is incorrect. Olanzapine is an atypical antipsychotic that can be used in manic patients with severe agitation and psychosis.

Answer E is incorrect. Reserpine depletes central and peripheral catecholamines and depresses sympathetic nerve function, resulting in vasodilation and sedation. This is a drug that can actually cause depression.

3. **The correct answer is A.** The patient has central diabetes insipidus, a disorder in which the kidneys fail to concentrate urine due to a lack of ADH (versus nephrogenic diabetes insipidus, in which ADH is present but the kidneys fail to respond). This diagnosis is evident from his low urine specific gravity with a high serum osmolality and the increase in urine specific gravity with administration of vasopressin. Desmopressin is an ADH analog that is used intranasally to treat central diabetes insipidus. Patients with nephrogenic diabetes insipidus would not respond to ADH analogs.

Answer B is incorrect. Fluid restriction is not indicated for, and is actually detrimental to, this patient due to the inability of his renal system to absorb water.

Answer C is incorrect. Hydrochlorothiazide is a diuretic used to treat nephrogenic diabetes insipidus. Desmopressin is the correct treatment for central diabetes insipidus, such as in this patient.

Answer D is incorrect. Insulin is used to treat type 1 diabetes mellitus and in the later stages of type 2 diabetes mellitus.

Answer E is incorrect. Metformin is a hypoglycemic drug used to treat type 2 diabetes mellitus.

4. **The correct answer is A.** Alzheimer's disease is the most likely diagnosis given the patient's age, presentation, and lack of strokelike symptoms or stepwise progression of illness. Other causes of dementia to consider would include vitamin B_{12} deficiency, thyroid dysfunction, syphilis, and hepatic encephalopathy. It is also unlikely that depression is the primary etiology of the patient's condition. Although this patient does not fulfill the criteria for depression at this point, depression is a significant comorbidity of Alzheimer's disease and should be repeatedly screened for and treated.

Answer B is incorrect. Gait disturbances are uncommon early in the course of Alzheimer's disease and would be much more common in other diagnoses, such as Parkinson's disease.

Answer C is incorrect. Stereotyped perseveration is another sign of frontotemporal dementia that is rare in Alzheimer's disease.

Answer D is incorrect. Causes of hyperprolactinemia in men include medications, primary hypothyroidism, and chest wall stimulation (from trauma or herpes zoster reactivation). The diagnosis of idiopathic hyperprolactinemia is made by exclusion of known causes. Forty percent of all pituitary tumors are prolactinomas.

Answer E is incorrect. Symmetric muscular weakness can occur in many neurologic diagnoses but is uncommon at this stage of Alzheimer's disease. It is, however, a characteristic sign of amyotrophic lateral sclerosis.

5. **The correct answer is C.** The axillary nerve wraps around the surgical neck of the humerus and is the nerve most often injured in an anterior dislocation of the shoulder. The axillary nerve innervates the deltoid muscle and sends a lateral cutaneous branch to the skin over the deltoid muscle.

Answer A is incorrect. The radial nerve runs in the humeral groove, and in a midshaft humeral break, one must be concerned about a radial nerve injury.

Answer B is incorrect. The median nerve can be compressed in the carpal tunnel and cause carpal tunnel syndrome. It may also be injured in the antecubital region during an elbow injury. It is generally not injured in a shoulder dislocation.

Answer D is incorrect. The medial cutaneous nerve arises from the medial cord of the brachial plexus and runs down the arm with the brachial artery to supply the medial cutaneous surface of the forearm.

Answer E is incorrect. The ulnar nerve arises from the medial cord of the brachial plexus and is injured when a person attempts to stop a fall by reaching up and grabbing hold of a branch or pole, or during birth when a baby is pulled out by its arm. It is not usually injured in shoulder dislocation injuries.

6. **The correct answer is A.** Patients with an L5–S1 disc herniation affecting the S1 nerve root can be expected to have pain and paresthesias and sensory loss over the back of the thigh, lateral posterior calf, and lateral foot with motor deficits of the gastrocnemius muscle with or without deficits in foot eversion. These patients can also demonstrate loss of the Achilles reflex, which is a test of the S1 root and gastrocnemius muscle.

Answer B is incorrect. Loss of the biceps reflex can occur with herniation involving the C5 or C6 nerve root and involves motor and sensory deficits in the upper extremities.

Answer C is incorrect. The patellar reflex can be lost with herniation affecting the L4 nerve root. This would also produce pain and sensory loss over the anterior thigh and inner shin, with motor deficits of the quadriceps muscle.

Answer D is incorrect. A disc herniation at the C5–6 or C6–7 level may result in the loss of the supinator reflex, with the former potentially involving the biceps reflex and the latter potentially affecting the triceps reflex.

Answer E is incorrect. The triceps reflex can be lost with herniation affecting the C7 nerve root. This would result in pain and paresthesias over the neck, lateral arm, and ring and index fingers, as well as in sensory loss over the radial forearm and index and middle fingers. C7 nerve root compression also involves motor loss of the triceps and extensor carpi ulnaris and can also involve loss of the supinator reflex.

7. **The correct answer is C.** The stroke syndrome described is the lateral medullary syndrome, also known as the posterior inferior cerebellar artery (PICA) syndrome or Wallenberg's syndrome. This syndrome results in numbness of the ipsilateral face and contralateral limbs, diplopia, dysarthria, and an ipsilateral Horner's syndrome. It classically results from a disruption of the PICA, which provides the blood supply for the dorsolateral quadrant of the medulla, including the nucleus ambiguus and the inferior surface of the cerebellum.

Answer A is incorrect. This vascular territory is supplied by the anterior inferior cerebellar artery. Disruption in blood flow typically causes ipsilateral deafness from involvement of the labyrinthine artery, ipsilateral facial weakness, and ataxia. It is the second most common brainstem stroke syndrome.

Answer B is incorrect. The cochlea and vestibular apparatus are perfused via the labyrinthine artery, and an isolated disruption of this end artery would result in isolated dysfunction of these two structures.

Answer D is incorrect. The internal capsule, caudate nucleus, putamen, and globus pallidus are perfused by the penetrating branches of the middle cerebral artery known as the lateral striate arteries. They are commonly involved with lacunar strokes.

Answer E is incorrect. The lateral geniculate body, globus pallidus, and posterior limb of the internal capsule are supplied by the anterior choroidal artery. Syndromes affecting this artery represent less than 1% of anterior circulation strokes and typically occur in the setting of symptomatic internal carotid artery occlusion.

8. **The correct answer is A.** The foramina of the trigeminal nerve divisions can be remembered with the mnemonic **S**tanding **R**oom **O**nly (SRO) for the **S**uperior orbital fissure, foramen **R**otundum, and foremen **O**vale, which transmit CN V_1, V_3, and V_3, respectively. This patient has a schwannoma of the mandibular di-

vision of the trigeminal nerve (CN V_3) as the nerve exits the skull through the foramen ovale. Compression of V_3 causes numbness over the ipsilateral jaw and lower face.

Answer B is incorrect. The maxillary division of the trigeminal nerve (CN V_2) exits the skull through the foramen rotundum and compression would cause decreased sensation over the cheek and middle face.

Answer C is incorrect. No cranial nerves exit through the foramen spinosum. The middle meningeal artery exits through this opening.

Answer D is incorrect. The jugular foramen transmits the glossopharyngeal (CN IX), vagus (CN X), and the spinal accessory nerve (CN XI).

Answer E is incorrect. CN III, IV, V_1, and VI exit the skull through the superior orbital fissure. Lesions of these nerves would lead to ipsilateral extraocular muscle paralysis and numbness of the ipsilateral forehead and upper face (CN V_1).

9. **The correct answer is C.** This patient presents with signs and symptoms consistent with amyotrophic lateral sclerosis (ALS), which affects both anterior horn cells in the spinal cord and upper motor neurons in the spinal cord. ALS results in a combination of upper and lower motor neuron signs, although the deficits may be asymmetric. More males are affected than females, and the incidence rises after age 40. Riluzole (Rilutek) is the only FDA-approved treatment for the disorder, and it prolongs life by only 3–6 months; it is thought to function by reducing the presynaptic release of glutamate.

Answer A is incorrect. Demyelination of axons in the dorsal columns and spinocerebellar tracts occurs in subacute combined degeneration of the spinal cord, which is also known as vitamin B_{12} neuropathy. It is associated with pernicious anemia and results in loss of vibration and position sense (dorsal columns) and arm/leg ataxia (spinocerebellar tracts).

Answer B is incorrect. Demyelination of axons in the posterior limb of the internal cap-

sule would cause contralateral spastic paralysis secondary to disruption of the descending fibers of the corticospinal tract, resulting in upper motor neuron signs.

Answer D is incorrect. Neuronal loss in the region of the anterior horn cells and posterior columns in the spinal cord occurs in Charcot-Marie-Tooth disease, also known as peroneal muscular atrophy. It results in loss of conscious proprioception (posterior columns) and lower motor neuron signs (anterior horn motor neurons).

Answer E is incorrect. Neuronal loss in the region of the anterior horn cells in the spinal cord occurs in poliomyelitis, an acute inflammatory viral infection that affects the lower motor neurons and results in a flaccid paralysis (pure lower motor neuron disease).

10. **The correct answer is B.** After an episode of meningitis has resolved, meningeal scarring can occur as a complication. In fact, scarring can be severe enough to decrease cerebrospinal fluid (CSF) absorption by arachnoid villi, thus causing hydrocephalus. A CT scan of this patient would show dilatation of the lateral and third ventricles with reduction of the extra-axial spaces. These findings suggest accumulation of CSF in the brain, leading to expansion of the cranial cavity and an increase in intracranial pressure. If left untreated, hydrocephalus can potentially lead to impairment of mental and muscular functions or even death.

Answer A is incorrect. Accumulation of blood in the subarachnoid space is usually due to trauma or a ruptured berry aneurysm.

Answer C is incorrect. Increased cerebrospinal fluid reabsorption would not cause hydrocephalus.

Answer D is incorrect. Rarely, hydrocephalus can result from increased production of cerebrospinal fluid by the choroid plexus. This mechanism is not usually a complication of meningitis.

Answer E is incorrect. Ventricular blockage can result in hydrocephalus; however, in this scenario such a mechanism is unlikely.

11. **The correct answer is D.** The area postrema of the medulla contains a chemoreceptor trigger zone that can initiate vomiting. The medulla also plays a role in cardiovascular and respiratory control and in brain stem reflexes.

    Answer A is incorrect. The midbrain helps regulate motor control, control of eye movements, and acoustic relay.

    Answer B is incorrect. The hypothalamus plays a role in autonomic and endocrine control.

    Answer C is incorrect. The pons plays a role in respiratory and urinary bladder control as well as in vestibular control of eye movements.

    Answer E is incorrect. The cerebellum regulates movement and posture and aids in motor learning.

12. **The correct answer is C.** The lateral striate arteries are sometimes referred to as the "arteries of stroke" and are penetrating branches of the middle cerebral artery that supply the internal capsule, caudate, putamen, and globus pallidus. Infarcts of this region frequently occur in the setting of long-standing hypertension and are known as lacunar infarcts.

    Answer A is incorrect. The anterior cerebral artery supplies the medial surface of the forebrain and supplies the leg-foot area of the motor and sensory homunculus.

    Answer B is incorrect. The anterior communicating artery connects the two anterior cerebral arteries and is the most common source of circle of Willis aneurysms, which can lead to bitemporal lower quadrantanopia.

    Answer D is incorrect. The posterior cerebral artery supplies the major blood supply to the midbrain and supplies the thalamus, the lateral and medial geniculate bodies, and the occipital lobe. Occlusion of this artery can result in contralateral hemianopia with macular sparing.

    Answer E is incorrect. The vertebral cerebral artery gives rise to two other arteries: the anterior spinal artery and the posterior inferior cerebellar artery. The former supplies the ante-rior two-thirds of the spinal cord and the latter supplies the dorsolateral medulla and inferior cerebellum.

13. **The correct answer is D.** The patient presents with classic signs of Wernicke-Korsakoff encephalopathy, which is associated with thiamine deficiency in chronic alcohol abusers. The classic signs are confusion, disorientation, anterograde amnesia, confabulation, oculomotor dysfunction, and motor ataxia. The lesion is located in the mamillary bodies.

    Answer A is incorrect. Lesions in the basal ganglia are associated with movement disorders.

    Answer B is incorrect. Lesions in Broca's area are associated with a motor aphasia with good comprehension.

    Answer C is incorrect. Lesions in the cerebellar vermis are associated with truncal ataxia and dysarthria.

    Answer E is incorrect. Lesions in Wernicke's area are associated with a sensory aphasia with poor comprehension.

14. **The correct answer is B.** Lumbar disc degeneration with enlargement of the facet joints can lead to lumbar spinal stenosis in the aging population. Spinal stenosis is characterized by neurogenic claudication—pain in the buttocks or back that is induced by walking or prolonged standing and relieved by rest. It can mimic vascular claudication symptoms, but the maximal pain is over the anterior thighs as opposed to the legs, as in typical claudication. Patients also have preserved lower extremity pulses without stigmata of peripheral vascular disease. Unlike patients with disc herniation, these patients have pain that is relieved by sitting and have negative leg raises bilaterally. Spinal stenosis can result in focal weakness and potentially alarming signs and should be aggressively imaged to rule out more ominous causes of back pain.

    Answer A is incorrect. Conus medullaris syndrome is a cord compression syndrome that produces perianal numbness and urinary retention with an atonic rectal sphincter, as opposed to the saddle anesthesia more typically found in the cauda equina syndrome, another cord compression syndrome.

Answer C is incorrect. The absence of positive straight leg raises and the improvement in symptoms with sitting are uncharacteristic of disc herniation syndromes.

Answer D is incorrect. Peripheral vascular disease (PVD), specifically atherosclerotic narrowing of the iliac and femoral arteries, can mimic symptoms of spinal stenosis. However, if this patient had PVD, her distal pulses would be reduced and her legs would most likely show evidence of stigmata associated with vascular disease.

Answer E is incorrect. Polymyalgia rheumatica (PMR) is a rheumatologic disorder associated with giant cell arteritis. It is characterized by symmetrical, aching proximal muscle pain that is typically most severe in the shoulder girdle, as well as stiffness in the morning and after inactivity. PMR is associated with an elevated erythrocyte sedimentation rate and C-reactive protein.

15. **The correct answer is B.** Motor innervation of the palatal arches and uvula is mediated by the vagus (X) nerve. Deviation of the uvula to one side implicates a lower motor neuron lesion contralateral to the side to which the uvula is deviating. An upper motor neuron vagus nerve lesion will cause the uvula to deviate toward the side of the lesion.

Answer A is incorrect. The glossopharyngeal nerve mediates taste, salivation, and swallowing, but injury would not cause any uvular, tongue, or palatal deviation.

Answer C is incorrect. The hypoglossal nerve mediates tongue movement. Injury to the left cranial nerve XII would result in deviation to that side because of the unopposed action of the opposite genioglossus muscle.

Answer D is incorrect. The glossopharyngeal nerve mediates taste, salivation, and swallowing, but injury would not cause any uvular, tongue, or palatal deviation.

Answer E is incorrect. A right-sided lower motor neuron injury to the vagus nerve would cause the uvula to deviate toward the intact (left) side.

Answer F is incorrect. The hypoglossal nerve mediates tongue movement. Injury to the right cranial nerve XII would result in deviation to that side because of the unopposed action of the opposite genioglossus muscle.

16. **The correct answer is B.** This patient is displaying signs of tardive dyskinesia, which is a complication of long-term antipsychotic therapy with the older agents. It is thought to result from increased dopamine receptor synthesis in response to long-term receptor blockade, which increases the sensitivity of dopamine at its receptors and causes the dopamine effects to disrupt the balance with cholinergic input. This leads to excessive involuntary movements. Of the drugs listed, fluphenazine, a first-line neuroleptic agent, would be the most likely agent to have caused this condition.

Answer A is incorrect. Clozapine, an atypical antipsychotic that modulates both serotonin and dopaminergic neurons in the central nervous system, has a much lower risk of tardive dyskinesia than typical antipsychotics such as haloperidol or fluphenazine, which affect dopaminergic neurons only.

Answer C is incorrect. Lithium is a mood stabilizer that is primarily used to treat episodes of mania in patients with bipolar disorder. It is not used to treat schizophrenia and does not cause tardive dyskinesia.

Answer D is incorrect. Risperidone, like clozapine, is an atypical antipsychotic that has a very low incidence of tardive dyskinesia in comparison to typical antipsychotics such as haloperidol, thioridazine, and fluphenazine.

Answer E is incorrect. Selegiline, a monoamine oxidase B inhibitor, is used to treat Parkinson's disease; it has no role in the treatment of schizophrenia.

17. **The correct answer is D.** This patient demonstrates many of the diagnostic features of multiple sclerosis, including optic neuritis and re-

current paresthesias. The pathologic hallmark of this disease consists of small gray plaques of demyelination present in the white matter of the central nervous system; microscopic pathology reveals gliosis and demyelination with associated lipid-laden macrophages.

Answer A is incorrect. Significantly enlarged blood vessels with duplication and fragmentation of the internal elastic lamina are evident in arteriovenous malformations.

Answer B is incorrect. Granulomatous inflammatory infiltrate of the adventitial and medial layers with fragmentation of the internal elastic lamina is consistent with inflammation of blood vessels as seen with arteritis. It does not describe blood vessel changes seen in multiple sclerosis.

Answer C is incorrect. Encephalitis due to infection with HIV is associated with white matter inflammation that includes multinucleate giant cells and mononuclear cells.

Answer E is incorrect. Spongiform degeneration and accumulation of proteinaceous material are associated with prion diseases such as Creutzfeldt-Jacob disease.

18. **The correct answer is A.** This patient suffers from Hirschsprung's disease. This disease develops when neural crest cells fail to migrate to the distal colon. Enteric neurons do not form in a segment of the rectosigmoid; these neurons are normally responsible for relaxation of the rectum to allow defecation. These patients present in infancy with abdominal distention, prolonged passage of meconium, absent or infrequent bowel movements, and poor nutrition/weight gain. The barium enema also suggests Hirschsprung's disease, as these patients typically have a narrow segment in the rectosigmoid with a massively dilated segment above this narrowing. A full-thickness biopsy showing absence of enteric neurons in the rectum and possibly sigmoid colon would provide a definitive diagnosis.

Answer B is incorrect. Motor function to the external anal sphincter is provided via the pudendal nerve. Defects in this nerve would lead to involuntary defecation with a full rectum.

Answer C is incorrect. The pelvic nerve regulates the defecation reflex, in which a full rectum brings about relaxation of the internal anal sphincter and constriction of the external anal sphincter, leading to the urge to defecate.

Answer D is incorrect. Sympathetic nerves stop colonic movements. Thus, absent sympathetic innervation would actually increase colonic movement.

Answer E is incorrect. The vagus nerve causes contractions in the proximal colon. The absence of the vagus effect on the colon would decrease defecation but would not lead to increased stool in the sigmoid colon.

19. **The correct answer is D.** A patient reporting "the worst headache of my life" along with the finding of blood that cannot be scraped from the surface of the brain is consistent with a subarachnoid hemorrhage, most commonly from a ruptured aneurysm. Blood trapped under (sub) the arachnoid mater cannot be scraped off when the dura mater is removed.

Answer A is incorrect. An epidural hemorrhage is generally caused by severe head trauma and damage to the middle meningeal artery. If the bony calvarium with the dura attached is removed, an epidural (above the dura) hemorrhage would be removed, and one would not see blood on the surface of the brain. The blood in an epidural hemorrhage is between the dura and the cranium.

Answer B is incorrect. The dura mater is a thick, fibrous structure of dense connective tissue without space for a significant amount of blood to pool. Blood collects either above or below the dura but not within it.

Answer C is incorrect. An intraparenchymal hemorrhage such as those caused by chronic hypertension would not appear as blood on the surface of the brain. It would likely be deeper in the brain, closer to the cerebral arteries. An intraparenchymal hemorrhage appears more like a bruise of the brain tissue and less like a frank pool of blood, as described in the vignette.

Answer E is incorrect. A subdural hemorrhage is defined as a hemorrhage under the dura mater that is caused by damage to bridging veins. There is a potential space between the dura mater and the arachnoid mater. When the calvarium is removed and the dura is adherent to the bony calvarium, this space is exposed, and any blood there should be readily scraped off. Blood that cannot be scraped off must be under still another layer, and the next layer under the dura is the arachnoid mater.

20. **The correct answer is D.** The basic theory of operant conditioning is that behavior can be modified through reward or punishment. Positive reinforcement is used to increase a desired behavior through a reward system. Negative reinforcement also supports a desired behavior, but instead of a reward, it is the removal of an aversive stimulus that increases the behavior. The flip side of operant conditioning is punishment, which suppresses an undesired behavior.

Answer A is incorrect. Aversive conditioning is a part of classical conditioning. Unwanted behaviors are paired with noxious and thus aversive stimuli.

Answer B is incorrect. Classical conditioning is learning in which a natural response is elicited by a conditioned stimulus that was previously presented in conjunction with an unconditioned stimulus. This is programming by association, not reward.

Answer C is incorrect. Learned helplessness is created through aversive conditioning, which is an example of classical conditioning.

Answer E is incorrect. Stimulus generalization is part of classical conditioning. This occurs when a new stimulus that is similar to an old stimulus elicits the same response.

21. **The correct answer is F.** This patient's history and physical exam findings are consistent with Bell's palsy, which is an acute peripheral facial nerve palsy of unknown cause. The symptoms seen in this patient can be easily understood if one remembers the different nerve fibers carried by the facial nerve (cranial nerve VII): af-ferent taste fibers from the anterior two-thirds of the ipsilateral tongue (decreased taste sensation), general touch and pain sensory fibers from a small area around the ipsilateral ear (retroauricular pain), and motor fibers to the muscles of facial expression (ipsilateral facial paralysis) and stapedius muscle (increased sensitivity to noise in the ipsilateral ear due to weakness of the stapedius muscle). This patient may also experience dryness in her ipsilateral (right) eye because the facial nerve carries parasympathetic fibers to the ipsilateral lacrimal gland, which provides lubrication to the eye. In addition, weakness of the facial muscles prevents complete eye closure, exacerbating the eye dryness. Patients with facial nerve paralysis should be given lubricating eye drops and instructed to tape their eye closed at night. While facial nerve paralysis can be caused by head trauma, AIDS, Lyme disease, sarcoidosis, or brainstem lesions, in most cases no cause is discovered and the diagnosis of Bell's palsy is made.

Answer A is incorrect. Decreased sensation of the left cheek could be caused by lesion of the left maxillary division of the trigeminal nerve (CN V_2); however, this patient shows signs of facial nerve palsy and shows no signs of trigeminal nerve involvement.

Answer B is incorrect. Decreased sensation on the right cheek could be caused by lesion of the right maxillary division of the trigeminal nerve (CN V_2); however, this patient shows signs of facial nerve palsy and shows no signs of trigeminal nerve involvement.

Answer C is incorrect. Lesion of the right vagus nerve would lead to deviation of the uvula and soft palate to the left; however, all signs and symptoms in this case suggest damage to the facial nerve (CN VII) and not the vagus nerve (CN X).

Answer D is incorrect. Unilateral lesions of the vagus nerve or nucleus ambiguus prevent elevation of the uvula on that side and thus cause the uvula and soft palate to deviate away from the side with the lesion due to unopposed action from the normal side. A lesion of the left vagus nerve would cause the uvula and soft palate to deviate to the right; however, the patient in this case has symptoms indicating palsy of the facial nerve (CN VII), not the vagus nerve (CN X).

Answer E is incorrect. The facial nerve carries sensory and motor fibers that innervate the ipsilateral face; thus, a lower motor nerve palsy of the facial nerve would cause dryness of the ipsilateral (right), not contralateral (left), eye.

22. **The correct answer is A.** Temporal lobe lesions or injuries can cause damage to the lower division of the geniculocalcarine tract, which is known as Meyer's loop. These radiations contain input from the inferior retinal quadrants and therefore represent the superior visual field quadrants. Since the lesion is behind the optic chiasm, the resulting deficit would be a contralateral upper quadrantanopia.

Answer B is incorrect. Left hemianopia with macular sparing would result from injury to the right visual cortex, which is located on the banks of the calcarine fissure.

Answer C is incorrect. Left lower quadrantanopia would result from injury to the neuronal radiations projecting to the superior bank of the calcarine sulcus.

Answer D is incorrect. Right upper quadrantanopia would result from injury to Meyer's loop on the left side, not the right side, since damage to the loop results in contralateral upper quadrantanopia.

Answer E is incorrect. Right hemianopia with macular sparing would result from injury to the left visual cortex.

Answer F is incorrect. Right lower quadrantanopia would result from injury to the neuronal projections to the superior bank of the calcarine sulcus on the left side, not the right side, since damage in this region results in contralateral lower quadrantanopia.

23. **The correct answer is B.** Humor is appreciating the amusing nature of an anxiety-provoking or adverse situation. The patient attempted to humiliate the doctor, but the situation is relayed to others in an amusing fashion. This is the only **mature** defense mechanism among the answer choices.

Answer A is incorrect. Dissociation is a temporary, drastic change in personality, memory, consciousness, or motor behavior that is used to avoid emotional stress. This is an immature defense mechanism.

Answer C is incorrect. Identification is an immature defense mechanism whereby a person models his behavior after someone that may have caused him stress or harm. For example, an abused child grows up to subsequently become an abuser himself.

Answer D is incorrect. Projection is the attribution of an unacceptable internal impulse to an external source. This is an immature defense mechanism.

Answer E is incorrect. Reaction formation is the process whereby a warded-off idea or feeling is replaced by an unconsciously derived emphasis on its opposite. This is an immature defense mechanism.

24. **The correct answer is A.** This specimen is taken from the patient's substantia nigra and demonstrates a typical melanin-containing neuron with pink-staining inclusions known as Lewy bodies. These are aggregations of the protein alpha-synuclein that are primarily seen in two neurologic diseases: Parkinson's disease and Lewy body dementia. Since this patient had no symptoms of dementia, the only remaining option is Parkinson's disease, which is characterized by resting tremor, cogwheel rigidity, bradykinesia, and postural instability.

Answer B is incorrect. Seizures are associated with many neurologic disorders but do not correlate with any particular histopathologic findings, especially Lewy bodies.

Answer C is incorrect. Myoclonic fasciculations are classically seen in Creutzfeldt-Jacob disease.

Answer D is incorrect. Symmetric muscle weakness is seen in Guillain-Barré syndrome and amyotrophic lateral sclerosis; Lewy bodies are not evident in either disease.

Answer E is incorrect. Tongue fasciculations are classically seen in degenerative neurologic diseases such as spinal muscular atrophy and amyotrophic lateral sclerosis.

25. **The correct answer is E.** The recurrent laryngeal nerve is the most commonly damaged nerve in thyroid surgery. It supplies all of the intrinsic laryngeal muscles except the cricothyroid muscle, which is innervated by the external laryngeal nerve. Injury will lead to paralysis of the vocal folds and hoarseness.

Answer A is incorrect. The accessory nerve supplies the pharyngeal constrictors, which constrict the pharynx during swallowing, and the palatopharyngeus and salpingopharyngeus muscles, which elevate the pharynx and larynx during swallowing and speaking.

Answer B is incorrect. The external laryngeal nerve is a branch of the superior laryngeal nerve and supplies motor innovation of the cricothyroid muscle. This nerve stretches and tenses the vocal folds, and injury may cause some hoarseness. This injury is less common than injury to the recurrent laryngeal nerve in thyroid surgery.

Answer C is incorrect. The glossopharyngeal nerve innervates the stylopharyngeus muscle, which elevates the pharynx and larynx when swallowing and speaking.

Answer D is incorrect. The internal laryngeal nerve is a branch of the superior laryngeal nerve, which supplies sensory and autonomic innervation to the larynx. Paralysis of this nerve causes anesthesia of the laryngeal mucosa.

26. **The correct answer is C.** Babinski's reflex is elicited when the plantar surface of the foot is firmly stroked. In response, the big toe dorsiflexes and the other toes fan out. This reflex usually disappears by the time an infant is 12 months of age but can reappear as a result of injury later in life.

Answer A is incorrect. At 1 month of age, infants should still have most if not all of the reflexes present at birth, including Babinski's, palmar, rooting, startle (Moro), and tracking.

Answer B is incorrect. At 6 months of age, infants usually retain Babinski's reflex but have lost the palmar, rooting, and startle reflexes.

Answer D is incorrect. By 24 months of age, Babinski's reflex should have disappeared. The presence of Babinski's reflex at this age should be considered abnormal.

Answer E is incorrect. By 48 months of age, Babinski's reflex should have disappeared. The presence of Babinski's reflex at this age should be considered abnormal.

27. **The correct answer is A.** This description of findings is consistent with the diagnosis of Gerstmann's syndrome, which results from damage to the visual association cortex (angular gyrus) and results in a cluster of four findings: (1) right-left confusion; (2) finger agnosia (inability to identify fingers by name); (3) agraphia without alexia (patients can read but not write); and (4) acalculia (difficulty with mathematical operations). Injury to the underlying visual radiations may also result in contralateral homonymous hemianopia or lower quadrantanopia.

Answer B is incorrect. Damage to the left posterior inferior frontal lobe could be expected to result in Broca's (expressive) aphasia and possibly brachiofacial weakness.

Answer C is incorrect. Damage to the left posterior superior temporal gyrus could be expected to result in Wernicke's (fluent/receptive) aphasia and may involve visual field deficits.

Answer D is incorrect. Injury to the left sylvian region may result in global aphasia as well as hemianopia and hemiplegia. Isolated posterior sylvian region involvement may result in conduction aphasia (poor repetition with good comprehension and fluent speech).

Answer E is incorrect. Injury to the left temporoparieto-occipital junction could result in transcortical sensory aphasia, which involves poor comprehension, good repetition, and nonfluent speech.

28. The correct answer is C. Patients with generalized anxiety disorder (GAD) have uncontrollable anxiety unrelated to a specific person, situation, or event. In order for the diagnosis to be made, the patient must have experienced uncontrollable anxiety or worry out of proportion to his or her life events for more days than not over the past 6 months or more. They also need three or more of the following symptoms: fatigability, irritability, distractibility, decreased sleep or quality of sleep, muscle tension, or restlessness. This patient complains of fatigue, insomnia, difficulty concentrating, and irritability in addition to generalized anxiety. Affected patients respond well to behavioral therapy and treatment with antidepressants and buspirone. Benzodiazepines can be used for short-term management but are not recommended for long-term management because of their addictive potential. GAD is often a chronic disease, but it can be controlled. Comorbid depression is common in GAD.

Answer A is incorrect. Adult attention-deficit/hyperactivity disorder (ADHD) is becoming recognized as an underdiagnosed condition; however, this patient has not developed the degree of impairment that would be expected with ADHD. Her complaints are of difficulty concentrating and irritability, which can be characteristic of ADHD, but she is not complaining of difficulty at work, which can be a hallmark of adult ADHD.

Answer B is incorrect. Patients with avoidant personality disorder are sensitive to rejection, socially inhibited, and timid with overwhelming feelings of inadequacy. There is a genetic association with anxiety disorders. This patient has a job as a public relations officer, which makes her unlikely to be suffering from a socially phobic personality disorder.

Answer D is incorrect. Patients with obsessive-compulsive disorder do display a fair amount of anxiety; however, that anxiety is diminished by the performance of certain tasks that must be completed.

Answer E is incorrect. Patients with social phobia disorder are anxious and nervous in social situations. This patient has a job with a significant social component in which she has been very successful.

29. The correct answer is B. This patient is suffering from attacks of vertigo that last for more than an hour, which may result from either Ménière's disease or migraine headaches. These can be distinguished based on the presence of auditory dysfunction. Ménière's disease is an idiopathic disorder that typically affects people between the ages of 30 and 60 and involves episodes of vertigo lasting for a period of hours with associated fluctuation and progressive low-frequency sensorineural hearing loss accompanied by aural fullness or pressure (tinnitus); the disease ultimately affects both ears in nearly half of patients. Ménière's disease is the result of an increase in the volume of the endolymphatic system (hydrops) secondary to malfunction of the endolymphatic sac, which is responsible for the filtration and excretion of endolymphatic fluid.

Answer A is incorrect. Damage to the cochlea could result in sensorineural hearing loss, as that seen in this patient, but would not result in vertigo.

Answer C is incorrect. Benign paroxysmal positional vertigo (BPPV) is another disease associated with vertiginous symptoms, wherein symptoms are caused by freely moving crystals of calcium carbonate within the semicircular canals. However, the episodes in BPPV last only seconds and are associated with nystagmus.

Answer D is incorrect. The utricle and saccule are responsible for reacting to acceleration and deceleration of the head rather than rotatory movement. Damage to these organs involves the feeling that one is tilted and/or their environment is tilted or even upside down. These patients tend to fall toward the side of the lesion.

Answer E is incorrect. Damage to the vestibulocochlear nerve would also result in sensorineural hearing loss, and potentially equilibrium disturbances, but would not present with the classic triad of Ménière's symptoms, nor would presentation include low-frequency sensorineural hearing loss. Patients with cranial nerve VIII lesions have impairment in the high-frequency range and exhibit problems with speech discrimination.

30. **The correct answer is A.** The genioglossus muscle is one of many muscles of the tongue required for lingual sounds; all are innervated by the hypoglossal nerve.

    Answer B is incorrect. The genioglossus muscle is required for lingual phonation; however, it is innervated by the hypoglossal nerve, not the vagus.

    Answer C is incorrect. The palatoglossus is the only muscle with the name "glossus" that is innervated by the vagus nerve (X). All other glossus muscles are innervated by the hypoglossal nerve (XII).

    Answer D is incorrect. This muscle/nerve pairing is the only other correct pairing. However, the palatoglossus muscle elevates the soft palate and plays little role in lingual sounds (lah).

    Answer E is incorrect. The styloglossus muscle is required for proper movement of the tongue; however, like all other glossus muscles with the exception of the palatoglossus, it is innervated by cranial nerve XII, the hypoglossal nerve. The glossopharyngeal nerve (IX) does not have somatic motor function; lesions affect somatic sensory and taste, not motor function of the tongue.

31. **The correct answer is E.** Guillain-Barré syndrome is an autoimmune disease mediated by antibodies that target components of Schwann cells in the peripheral nervous system (PNS). Schwann cells are flattened cells with cytoplasm that contain a flattened nucleus, a small Golgi apparatus, and a few mitochondria. These cells form both myelinated and unmyelinated coverings over axons of the PNS. Schwann cells myelinate neurons in the peripheral nervous tissue; however, they do not myelinate axons of the central nervous system (CNS). Guillain-Barré syndrome normally presents with ascending weakness or paralysis, most often 2–4 weeks after a respiratory or gastrointestinal infection. *Campylobacter jejuni* in particular is very strongly associated with the disease. About 25% of patients require respiratory support as the paralysis ascends over hours to days, but symptoms usually subside over the ensuing weeks. Current treatment options include intravenous immunoglobulin or plasmapheresis, both of which diminish autoantibody levels. Corticosteroids are not effective.

    Answer A is incorrect. Lower motor neurons are not directly targeted by the autoantibodies in Guillain-Barré syndrome; however, the loss of myelin leads to the lower motor neuron dysfunction and degeneration that are responsible for the disease symptoms.

    Answer B is incorrect. Upper motor neurons are not targeted by autoantibodies in Guillain-Barré syndrome. Upper motor neurons can degenerate after infection by the poliovirus—the resulting asymmetric paralysis can lead to permanent paralysis. The Salk (dead) and Sabin (live) vaccines both inoculate against this infection.

    Answer C is incorrect. Muscle is not directly targeted in this condition, although it does atrophy in response to denervation. Myasthenia gravis is an autoimmune disorder in which autoantibodies target acetylcholine receptors at the neuromuscular junction. The disease most often presents with muscle weakness intensified by muscle use, particular in the extraocular and facial muscles. Treatment includes drugs that block acetylcholinesterase, such as pyridostigmine.

    Answer D is incorrect. Oligodendrocytes function in electrical insulation and in myelin production in the central nervous system, but not the peripheral nervous system. These cells are destroyed in multiple sclerosis, which is considered by many to be an autoimmune condition. Oligodendrocyte myelin differs in composition to the myelin of Schwann cells, however, and is not targeted in Guillain-Barré syndrome.

32. The correct answer is C. This patient is presenting with progressive multifocal leukoencephalopathy (PML), which is caused by the JC virus in patients with AIDS. PML is a reactivation of a dormant virus to which the patient has previously been exposed. Initial findings include neurological deficits of speech, memory, and coordination. Vision problems are also common. The disease causes a very rapid decline in neurological function resulting in coma and death. The 3-week course for this patient is not uncommon. The disease causes multiple areas of demyelination throughout the white matter of the central nervous system. There is no specific treatment for PML, but some patients have shown some clinical improvement with the initiation of highly active antiretroviral therapy.

Answer A is incorrect. *Cryptococcus neoformans* is a common cause of meningitis in patients with HIV/AIDS. The classic meningitis triad of fever, headache, and nuchal rigidity are usually present. Abnormalities on cerebrospinal fluid examination would also be present.

Answer B is incorrect. Herpes simplex virus can cause temporal lobe encephalitis in patients with HIV/AIDS. It is also seen in the general population but at a lower frequency. Rapid onset of fever and focal neurological deficits are the most common presenting features. Deficits often stem from damage to the temporal lobe and can include memory problems, personality changes, and potentially seizures.

Answer D is incorrect. *Pneumocystis jiroveci* (formerly *carinii*) is a common cause of pneumonia in patients with HIV whose CD4 counts are < 200 cells/μL. On x-ray of the chest, the classic picture is one of "ground glass," although other radiological features are also common.

Answer E is incorrect. Toxoplasmosis is the most common cause of encephalitis in patients with HIV/AIDS and is seen mostly in patients with a CD4 count < 100 cells/μL. The most common manifestation of toxoplasmosis is seizures and headache, although other focal neurological deficits may be seen. The classic radiological picture is one or more ring-enhancing lesions with surrounding edema.

33. The correct answer is A. The history, physical exam, and MRI findings are consistent with the diagnosis of syringomyelia, which may be primary (Arnold-Chiari malformation) or acquired as a result of trauma, tumor, or inflammation. Arnold-Chiari malformations involve downward herniation of the cerebellar tonsils into the foramen magnum and are often associated with syringomyelia. Type II Arnold-Chiari malformations are always associated with spina bifida, whereas type I malformations are not. Therefore, a type I malformation is the most appropriate diagnosis. Syringomyelia consists of an enlargement of the central canal of the spinal cord, most commonly occurring at C8–T1. Crossing fibers of the spinothalamic tract are damaged (loss of pain and temperature sensation) with preserved dorsal column function (intact position and vibration sense).

Answer B is incorrect. Type II Arnold-Chiari malformations are associated with spina bifida; type I Arnold-Chiari malformations have no such association. Although both types are associated with syringomyelia, the fact that the patient has no prior medical history of spina bifida means that this patient has a type I malformation.

Answer C is incorrect. Communicating hydrocephalus occurs as a result of a blockage of cerebrospinal fluid outside the brain and is typically associated with malfunctioning arachnoid villi. This diagnosis would show ventricular enlargement on MRI.

Answer D is incorrect. Congenital aqueductal stenosis is a common cause of congenital hydrocephalus and would present very early in life.

Answer E is incorrect. Dandy-Walker syndrome is a congenital noncommunicating hydrocephalus typically associated with a cluster of abnormal findings that include abnormal formation of the cerebellar vermis. This condition leads to obstruction of the outlet foramina of Luschka and Magendie.

34. **The correct answer is B.** In zero-order elimination, the concentration of a drug decreases linearly with time. If the concentrate ion of the drug was 50 μg/mL and 30 μg/mL at 1 and 2 hours, respectively, then the rate of elimination is 20 μg/mL/hr. Therefore, at 3 hours there would be 10 μg/mL remaining.

    Answer A is incorrect. Calculation error.

    Answer C is incorrect. Calculation error.

    Answer D is incorrect. Calculation error.

    Answer E is incorrect. Calculation error.

35. **The correct answer is D.** Tranylcypromine is a nonselective monoamine oxidase inhibitor and may lead to serotonin syndrome if taken with selective serotonin reuptake inhibitors (SSRIs) due to an overall increase in serotonin. Serotonin syndrome is characterized by mental status changes, autonomic changes (e.g., fever, diaphoresis, tachycardia), and neuromuscular changes (e.g., tremor or rigidity).

    Answer A is incorrect. Citalopram is a selective serotonin reuptake inhibitor associated with anxiety, insomnia, tremor, and nausea.

    Answer B is incorrect. Lithium intake has been associated with tremor, hypothyroidism, and nephrogenic diabetes insipidus.

    Answer C is incorrect. Nortriptyline is a tricyclic antidepressant associated with the "3 C's": Convulsions, Coma, and Cardiotoxicity.

    Answer E is incorrect. Trazodone is a heterocyclic associated with sedation, nausea, priapism, and postural hypotension.

36. **The correct answer is D.** A midshaft fracture of the humerus could cause injury to the structures found in the radial groove: the radial nerve and the deep brachial artery.

    Answer A is incorrect. The anterior and posterior circumflex humeral artery would be damaged by injury to the surgical neck of the humerus.

Answer B is incorrect. The axillary nerve is damaged by injury to the surgical neck of the humerus.

Answer C is incorrect. The median nerve is damaged by injury to the distal end of the humerus.

Answer E is incorrect. The ulnar nerve can be damaged by injury to the medial epicondyle of the humerus.

37. **The correct answer is A.** The patient is exhibiting extrapyramidal adverse effects associated with neuroleptic use. Of the choices listed, only chlorpromazine is a neuroleptic. Typical antipsychotics work by decreasing the amount of dopamine available in the brain; the extrapyramidal adverse effects are the result of blocking the dopamine receptors.

    Answer B is incorrect. Imipramine is a tricyclic antidepressant associated with the "3 C's": Convulsions, Coma, and Cardiotoxicity.

    Answer C is incorrect. Lithium intake has been associated with tremor, hypothyroidism, and nephrogenic diabetes insipidus.

    Answer D is incorrect. Sertraline is a selective serotonin reuptake inhibitor associated with anxiety, insomnia, tremor, and nausea. It may lead to serotonin syndrome that may be characterized by a progression of headaches, dizziness, vomiting, coma, and death if taken with monoamine oxidase inhibitors.

    Answer E is incorrect. Trazodone is a heterocyclic associated with sedation, nausea, priapism, and postural hypotension.

38. **The correct answer is A.** This description is consistent with Broca's (expressive) aphasia, which is classically characterized by both comprehension without fluency and difficulty finding certain words. This aphasia is consistent with damage to the dominant inferior frontal gyrus. In contrast to patients with Wernicke's aphasia, Broca's patients have insight into their condition.

    Answer B is incorrect. Conduction aphasia results from damage to the arcuate fasciculus, which connects Brodmann's speech area with Wernicke's speech area. It is characterized by fluent speech with intact comprehension but poor repetition.

Answer C is incorrect. Global aphasia results from perisylvian lesions that encompass both Broca's and Wernicke's areas. Clinically, a combination of symptoms from both Broca's and Wernicke's aphasia results.

Answer D is incorrect. Thalamic aphasia involves fluent paraphasic speech with preserved comprehension and repetition. It can closely resemble a thought disorder of schizophrenic patients.

Answer E is incorrect. Transcortical motor aphasia is similar to Broca's aphasia but involves preserved repetition with good comprehension and nonfluent speech.

Answer F is incorrect. Transcortical sensory aphasia is similar to Wernicke's aphasia but involves preserved repetition with fluent speech and poor comprehension.

Answer G is incorrect. Wernicke's aphasia is a fluent aphasia that consists of impaired comprehension and repetition with marked paraphasia.

39. **The correct answer is A.** Physostigmine antagonizes the action of anticholinergics, which block the postsynaptic receptor sites of acetylcholine. Physostigmine reversibly inhibits the destruction of acetylcholine by acetylcholinesterase, thereby increasing the concentration of acetylcholine at sites of cholinergic transmission and counteracting the effects of the anticholinergics.

Answer B is incorrect. Bethanechol is a direct acetylcholine receptor agonist that acts more potently at muscarinic than at nicotinic receptors. It has little susceptibility to cholinesterase. Bethanechol is indicated for use with neurogenic ileus and urinary retention.

Answer C is incorrect. Echothiophate is an organophosphate cholinesterase inhibitor and therefore also acts to increase available acetylcholine. Because it is more stable in aqueous

solution than other organophosphates, it is indicated for use in glaucoma.

Answer D is incorrect. Neostigmine is also an anticholinergic antagonist. Like physostigmine, it would increase levels of acetylcholine by inhibiting the action of acetylcholinesterase in the synapse.

Answer E is incorrect. Pralidoxime is used to rescue the activity of cholinesterases following organophosphate poisoning. It therefore decreases levels of acetylcholine in the synapse. However, because it acts specifically to break the cholinesterase-phosphate bond created by the organophosphate, it has no effect in the absence of the organophosphate poison.

40. **The correct answer is A.** This patient is suffering from cluster headaches, which are repetitive headaches that occur for weeks to months at a time with intervening periods of remission. Men are affected more than women, with a peak incidence in persons 25–50 years old. Attacks begin without any prodromal symptoms, typically around the eye or temple, and are excruciating in quality. They are always unilateral and may last for minutes to hours, with a mean duration of 45 minutes. In contrast to patients with migraines, who favor remaining in a dark, quiet room, cluster headache patients typically prefer to stay active. Treatment is difficult because of the short duration of symptoms, but effective options include oxygen, intranasal lidocaine, and triptans. Prophylaxis may consist of treatment with prednisone, verapamil, or methysergide for 1–2 months.

Answer B is incorrect. Medication-overuse headaches are secondary to excessive use of analgesia and may occur in patients who have tension, migraine, or cluster headaches. The diagnosis should be considered in patients who have frequent or daily headaches despite the use of medications. Although this patient is taking over-the-counter medications, the periodicity of the headaches precludes the regular administration of analgesia, which would be necessary for the consideration of this diagnosis.

Answer C is incorrect. Migraine headaches can be preceded by prodromal symptoms and can also be bilateral in nature. Typically, the headaches gain in severity and can last from 10–12 hours. They may be associated with nausea and vomiting. Frequently, such patients have a family history of migraine. Effective treatment involves use of triptans.

Answer D is incorrect. A headache induced by temporomandibular joint dysfunction syndrome is a result of masticatory system dysfunction and frequently presents with unilateral ear or auricular pain radiating to the jaw. The pain is deep and continuous, is most severe in the morning, and can be associated with jaw dysfunction. Treatment is aimed at the underlying joint malfunction.

Answer E is incorrect. Tension headaches are the most common headache syndrome but typically present with pain that is bifrontal and "squeezing." They may be accompanied by nausea but not by vomiting or photophobia and are not preceded by prodromal symptoms. Acetaminophen and nonsteroidal anti-inflammatory drugs are typically effective for relief.

41. **The correct answer is B.** Patients with disorganized schizophrenia have disorganized speech and behavior as well as an inappropriate affect. They are frequently childlike. They are usually incapable of mustering complete delusions. This subtype is associated with a poor long-term prognosis.

Answer A is incorrect. Patients with catatonic schizophrenia are characterized by extreme stupor (most famously "waxy flexibility"), bizarre voluntary movements, and echolalia or echopraxia. This subtype is uncommon.

Answer C is incorrect. Patients with paranoid schizophrenia are characterized primarily by their delusions and hallucinations. They can frequently be quite angry and aggressive. In general, they are not as disorganized as other subtypes of schizophrenia.

Answer D is incorrect. Patients with residual schizophrenia have met the diagnostic criteria for schizophrenia in the past but are no longer actively psychotic (i.e., not actively delusional). These patients still retain some bizarre behavior patterns, bizarre speech patterns, or negative symptoms such as flat affect, social withdrawal, thought blocking, or lack of motivation.

Answer E is incorrect. Patients with undifferentiated schizophrenia show characteristics that are not exclusive to any one subtype. This is the most common presentation of schizophrenia.

42. **The correct answer is C.** The pudendal nerve arises from S2, S3, and S4 of the sacral plexus and innervates the structures of the perineum, including sensation of the genitalia. It runs with the pudendal artery through the greater sciatic foramen. A pudendal nerve block can alleviate perineal pain during childbirth; however, it will not affect pain from contractions.

Answer A is incorrect. The inferior gluteal nerve arises from L5, S1, and S2 of the sacral plexus and innervates the gluteus maximus. Numbing this nerve would not effectively relieve perineal pain from childbirth.

Answer B is incorrect. The obturator nerve arises from the lumbar plexus in the abdomen and enters the pelvis deep to the psoas major. Numbing this nerve would affect the muscles of the medial thigh and would not effectively relieve perineal pain from childbirth.

Answer D is incorrect. The sciatic nerve is the largest to the lower extremities, arising from L4 through S3. It passes through the greater sciatic foramen inferior to the piriformis. Numbing this nerve would not effectively relieve perineal pain from childbirth.

Answer E is incorrect. The superior gluteal nerve arises from L4, L5, and S1 of the sacral plexus and innervates the gluteus medius and minimus muscles. Numbing this nerve would not effectively relieve perineal pain from childbirth.

43. The correct answer is D. This classic drug response, called epinephrine reversal, is a favorite subject on the Step 1 examination. Epinephrine, a nonselective α- and β-adrenergic agonist, increases blood pressure. The unknown drug is an α-adrenergic antagonist such as phentolamine, which blocks epinephrine's vasoconstrictive action on arterioles. Subsequent administration of epinephrine produces only β-receptor stimulation, which causes vasodilation in skeletal muscle and leads to a decrease in blood pressure.

Answer A is incorrect. An acetylcholinesterase inhibitor should not affect the subsequent administration of epinephrine.

Answer B is incorrect. A nicotinic ganglionic blocker may prevent a potential decrease in heart rate due to baroreceptor reflexes, but epinephrine would still cause an increase in blood pressure because its access to end-organ receptors would be unaltered.

Answer C is incorrect. A nonselective α agonist would only enhance epinephrine's effect on blood pressure by activating its own pressor effect via α receptors.

Answer E is incorrect. A nonselective β-receptor antagonist would enhance epinephrine's increase in blood pressure. After administration of a β antagonist such as propranolol, epinephrine would produce only α-receptor stimulation, which would increase blood pressure.

44. The correct answer is A. Cluster C personality disorders include avoidant, obsessive-compulsive, and dependent; patients with these disorders are characterized as anxious or worried and have abnormal fears about relationships, separation, and control. There is a genetic association with anxiety disorders. Patients with avoidant personality disorder are sensitive to rejection, socially inhibited, and timid, with overwhelming feelings of inadequacy.

Answer B is incorrect. Patients with dependent personality disorder are submissive and clinging; they have low self-esteem and have an excessive need to be taken care of.

Answer C is incorrect. Patients with histrionic personality disorder display excessive emotionality, somatization, and attention-seeking and sexually provocative behavior.

Answer D is incorrect. Patients with narcissistic personality disorder are grandiose and have a sense of entitlement. They frequently demand the best of everything, including physicians and health care.

Answer E is incorrect. Patients with schizoid personality disorder exhibit voluntary social withdrawal and have limited emotional expressions.

Answer F is incorrect. Patients with schizotypal personality disorder demonstrate interpersonal awkwardness, odd thought patterns, and an odd appearance.

45. The correct answer is D. Neuroblastoma is the most commonly occurring tumor of the adrenal medulla in children, but it can occur anywhere along the sympathetic chain. This rapidly growing tumor is also the most common malignant solid tumor outside of the cranium in children. Wide metastasis and elevated urinary catecholamines are common in these patients. Children diagnosed at an age younger than 1 year have an improved prognosis; in fact, tumors can regress spontaneously in younger patients. The tumors frequently demonstrate areas of necrosis, hemorrhage, and calcification. Microscopic examination reveals malignant small cells in a pseudorosette pattern around nerve fibrils. Amplification of the n-*myc* oncogene can be seen in neuroblastoma. In fact, the greater the gene amplification, the more aggressive the tumor.

Answer A is incorrect. The *bcl-2* oncogene is associated with follicular and undifferentiated lymphomas.

Answer B is incorrect. The c-*myc* oncogene is associated with Burkitt's lymphoma.

Answer C is incorrect. The *erb*-B2 oncogene is associated with breast, ovarian, and gastric carcinomas.

Answer E is incorrect. The *ras* oncogene is associated with a number of cancers, including colon carcinoma.

46. **The correct answer is B.** Children with attention-deficit/hyperactivity disorder demonstrate persistent symptoms of inattention, hyperactivity, and impulsivity that have persisted for at least 6 months and are maladaptive and disruptive to the child's life. These children are often difficult to control in the classroom.

    Answer A is incorrect. Patients with antisocial personality disorder show a disregard for and violation of the rights of others, including a proclivity for criminal behavior. This is the only personality disorder with an age limit— patients must be above the age of 18. Minors with similar behavior are considered to have conduct disorder. This is the only conduct disorder in which males outnumber females.

    Answer C is incorrect. Bipolar disorder can be diagnosed in children; however, this patient is not exhibiting characteristics of bipolar disorder. This child is not experiencing cyclical changes in mood, although irritability can be a component of childhood depression.

    Answer D is incorrect. Conduct disorder can exist in children with attention-deficit/hyperactivity disorder, but at this point the patient is not exhibiting diagnostic characteristics such as aggression, destruction of property, deceitfulness, and serious violations of rules.

    Answer E is incorrect. Oppositional defiant disorder can also exist in children with attention-deficit/hyperactivity disorder, but the patient's mother is not complaining of characteristics of that disorder, which include frequent outbursts of temper, argumentative behavior, and defiance.

47. **The correct answer is E.** Spina bifida occulta is caused by failure of the posterior vertebral arches to close. Generally, there are no associated clinical abnormalities.

    Answer A is incorrect. Anencephaly occurs when the cephalic end of the neural tube fails to close, resulting in the absence of a major portion of the brain, skull, and scalp. Infants with this disorder are born without a forebrain and a cerebrum. The remaining brain tissue is often exposed.

    Answer B is incorrect. Meningocele occurs when there is herniation of the meninges through the spinal canal defect (i.e., subarachnoid space).

    Answer C is incorrect. Meningomyelocele occurs when there is herniation of the meninges and spinal cord through the spinal canal defect (i.e., subarachnoid space and spinal cord).

    Answer D is incorrect. Spina bifida cystica is caused by the failure of the posterior vertebral arches to close, along with external protrusion of a saclike structure. This is further classified according to the extent of neural involvement (e.g., meningocele, meningomyelocele, or myelomeningocele).

48. **The correct answer is A.** The description is consistent with internuclear ophthalmoplegia, which consists of medial rectus palsy on attempted lateral conjugate gaze with associated monocular horizontal nystagmus in the abducting eye with preserved convergence. It results from damage to the ipsilateral medial longitudinal fasciculus, which is the connection between the abducent and oculomotor nuclei, so that the two nerves' actions become unlinked. The third nerve and medial rectus muscle function normally in convergence but not during actions that require conjugate eye movements. In young patients, it is most commonly the result of central nervous system infection or multiple sclerosis, whereas in older patients it is more commonly the result of vascular disease.

    Answer B is incorrect. Although internuclear ophthalmoplegia involves medial rectus palsy on attempted lateral conjugate gaze, it is distinguished from pure medial rectus damage by observation of the eyes at rest. In medial rectus palsy, the affected eye looks "down and out" while at rest.

Answer C is incorrect. Pupillary light-near dissociation is also known as Argyll-Robertson pupil and is an absent miotic reaction to light with preserved accommodation. This condition can occur in neurosyphilis, diabetes, and systemic lupus erythematosus.

Answer D is incorrect. A relative afferent pupillary defect is also known as a Marcus Gunn pupil. It results from a lesion in the afferent limb of the pupillary light reflex and can be seen in the retrobulbar neuritis of multiple sclerosis. It would not result in medial rectus palsy on attempted lateral conjugate gaze.

Answer E is incorrect. A pure sixth-nerve palsy would have almost the opposite effect of this scenario and would cause a lateral rectus palsy as opposed to a medial rectus palsy.

49. **The correct answer is B.** Neurofibromatosis type 1 (NF1), or von Recklinghausen's disease, is one of the most common inherited disorders, with an incidence of 1 in 4000. The clinical hallmarks of the disease include café au lait spots, neurofibromas, and Lisch's nodules (pigmented hamartomas) of the iris. Neurofibromin, the NF1 gene product, is defective in this condition.

Answer A is incorrect. Brushfield's spots are found in the irises of patients with Down's syndrome.

Answer C is incorrect. Macro-orchidism, or large testicles, is an associated physical finding of fragile X syndrome.

Answer D is incorrect. Mitral valve prolapse is associated with adult polycystic kidney disease and Marfan's syndrome.

Answer E is incorrect. Tendon xanthomas, which present as raised yellow plaques full of lipid-laden macrophages, are found in patients with familial hypercholesterolemia.

50. **The correct answer is D.** Guillain-Barré syndrome is a demyelinating disease of peripheral nerves causing acute and progressive weakness. A major complication of Guillain-Barré syndrome is respiratory paralysis leading to hypoventilation. Hypoventilation leads to an inability of the lungs to excrete the carbon dioxide the body produces, leading to retention of carbon dioxide. This causes a drop in pH and a compensatory retention of bicarbonate. These acid-base abnormalities are consistent with respiratory acidosis. Hypoventilation (from a variety of etiologies) is a primary cause of respiratory acidosis.

Answer A is incorrect. An increase in anions would be consistent with anion-gap metabolic acidosis. Metabolic acidosis is indicated by the presence of low pH with low plasma bicarbonate and low carbon dioxide and an increased anion gap, measured by ($[Na^+] - [Cl^-] - [HCO_3^-]$), which is normally 10–16 mEq/L. The main causes are lactic acidosis, diabetic ketoacidosis, and renal failure.

Answer B is incorrect. Non–anion-gap metabolic acidosis is the presence of low pH with low plasma bicarbonate without an elevated anion gap. The cause is generally gastrointestinal losses of bicarbonate (i.e., diarrhea, biliary drains, emesis, nasogastric tube losses). Another important and common cause of a metabolic non–anion-gap acidosis is the presence of an ileal conduit or bladder reconstruction from colonic tissue. The gastrointestinal tissue absorbs Cl^- from the urine in exchange for bicarbonate. Other causes include renal tubular acidosis, or hypochloremia.

Answer C is incorrect. Metabolic alkalosis would present with a high pH, a high bicarbonate, and (with respiratory compensation) a high carbon dioxide. The causes of metabolic alkalosis include vomiting, diuretic therapy, and chloride restriction. The compensation is hypoventilation.

Answer E is incorrect. Respiratory alkalosis can be caused only by an increase in ventilation, leading to excessive loss of carbon dioxide that is balanced by an increased excretion of bicarbonate. Hence, a low carbon dioxide and low bicarbonate indicate respiratory alkalosis. This is caused by hyperventilation.

CHAPTER 12

Renal

1. Patients with renal artery stenosis may present with very high blood pressures due to increased renin secretion. Which of the following structures in the kidney is responsible for sensing inadequate perfusion and secreting renin?

   (A) Afferent arteriole
   (B) Collecting duct
   (C) Distal convoluted tubule
   (D) Efferent arteriole
   (E) Loop of Henle

2. A 48-year-old man is hospitalized for shock after massive blood loss in a motor vehicle accident. On the patient's second day in the hospital, his blood urea nitrogen and creatinine levels begin to rise and he develops pitting edema to his knees. A subsequent urinalysis shows numerous granular casts. Which of the following is the most appropriate treatment?

   (A) Angioplasty
   (B) Broad-spectrum antibiotics
   (C) Corticosteroids
   (D) Fluids and dialysis
   (E) Use of ultrasound to remove blockage

3. A 50-year-old man with a history of large bowel obstruction is diagnosed with colon cancer and undergoes resection of his colon. He returns to his physician for his regular checkup and complains that in the past 3 weeks he has not been feeling well and has noticed significant swelling of his legs. On physical examination, the physician notes 2+ pitting edema and a blood pressure of 155/94 mm Hg. Urinalysis shows 4+ protein with no RBCs or casts. Which of the following would most likely be present on a kidney biopsy from this patient?

   (A) A spike-and-dome pattern of deposition on electron microscopy
   (B) A tram-track pattern on electron microscopy
   (C) A tram-track pattern on light microscopy

   (D) Lumpy subepithelial deposits on light microscopy
   (E) Nonlinear mesangial staining with IgA immunofluorescence

4. Respiratory acidosis is a major complication in morphine overdoses. Which of the sets of laboratory data in the table correspond to a pure respiratory acidosis?

Choice	pH	P_{CO_2} (mm Hg)	HCO_3^- (mEq/L)	Na^+ (mEq/L)	Cl^- (mEq/L)
A	7.2	42	15	140	89
B	7.2	42	15	140	114
C	7.2	68	15	140	104
D	7.2	68	25	140	104
E	7.4	68	12	140	89
F	7.6	42	20	140	104
G	7.6	68	18	140	104

   (A) A
   (B) B
   (C) C
   (D) D
   (E) E
   (F) F
   (G) G

5. Monitoring acid-base status is very important in individuals with kidney pathology. Which of the following diuretics causes metabolic alkalosis?

   (A) Acetazolamide and potassium-sparing diuretics
   (B) Loop diuretics and acetazolamide

(C) Loop diuretics and potassium-sparing diuretics

(D) Loop diuretics and thiazides

(E) Thiazides and acetazolamide

(F) Thiazides and potassium-sparing diuretics

6. A 25-year-old man comes to the emergency department with bloody sputum. A few weeks later he progresses to renal failure with significant hematuria and hypertension. A renal biopsy shows linear immunofluorescence. Which of the following types of hypersensitivity reaction is this patient experiencing?

(A) Type I hypersensitivity

(B) Type II hypersensitivity

(C) Type III hypersensitivity

(D) Type IV hypersensitivity

(E) Type V hypersensitivity

7. Acid-base disturbances are seen frequently in the clinical setting. Knowing the most common causes of these disorders is imperative. Which of the following is a cause of metabolic acidosis?

(A) Diarrhea

(B) Loop diuretics

(C) Massive volume loss with hypokalemia

(D) Thiazide diuretics

(E) Vomiting

8. A 28-year-old woman who is 6 months pregnant presents to the emergency department with a temperature of 38.2° C (100.8° F) and complaints of chills and pain on her right side, which she locates by pointing to the area above her right iliac crest. She has a history of recurrent urinary tract infections. During the examination, the physician taps on the area over the junction of the lower ribs and the thoracic vertebrae. The patient winces and pulls away in pain. Urinalysis indicates white blood cell casts in the urine. Which of the following is the most likely diagnosis?

(A) Abdominal aortic aneurysm

(B) Compression fracture of lower thoracic vertebrae

(C) Localized cystitis

(D) Premature labor

(E) Pyelonephritis

9. A 64-year-old man presents to his primary care physician for a routine physical. He is in good health, smokes half a pack of cigarettes a day, and has no concomitant medical problems, but he tells the physician that he has been diagnosed with hypertension in the past. In the course of his physical examination, the physician notes a blood pressure of 160/100 mm Hg and 1+ pitting edema to his knees. He also notes bilateral bruits heard best from the costophrenic angle at approximately T11. Which of the following is contraindicated in this patient's care?

(A) Angioplasty

(B) Angiotensin-converting enzyme inhibitor

(C) Diuretics

(D) Smoking cessation

(E) Surgical management

10. A 2-month-old infant is found to have a horseshoe kidney. Which structure prevents this abnormal kidney from being appropriately located?

(A) Aorta

(B) Celiac trunk

(C) Inferior mesenteric artery

(D) Inferior vena cava

(E) Superior mesenteric artery

11. A 23-year-old man is being treated with chemotherapy for leukemia when he develops severe intermittent left flank pain. Three days later, the patient begins to experience acute renal failure. His fractional excretion of sodium is calculated to be > 4% with urine osmolality of > 350 mOsm/kg. Blood and urine cultures are negative for bacteria and eosinophilia. A renal stone is suspected, but an abdominal radiograph fails to locate any pathology. Which of the following is the most likely location of the lesion causing this patient's renal failure?

(A) Glomeruli

(B) Interstitium of the kidney

(C) Kidney tubules

(D) Left ureter

(E) Urethra

12. A 68-year-old white woman recovering from a total hip replacement following a fall at home is administered ketorolac for the management of pain. Twenty-four hours later, her urine production decreases and her serum blood urea nitrogen and creatinine levels rise to 64 mg/dL and 2.5 mg/dL, respectively. Which of the following describes the mechanism through which nonsteroidal anti-inflammatory drugs such as ketorolac can cause acute renal failure?

(A) Inhibition of renal prostaglandin production and constriction of the afferent arteriole

(B) Inhibition of renal prostaglandin production and constriction of the efferent arteriole

(C) Inhibition of renal prostaglandin production and significant dilation of glomerular efferent arterioles

(D) Stimulation of renal prostaglandin production and reflex arteriolar vasoconstriction

(E) Stimulation of renal prostaglandin production and reflex arteriolar vasodilation

13. A 56-year-old man with a 60–pack-year smoking history and normal fluid intake presents to his physician with 2 months of fatigue and weakness accompanied by cough and mild dyspnea. The patient's vital signs are normal, but a lower left lobe mass is noted on x-ray of the chest. Biopsy leads to the diagnosis of small cell carcinoma. Relevant laboratory studies are as follows:

Plasma Na^+: 125 mEq/L
Plasma K^+: 3.9 mEq/L
Plasma CO_2: 24 mEq/L
Plasma osmolality: 253 mOsm/L
Urine Na^+: 48 mEq/L
Urine osmolality: 280 mOsm/L

The hormone most likely responsible for this patient's abnormal laboratory values has which of the following direct effects?

(A) Activation of G protein–coupled receptors in the adrenal cortex elevates cAMP levels and leads to increased production and secretion of corticosteroids

(B) Activation of G protein–coupled receptors in the hypothalamus results in elevated cAMP levels and inhibition of hypothalamic-induced thirst mechanism

(C) Activation of V2 receptors leads to an increase in total peripheral resistance; activation of V1 receptors results in the concentration of urine

(D) Activation of V2 receptors results in the insertion of aquaporins into the collecting duct; activation of V1 receptors leads to a decrease in total peripheral resistance

(E) Activation of V2 receptors results in the insertion of aquaporins into the renal collecting duct; activation of V1 receptors leads to an increase in total peripheral resistance

(F) Cleavage of angiotensinogen to angiotensin I leads to an increase in both aldosterone levels and total peripheral resistance

14. A 24-year-old man who is in the hospital for treatment of a severe gram-negative infection subsequently becomes oliguric. He is also having difficulty hearing the hospital staff. Laboratory studies show elevated blood urea nitrogen (BUN) and plasma creatinine levels. Which of the following antibiotics is the most likely cause of this patient's symptoms?

(A) Chloramphenicol
(B) Doxycycline
(C) Erythromycin
(D) Gentamicin
(E) Imipenem

15. A 64-year-old man who is taking common medications for hypertension, hypercholesterolemia, and coronary artery disease comes to the emergency department because of blood in his urine, nausea, and vomiting. Urinalysis shows reddish-colored urine with no RBCs, but with granular casts and protein. A basic metabolic panel shows highly elevated BUN and creatinine levels with a blood urea nitrogen:creatinine ratio of 10:1, and severe uremia. He is declared to be in acute renal failure and placed on dialysis. This patient has recently started a new drug for his coronary artery dis-

ease. Which of the following is the most likely cause of this patient's renal failure?

(A) A β-blocker
(B) A nonsteroidal anti-inflammatory drug (NSAID)
(C) A statin drug
(D) An autoimmune reaction
(E) Trauma

16. A 35-year-old woman presents to the emergency department after experiencing the acute onset of right flank pain and fever. Laboratory results show white cell casts in the urine. Which of the following is the most prominent cell type found in the infiltrate of the involved organ?

(A) Macrophage
(B) Monocyte
(C) Plasma cell
(D) Polymorphonuclear leukocytes
(E) T lymphocyte

17. A previously healthy 20-year-old college student presents to the student health office complaining of a 1-week history of fatigue and dark-colored urine. On physical examination, his blood pressure is 155/90 mm Hg and his serum creatinine level is 4.4 mg/dL. Urinalysis shows 3+ blood and red cell casts without protein, glucose, or ketones. A kidney biopsy shows crescentic changes of the glomerulus. Which of the following is the most likely diagnosis?

(A) Diabetic nephropathy
(B) Membranoproliferative glomerulonephritis
(C) Minimal change disease
(D) Rapidly progressive glomerulonephritis
(E) Systemic lupus erythematosus

18. A 22-year-old college student is brought to the emergency department after he began complaining of ants crawling over his body and his friends noted increasing agitation and threatening gestures. On physical examination he is febrile, restless, and tachycardic, and his pupils are markedly dilated. Appropriate treatment

would most likely include which of the following?

(A) Acidifying urine to increase renal clearance
(B) Alkalinizing urine to increase renal clearance
(C) Treating with flumazenil
(D) Treating with naloxone
(E) Treating with water to dilute drug effects

19. A 19-year-old woman with a severe gastrointestinal infection presents to the emergency department with a 5-day history of vomiting and diarrhea. She is acutely dehydrated. Laboratory studies show a pH of 7.38, a CO_2 level of 37 mm Hg, and an HCO_3^- level of 25 mEq/L. Which of the following statements is most accurate regarding this patient's acid-base status?

(A) She has a metabolic acidosis
(B) She has a mixed metabolic alkalosis and metabolic acidosis
(C) She has a mixed respiratory alkalosis and respiratory acidosis
(D) She has a respiratory alkalosis
(E) She has no acid-base disturbances

20. A 59-year-old woman with type 2 diabetes mellitus comes to her primary care physician for a routine visit. Her creatinine level has been slowly increasing over the last decade due to poor compliance with her medical regimen. If her renal disease were to progress, she would be at risk for developing which of the following conditions?

(A) Bacteriuria
(B) Hypokalemia
(C) Hypotension
(D) Metabolic alkalosis
(E) Osteomalacia
(F) Polycythemia

21. A 16-year-old boy comes to the physician with a 1-year history of intermittent, painless hematuria without dysuria or increased frequency of micturition. He says he has also had several respiratory infections and adds that the hematuria increased within several days of the infections. Which of the following is most likely to be found if the boy is diagnosed with IgA nephropathy (Berger's disease)?

(A) IgA mesangial deposition
(B) Increased antistreptolysin O titer
(C) Lumpy-bumpy electron-dense deposits
(D) Proteinuria exceeding 3.5 gm/24 hr
(E) Subepithelial IgA deposits

22. A 34-year-old woman comes to the hospital to deliver a full-term infant. The labor is complicated by an amniotic fluid embolism, and subsequent blood tests show the presence of fibrin split products. The next day the patient abruptly develops anuria, gross hematuria, and flank pain accompanied by rapidly increasing blood urea nitrogen and creatinine levels and a new cardiac friction rub. The patient's CT scan demonstrates hypodensities within the renal cortex. Which of the following is the correct treatment?

(A) Aggressive fluid support
(B) Biopsy to evaluate for malignancy
(C) Broad-spectrum antibiotics
(D) Dialysis
(E) No treatment is necessary at this time

23. A 40-year-old man presents to his physician with sharp, sudden, sporadic pain in his lower back and some hematuria. His physical examination is unremarkable, with normal blood pressure and absence of any palpable masses in the abdomen but some flank pain. A plain film of the pelvis does not show any renal calculi. Which of the following is the most likely cause of this man's symptoms?

(A) Hyperparathyroidism
(B) Hyperuricemia
(C) Prostate cancer
(D) *Proteus vulgaris* infection
(E) Staphylococcal infection

24. What is the primary driving force for calcium reabsorption in the thick ascending loop of Henle?

(A) A functioning sodium-potassium-chloride triple transporter
(B) Action of parathyroid hormone
(C) Maintenance of negative charge in the lumen
(D) Sodium-calcium cotransport
(E) Volume contraction

25. A routine urine analysis in a 6-year-old child shows the presence of protein. Follow-up studies show gross proteinuria (2 mg/dL) with lipoid sediment and mild hypoalbuminemia (3.2 mg/dL). Which of the following statements most accurately describes the renal corpuscle?

(A) Molecules greater then 69,000 Da cross the renal corpuscle
(B) Most Na^+ ions are reabsorbed by the renal corpuscle
(C) Negatively charged molecules are more likely to cross the renal corpuscle
(D) Renin gets released by the renal corpuscle
(E) The renal corpuscle contains large proteoglycan molecules

26. A 56-year-old woman who has been taking cefoxitin for treatment of *Klebsiella* pneumonia is found to still have *Klebsiella* organisms in her blood 1 week after beginning treatment. Another drug is added to the patient's regimen. Two days later, the following laboratory values are obtained:

Na^+: 141 mEq/L
K^+: 4.3 mEq/L
Cl^-: 102 mEq/L
HCO_3^-: 24 mEq/L
Blood urea nitrogen: 65 mg/dL
Creatinine: 4.4 mEq/L

Which of the following medications was most likely added to this patient's regimen?

(A) Azithromycin
(B) Aztreonam
(C) Clindamycin
(D) Piperacillin
(E) Tobramycin

27. A 32-year-old woman finishes running a marathon. She drinks 6 L of water in an attempt to replace the fluid she lost during the race. Drinking excessive water after prolonged strenuous exercise causes which of the following?

(A) Decreased urine osmolarity
(B) Increased hormonal secretion from the posterior pituitary
(C) Increased plasma osmolarity
(D) Increases in aquaporin transport in the distal tubule and collecting duct
(E) Stimulation of osmoreceptors in the hypothalamus

28. ADH has its effects in the collecting ducts of the kidney. Which of the following best characterizes ADH activity?

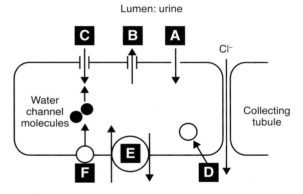

Lumen: urine

Reproduced, with permission, from USMLERx.com.

(A) Binds and blocks A
(B) Binds and blocks C
(C) Binds at F and activates G$_i$–cyclic adenosine monophosphate cascade
(D) Binds at F and activates G$_s$–cyclic adenosine monophosphate cascade
(E) Stimulates D

29. A 49-year-old man poisons his wife with antifreeze. She is taken to a nearby hospital, where all efforts to detoxify her and prevent cardiopulmonary arrest fail. The medical examiner's report states that the woman had high serum levels of ethylene glycol. A biopsy of her kidney shows diffuse tubular necrosis. Which of the following would have been her plasma

blood urea nitrogen:creatinine (BUN:Cr) ratio and urine output prior to her death?

(A) 10–15:1 with low urine output
(B) < 15:1 with normal urine output
(C) 15–20:1 with normal urine output
(D) > 15:1 with low urine output
(E) > 20:1 with normal urine output
(F) > 20:1 with low urine output

30. A medical student is doing research to measure the effects of newly bioengineered molecules on the function of the glomerulus. Which of the following mechanisms are likely to result in an overall increase in renal blood flow?

(A) Stimulation of afferent α-adrenergic receptors alone
(B) Stimulation of afferent angiotensin II receptors alone
(C) Stimulation of angiotensin II receptors and opening of vascular smooth muscle stretch-activated calcium channels
(D) Stimulation of renal α-adrenergic and angiotensin II receptors
(E) Stimulation of renal dopamine and bradykinin receptors

31. An 18-year-old woman presents to the emergency department with a 3-day history of worsening fever and redness in her right foot. On examination, the patient is found to have erythema around a puncture wound in her foot. The patient is admitted to the hospital and given IV penicillin and nonsteroidal anti-inflammatory drugs, which decrease the erythema, pain, and swelling. Three days later the patient develops new onset of weakness, fatigue, rash, and fever. Significant laboratory findings include a blood urea nitrogen level of 45 mg/dL and a creatinine level of 2.8 mg/dL. Urinalysis shows WBC casts, eosinophils, and a fractional excretion of sodium of 2.5%. Which of the following is the most likely cause of her new onset of illness?

(A) Intravenous antibiotics
(B) NSAIDs
(C) Poststreptococcal glomerulonephritis
(D) Systemic lupus erythematosus
(E) Urolithiasis

32. Diuretics are medications that increase the amount of urine flow by inhibiting transport proteins or enzymes in the nephron. Which of the following diuretics will also decrease the amount of calcium excreted from the kidney?

   (A) Acetazolamide
   (B) Amiloride
   (C) Furosemide
   (D) Hydrochlorothiazide
   (E) Spironolactone

33. During gynecologic surgery, it is always necessary to identify and isolate the ureters to prevent damage to these important structures during a procedure. Which of the following best describes the course of the ureters in the female pelvis?

   (A) Anterior to both the external iliac and uterine arteries
   (B) Anterior to the external iliac artery and posterior to the uterine artery
   (C) Posterior to both the external iliac and uterine arteries
   (D) Posterior to the external iliac artery and anterior to the uterine artery
   (E) Running along with the ovarian artery

34. The nephrotic syndrome is characterized by severe proteinuria, decreased serum albumin level, and edema. The glomerular basement membrane is essential for maintaining serum oncotic pressure balance. In nonpathologic states, albumin is not filtered across the glomerular basement membrane for which of the listed reasons?

   (A) A combination of small pore size and negative charge prevents albumin filtration
   (B) A combination of small pore size and positive charge prevents albumin filtration
   (C) Albumin is freely filtered across the basement membrane but is readily reabsorbed along the nephron
   (D) The positive charge of the basement membrane repels albumin
   (E) The small size of the glomerular basement membrane pores excludes albumin molecules

35. A 54-year-old homeless woman is found unconscious on the street. Upon admission to the emergency department, her laboratory tests show the following:

   Na^+: 137 mEq/L
   K^+: 3.3 mEq/L
   Cl^-: 112 mEq/L
   HCO_3^-: 15 mEq/L
   Arterial blood gas on room air: pH 7.28
   Partial carbon dioxide pressure: 28 mm Hg
   Partial oxygen pressure: 90 mm Hg

   Which of the following caused her acidosis?

   (A) An aspirin overdose
   (B) Diabetic ketoacidosis
   (C) Severe diarrhea
   (D) Severe underperfusion of her peripheral muscles
   (E) Uremia

36. A patient with hepatocellular carcinoma develops severe ascites such that 3–5 L of fluid must be drained from her peritoneal cavity every 3 days. This procedure may have detrimental effects on kidney function that necessitates monitoring of glomerular filtration rate. Laboratory values are as follows:

   Creatinine clearance: 120 mg/mL
   Glomerular capillary hydrostatic pressure: 40 mm Hg
   Plasma inulin: 1.5 mg/mL
   Urinary inulin: 50 mg/mL

   Which of the following is her urine flow rate?

   (A) 1.6 mL/min
   (B) 3.6 mL/min
   (C) 4.5 mL/min
   (D) 36 mL/hr
   (E) 450 mL/day

37. A diet high in sodium can contribute to hypertension. Which of the following is a renal response to increased sodium intake?

   (A) Decrease in atrial natriuretic peptide and constriction of glomerular afferent arterioles

(B) Decreased sympathetic activity and dilation of afferent arterioles

(C) Increase in atrial natriuretic peptide and dilation of glomerular afferent arterioles

(D) Increase in the renin-angiotensin-aldosterone axis

(E) Increased plasma oncotic pressure

38. Mannitol, an osmotic diuretic, is sometimes used to lower intracranial pressure. Where along the nephron is the primary site of action of mannitol?

(A) Collecting tubule
(B) Distal tubule
(C) Loop of Henle
(D) Proximal tubule
(E) Thick ascending limb of loop of Henle

39. An 18-year-old African-American man has had increasing lethargy, proteinuria, and edema following a bout of the flu 3 weeks ago. At that time, the patient visited his primary care physician, who prescribed corticosteroids for 3 weeks without improvement of his condition. His physician then referred him to a nephrologist, who performed a renal biopsy and diagnosed him with focal segmental glomerulosclerosis. Which of the following was the most likely histologic description in this patient's biopsy report?

(A) Entire glomerular tufts show obliterated capillaries; > 50% of glomeruli affected

(B) Entire glomerular tufts show obliterated capillaries with cellular proliferation

(C) Parts of the glomerular tufts show obliterated capillaries; < 50% of glomeruli affected

(D) Parts of the glomerular tufts show obliterated capillaries; > 50% of glomeruli affected

(E) Parts of the glomerular tufts show obliterated capillaries with cellular proliferation

40. Mr. Jones has type 1 diabetes mellitus and forgot to take his insulin. Although his serum glucose level begins to rise rapidly, sugars are not detectable in his urine for hours. Which molecules are responsible for this phenomenon?

(A) Glucose-chloride cotransporters in the thick ascending limb

(B) Negatively charged proteins in the glomerular wall

(C) Occludin proteins in the tight junctions of glomerular capillary endothelial cells

(D) Sodium-glucose cotransporters in the proximal tubule

(E) Sodium-potassium exchange pump in the distal convoluted tubule

41. The peritoneum is a continuous serous membrane that lines the abdominopelvic cavity and invests many organs. Which of the following organs are retroperitoneal in their location?

(A) Kidney
(B) Liver
(C) Spleen
(D) Stomach
(E) Transverse colon

42. Shock is defined as a metabolic state in which oxygen delivery inadequately meets oxygen demand. The mechanisms for shock include pump failure, blood volume loss, obstruction to blood flow, and increased venous capacity. Which of the following is a sign or symptom associated with shock?

(A) Bradycardia
(B) Hypertension
(C) Orthopnea
(D) Polyuria
(E) Tachycardia

43. A 43-year-old man has had type 1 diabetes mellitus for 30 years. He uses insulin to treat his diabetes, but his blood glucose levels are poorly controlled. Over the years, he has developed painful peripheral neuropathy and a non-healing diabetic foot ulcer. Which of the following would be found on a biopsy of this man's kidney?

(A) Crescent-shaped lesions in the glomeruli
(B) Nodular glomerular changes
(C) Proliferation of the mesangial membranes
(D) Segmental sclerosis and hyaline casts
(E) Tram-track appearance on light microscopy

44. Angiotensin II stimulates the Na^+-H^+ exchanger in the proximal tubule. How does this affect the handling of HCO_3^- and H^+ in the proximal tubule?

(A) Decreased net HCO_3^- reabsorption, decreased net H^+ secretion

(B) Increased net HCO_3^- reabsorption, increased net H^+ secretion

(C) Increased net HCO_3^- reabsorption, no effect on net H^+ secretion

(D) No effect on net HCO_3^- reabsorption, increased net H^+ secretion

(E) No effect on net HCO_3^- reabsorption, no effect on net H^+ secretion

45. A 67-year-old man with a history of hypertension has a severe heart attack while walking to his car after a night drinking with his friends. When he arrives at the emergency department, he is pale and cold and his friends notice that "he seems to be sweating a lot." He is tachycardic and hypotensive, and is admitted to the cardiac intensive care unit. The next day, he has low urine output, his blood urea nitrogen level is 35 mg/dL, his creatinine level is 1.3 mg/dL, and his blood pressure is 85/55 mm Hg. His baseline blood pressure due to his hypertension was around 145/90 mm Hg. Which of the following is the most likely cause of his low urine input?

(A) A blockage of the ureters or urethra

(B) Acute tubular necrosis

(C) Decrease in perfusion of the kidney

(D) Ethanol-induced reduction in urine output

(E) Low urine output is normal in times of stress

46. A 13-year-old boy is brought to the emergency department with periorbital edema, hypertension, and tea-colored urine. His parents say that he had a sore throat about 3 weeks ago. Urinalysis shows RBCs with casts. A positive antistreptolysin O titer and decreased levels of complement are also noted. What findings would be expected in this patient's glomeruli?

(A) Linear subendothelial pattern

(B) Mesangial deposits

(C) Subendothelial deposits in a "spike-and-dome" pattern

(D) Subendothelial humps

(E) Subepithelial humps

(F) Granular subendothelial deposits

47. Two weeks after beginning diuretic therapy to control essential hypertension, a patient presents to his physician for a checkup. Physical examination reveals a blood pressure of 130/85 mm Hg. Laboratory tests show a pH of 7.48, partial arterial carbon dioxide pressure of 50 mm Hg, and a bicarbonate level of 41 mEq/L. Which of the following scenarios is most probable in this patient?

(A) Acetazolamide-induced metabolic alkalosis

(B) Acetazolamide-induced respiratory alkalosis

(C) Furosemide-induced respiratory alkalosis

(D) Hydrochlorothiazide-induced metabolic alkalosis

(E) Hydrochlorothiazide-induced respiratory alkalosis

(F) Spironolactone-induced metabolic alkalosis

48. A 17-year-old girl develops severe diarrhea after eating an undercooked hamburger at a family picnic. After 3 days of experiencing diarrhea, she presents to the emergency department with moderate dehydration and orthostatic hypotension. Which of the following acid-base states is most probable in this patient?

(A) Anion-gap metabolic acidosis

(B) Metabolic alkalosis

(C) Non—anion-gap metabolic acidosis

(D) Normal

(E) Respiratory acidosis

(F) Respiratory alkalosis

49. An 8-year-old girl presents to the emergency department complaining of frequent urination, constant thirst, and new, strange "staining" of her teeth. She recently had a cold, and her pediatrician prescribed an antibiotic that she said may hurt her kidneys. She did not bring the bottle with her. Which of the following medications was this patient most likely prescribed?

(A) Demeclocycline
(B) Neomycin
(C) Norfloxacin
(D) Penicillin G
(E) Vancomycin

50. Which of the reasons below describes why celecoxib would be contraindicated in a patient who is severely dehydrated?

(A) Due to its effects on platelet function
(B) Due to its effects on the arterioles of the kidney
(C) Due to its effects on the gastrointestinal mucosa
(D) Due to its effects on the production of inflammatory cytokines
(E) It would not be contraindicated

HIGH-YIELD SYSTEMS

Renal

1. **The correct answer is A.** The juxtaglomerular (JG) cells in the afferent arteriole and the macula densa in the distal convoluted tubule together make up the juxtaglomerular apparatus, which is responsible for controlling renal blood flow via renin release. In renal artery stenosis, the blood flow to the kidney is low. This low pressure is detected by JG cells in the afferent arteriole that secrete renin to raise blood pressure and renal perfusion through the renin-angiotensin system.

Answer B is incorrect. The collecting duct is strongly influenced by hormones such as ADH and aldosterone and aids in concentrating or diluting urine. It does not have a role in sensing perfusion pressure or secreting renin.

Answer C is incorrect. The distal convoluted tubule contains the macula densa cells that sense low Na^+ flow inside the nephron, another sign that the kidney is not well perfused. The macula densa cells are in intimate contact with the juxtaglomerular (JG) cells, and although the macula densa cells help in sensing low perfusion, it is the JG cells that actually secrete renin.

Answer D is incorrect. The efferent arteriole carries blood flow away from the glomerulus. The juxtaglomerular cells that sense blood pressure are in the afferent arteriole. The words *afferent* and *efferent* are also used in nerves, and it may help to remember the mnemonic **SAME** (**S**ensory **A**fferent, **M**otor **E**fferent) to remember the direction of flow in the afferent (toward the kidney) and efferent (away from the kidney) systems.

Answer E is incorrect. The loop of Henle is primarily responsible for concentrating urine, not for sensing perfusion or secreting renin.

2. **The correct answer is D.** This man's history indicates that he is suffering from acute tubular necrosis secondary to ischemia of the epithelial cells of the proximal convoluted tubule. These cells, given their high metabolic rate, are particularly sensitive to a drop in blood pressure such as that experienced in hemorrhagic shock. In this patient, the immediate therapeutic plan is to correct the fluid and electrolyte imbalance. The fluid replacement should include both crystalloid (e.g., normal saline, lactated Ringer's) and blood products due to the severity of blood loss. If recovery of renal function is delayed or if the kidneys never fully recover, dialysis is indicated. The epithelium will usually regenerate in a few weeks.

Answer A is incorrect. Angioplasty is a minimally invasive procedure that involves eliminating the renal artery occlusion by placing intravascular stents in the renal artery and thereby restoring proper blood flow to the kidney. This patient is not suffering from acute renal failure due to stenosis/occlusion of the renal artery, so angioplasty is not indicated as an appropriate treatment.

Answer B is incorrect. Broad-spectrum antibiotics are indicated in cases of shock due to sepsis or in pyelonephritis. This patient is in hemodynamic shock caused by massive blood loss. Since there is no infection, antibiotics will not be beneficial. Additionally, because the patient is experiencing renal failure, any drug that is metabolized by the kidney should be used with caution.

Answer C is incorrect. Immune-mediated disease can also cause acute renal failure. Corticosteroids are indicated in immune-mediated disease. Since that is not the mechanism of this patient's renal failure, it is not indicated.

Answer E is incorrect. This treatment is reserved primarily for renal stones obstructing the outflow of urine and causing postrenal acute renal failure.

3. **The correct answer is A.** This vignette describes a nephrotic syndrome. Spike-and-dome deposits are only found in membranous glomerulonephritis. Membranous glomerulonephritis is an immune complex–mediated disease. Patients with this disease normally pre-

sent with a nephrotic picture of generalized edema due to massive loss of albumin and proteins. Immunofluorescence shows a granular pattern of IgG and complement along the basement membrane and a spike-and-dome appearance on electron microscopy. Membranous glomerulonephritis is the most common cause of adult-onset nephrotic syndrome.

Answer B is incorrect. This is a finding of membranoproliferative glomerulonephritis, an uncommon autoimmune renal disorder that normally affects young individuals (8–30 years of age). The diagnosis is based on a histologic presentation that includes mesangial proliferation and a tram-track appearance on light microscopy.

Answer C is incorrect. This is a finding of Alport's syndrome, a heterogeneous (although most commonly X-linked) genetic disorder with either absent or mutated collagen IV, which leads to a nephritic renal disease, as well as nervous system and ocular disorders.

Answer D is incorrect. This is a description of the findings in acute poststreptococcal glomerulonephritis, an autoimmune disease most frequently seen in children. It normally presents a few weeks after a streptococcal infection with peripheral and periorbital edema, dark urine, and proteinuria. These symptoms are caused by circulating antistreptococcal antibody-antigen complexes that deposit in the glomerular basement membrane, leading to complement activation and glomerular damage.

Answer E is incorrect. This is the main finding in IgA nephropathy (Berger's disease). This disease presents within several days of an infection (as opposed to poststreptococcal glomerulonephritis, which presents weeks after) with a nephritic picture due to IgA deposition in the mesangium. It is the most common global nephropathy, but it is a mild disease with minimal clinical significance.

4. **The correct answer is D.** Hypoventilation causes an inability on the part of the lungs to excrete the CO_2 the body produces, leading to retention of CO_2. This causes a drop in pH and a compensatory retention of bicarbonate.

These acid-base abnormalities are consistent with respiratory acidosis. Hypoventilation (from a variety of etiologies) is a primary cause of respiratory acidosis.

Answer A is incorrect. An increase in anions would be consistent with anion-gap metabolic acidosis. Metabolic acidosis is indicated by the presence of low pH with low plasma bicarbonate and low carbon dioxide and an increased anion gap, measured by ($[Na^+] - [Cl^+] - [HCO_3^-]$), which is normally 10–16 mEq/L. The main causes are lactic acidosis, diabetic ketoacidosis, and renal failure.

Answer B is incorrect. Non–anion-gap metabolic acidosis is the presence of low pH with low plasma bicarbonate without an elevated anion gap. The cause is generally gastrointestinal losses of bicarbonate (i.e., diarrhea, biliary drains, emesis, nasogastric tube losses). Another important and common cause of a metabolic non–anion-gap acidosis is the presence of an ileal conduit or bladder reconstruction from colonic tissue. The gastrointestinal tissue absorbs Cl^- from the urine in exchange for bicarbonate. Other causes include renal tubular acidosis, or hypochloremia.

Answer C is incorrect. The pH is this answer is low, which corresponds to an acidosis. The P_{CO_2} is high, which is consistent with a respiratory acidosis, however the HCO_3^- is low, which is consistent with a metabolic acidosis. Thus, this patient has a mixed respiratory and metabolic acidosis.

Answer E is incorrect. The pH in this instance is normal, while there is an increased anion gap. An anion gap usually indicates that the patient has an acidosis. Since the pH of the blood is normal and not lowered, it indicates that this is a mixed acid-base disorder, in which a metabolic or respiratory alkalosis is counteracting a metabolic anion-gap acidosis.

Answer F is incorrect. Respiratory alkalosis can be caused only by an increase in ventilation leading to excessive loss of carbon dioxide, which is balanced by an increased excretion of bicarbonate. Hence, a high pH, a low CO_2, and a low bicarbonate indicate respiratory alkalosis. This is caused by hyperventilation.

Answer G is incorrect. Metabolic alkalosis would present with a high pH, a high bicarbonate, and (with respiratory compensation) a high CO_2. The causes of metabolic alkalosis include vomiting, diuretic therapy, and chloride restriction. The compensation is hypoventilation.

5. **The correct answer is D.** Thiazides and furosemide lead to metabolic alkalosis. There are two components to the development of metabolic alkalosis: volume depletion and electrolyte imbalance; specifically hypochloremia and hypokalemia. Volume contraction leads to increased sodium reabsorption and bicarbonate retention. The diuretic-induced hypochloremia and hypokalemia lead to persistence of the alkalosis because the hypokalemia causes hydrogen to be exchanged for sodium rather than potassium at the distal convoluted tubule.

Answer A is incorrect. Neither potassium-sparing diuretics nor acetazolamide cause metabolic alkalosis. Potassium-sparing diuretics cause metabolic acidosis by inhibiting sodium-hydrogen exchange channels, and acetazolamide promotes the loss of bicarbonate in the urine, causing metabolic acidosis.

Answer B is incorrect. Acetazolamide inhibits the enzyme carbonic anhydrase, which is important in the reabsorption of sodium, bicarbonate, and chloride at the proximal tubule. Since it promotes the loss of bicarbonate in the urine, it tends to cause metabolic acidosis.

Answer C is incorrect. The potassium-sparing diuretics, such as spironolactone, inhibit aldosterone-sensitive sodium channels that excrete hydrogen or potassium in exchange for sodium. Inhibition of these channels may lead to hyperkalemia and metabolic acidosis.

Answer E is incorrect. Thiazides do cause metabolic alkalosis by causing volume depletion, hypochloremia, and hypokalemia. However, acetazolamide promotes the loss of bicarbonate in the urine, causing metabolic acidosis.

Answer F is incorrect. Thiazides do cause metabolic alkalosis by causing volume deple-

tion, hypochloremia, and hypokalemia. However, potassium-sparing diuretics cause metabolic acidosis by inhibiting sodium-hydrogen exchange channels.

6. **The correct answer is B.** This patient has Goodpasture's syndrome, which is an autoimmune disease involving the formation of antibodies to the alveolar and glomerular basement membranes. This is an example of a type II hypersensitivity reaction in which antibody binds to antigen on a cell, leading to lysis by complement or phagocytosis. It is one of the several forms of rapidly progressive (or crescentic) glomerulonephritis. Patients are usually men in their 20s presenting with a history of hemoptysis and nephritic renal failure that is associated with crescent formation. Since the damage in this disease is caused by the actions of antibodies to the basement membrane, diagnosis is made by immunofluorescence, which shows a smooth linear staining along the basement membrane.

Answer A is incorrect. Type I hypersensitivity reactions are those in which antigen cross-links preformed IgE on presensitized mast cells and basophils, triggering the release of vasoactive amines. Examples of this type of reaction are asthma and anaphylaxis.

Answer C is incorrect. Type III hypersensitivity reactions are those involving immune complex deposition. Antigen-antibody complexes are deposited and activate complement, which attracts neutrophils, which then release lysosomal enzymes. Serum sickness and Arthus reaction are variants of the type III hypersensitivity reaction. Examples include rheumatoid arthritis and polyarteritis nodosa.

Answer D is incorrect. Type IV hypersensitivity reactions are delayed cell-mediated reactions. Sensitized T-lymphocytes encounter antigen and then release lymphokines, which leads to macrophage activation. Examples include skin tests for tuberculosis and transplant rejection.

Answer E is incorrect. There is no such thing as a type V hypersensitivity reaction.

7. **The correct answer is A.** Metabolic alkalosis presents with a high pH, a high bicarbonate, and (with respiratory compensation) a high CO_2. The causes of metabolic alkalosis include vomiting, diuretic therapy, and chloride restriction. The compensation is hypoventilation. Diarrhea causes a non–anion-gap metabolic acidosis. Bicarbonate lost in the gastrointestinal tract gets exchanged for chloride, which is why gastrointestinal losses result in a hyperchloremic non–anion-gap acidosis. So while there is a generation of anions, they are anions that are counted in normal electrolyte measurements. Therefore, gastrointestinal losses do not result in an increase in unmeasured anions (i.e., an anion gap); instead, it would manifest as a low pH with low plasma bicarbonate without an elevated anion gap. Other causes are renal tubular acidosis and hypochloremia.

Answer B is incorrect. Loop diuretics such as furosemide can lead to metabolic alkalosis. There are three components to the development of the metabolic alkalosis: volume depletion, electrolyte imbalance (specifically leading to hypochloremia and hypokalemia), and secondary aldosteronism. Volume contraction leads to increased sodium reabsorption and increased bicarbonate threshold. The diuretic-induced hypochloremia and hypokalemia lead to the persistence of the alkalosis. A drop in intravascular volume causes activation of the renin-angiotensin-aldosterone system and an increase in aldosterone levels. With persistent hypokalemia, hydrogen is preferentially excreted instead of potassium at the distal convoluted tubule in exchange for sodium.

Answer C is incorrect. Volume contraction with hypokalemia is seen in both vomiting and excessive diuretic use.

Answer D is incorrect. Thiazide diuretics can lead to metabolic alkalosis through the same mechanism as loop diuretics: volume depletion, electrolyte imbalance, and increased aldosterone.

Answer E is incorrect. The loss of hydrochloric acid due to vomiting leads to a transient increase in pH. The kidney responds by excretion of sodium and/or potassium bicarbonate. As the vomiting persists, the alkalemic and dehydrated patient tries to conserve sodium through activation of the renin-angiotensin-aldosterone system. Therefore, while bicarbonate excretion persists due to the alkalosis, it is primarily excreted with potassium rather than sodium due to the dehydration. Compensating by conserving sodium and excreting bicarbonate at the expense of potassium soon fails because in the presence of severe hypokalemia, the kidney begins to exchange hydrogen ions in the distal convoluted tubule in order to conserve potassium. Therefore, acidic urine in the setting of volume contraction and alkalosis is primarily due to the loss of potassium.

8. **The correct answer is E.** Pyelonephritis is infection of the kidneys by an ascending infection from the lower urinary tract, most often caused by *Escherichia coli* from the periurethral/perianal area. The classic symptoms are fever, chills, flank pain, and costovertebral angle tenderness, all of which are demonstrated by this patient. Pregnancy is a predisposing factor for urinary tract infections, a recurring problem in this patient. Casts indicate that the origin of the white blood cells is the kidney, which confirms the clinical suspicion of pyelonephritis.

Answer A is incorrect. An abdominal aortic aneurysm may present with back and abdominal pain and/or pulsations of the abdomen. This condition may often be asymptomatic for years as the dilation of the aorta worsens. Fever and urinary casts would not be a part of the clinical picture.

Answer B is incorrect. A compression fracture may also cause back pain and tenderness over the costovertebral angle, but in conjunction with the other symptoms and findings, this is not the best answer.

Answer C is incorrect. Localized cystitis is not usually accompanied by systemic symptoms, such as fever. However, cystitis may be present in conjunction with the pyelonephritis, as it is an ascending infection. Symptoms of cystitis include urinary frequency and dysuria. Casts would not be seen if the infection were localized to the urinary bladder.

Answer D is incorrect. Premature labor involves regular uterine contractions that dilate the cervix. The labor does not cause fever, but back pain may be present.

9. **The correct answer is B.** This patient is most likely suffering from bilateral renal artery stenosis. Stenosis of the renal arteries leads to a decrease in perfusion of the kidney and therefore a drop in intraglomerular pressure and glomerular filtration rate (GFR). The underperfused kidneys respond by the activation of the renin-angiotensin-aldosterone system. With angiotensin-converting enzyme (ACE) inhibitors, the vasoconstrictive effect of angiotensin II on the ability of the efferent arterioles to increase effective GFR will be abolished. ACE inhibitors should be avoided in patients with renal stenosis due to deterioration of renal function.

Answer A is incorrect. Angioplasty is a minimally invasive procedure that involves eliminating the occlusion by placing intravascular stents in the renal artery, thereby restoring blood flow to the kidney. This form of therapy is the primary indication for renal stenosis in symptomatic patients. Patency rates after angioplasty are strongly dependent on the size of the vessel treated and the quality of inflow and outflow through the vessel.

Answer C is incorrect. In patients with bilateral renal artery stenosis leading to hypertension, both kidneys will be underperfused, so both kidneys will retain sodium and water by activation of the renin-angiotensin-aldosterone system. Diuretics can counteract this effect and control blood pressure; therefore, this treatment is indicated.

Answer D is incorrect. Smoking is a risk factor for developing atherosclerotic plaques that may occlude vessels such as the renal arteries. Quitting may lower the rate of atherosclerotic buildup. This recommendation is indicated in this patient.

Answer E is incorrect. Surgery is another therapeutic option for renal stenosis. It is particularly indicated if angioplasty cannot be performed, as in completely occluded renal vessels.

10. **The correct answer is C.** A horseshoe kidney forms when the inferior poles of two kidneys fuse during development. As the kidneys rise from the pelvis, they get trapped under the inferior mesenteric artery and cannot rise to the normal level in the abdomen. These patients are typically asymptomatic if they have no other abnormalities.

Answer A is incorrect. The aorta would not obstruct the path of a rising horseshoe kidney during development.

Answer B is incorrect. The celiac trunk leaves the aorta at a level above the location of normally developed kidneys, and thus cannot be responsible for the low location of a horseshoe kidney.

Answer D is incorrect. The inferior vena cava would not obstruct the path of a rising horseshoe kidney during development.

Answer E is incorrect. The superior mesenteric artery leaves the aorta at the level where normally developing kidneys are located, and thus it cannot be responsible for the low level of a horseshoe kidney.

11. **The correct answer is E.** The calculated fractional excretion of sodium of > 4% and the urine osmolality of > 350 mOsm/kg indicate that this is postrenal failure due to obstruction. Uric acid stones are formed from a metabolite of nucleic acid turnover, which is increased in the setting of cell destruction (e.g., tumor lysis syndrome, as seen in this case). These stones are often seen in the setting of diseases with increased cell proliferation and turnover, such as leukemia and myeloproliferative disorders. Uric acid stones are radiolucent. Other causes of postrenal obstruction include neoplasia and benign prostatic hyperplasia.

Answer A is incorrect. Kidney failure as a result of glomerular dysfunction presents with a prerenal azotemia. There is an effective decrease in glomerular filtration rate, and Na^+/H_2O are retained by the kidney. The fractional excretion of sodium in prerenal failure is normally less than 1% with an osmolality that is > 500 mOsm/kg.

Answer B is incorrect. Acute interstitial disease of the kidney is commonly caused by an allergic reaction to medicine (e.g., penicillin, nonsteroidal anti-inflammatory drugs) or infection. In an acute setting, it presents with an intrinsic renal picture as is seen in this patient. In the setting of an infection, urine cultures are usually positive; in the setting of an allergic reaction, eosinophilia is common.

Answer C is incorrect. Kidney failure as a result of tubular dysfunction presents with an intrinsic renal picture. This is most commonly due to acute tubular necrosis or ischemia/toxins. Patchy necrosis leads to debris obstructing the tubules and fluid backflow, leading to a drop in glomerular filtration rate. The fractional excretion of sodium in intrinsic renal failure is normally > 2% with an osmolality that is > 350 mOsm/kg (similar to postrenal). However, the presentation of severe intermittent flank pain is consistent with a kidney stone.

Answer D is incorrect. Postrenal obstruction can only cause acute renal failure with bilateral obstruction. Unilateral obstruction will cause severe pain, but not renal failure.

12. **The correct answer is A.** Renal prostaglandin synthesis produces a vasodilatory effect on the afferent arterioles that counteracts the effects of vasoconstriction produced by angiotensin II and thereby protects the glomerular filtration rate (GFR). NSAIDs inhibit renal prostaglandin synthesis, resulting in an inability of afferent arterioles to dilate. Without adequate afferent arteriolar vasodilation, GFR is reduced and acute renal failure ensues.

Answer B is incorrect. Inhibition of prostaglandin synthesis causes excessive vasoconstric-

tion of the afferent arterioles, leading to decreased glomerular filtration rate (GFR). Constriction of the efferent arteriole would serve to increase GFR.

Answer C is incorrect. Prostaglandins act to dilate the afferent arterioles, with less significant effect on the efferent arterioles.

Answer D is incorrect. NSAIDs act to inhibit, not stimulate, renal prostaglandin synthesis, leading to excessive constriction of the afferent arteriole and decreases in glomerular filtration rate.

Answer E is incorrect. NSAIDs act to inhibit, not stimulate, renal prostaglandin synthesis, leading to excessive constriction of the afferent arteriole and decreases in glomerular filtration rate.

13. **The correct answer is E.** In healthy people, osmoreceptors in the wall of the third ventricle sense increased body fluid osmolarity and trigger the release of ADH from the posterior pituitary. ADH exerts its main effects on the V2 receptors located in the principal cells of the late distal tubule and collecting duct, where a G_s protein-coupled mechanism directs the insertion of aquaporin water channels into the luminal wall. These channels are permeable only to water and result in a reabsorption of water, concentration of urine, and dilution of body fluids. Activation of the V1 receptor found in the vascular smooth muscles results in activation of G_q protein second-messenger cascade and contraction of vascular smooth muscle, leading to an increase in total peripheral resistance. In patients with the syndrome of inappropriate ADH secretion (SIADH), which can be caused by central nervous system disturbances (e.g., stroke, hemorrhage, infection), small-cell lung carcinoma, intracranial neoplasms, and occasionally by pancreatic tumors, the unregulated release of ADH leads to the persistent excretion of concentrated urine high in sodium. This causes hyponatremia and decreased serum osmolality without potassium or acid-base disturbances.

Answer A is incorrect. ACTH is secreted by

the anterior pituitary in response to the presence of corticotropin releasing hormone produced in the hypothalamus. It can also be secreted by pituitary tumors or small-cell lung carcinomas, but would present with Cushing's syndrome (hypertension, weight gain, buffalo hump, truncal obesity, striae, hyperglycemia, and osteoporosis) rather than hyponatremia.

Answer B is incorrect. Neuronal signals from the osmoreceptors of the third ventricle stimulate the production of ADH as well as stimulate the sensation of thirst.

Answer C is incorrect. V2 receptors are coupled to the insertion of aquaporins; V1 receptors are coupled to the contraction of vascular smooth muscle.

Answer D is incorrect. Activation of V1 receptors leads to an increase in total peripheral resistance.

Answer F is incorrect. Renin is secreted by smooth muscle cells in the afferent arteriole and acts to cleave angiotensinogen to angiotensin I. This activates the renin-angiotensin-aldosterone axis, leading to increased salt and water retention. A patient with persistent activation of this axis would present primarily with hypertension and edema with relatively low urine sodium levels.

14. **The correct answer is D.** This patient is in the early stages of renal failure with symptoms of oliguria and elevated BUN and creatinine levels. Combined with the patient's reduced hearing, these symptoms represent the ototoxicity and nephrotoxicity seen with aminoglycoside administration. Gentamicin is a type of aminoglycoside.

    Answer A is incorrect. Chloramphenicol toxicity is associated with anemia, aplastic anemia, and gray baby syndrome.

    Answer B is incorrect. Doxycycline toxicity includes gastrointestinal distress, tooth discoloration and inhibition of bone growth in children, and photosensitivity reactions.

    Answer C is incorrect. Erythromycin toxicity

includes gastrointestinal discomfort, acute cholestatic hepatitis, eosinophilia, and skin rashes. It is not generally associated with nephrotoxicity.

Answer E is incorrect. Imipenem is a broad-spectrum antibiotic that can cause gastrointestinal distress, skin rash, and seizures at higher doses.

15. **The correct answer is C.** This man is suffering from acute tubular necrosis (ATN), which is shown by the granular casts in his urine. A documented adverse effect of statin drugs is that they can cause rhabdomyolysis—the destruction of skeletal muscle with subsequent excretion of myoglobin by the kidneys. Myoglobin is nephrotoxic and, in significant amounts, may lead to ATN (also a common complication of crush injuries). There is no hemoglobin in the urine; myoglobin is causing the urine to turn red.

    Answer A is incorrect. β-Blockers do not cause acute tubular necrosis.

    Answer B is incorrect. An NSAID could cause prerenal failure in the setting of hypotension (NSAIDs decrease prostaglandins in the efferent arterioles and therefore can decrease glomerular filtration rate in a hypotensive setting, which can lead to acute tubular necrosis). This, however, would not account for the myoglobinuria.

    Answer D is incorrect. Hemolytic-uremic syndrome or thrombotic thrombocytopenic purpura could cause acute renal failure, but there is no other evidence of this type of process.

    Answer E is incorrect. A crush injury could cause this scenario, but any injury large enough to cause kidney failure would certainly be noticeable to the patient and/or doctors.

16. **The correct answer is D.** The presence of white cell casts in the urine indicates that this is acute pyelonephritis and not just a lower urinary tract infection (UTI). Pyelonephritis is an acute infection of the renal parenchyma that

most often results from an ascending progression of a UTI from the bladder. This most frequently involves *Escherichia coli*. Other clinical manifestations of a UTI include dysuria, urinary frequency, hematuria, bacteriuria, and pyuria. If white blood cell casts are seen, implying involvement of the kidney, the clinician can be sure that the UTI has ascended, making it a case of pyelonephritis. Acute pyelonephritis, like most acute phases of inflammation, is characterized by a predominance of polymorphonuclear leukocytes.

Answer A is incorrect. After 2–3 days, neutrophils are replaced by monocytes, macrophages, plasma cells, and lymphocytes as part of chronic inflammation. Macrophages are longer lived than neutrophils and are capable of proliferating and phagocytosing larger particles.

Answer B is incorrect. A monocyte has a kidney-shaped nucleus and differentiates into a macrophage in tissue; it is seen in chronic inflammation.

Answer C is incorrect. A plasma cell has a clock-faced chromatin distribution. B lymphocytes differentiate into plasma cells, which then produce large amounts of antibody. They are a component of humoral immunity.

Answer E is incorrect. T lymphocytes are the key component of cell-mediated immunity and are not the primary cell in acute inflammation.

17. **The correct answer is D.** Rapidly progressive (crescentic) glomerulonephritis (RPGN) is a renal disease with a rapid course (weeks to months) to renal failure. It is characterized by extensive capillary damage leading to accumulation of cells and fibrinous changes in Bowman's space, together with the characteristic "crescent" seen on biopsy. Renal insufficiency is present at diagnosis in almost all cases. The urinalysis typically reveals a nephritic picture of hematuria, red cell casts, and a variable degree of proteinuria. RPGN is a heterogeneous autoimmune disease caused by anti–glomerular basement membrane (as in Goodpasture's syndrome) immune complex deposition or by

the progression of the ANCA-positive vasculitides (e.g., Wegener's granulomatosis).

Answer A is incorrect. Diabetic nephropathy is the most common cause of kidney failure in the United States. The histologic morphology is characterized by an increase in mesangial matrix and marked nodular accumulations known as Kimmelstiel-Wilson nodules with diffuse glomerulosclerosis. Urinalysis would show glucose if this were the etiology.

Answer B is incorrect. Membranoproliferative glomerulonephritis is an uncommon autoimmune disorder that affects young individuals (8–30 years old). The diagnosis is based on the histologic finding of mesangial proliferation and thickening of the capillary walls with mesangial interposition, which creates a tram-track appearance on light microscopy.

Answer C is incorrect. Minimal change disease is the most common cause of nephrotic syndrome in children. It usually presents as massive proteinuria and hyperlipidemia secondary to disruption of the epithelial foot process, which decreases the ability of the kidney to retain serum proteins, such as albumin. The primary histopathologic finding is diffuse epithelial foot process fusion on electron microscopy.

Answer E is incorrect. Systemic lupus erythematosus (SLE) is a chronic autoimmune disease that affects multiple organ systems, including the kidney. SLE affects young adults (women more than men) and usually presents with a combined nephritic and nephrotic picture. Histologically, SLE kidneys have a peculiar wire-loop appearance with subendothelial basement membrane deposits.

18. **The correct answer is A.** This patient is suffering an acute overdose of amphetamine. He should be treated with ammonium chloride to acidify his urine and increase renal clearance of the weak base. This phenomenon, called ion trapping, occurs because increasing the ratio of ionized to nonionized drug species in the renal tubule allows more of the drug to be retained in the urine and excreted. Weak bases in acidic environments have high ratios of ion-

ized species, which are water soluble and do not cross membranes. When urine is acidified, the levels of ionized amphetamine are high, and therefore more drug is trapped in the renal tubule.

Answer B is incorrect. Alkalinization with bicarbonate is used to increase renal clearance of weak acids such as phenobarbital, methotrexate, tricyclic antidepressants, and aspirin.

Answer C is incorrect. Flumazenil is a treatment for acute benzodiazepine overdose.

Answer D is incorrect. Naloxone is a treatment for opioid overdose.

Answer E is incorrect. Treatment with water would have no effect on this patient's acute intoxication.

19. **The correct answer is B.** While this patient's pH, bicarbonate, and carbon dioxide levels are all very close to normal, it is always important to look more closely before concluding that there is no disorder. Vomiting is a common cause of a metabolic alkalosis, while diarrhea is a common cause of non–anion-gap metabolic acidosis. The patient has had gastrointestinal symptoms that have led to acute dehydration, which indicates that these symptoms are probably quite severe. Therefore, it is more likely that she has a mixed acid-base disorder than no electrolyte imbalances at all.

Answer A is incorrect. Non–anion-gap metabolic acidosis is the presence of a low pH with a low plasma bicarbonate level and without an elevated anion gap. The cause is generally diarrhea, renal tubular acidosis, or hypochloremia.

Answer C is incorrect. While a mixed respiratory disorder could lead to this electrolyte profile, the patient has no respiratory pathology. Therefore, it is more likely that her acid-base status is being determined by a metabolic process.

Answer D is incorrect. Respiratory alkalosis can be caused only by an increase in ventilation leading to excessive loss of CO_2, which is balanced by an increased excretion of bicar-

bonate. Hence, a high pH and low CO_2 and bicarbonate levels indicate respiratory alkalosis.

Answer E is incorrect. Although this patient's pH, bicarbonate, and carbon dioxide levels are close to normal, the gastrointestinal symptoms (vomiting, diarrhea) suggest that she has a mixed acid-base disorder than no electrolyte imbalances at all.

20. **The correct answer is E.** Chronic renal failure is a common complication in noncompliant diabetic patients. Chronic renal failure results in the progressive loss of renal function, eventually leading to end-stage renal disease. In chronic renal failure, the kidneys are unable to keep up their normal excretory, metabolic, and endocrine functions. The abnormalities include accumulation of toxins, underproduction of hormones (vitamin D and erythropoietin), and increased release of renin. Symptoms and clinical abnormalities associated with chronic renal failure include edema, hyperkalemia, metabolic acidosis, hyperphosphatemia, hypocalcemia, renal osteodystrophy, hypertension, pulmonary edema, congestive heart failure, uremia, anemia, nausea, vomiting, peripheral neuropathy, and pruritus. The pathogenesis of osteomalacia in patients with chronic renal disease is caused by failure of the kidney to turn $25(OH)D$ into the active form $1,25(OH)_2D$. Without active vitamin D, there is impaired mineralization of bone, leading to renal osteodystrophy.

Answer A is incorrect. Bacteriuria is the presence of bacteria in the urine. This is associated with urinary tract infections, not renal failure.

Answer B is incorrect. In end-stage renal disease, the kidneys are unable to regulate and excrete potassium, leading to hyperkalemia, not hypokalemia. Cardiac arrhythmias are a common complication of hyperkalemia.

Answer C is incorrect. Hypotension is not caused by renal failure. Excess retention of sodium and water leads to fluid overload and results in hypertension, congestive heart failure, and pulmonary edema.

Answer D is incorrect. Metabolic acidosis,

not alkalosis, occurs due to a decrease in acid secretion and a decrease in bicarbonate production.

Answer F is incorrect. Anemia, not polycythemia, will result in renal failure as the kidneys become unable to produce erythropoietin. Some renal cancers can lead to over-expression of erythropoietin and lead to polycythemia, but renal failure leads to anemia.

21. **The correct answer is A.** IgA nephropathy (Berger's disease) presents within several days of an infection (as opposed to poststreptococcal glomerulonephritis, which presents weeks after) with a nephritic picture due to IgA deposition in the mesangium. It is the most common global nephropathy, but it is a mild disease. It is common in children and presents as a recurrent hematuria with minimal clinical significance. On immunofluorescence, it presents with nonlinear mesangial deposits of IgA. Treatment is with angiotensin-converting enzyme inhibitors and corticosteroids. Patients with IgA nephropathy have a risk of recurrence of the disease.

Answer B is incorrect. Increased antistreptolysin O titers are associated with acute poststreptococcal glomerulonephritis rather than IgA nephropathy (Berger's disease). The classic findings include RBCs and casts in the urine (causing the tea-colored appearance), elevated antistreptolysin O titers, decreased complement levels, and "lumpy-bumpy" electron-dense deposits in the glomerulus.

Answer C is incorrect. Acute poststreptococcal glomerulonephritis is an autoimmune disease most frequently seen in children. It normally presents a few weeks after a streptococcal with a nephritic picture of peripheral and periorbital edema, dark urine, and proteinuria. These symptoms are caused by circulating antistreptococcal antibody-antigen complexes that deposit in the glomerular basement membrane, leading to complement activation and glomerular damage. The classic findings are RBCs and casts in the urine (which cause the characteristic tea-colored urine), a positive an-

tistreptolysin O titer, decreased levels of complement, and "lumpy-bumpy" electron-dense deposits in the subepithelium of the glomerulus. Recovery is spontaneous and treatment is supportive.

Answer D is incorrect. IgA nephropathy usually presents with a nephritic picture, which does not involve the massive proteinuria that is seen in nephrotic syndromes.

Answer E is incorrect. IgA deposition in Berger's disease is primarily in the mesangium and not the subepithelium.

22. **The correct answer is D.** This patient has diffuse cortical necrosis: generalized infarctions of the cortices of both kidneys, which is a common complication of disseminated intravascular coagulation (DIC). DIC commonly occurs after a complication of pregnancy such as amniotic fluid embolus and placental abruption, and affected patients develop the abrupt onset of the triad of anuria, gross hematuria, and flank pain. The diagnosis can usually be established by ultrasonography, which will demonstrate hypodense areas in the renal cortex. Although many patients can be sustained on dialysis, only 20–40% have partial recovery of kidney function. Indications for acute dialysis in DIC include (1) acidosis refractory to bicarbonate, (2) severe electrolyte abnormalities refractory to medical intervention (especially high K^+ levels), (3) intoxication with some drugs, (4) volume overload refractory to diuretics, and (5) uremic symptoms (e.g., cardiac friction run, altered mental status). The fact that this patient has a new-onset pericardial friction rub indicates uremia and makes dialysis imperative.

Answer A is incorrect. Aggressive fluid support is not beneficial for kidney recovery after the development of diffuse cortical necrosis. The kidney has been severely damaged by the microthrombi of disseminated intravascular coagulation. Aggressive fluid resuscitation is contraindicated due to (1) the lack of hypotension and (2) the renal failure. Fluids will only cause volume overload if they cannot be excreted.

Answer B is incorrect. While renal malignancy can cause hematuria, it is less likely to cause renal failure. In this case a biopsy to look for renal malignancy is not necessary because the cause of the patient's symptoms is already known. The first treatment should be dialysis to counteract renal failure and allow any remaining renal tissue to recover.

Answer C is incorrect. Broad-spectrum antibiotics are indicated in cases of shock due to sepsis. This patient has disseminated intravascular coagulation caused by an amniotic embolus, and since there is no infection, antibiotics will not be beneficial. Additionally, as the patient is experiencing renal failure, any antibiotic that is renally metabolized should be renally dosed to account for the patient's creatinine clearance rate.

Answer E is incorrect. This patient is in severe acute renal failure. Failure to treat will result in death.

23. **The correct answer is B.** Normally, hyperuricemia leads to kidney stones that are radiolucent and therefore not seen on x-ray. These stones are often seen in the setting of diseases with increased cell proliferation and turnover, such as leukemia and myeloproliferative disorders. Remember that uric acid is a metabolite of nucleic acid turnover, which is heightened in the setting of cell destruction.

Answer A is incorrect. Calcium stones are the most common cause of kidney stones (80–85%). Therefore, states that lead to increased calcium (e.g., hyperparathyroidism, destructive bone diseases) can lead to their formation. The stones are made of calcium oxalate or calcium phosphate and are radiopaque. Other risk factors are increased vitamin D and milk-alkali syndrome.

Answer C is incorrect. Prostate cancer commonly sends metastases to the bone, the destruction of which leads to a hypercalcemic state and the production of radiopaque calcium-based stones.

Answer D is incorrect. Urinary tract infection with urease-positive microorganisms such as

Proteus vulgaris and *Staphylococcus saprophyticus* can form large struvite calculi (ammonium, magnesium, and phosphate) that are radiopaque. This is the second most common cause of kidney stones.

Answer E is incorrect. Urinary tract infection with urease-positive microorganisms such as *Staphylococcus saprophyticus* can form large struvite calculi that are radiopaque.

24. **The correct answer is A.** Calcium is reabsorbed in three areas along the nephron: the proximal tubule, the thick ascending loop, and the distal tubule. In the proximal tubule, calcium reabsorption is coupled to sodium reabsorption. In the thick ascending loop, calcium reabsorption is dependent on the function of the sodium-potassium-chloride triple transporter. In the distal tubule, calcium reabsorption is not coupled to sodium reabsorption but is controlled by parathyroid hormone. Normally, the triple-transporter gradient is maintained by the basolateral sodium-potassium ATPase. As sodium exits and potassium enters, the sodium-generated driving force for triple-transporter function is created. The potassium that enters from the basolateral (through the ATPase) and luminal (through the triple transporter) cell surfaces are passed passively through both the basolateral and luminal membranes by specific channels. Because the triple transporter brings in two cations and two anions and the ATPase exchanges one cation for one anion, the potassium exiting the luminal membrane creates an electronegative environment inadverse the cell. The triple-transport function is therefore said to be electrogenic. This +7-mV positive luminal charge difference drives the reabsorption of calcium (and magnesium) by a paracellular route.

Answer B is incorrect. Parathyroid hormone controls calcium reabsorption in the distal tubule.

Answer C is incorrect. The triple transporter maintains a lumen positive charge; positive ions are reabsorbed to maintain electroneutrality.

Answer D is incorrect. Sodium and calcium are not cotransported in the thick ascending loop of Henle.

Answer E is incorrect. Volume contraction increases calcium (and sodium) reabsorption in the proximal tubule.

25. **The correct answer is E.** Minimal change disease results from a dysfunction of the glomerular filtration barrier that prevents protein and other macromolecules from entering the proximal tubule. Endothelial cells, basal lamina, and the diaphragm serve as a tripartite filtration barrier for fluid flowing from the glomerular capillaries into Bowman's space. Part of this barrier is composed of large negatively charged proteoglycans, such as heparan sulfate, that prevent the passage of smaller negatively charged proteins, such as albumin. In minimal change disease, damage to epithelial cells reduces production of these and other molecules that are critical components of the filtration barrier; the result is albumin and other small proteins are released into the urine.

Answer A is incorrect. Molecules > 69,000 Da are trapped by the basal lamina and cannot cross.

Answer B is incorrect. Most Na^+ ions are reabsorbed in the proximal convoluted tubule, not by the glomerular filtration barrier.

Answer C is incorrect. The filtration barrier has negatively charged components that prevent negatively charged macromolecules from crossing.

Answer D is incorrect. Renin gets released at low Na^+ concentrations; however, it is the macula densa, not the glomerulus, that detects low Na^+ concentrations, stimulating juxtaglomerular cells to release the enzyme renin.

26. **The correct answer is E.** On its own, tobramycin, an aminoglycoside, can cause nephrotoxicity. However, when combined with a cephalosporin (such as cefoxitin), the nephrotoxic effects are greatly increased. Renal failure is reflected by the elevated creatinine level.

Answer A is incorrect. Azithromycin is not an appropriate treatment for *Klebsiella pneumoniae* infection and is not associated with nephrotoxicity.

Answer B is incorrect. Aztreonam is not associated with nephrotoxicity.

Answer C is incorrect. Clindamycin can cause pseudomembranous colitis but does not cause nephrotoxicity.

Answer D is incorrect. Piperacillin is associated with hypersensitivity reactions and not nephrotoxicity.

27. **The correct answer is A.** Drinking water after exercise has the effect of diluting body fluids and causing a decrease in plasma osmolarity. The body's response is to decrease urine osmolarity and increase urine volume. Rapid ingestion of large volumes of water can lead to hyponatremia and cause severe harm as brain cells swell as fluid moves from the extracellular to the intracellular fluid compartments.

Answer B is incorrect. ADH and oxytocin are the two hormones secreted by the posterior pituitary. Neither hormone would be secreted in response to volume expansion and decreased plasma osmolarity, and ADH secretion would specifically be decreased.

Answer C is incorrect. When ingested water is distributed throughout the body fluids, plasma osmolarity decreases.

Answer D is incorrect. Inhibition of ADH secretion has the effect of reducing the number of aquaporin molecules that are mobilized in the principal cells of the late distal tubule and collecting duct. This acts to decrease water resorption and dilute the urine.

Answer E is incorrect. In hypo-osmolar states, the osmoreceptors of the hypothalamus are inhibited and result in suppression of thirst as well as inhibited secretion of ADH.

28. **The correct answer is D.** ADH binds the V_2 receptors on the basolateral adverse of the principal cell and activates a G_s–cyclic adeno-

sine monophosphate cascade that mobilizes aquaporin molecules to the luminal surface.

Answer A is incorrect. Binding and blocking A is the site and activity of triamterene.

Answer B is incorrect. ADH action is on the basolateral, not the luminal adverse.

Answer C is incorrect. ADH is coupled to G_s, not G_i.

Answer E is incorrect. Stimulation at D is the activity of aldosterone.

29. **The correct answer is A.** The important point of this question is that this woman died in renal failure, which is indicated by the diffuse tubular necrosis seen on autopsy. Tubular necrosis indicates acute renal failure, which can be secondary to ischemia, crush injuries (causing myoglobinuria), or a variety of toxins (in this case ethylene glycol, which results in a profound metabolic anion-gap acidosis). If the rest of the organ systems can be supported, individuals with acute tubular necrosis (ATN) usually recover in 2–3 weeks with supportive dialysis. To calculate this woman's BUN:Cr ratio and urine output before her death, one has to figure out what type of renal failure she had: prerenal, intrarenal, or postrenal. ATN is an intrarenal process, and intrarenal damage is marked by a decline in glomerular filtration rate, and BUN and plasma Cr concentrations increase in proportion to one another, thus the ratio remains below 15:1. In ATN. Also, because the kidney is damaged in ATN, it is unlikely that it will be able to reabsorb sodium and to concentrate the urine. Thus, the fraction of excreted sodium is usually > 2%. Renal failure is also associated with low urine output. Therefore, this patient's renal function prior to death most likely showed a BUN:Cr ratio of < 15:1 and low urine output.

Answer B is incorrect. A BUN:Cr ratio of < 15:1 is consistent with intrarenal disease, as this patient had; however, the patient would not have normal urine output, so this answer is incorrect.

Answer C is incorrect. A BUN:Cr ratio of 15–20:1 is consistent with postrenal, not in-

trarenal, disease. Additionally, renal failure is not associated with normal urine output.

Answer D is incorrect. A BUN:Cr ratio of 15–20:1 with low urine output is consistent with postrenal causes of renal failure. Prostatic disease and urethral stones can cause urinary obstruction, leading to acute renal failure. Postrenal disease is manifested by low urine output and a fractional excretion of sodium of > 4%.

Answer E is incorrect. A BUN:Cr ratio of > 20:1 describes a prerenal, not intrarenal, cause of acute renal failure. Also, patients in renal failure do not have normal urine output.

Answer F is incorrect. A BUN:Cr ratio of > 20:1 is indicative of prerenal disease. Prerenal disease is characterized by decreased blood flow to the kidneys, but the parenchyma is normal. The kidneys, sensing low body volume, will avidly hold on to sodium, resulting in a fractional excretion of sodium of < 1%. Also, because more water is reabsorbed proximally in prerenal disease, the tubular concentration of urea increases, leading to an increase in urea reabsorption and a subsequent rise in BUN that is out of proportion to the rise in creatinine. The result is a BUN:Cr ratio of > 20:1. Again, because kidneys in patients with prerenal disease are underperfused, they are trying to hold on to water, resulting in decreased urine output.

30. **The correct answer is E.** Renal blood flow is determined by the equation: flow = change in pressure/resistance. In the kidney, resistance is provided by the glomerular afferent and efferent arterioles. These arterioles can be modified by a number of endogenous substances and physiologic actions. Dopamine has a selective action such that low levels dilate cerebral, cardiac, splanchnic, and renal arterioles. Similarly, bradykinin induces the vasodilation of arterioles. The combined actions of these substances act to reduce resistance and thus increase renal blood flow.

Answer A is incorrect. Stimulation of afferent α_1-adrenergic receptors acts to vasoconstrict the arteriole.

Answer B is incorrect. Stimulation of afferent angiotensin II receptors acts to vasoconstrict the arteriole.

Answer C is incorrect. In autoregulation of renal blood flow, the myogenic hypothesis suggests that increased stimulation of stretch-activated calcium channels in the vascular smooth muscle causes an increase in intracellular calcium and a contraction of the muscle. This increase in resistance produces a reduction in flow.

Answer D is incorrect. α_1-Adrenergic receptors are found on both the afferent and efferent arterioles, but there are far more receptors on the afferent vessels. Angiotensin II (AT II) is a potent constrictor of both afferent and efferent arterioles, but the efferent arterioles are more sensitive to low levels of AT II. Activating both receptors causes vasoconstriction, thereby increasing vascular resistance and decreasing flow.

31. **The correct answer is A.** The patient's urinalysis indicates that her renal failure is intrarenal in origin (shown by her fractional excretion of sodium of between 2% and 4%) and that interstitial nephritis is occurring (as seen by the WBC casts). Allergic interstitial nephritis is an inflammatory process that results in infiltration of the interstitium of the kidney with polymorphonuclear leukocytes and lymphocytes. The cause of interstitial nephritis is usually an allergic reaction to medications, but infections and immunologic disorders occasionally precipitate the disorder. Medications commonly associated with allergic reaction include penicillins (particularly methicillin and nafcillin), cephalosporins, and sulfonamides. Clinical findings include fever, rash, and eosinophilia. The most likely culprit in this case is the penicillin she was given for the foot infection.

Answer B is incorrect. NSAIDs could cause acute tubular necrosis in the setting of low renal blood flow, as they can cause the arterioles in the kidney to constrict. This, however, would most likely lead to an ischemic picture, not an allergic one, and there would be no eosinophilia. While there have been instances

of NSAIDs resulting in an allergic picture, it usually occurs in people with allergies to NSAIDs and is rarer than this reaction to penicillin.

Answer C is incorrect. Poststreptococcal glomerulonephritis is a type of immune-complex glomerulonephritis. This condition usually presents about 10 days after pharyngitis or 2 weeks after skin infection and is usually seen in children. Most patients test positive for antistreptolysin O, which can be helpful in making the diagnosis. While this is possible given her skin infection, it classically presents with a nephritic picture. Eosinophils and rash would not be seen.

Answer D is incorrect. Systemic lupus erythematosus (SLE) is a chronic autoimmune disease that affects multiple organ systems, including the kidney. SLE affects young adults (women almost three times more than men) and usually presents with a glomerular nephritis rather than with interstitial nephritis. Eosinophilia is not typically found in lupus nephropathy.

Answer E is incorrect. Urolithiasis (kidney stones) will present with postrenal failure and a fractional excretion of sodium of > 4%. The complications of urolithiasis are hydronephrosis due to obstruction and interstitial nephritis if the stone is secondary to a bacterial infection. On clinical presentation, some patients present with excruciating flank pain.

32. **The correct answer is D.** Hydrochlorothiazide is a diuretic that inhibits NaCl reabsorption at the distal tubule and also reduces the excretion of calcium.

Answer A is incorrect. Acetazolamide inhibits carbonic anhydrase at the proximal convoluted tubule to cause increased excretion of HCO_3^-. It has no effect on calcium excretion.

Answer B is incorrect. Amiloride is also a potassium-sparing diuretic that directly inhibits the Na^+ reabsorption transport ion at the cortical collecting duct and thus reduces the K^+ secretion at the same site. Amiloride has no effect on calcium excretion.

Answer C is incorrect. Furosemide is a loop diuretic that reduces the medullary concentration gradient by inhibiting the cotransport ions (Na^+, K^+, and $2Cl^-$) in the thick ascending loop of Henle. It increases calcium excretion from the kidney.

Answer E is incorrect. Spironolactone is a potassium-sparing diuretic that functions as an aldosterone antagonist so that Na^+ reabsorption and K^+ secretion are inhibited at the cortical collecting duct. It does not affect calcium excretion.

33. **The correct answer is B.** The ureter crosses the iliac artery anteriorly at its bifurcation. It then continues into the pelvis, where is passes posteriorly to the uterine artery. One way to remember the location of the ureter with relation to the uterine artery is "water under the bridge."

    Answer A is incorrect. The ureter does cross over (anterior to) the iliac artery but crosses the uterine artery posteriorly.

    Answer C is incorrect. The ureter does cross the uterine artery on the posterior aspect, but it passes over (anterior to) the iliac artery.

    Answer D is incorrect. The ureter crosses over (anterior to) the iliac artery and under (posterior to) the uterine artery.

    Answer E is incorrect. The ovarian artery is found posterior to the psoas muscle, while the ureter runs along the anterior surface of the psoas muscle.

34. **The correct answer is A.** The glomerular basement membrane is composed of endothelial fenestrae with filtration slits lined with anionic glycoproteins on the lamina rara interna and externa. The small diameter of the filtration slits partially blocks albumin filtration, but the charge selectivity of the barrier provides the largest obstacle to filtration by electrostatically repelling the negatively charged albumin molecules.

    Answer B is incorrect. This choice is incorrect, as the filtration slits are lined with nega-

tively charged anionic glycoproteins and are not positively charged.

Answer C is incorrect. Albumin is neither freely filtered nor absorbed in the glomerulus.

Answer D is incorrect. Neither the basement membrane nor albumin is positively charged.

Answer E is incorrect. The size selectivity of the endothelial filtration slits provides an obstacle to albumin filtration, but size selectivity alone does not account for the complete absence of albumin filtration in nonpathologic states.

35. **The correct answer is C.** To understand the metabolic abnormality of this woman, one must first look at the pH and then the HCO_3^- and P_{CO_2}. Her pH is 7.28, and so she is suffering from a form of acidosis. Metabolic acidosis is the presence of low pH with low plasma HCO_3^- level; her level is 15 mEq/L (normal = 23 mEq/L), thus she is suffering from metabolic acidosis. In an attempt to regulate pH, the respiration rate changes; here her P_{CO_2} is 28 mm Hg (normal is 40 mm Hg), thus her lungs are blowing off more CO_2 in order to raise the pH. The causes of metabolic acidosis are events that either increase acid levels (e.g., diabetic ketoacidosis, uremia, hypovolemic shock) or decrease the amount of base present (e.g., diarrhea, kidney failure). Metabolic acidosis can be further subdivided into non–anion-gap and anion-gap metabolic acidosis. The serum anion gap ($[Na^+] - [Cl^-] - [HCO_3^-]$) normally is within 10–16 mEq/L. If the primary cause of acidosis is a loss of HCO_3^-, there will be an increase in Cl^- and the anion gap will be normal, as seen in the case of severe diarrhea. However, in the case of high serum anion gap, the metabolic acidosis is caused by an increase of an "unmeasured" anion (e.g., lactate in the case of lactic acidosis): $(Na^+) - (Cl^-) - (HCO_3^-)$ = unmeasured anions – unmeasured cations. In this case the patient's anion gap is $137 - 112 - 15 = 10$, thus she has a non–anion-gap acidosis. Of the answers listed, only diarrhea can cause a non—anion-gap acidosis.

Answer A is incorrect. Salicylate overdose is one of the causes of anion-gap acidosis (ingested salicylic acid is the unmeasured anion). Note that severe salicylate toxicity can cause respiratory depression, which would cause a high $PaCO_2$.

Answer B is incorrect. Diabetic ketoacidosis causes a severe anion-gap acidosis (the unmeasured anions in this case are ketoacids). One way to remember all of the causes of anion-gap acidosis is the mnemonic **MUDPILES**: Methanol, Uremia, Diabetic ketoacidosis, Paraldehyde or Phenformin, Iron tablets or Isoniazid, Lactic acidosis, Ethylene glycol, Salicylates.

Answer D is incorrect. Underperfusion causes anion-gap acidosis (the anion in this case is lactic acid). The patient has a non–anion-gap acidosis, so this answer is incorrect.

Answer E is incorrect. Uremia indicates renal failure. The inability of the kidney to excrete organic acids leads to an anion-gap acidosis.

36. **The correct answer is B.** Inulin is freely filtered across the glomerular capillary wall and is neither reabsorbed nor secreted. It is therefore used to calculate the glomerular filtration rate (GFR), otherwise known as clearance of inulin. Creatinine clearance can also be used as a physiologic approximation of GFR. GFR is calculated as: urinary concentration of inulin × urinary flow rate/plasma concentration of inulin. Using this equation, urine flow rate = GFR × plasma concentration of inulin/urinary inulin concentration = 120 mL/min × 1.5 mg/mL ÷ 50 mg/mL = 3.6 mL/min. Note that glomerular capillary hydrostatic pressure listed in the table of laboratory values is a distracter that is not used in the equation.

Answer A is incorrect. This answer underestimates the patient's urine flow rate, which is 3.6 mL/min.

Answer C is incorrect. This answer overestimates the patient's urine flow rate, which is 3.6 mL/min.

Answer D is incorrect. This answer translates into a value of 0.6 mL/min, which underesti-

mates the patient's urine flow rate, which is 3.6 mL/min.

Answer E is incorrect. This answer translates into a value of 0.3 mL/min, which underestimates the patient's urine flow rate, which is 3.6 mL/min.

37. **The correct answer is B.** Increased sodium intake leads to volume expansion and increased stretch in baroreceptors located in the afferent arteriole. The baroreceptor response to increased plasma volume is decreased sympathetic activity producing vasodilation of glomerular afferent arterioles. This increases the glomerular filtration rate while also decreasing sodium reabsorption in the proximal tubule.

Answer A is incorrect. Atrial natriuretic peptide is secreted by the atria in response to increased extracellular fluid volume and causes dilation, not constriction, of the glomerular afferent arterioles.

Answer C is incorrect. Atrial natriuretic peptide (ANP) is secreted by the atria in response to increased extracellular fluid volume and causes dilation of the glomerular afferent arterioles. This is a physiologic response to sodium intake and volume expansion; however, the kidney is not involved in ANP release.

Answer D is incorrect. Increased plasma sodium and water leads to increased sodium chloride delivery to the macula densa, leading to suppression of renin release by the juxtaglomerular apparatus.

Answer E is incorrect. Increased extracellular fluid volume dilutes the existing proteins, resulting in a decrease in plasma oncotic pressure.

38. **The correct answer is C.** Mannitol is an osmotic diuretic. Osmotic diuretics are filtered but not reabsorbed and thus serve to increase the osmolarity of tubular fluid, drawing water into the lumen and increasing urine production. Although osmotic diuretics are functional at many locations along the nephron, their primary site of action is in the descending loop of

Henle, where the tubule is permeable to water but impermeable to solutes.

Answer A is incorrect. The collecting tubule is the site of action for potassium-sparing diuretics.

Answer B is incorrect. The distal tubule is the site of action for thiazide diuretics.

Answer D is incorrect. The proximal tubule is the primary site of action for carbonic anhydrase inhibitors such as acetazolamide.

Answer E is incorrect. The thick ascending limb of the loop of Henle is the site of action for furosemide and other loop diuretics.

39. **The correct answer is C.** Focal segmental glomerulosclerosis is a nephrotic disease and generally presents in African-Americans between 18–30 years of age; it is three to four times more common in men than in women. Other risk factors include obesity and HIV-positive status. Nephrotic syndrome is a renal disorder that is characterized by massive proteinuria (> 3.5 g/24 hr protein in urine). This is due to hypoalbuminemia, generalized edema, and hyperlipidemia (thought to be secondary to elevated hepatic activity, which is meant to replace the lost albumin and clotting factors). Simply put, this is considered a "leaky" kidney without active inflammation. The name of the disease describes the pattern of glomerular damage, which is glomerular sclerosis (obliteration of capillary lumen) with focal (< 50% of glomeruli affected) and segmental (only parts of glomerulus effected) patterns. The cause of focal segmental glomerulosclerosis is unknown. Typically, it is resistant to steroid treatment.

Answer A is incorrect. Focal segmental glomerulosclerosis means that < 50% of the glomeruli are affected (focal) and that only parts of the glomerular tuft are affected (segmental). This answer is not consistent with this definition.

Answer B is incorrect. Focal segmental glomerulosclerosis means that < 50% of the glomeruli are affected (focal) and that only parts of the glomerular tuft are affected (seg-

mental). This answer is not consistent with this definition.

Answer D is incorrect. Focal segmental glomerulosclerosis means that < 50% of the glomeruli are affected (focal) and that only parts of the glomerular tuft are affected (segmental). This answer is not consistent with this definition.

Answer E is incorrect. There is no cellular proliferation seen in focal segmental glomerulosclerosis.

40. **The correct answer is D.** Glucose is reabsorbed from the proximal tubule by a sodium-glucose cotransport system. These transporters are able to handle filtered glucose concentrations in the healthy physiologic range. Glucose transporters are able to reabsorb all glucose up to 200 mg/dL. At 200 mg/dL, however, the transporters begin to become saturated and glucose starts to spill into the urine. At 350 mg/dL, all transporters are occupied and all filtered glucose above that concentration is excreted. Glucose will therefore not begin to spill into Mr. Jones's urine until his glucose level is elevated to at least 200 mg/dL.

Answer A is incorrect. Glucose is normally resorbed completely by the proximal tubule. There are no glucose transporters elsewhere in the renal tubules.

Answer B is incorrect. Negatively charged proteins in the glomerular wall help form the glomerular filtration barrier. In particular, they impede the filtration of large negatively charged molecules such as albumin and other plasma proteins. Glucose, a small neutral molecule, is not affected by this barrier.

Answer C is incorrect. Glomerular capillaries are made up of fenestrated epithelial cells that do not contain tight junctions. Tight junctions are normally found in the blood-brain barrier of the brain and retina.

Answer E is incorrect. The sodium-potassium exchange pump indirectly provides the energy for glucose resorption in the proximal convoluted tubule; the sodium gradient is necessary for the sodium-glucose cotransporters to function. Glucose is only resorbed in the proximal tubule, not in the distal tubule.

41. **The correct answer is A.** The kidneys are located between the parietal peritoneum and the posterior abdominal wall. They are retroperitoneal organs only partially covered by the parietal peritoneum anteriorly. Retroperitoneal organs (i.e., the duodenum, descending colon, ureters, pancreas, and aorta) lie outside the peritoneal cavity. The peritoneal cavity is a potential space with no organs except for a thin film of peritoneal fluid that lubricates its surface. Intraperitoneal organs are invaginated into this closed sac (peritoneum) and are not literally within the cavity itself.

Answer B is incorrect. The liver, the largest gland in the body, weighs approximately 1500 g. It lies mainly in the right upper quadrant inferior to the diaphragm. Functions of the liver include glycogen storage, secretion of bile, and detoxification of chemicals. The liver is not retroperitoneal in its location.

Answer C is incorrect. The spleen, one of the major lymphatic organs, is located intraperitoneally in the left upper quadrant.

Answer D is incorrect. The stomach is the expanded part of the digestive tract between the esophagus and the small intestine. The stomach is an intraperitoneal organ, not a retroperitoneal one.

Answer E is incorrect. The transverse colon is the largest and most mobile part of the large intestine. It spans the abdomen from the right colic flexure to the splenic flexure, where it folds inferiorly to become the descending colon. In contrast to the ascending and descending colon, the transverse colon passes intraperitoneally.

42. **The correct answer is E.** Tachycardia is one of the responses to shock. This is an attempt to compensate for the underperfusion of tissues by increasing heart rate, one of the components of cardiac output.

Answer A is incorrect. The immediate hypotension of shock is compensated for by an increase in heart rate, rather than a decrease.

Answer B is incorrect. Shock is associated with hypotension because of the loss, or perceived loss, of blood volume.

Answer C is incorrect. In response to shock, a patient is described as having tachypnea, or very rapid breathing, in an attempt to compensate for the underperfusion. This occurs regardless of the body position, whereas orthopnea occurs while lying down.

Answer D is incorrect. The body compensates for the real or perceived hypovolemic state by reducing urine output, leading to oliguria.

43. **The correct answer is B.** In diabetic nephropathy, diagnostic tests are important in the treatment and control of the progression of the disease. The histologic morphology is characterized by an increase in mesangial matrix by marked nodular accumulations known as Kimmelstiel-Wilson nodules and diffuse glomerulosclerosis.

Answer A is incorrect. Rapidly progressive (crescentic) glomerulonephritis is a renal disease that has a rapid course (weeks to months) to renal failure. It is characterized by extensive capillary damage that leads to accumulation of cells and fibrinous changes in Bowman's space, leading to the characteristic "crescent" seen on biopsy.

Answer C is incorrect. Membranoproliferative glomerulonephritis is an uncommon autoimmune renal disorder that normally affects young individuals (8–30 years of age). The diagnosis is based on a histologic presentation that includes mesangial proliferation, thickening of the peripheral capillary walls by subendothelial immune deposits, and mesangial interposition into the capillary wall, giving rise to a tram-track appearance on light microscopy.

Answer D is incorrect. Focal segmental glomerulosclerosis is a nephrotic disease and generally presents in young, hypertensive African-American males (obesity and HIV-positive status are also risk factors). The name of the disease describes the pattern of glomerular damage, which is glomerular sclerosis (obliteration of capillary lumen) with focal patterns (some glomeruli affected) and segmental patterns (only parts of glomerulus).

Answer E is incorrect. Membranoproliferative glomerulonephritis is characterized by a tram-track appearance on light microscopy due to mesangial interposition into the capillary wall.

44. **The correct answer is C.** Angiotensin II (AT II) increases the activity of the Na^+-H^+ exchanger in the proximal tubule to facilitate salt and water resorption. As a result, increased H^+ is pumped into the tubular lumen. Luminal H^+ is then returned to the tubular cell in the process of HCO_3^- resorption as H^+ and HCO_3^- join and form water and carbon dioxide after catalysis by brush-border carbonic anhydrase. Water and carbon dioxide diffuse back into the tubular cell and again liberate H^+ and HCO3- after carbonic anhydrase catalysis. Here, the HCO_3^- is transported into the bloodstream while the H^+ is free to participate in another round of HCO_3^- resorption via the Na^+-H^+ exchanger. Thus, the net result of increased Na^+-H^+ exchange is an increase in HCO_3^- resorption and no net change in H^+ secretion. Increased HCO_3^- reabsorption after AT II stimulation accounts for the contraction alkalosis that occurs as a result of volume depletion.

Answer A is incorrect. Increased Na^+-H^+ exchange in the proximal tubule leads to increased delivery of H^+ to the tubular lumen, which is then used to shuttle HCO_3^- back into the tubular cell. Hence, HCO_3^- resorption is increased while net H^+ secretion remains unchanged.

Answer B is incorrect. Increased Na^+-H^+ exchange in the proximal tubule leads to increased delivery of H^+ to the tubular lumen. However, there is no net increase in H^+ secretion, as the H^+ in the lumen is returned to the tubular cell in the process of HCO_3^- resorption.

Answer D is incorrect. Increased Na^+-H^+ exchange in the proximal tubule leads to increased delivery of H^+ to the tubular lumen, which is then used to shuttle HCO_3^- back into the tubular cells. Hence, HCO_3^- resorption is increased while net H^+ secretion remains unchanged. There is no net increase in H^+ secretion, as the H^+ in the lumen is returned to the cell in the process of HCO_3^- resorption.

Answer E is incorrect. Increased Na^+-H^+ exchange in the proximal tubule leads to increased delivery of H^+ to the tubular lumen, which is then used to shuttle HCO_3^- back into the tubular cells. Hence, HCO_3^- resorption is increased while net H^+ secretion remains unchanged.

45. **The correct answer is C.** This patient is in cardiogenic shock, which is shown by his hypotension with a systolic blood pressure of < 90 mm Hg. This has led to a loss of perfusion in his kidneys, which has, in turn, led to prerenal failure. Prerenal failure is defined by a blood urea nitrogen/creatinine (BUN:Cr) ratio of > 20:1. When the glomerular filtration rate drops, there is an increase in sodium and water reabsorption in the proximal tubule. This leads to an increase in tubular urea concentration, which favors increased reabsorption of urea. This will raise the BUN (remember, this is urea in the blood) and therefore, the BUN:Cr ratio will rise.

Answer A is incorrect. Blockage of the ureters is a postrenal cause of renal failure. It would present with pain on urination and is unlikely in the setting of cardiogenic shock.

Answer B is incorrect. This patient's blood urea nitrogen/creatinine (BUN:Cr) ratio of > 20:1 indicates that this is a prerenal process, not an intrarenal one. An acute tubular necrosis would present with renal failure in the setting of a BUN:Cr ratio of 10–15:1 with many hyaline casts and cellular debris in the urine.

Answer D is incorrect. Ethanol actually causes diuresis. By inhibiting the release of antidiuretic hormone from the posterior pituitary, alcohol consumption leads to increased urine output. The volume load that accompanies alcohol ingestion also contributes to increased urine output.

Answer E is incorrect. Urine output is controlled mainly by two factors: the hydration state of the body and the level of kidney function. Therefore, low urine output is seen only in the setting of dehydration or kidney dysfunction. Stress by itself will not cause low urine output unless it is coupled with dehydration or an acute renal disease process.

46. **The correct answer is E.** Acute poststreptococcal glomerulonephritis is an autoimmune disease most frequently seen in children. Under light microscopy, the glomeruli appear enlarged and hypercellular, with neutrophils and subepithelial immune complex depositions described as "lumpy-bumpy." Under electron microscopy, the large irregular deposits are observed in the subepithelium of the glomerulus. This condition normally presents a few weeks after a streptococcal infection with peripheral and periorbital edema, dark urine, and proteinuria. These symptoms are caused by circulating antistreptococcal antibody-antigen complexes that deposit in the glomerular basement membrane, leading to complement activation and glomerular damage. The classic findings are RBCs and casts in the urine (which cause the characteristic tea-colored urine), a positive antistreptolysin O titer, and decreased levels of complement.

    Answer A is incorrect. Linear subendothelial patterns are seen in vasculitides such as Goodpasture's syndrome.

    Answer B is incorrect. Mesangial deposits are usually seen in IgA nephropathy.

    Answer C is incorrect. A "spike-and-dome" pattern of deposition is a pattern seen in membranous glomerulonephritis.

    Answer D is incorrect. Subendothelial humps are usually seen in membranoproliferative glomerulonephritis.

    Answer F is incorrect. Granular subendothelial deposits are usually seen in systemic lupus erythematosus.

47. **The correct answer is D.** Hydrochlorothiazide and furosemide cause metabolic alkalosis.

Note that the laboratory values have elevated pH, partial arterial carbon dioxide pressure, and bicarbonate, indicating a metabolic alkalosis with partial respiratory compensation. Both thiazides and loop diuretics inhibit sodium uptake and thus increase distal delivery of sodium to the late distal tubule and collecting duct. An increased amount of sodium is taken into these distal cells from the luminal surface and exchanged for potassium and protons to maintain electroneutrality. This creates a condition of hypokalemia (too little potassium in the blood), kaluresis (urination of excess potassium), and excess urinary acid secretion. This loss of acid promotes metabolic alkalosis. In addition, hypokalemia induces the movement of potassium from its vast storehouse within tissues to the extracellular compartment in exchange for protons. This movement of potassium from tissues into blood and protons from the blood into tissues further promotes metabolic alkalosis.

Answer A is incorrect. Acetazolamide impairs reuptake of bicarbonate and secretion of acid in the proximal tubule. The loss of bicarbonate in the urine leads to metabolic acidosis.

Answer B is incorrect. Diuretics do not cause respiratory alkalosis.

Answer C is incorrect. Diuretics do not cause respiratory alkalosis.

Answer E is incorrect. Diuretics do not cause respiratory alkalosis.

Answer F is incorrect. Spironolactone inhibits the absorption of sodium in the distal convoluted tubule and proximal collecting duct, resulting in a decrease in secretion of other cations (potassium and protons) into the lumen. Decreased acid secretion can result in metabolic acidosis.

48. **The correct answer is C.** Metabolic acidosis is the presence of low pH with low plasma bicarbonate. The cause is generally either an increase in acid (e.g., diabetic ketoacidosis, hypovolemic shock via generation of lactic acid) or a decrease in base (e.g., diarrhea, kidney failure). Metabolic acidosis can be further subdi-

vided into non–anion-gap and anion-gap metabolic acidosis. Serum anion gap ($[Na^+] - [Cl^-] - [HCO_3^-]$) is normally within 10–16 mEq/L. If the primary cause of acidosis is a loss of HCO_3^-, there will be an increase in Cl^- and the anion gap will be normal, as seen in the case of severe diarrhea. However, in the case of high serum anion gap, the metabolic acidosis is caused by an increase of an "unmeasured" anion such as lactate (e.g., lactic acidosis).

Answer A is incorrect. The patient's anion gap will be normal. The primary cause of her metabolic acidosis is loss in HCO_3^- due to her diarrhea. As stated above, increased anion-gap metabolic alkalosis is caused by an increase in "unmeasured" anion. A useful mnemonic is **MUDPILES**—**M**ethanol, **U**remia, **D**iabetic ketoacidosis/EtOH ketoacidosis, **P**araldehyde, **I**NH/**I**ron toxicity, **L**actic acidosis, **E**thylene glycol, and **S**alicylates. Rhabdomyolysis is also a cause of metabolic acidosis but traditionally is not included in this mnemonic.

Answer B is incorrect. Metabolic alkalosis is the presence of high pH with increased plasma bicarbonate. This occurs with addition of alkaline compounds (antacid ingestion) or loss of acid (vomiting). This would not be caused by diarrhea.

Answer D is incorrect. In severe diarrhea with significant loss of fluids and electrolytes, especially bicarbonate, it is unlikely that the patient will have a normal acid-base state.

Answer E is incorrect. Respiratory acidosis is the presence of low pH due to a decrease in ventilation and an increase in serum CO_2. This occurs in cases of inadequate ventilation (e.g., depressed respiration by drugs or neurologic injury) or impaired gas exchange (e.g., pulmonary edema). This would not be caused by diarrhea.

Answer F is incorrect. Respiratory alkalosis is the presence of high pH due to an increase in ventilation leading to a decrease in serum CO_2. This occurs in cases of increased respiratory drive (e.g., by drugs or central nervous system disorders, anxiety, and fear). This would not be caused by diarrhea.

49. **The correct answer is A.** Demeclocycline is a tetracycline that is associated with nephrotoxicity, hepatotoxicity, and tooth discoloration.

Answer B is incorrect. Neomycin is an aminoglycoside that is associated with nephrotoxicity, ototoxicity, and a myasthenialike syndrome.

Answer C is incorrect. Norfloxacin is a fluoroquinolone and is associated with tendinitis and tendon rupture.

Answer D is incorrect. Penicillin is associated with hypersensitivity reactions and hemolytic anemia in sensitive individuals.

Answer E is incorrect. Vancomycin is associated with nephrotoxicity, ototoxicity, and thrombophlebitis. It is also known to cause a diffuse flushing known as "red man" syndrome.

50. **The correct answer is B.** When the amount of fluids in the body contracts, the body attempts to compensate by releasing angiotensin II, a potent vasoconstrictor. In order to protect the kidney from losing its perfusion due to this vasoconstriction, the kidney simultaneously releases prostaglandins at both the afferent and efferent arterioles, where they act as vasodilators. By inhibiting cyclooxygenase (COX)-1 and/or COX-2 enzymes, the pathway that produces the prostaglandins that keep the kidneys perfused becomes blocked, leading to decreased blood flow to the kidneys and resulting in a prerenal cause of renal failure. Celecoxib is a selective COX-2 inhibitor that affects the arterioles of the kidney and can cause renal failure in dehydrated patients.

Answer A is incorrect. Inhibition of the cyclooxygenase (COX)-2 enzyme will lead to a decrease in the production of thromboxane, causing a decrease in platelet aggregation. Thus, COX-2 inhibitors are used to prevent thrombosis in patients with a history of myocardial infarction or in patients with an increased likelihood of clotting. This effect is not contraindicated in the context of volume contraction.

Answer C is incorrect. Celecoxib is a selective cyclooxygenase (COX)-2 inhibitor that is effective because it spares the gastric mucosa the damaging effects of COX-1 inhibition.

Answer D is incorrect. Inhibition of the COX-2 enzyme will lead to a decrease in the production of prostaglandins, thromboxane, and prostacyclins, which affect platelet function and small vessel diameter. This effect is not contraindicated in the context of volume contraction.

Answer E is incorrect. Ibuprofen and other NSAIDs are contraindicated in dehydrated patients. NSAIDs reduce the kidneys' ability to maintain renal blood flow in times of volume depletion. In situations such as dehydration, there is an increased risk in developing prerenal disease; when NSAIDs are added to the situation the risk increases.

CHAPTER 13

Reproductive

1. A 53-year-old woman experiences hot flashes associated with menopause. She calls her primary care physician to ask for advice about the risks and benefits of hormone replacement therapy. Which of the following is a potential benefit of hormone replacement therapy?

(A) Decreased risk of breast cancer
(B) Decreased risk of deep venous thrombosis
(C) Decreased risk of hip fracture
(D) Decreased risk of myocardial infarction
(E) Decreased risk of stroke

2. A 32-year-old woman who is at 30 weeks of gestation presents to the emergency department with vaginal bleeding and painful abdominal cramps. Her blood pressure is 125/80 mm Hg. A urinalysis shows no protein, leukocytes, or bacteria with few RBCs. A peripheral blood smear shows a decreased number of normocytic, normochromatic RBCs with many schistocytes. Which of the following is the most likely diagnosis?

(A) Abruptio placentae
(B) Amniotic fluid embolism
(C) Hydrops fetalis
(D) Placenta previa
(E) Preeclampsia

3. A previously healthy 25-year-old sexually active man comes to the physician because of a painful genital rash for the past 5 days. Physical examination reveals grouped vesicles on an erythematous base. Tzanck smear shows multinucleated giant cells. Which of the following mechanisms is involved in the pathogenesis of this patient's infective agent?

(A) Direct invasion into the bloodstream
(B) Invasion of CD4+ cells
(C) Migration to the central nervous system by retrograde axonal transport
(D) Migration to the peripheral nervous system by anterograde axonal transport
(E) Migration to the peripheral nervous system by retrograde axonal transport

4. A 23-year-old sexually active woman presents to her physician with a high temperature, pelvic pain, purulent cervical discharge, and cervical motion tenderness. A Gram's stain prepared from a swab of the discharge is shown in the micrograph. Which of the following is the most likely infectious organism?

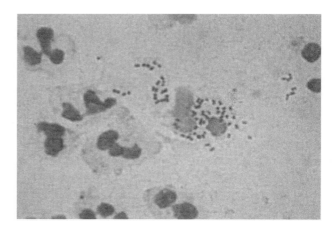

Reproduced, with permission, from Wolff K, Johnson RA, Suurmond D. *Fitzpatrick's Color Atlas & Synopsis of Clinical Dermatology*, 5th ed. New York: McGraw-Hill, 2005: Fig 27.15.

(A) *Candida albicans*
(B) *Chlamydia trachomatis*
(C) *Gardnerella vaginalis*
(D) *Neisseria gonorrhoeae*
(E) *Trichomonas vaginalis*

5. A woman who is 31 weeks pregnant comes to the emergency department with symptoms of preeclampsia. The presence of which of the following signs would change this initial diagnosis?

(A) Edema
(B) Hyperreflexia
(C) Hypertension
(D) Proteinuria
(E) Seizure

6. CT imaging of the pelvis performed on a 29-year-old African-American woman with dysmenorrhea reveals uterine masses similar to those seen in the image. Biopsy shows a whorled pattern of smooth muscle. These masses are most commonly associated with which of the following conditions?

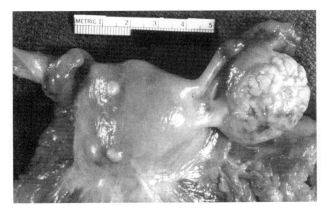

Image courtesy of PEIR Digital Library (http://peir.net).

(A) Enlargement with menopause
(B) Enlargement with pregnancy
(C) Formation of chocolate cysts
(D) Malignant transformation
(E) Necrosis and hemorrhage

7. If the hypothalamus were destroyed, levels of which hormone would rise?

(A) ADH
(B) Growth hormone
(C) Luteinizing hormone
(D) Oxytocin
(E) Prolactin
(F) Testosterone
(G) Thyroid-releasing hormone

8. A patient with a testicular tumor has blood work done that shows a serum α-fetoprotein level of 30 μg/mL (normal <10 μg/mL). Which of the following is the most likely age range of this patient?

(A) Infancy to 3 years
(B) 10–20 years

(C) 20–30 years
(D) 30–40 years
(E) 40–50 years

9. A 25-year-old woman with a history of recurrent upper respiratory infections (URIs) presents to her physician with her fifth URI in the past year. She mentions that she may be getting sick due to increased stress at home; she and her husband have been trying to conceive unsuccessfully for several years. The patient's WBC count, immunoglobulin, and platelet levels are all within normal limits. Which organizational unit represents the structure most likely to be defective in this patient?

(A) Central pair with nine peripheral pairs of microtubules
(B) Collagen α chains in triplets
(C) Multilobular nucleus with enzyme-filled granules
(D) Numerous adjoining e-cadherin molecules with actin filaments
(E) Two longer heavy chains and two shorter light chains linked by disulfide bonds

10. A young couple is having trouble conceiving and decides to undergo in vitro fertilization. The woman begins treatment to stimulate ovulation prior to ova collection and fertilization. Which of the following hormones is most directly responsible for ovulation?

(A) Estrogen
(B) Follicle-stimulating hormone
(C) Gonadotropin-releasing hormone
(D) Human chorionic gonadotropin
(E) Luteinizing hormone
(F) Progesterone

11. A 57-year-old woman is scheduled for elective hysterectomy. Severing which of the following structures during surgery would disrupt the most blood flow to the ipsilateral ovary?

(A) Cardinal ligament
(B) Fallopian tube
(C) Round ligament
(D) Suspensory ligament
(E) Ureter

12. Which of the following is the function of the androgen-binding globulin?

    (A) Spermatocyte maturation
    (B) Testosterone transport
    (C) To bind inhibin
    (D) To convert testosterone into estrogen
    (E) To inhibit androgen secretion

13. A 23-year-old woman who works as a prostitute comes to the clinic for a follow-up appointment because the results of her Pap smear showed a high-grade squamous intraepithelial lesion. Which of the following strains of the human papillomavirus is this condition most often associated with?

    (A) Strains 1 and 2
    (B) Strains 6 and 11
    (C) Strain 8
    (D) Strains 16 and 18
    (E) Strain L1-3

14. Following a normal pregnancy and labor, a baby is born to a young couple. The baby cries immediately and has Apgar scores of 9 at both 1 and 5 minutes. While examining the baby, the pediatrician at the delivery notes that the baby has some labial scrotal fusion and a phallus-like organ. The baby is also noted to be hypotensive and hypovolemic. Genotyping is done and the baby is found to be 46,XX. Which of the following is the most likely cause of the patient's pseudohermaphroditism?

    (A) 11-β-Hydroxylase deficiency
    (B) 17-β-Hydroxylase deficiency
    (C) 21-β-Hydroxylase deficiency
    (D) Mutation in the androgen receptor gene
    (E) 5-α-Reductase deficiency

15. A 50-year-old woman tells her physician that she is concerned about her risk for developing endometrial cancer. Which of the following factors poses the largest risk for developing endometrial cancer?

    (A) Alcoholism
    (B) Early sexual activity
    (C) Low-fiber diet
    (D) Multiparity
    (E) Prolonged unopposed estrogen use

16. A 27-year-old woman presents to her primary care physician with breast pain, nonbloody nipple discharge, and multiple bilateral breast masses. She denies any history of breast cancer in her family. Which of the following characteristics would most likely confirm that a breast mass is benign?

    (A) Central necrosis
    (B) Lymphocytic infiltration
    (C) Lymphatic involvement
    (D) Overlying eczema
    (E) Sclerosis

17. A 57-year-old man with erectile dysfunction has cavernosography prior to surgery. Cavernosography demonstrates a leak from the dorsal vein to the saphenous vein. Which of the following is the most likely cause of this patient's impotence?

    (A) Arterial insufficiency
    (B) Hormonal impotence
    (C) Psychogenic impotence
    (D) Somatosensory defect
    (E) Venous outflow

18. A 26-year-old primigravida presents to her obstetrician for a checkup 1 week after undergoing a cesarean section. The cesarean section was performed because of failure to progress. She says that she has been crying a lot over the past week and is worried that it is not normal to feel like this. Which of the following symptoms would make one more suspicious about postpartum depression instead of postpartum blues?

    (A) Anxiety about the infant
    (B) Easily fatigued
    (C) Easily irritated
    (D) Emotional lability
    (E) Feeling hopeless

19. A couple comes to the clinic for ultrasound testing during the woman's 15th week of pregnancy. She wants to know when the technician can tell them the gender of their baby. Which of the following hormones causes the prenatal differentiation of the external genitalia in males?

(A) Dihydrotestosterone
(B) Estradiol
(C) Follicle-stimulating hormone
(D) Luteinizing hormone
(E) Testosterone

20. A 46,XY infant is born with a nonsense mutation in the *SRY* gene. Which of the following will be the symptomatic manifestation of this mutation?

    (A) Female pseudohermaphrodite
    (B) Male pseudohermaphrodite
    (C) Normal female development
    (D) Normal male development
    (E) True hermaphrodite

21. Biopsy of a bilateral ovarian mass reveals round, mucin-secreting cells, as seen in the image. Which of the following other physical findings might be found in a patient with this condition?

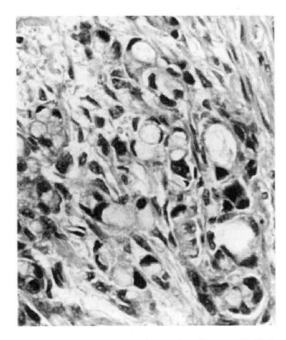

Reproduced, with permission, from Chandrasoma P, Taylor CR. *Concise Pathology*, 3rd ed. New York: McGraw-Hill, 1998: Fig. 52-16.

    (A) Galactorrhea
    (B) Melena
    (C) Palpable gallbladder

(D) Pearly papules on face
(E) Supraclavicular lymphadenopathy

22. A 25-year-old married woman who has been trying to become pregnant for the past 5 months presents to the emergency department with sudden and severe abdominal pain. Ultrasonography shows a mass in her left fallopian tube with free fluid in the cul-de-sac. Previous infection by which of the following agents most likely put this patient at a higher risk for developing this complication?

    (A) *Chlamydia trachomatis*
    (B) *Escherichia coli*
    (C) Herpes simplex virus
    (D) Human papilloma virus
    (E) *Streptococcus agalactiae*

23. A woman in her seventh month of pregnancy asks her obstetrician why her breasts are enlarging. In which of the following locations is the hormone responsible for breast milk production synthesized?

    (A) Adenohypophysis
    (B) Corpus luteum
    (C) Hypothalamus
    (D) Placenta
    (E) Syncytiotrophoblast

24. A healthy woman presents to the physician for a checkup. Her physical examination is unremarkable, and laboratory studies are all within normal limits. She expresses concern about "inheriting" breast cancer because she had an aunt who recently died of the disease. The gene that would most likely indicate an inheritable form of breast cancer in this patient is located on which of the following chromosomes?

    (A) 3
    (B) 5
    (C) 11
    (D) 17
    (E) 18
    (F) 22

25. A 14-year-old boy is brought to the clinic by his parents who are concerned because he has not yet begun puberty. Laboratory results indicate hypogonadism secondary to failure of the hypothalamic-pituitary-gonadal axis. Which of the following are possible adverse effects of the treatment for this patient's condition?

(A) Decreased serum LDL levels
(B) Growth of scalp hair
(C) Increased spermatogenesis
(D) Nausea and vomiting
(E) Premature closing of the epiphyseal plates

26. A 26-year-old woman presents to her gynecologist with a purulent vaginal discharge, lower abdominal pain, and fever. She reports having unprotected sexual intercourse about 1 month ago. On physical examination, she demonstrates cervical motion tenderness. Which of the following is the most likely cause of this patient's infection?

(A) *Candida albicans*
(B) *Chlamydia trachomatis*
(C) *Gardnerella vaginalis*
(D) *Streptococcus agalactiae* (group B strep)
(E) *Trichomonas vaginalis*

27. A 34-year-old woman with lupus who is 35 weeks pregnant comes to the emergency department because she is unable to walk due to swelling of her legs. Physical examination shows a temperature of 36.5° C (97.7° F), a pulse of 95/min, and a blood pressure of 150/90 mm Hg. The patient complains of a severe headache but has no other symptoms. Which of the following tests would aid in the initial diagnosis of this patient?

(A) Electroencephalogram
(B) Liver panel
(C) Papanicolaou smear
(D) Peripheral blood smear
(E) Urinalysis

28. An 80-year-old woman sustains a broken hip after a minor fall from a chair. The only medications she takes are multivitamins. Which of the following is the most likely hormonal profile of this woman?

Choice	Estrogen	Luteinizing Hormone	Follicle-Stimulating Hormone	Gonadotropin-Releasing Hormone
A	↓	↓	↓	↑
B	↓	↓	↓	↓
C	↓	↑	↑	↑
D	↑	↑	↑	↑
E	↑	↑	↑	↓

(A) A
(B) B
(C) C
(D) D
(E) E

29. A 23-year-old woman comes to the physician with vaginal candidiasis and is placed on an antifungal medication. Shortly thereafter, she experiences amenorrhea. Which of the following antifungal drugs did this patient use?

(A) Amphotericin B
(B) Fluconazole
(C) Flucytosine
(D) Ketoconazole
(E) Itraconazole

30. A 26-year-old man presents to an urologist after he and his wife failed to conceive for 14 months. His testosterone levels are normal, and initial semen analysis shows significantly decreased volume and no detectable sperm. A testicular fine-needle biopsy, however, demonstrates normal sperm motility and normal sperm morphology. His past surgical history includes an inguinal repair. Which of the following is the most likely cause of the patient's infertility?

(A) Disordered sperm transport
(B) Primary gonadal deficiency
(C) Secondary hypogonadism
(D) Sperm dysfunction
(E) Y-chromosome abnormality

31. A 73-year-old patient has been hospitalized for 6 days due to complications from surgery. The patient had a urinary catheter in place, which was removed on the fourth hospital day. Now she is complaining of painful and frequent urination and has a fever of 38.9° C (102° F). Urinalysis results are positive for nitrites and leukocyte esterase. A urine culture grows a gram-negative rod that produces a red pigment. Which of the following organisms is the most likely cause of this patient's symptoms?

(A) *Candida albicans*
(B) *Escherichia coli*
(C) *Klebsiella pneumonia*
(D) *Proteus mirabilis*
(E) *Pseudomonas aeruginosa*
(F) *Serratia marcescens*
(G) *Staphylococcus saprophyticus*

32. A 25-year-old woman comes to her physician complaining of cyclic dysmenorrhea and pain with intercourse. A sonogram reveals bilateral adnexal masses, and a laparoscopy shows chocolate cysts. This patient at risk for developing which of the following conditions?

(A) Abnormal vagina bleeding
(B) Carcinoma
(C) Infertility
(D) Masculinization
(E) Obesity

33. A new mother calls her obstetrician to say that she is having trouble breast-feeding. She is unable to produce enough milk to sate her baby even though her breasts are aching with stored milk. What medication can be prescribed to aid in milk letdown?

(A) ADH
(B) Human chorionic gonadotropin
(C) Oxytocin
(D) Somatostatin
(E) Somatotropin

34. During hernia surgeries, it is important to isolate important structures in the inguinal canal so that they do not become damaged and cause a functional deficit. Which of the following structures lies inside the inguinal canal but outside of the spermatic cord?

(A) Ductus deferens
(B) Ilioinguinal nerve
(C) Pampiniform plexus
(D) Testicular artery
(E) Testicular lymphatic vessels

35. A 2-month-old boy is brought to the pediatrician by his mother for a well-baby visit for the first time since his birth. On examination, the doctor notes that the patient has cryptorchidism, with both testicles remaining undescended. This patient is at increased risk for developing which of the following conditions?

(A) Hypogonadotropic hypogonadism
(B) Indirect inguinal hernia
(C) Retractile testis
(D) Testicular cancer
(E) Torsion of the spermatic cord

36. A 45-year-old man presents to his physician complaining of erectile dysfunction. Which of the following is the mechanism of action of the oral agents approved for the treatment of erectile dysfunction?

(A) Androgen supplementation
(B) Antiandrogen action via receptor site interference
(C) Binding to G proteins to stimulate adenylyl cyclase
(D) Inhibition of cyclic adenosine monophosphate (cAMP) phosphodiesterase
(E) Inhibition of cyclic guanosine monophosphate (cGMP) phosphodiesterase

37. A 35-year-old man comes to the physician complaining of painful vesicles that have erupted on his genitals. On further questioning, he admits to unprotected sex with multiple partners. To confirm the diagnosis, the physician performs a Tzanck test. Results are shown in the image. Which of the following is the pathognomonic finding on this patient's Tzanck smear?

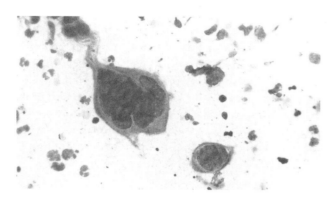

Reproduced, with permission, from Wolff K, Johnson RA, Suurmond D. *Fitzpatrick's Color Atlas & Synopsis of Clinical Dermatology*, 5th ed. New York, McGraw-Hill, 2005: 801.

(A) A multinucleated giant cell
(B) Auer rods
(C) Call-Exner bodies
(D) Cowdry A Inclusions
(E) Mallory bodies

38. A woman at 32 weeks of gestation comes to the emergency department with painless vaginal bleeding. Her temperature is 37.1° C (98.8° F), her pulse is 76/min, and her blood pressure is 126/90 mm Hg. The fetal heart rate is 155/min. She has no other symptoms. Urinalysis shows no blood cells or bacteria and a normally elevated β-human chorionic gonadotropin (β-hCG). Which of the following diagnoses should the emergency department physician consider before performing an examination?

(A) Abruptio placentae
(B) Eclampsia
(C) Hydatidiform mole
(D) Placenta previa
(E) Preeclampsia

39. Abnormal opening of the urethra on the ventral penis is caused by the failure of a certain urogenital structure to complete normal development in the fetus. This structure is present in both male and female infants, but has a different fate in each. What structure in the female infant is derived from the fetal structure described here?

(A) Glans clitoris
(B) Greater vestibular glands (of Bartholin)
(C) Labia majora
(D) Labia minora
(E) Urethral and paraurethral glands (of Skene)
(F) Vestibular bulbs

40. Thirty percent of births in the United States are the result of unintended pregnancies despite widespread contraception use. Oral contraceptive pills are the most widely used form of hormonal contraception. Which of the following is an absolute contraindication for oral contraceptive pill use?

(A) Anticonvulsant drug therapy
(B) Cervical cancer
(C) Coronary heart disease
(D) Hypertension
(E) Previous thromboembolic event

41. Vasectomy involves bilateral excision of a segment of the ductus deferens. Sperm can no longer pass to the urethra and therefore degenerate in the epididymis and ductus deferens. Which of the following anatomical structures crosses directly posterior to the ductus deferens?

(A) Efferent ductules
(B) Spermatic cord
(C) Sympathetic nerve fibers
(D) Testicular artery
(E) Ureter

42. A 38-year-old nulliparous woman comes to the physician for an annual check-up. She reports a 10-pack-year smoking history and a family history of early mastectomy. Physical examination is notable for a scaly patch on her right nipple. On palpation, there is a firm mass and a clear discharge from the nipple. Which of the following would most likely be seen on a histological examination of this mass?

(A) Intralobular clusters of tumor cells
(B) Large cells with clear halos
(C) Lymphocytic infiltration
(D) Necrosis
(E) Pools of mucous
(F) Proliferation of normal epithelial cells
(G) Proliferation of normal glands and ducts

43. A 30-year-old woman finds a lump in her breast during a self-examination. A biopsy indicates malignancy, and a lumpectomy is performed. The pathology report states that the malignant tissue is a primary breast cancer that is Her-2/neu-positive, but estrogen and progesterone receptor-negative. Which of the following is a reason why this woman is not a candidate for tamoxifen?

(A) Tamoxifen causes severe hypersensitivity reactions
(B) Tamoxifen exacerbates osteoporosis
(C) Tamoxifen increases the risk of heart disease
(D) Tamoxifen is not effective in estrogen receptor–negative tumors
(E) Tamoxifen is not effective orally

44. The prostate is a walnut-sized gland located between the urogenital diaphragm and the bladder. Which of the following is the main purpose of the prostate in the normal adult male?

(A) Production of an enzyme that liquefies semen after ejaculation
(B) Production of seminal fluid
(C) Spermatogenesis
(D) To mediate erectile function
(E) To provide space for sperm maturation and storage

45. An infant is born with ambiguous genitalia. On initial laboratory testing, the infant has a testosterone level of 482 ng/dL (normal 437–707 ng/dL), an estrogen level of 12 pg/mL (normal 10–60 pg/mL) and a luteinizing hormone level of 8 U/L (normal 7–24 U/L). Testes are present. At puberty, the genitalia will become masculinized. Which of the following disorders does this infant have?

(A) 5-α-Reductase deficiency
(B) Double Y syndrome
(C) Female pseudohermaphroditism
(D) Testicular feminization syndrome
(E) True hermaphroditism

46. During a nephrectomy, the renal artery and vein must be ligated close to the hilum so important vessels to other organs are spared. Into which of the following locations do the right and left testicular/ovarian veins drain?

(A) Right = inferior vena cava, left = inferior mesenteric vein
(B) Right = inferior vena cava, left = inferior vena cava
(C) Right = inferior vena cava, left = left renal vein
(D) Right = right renal vein, left = inferior vena cava
(E) Right = right renal vein, left = left renal vein

47. A 22-year-old obese woman presents to her gynecologist with amenorrhea and hirsutism. Ultrasonography reveals polycystic ovaries. Which of the following is a likely pathophysiologic mechanism of this disorder?

(A) Decreased estrogen
(B) Decreased testosterone
(C) Excess follicle-stimulating hormone
(D) Excess luteinizing hormone
(E) Excess progesterone

48. A 23-year-old woman is brought to the emergency department with vaginal bleeding. The patient says that she is in her ninth week of pregnancy. Laboratory studies show a human chorionic gonadotropin (hCG) level of 153 IU/L. The sample shown in the image is retrieved from the patient's uterus. There are no recognizable fetal parts. Which of the following describes the most likely genotype and parental source of DNA in this mass?

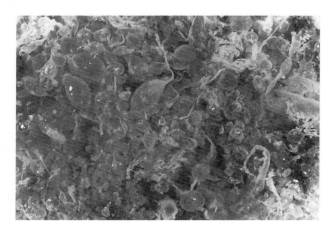

Image courtesy of Armed Forces Institute of Pathology.

(A) 46,XX; maternal
(B) 46,XX; paternal
(C) 46,XX; maternal and paternal
(D) 69,XXX; maternal and paternal
(E) 69,XXY; maternal and paternal

49. The placenta produces a hormone immediately following fertilization. Which of the following is the action of this hormone?

(A) To increase the threshold for uterine contraction
(B) To initiate parturition
(C) To stimulate lactation
(D) To stimulate the corpus luteum to produce estriol and progesterone
(E) To stimulate the growth of breasts during the pregnancy

50. A 38-year-old woman comes to the physician complaining of vaginal burning and itching. On physical examination, a yellowish vaginal discharge and inflammation of the walls of the vagina and vulva are observed. A culture indicates that this patient's infection is caused by a fungus. Which of the following symptoms would most likely be present in an individual infected with this type of fungus?

(A) Blood-tinged sputum, loss of appetite, weight loss, painful red rash on the legs, and change in mental status
(B) Chronic lung disease resembling tuberculosis
(C) Lung cavity lesions
(D) Meningoencephalitis
(E) Thrush, diaper rash, disseminated infection, chronic mucocutaneous disease

1. **The correct answer is C.** Menopause occurs when a woman has no menstrual cycles for one year. The 2–8 years leading up to this time are called perimenopause. During this time, hormones fluctuate tremendously, eventually leading to a decrease in estrogen, an increase in follicle-stimulating hormone, an increase in luteinizing hormone, and an increase in gonadotropin-releasing hormone. Associated symptoms include hot flashes, vaginal atrophy, osteoporosis, and coronary artery disease. (Remember, menopause causes **HAVOC: H**ot flashes, **A**trophy of the **V**agina, **O**steoporosis, and **C**oronary artery disease.) Combinations of estrogen and progestin are used as hormone replacement therapy (HRT) to decrease hot flashes, vaginal dryness, mood swings, and postmenopausal osteoporosis. The Women's Health Initiative, begun in 1991 to study the effects of HRT on heart disease, ended 3 years early in 2002 because the risks of HRT were found to outweigh any potential benefit. These risks include increased risk of breast cancer, increased risk of stroke, increased risk of myocardial infarction in the first year after starting therapy, and increased risk of deep venous thrombosis and pulmonary embolism. Possible benefits include decreased risk of hip fracture and decreased risk of colorectal cancer.

Answer A is incorrect. The risk of breast cancer is increased by 26% in women receiving hormone replacement therapy.

Answer B is incorrect. The risk of deep venous thrombosis and pulmonary embolism is doubled in women receiving hormone replacement therapy.

Answer D is incorrect. The risk of myocardial infarction is increased by 29% in women receiving hormone replacement therapy.

Answer E is incorrect. The risk of stroke is increased by 41% in women receiving hormone replacement therapy.

2. **The correct answer is A.** Abruptio placentae is premature separation of the placenta during the third trimester, resulting in painful vaginal bleeding, uterine contractions, and possible fetal death secondary to decreased blood flow. This complication of pregnancy may be associated with disseminated intravascular coagulation secondary to hemorrhage, illustrated in this patient by the partially hemolyzed schistocytes.

Answer B is incorrect. Amniotic fluid embolism is also referred to as anaphylactoid syndrome of pregnancy and is characterized by hypoxia, respiratory distress, cardiogenic shock, and disseminated intravascular coagulation. It occurs with tearing of maternal vessels and can result in maternal respiratory distress.

Answer C is incorrect. Hydrops fetalis is diagnosed with two or more of the following findings: fetal skin edema, pleural effusion, pericardial effusion, or ascites. It can be a complication of parvovirus B19 infection but is not associated with hemolysis or vaginal bleeding.

Answer D is incorrect. Placenta previa is atypical implantation of the placenta inferiorly, partially or completely covering the cervical os. This can present with painless bleeding, especially near the time of delivery, and cervical dilatation. This condition is not associated with infection or hemolysis.

Answer E is incorrect. Preeclampsia usually presents during the third trimester of pregnancy with hypertension, proteinuria, and edema. It can also be associated with **HELLP** syndrome (**H**emolysis, **E**levated **L**iver function tests, and **L**ow **P**latelets). This patient does not have hypertension or proteinuria. Few RBCs in the urine are normal, considering vaginal bleeding.

3. **The correct answer is E.** The grouped vesicles along with a Tzanck smear positive for multinucleated giant cells indicate that this young man has an active herpes infection. Herpes simplex virus is an enveloped virus with a double-stranded linear DNA genome. After the primary outbreak, the virus travels in a retro-

grade fashion along the axon via microtubular-dependent transport. Once it reaches the neuronal soma in the peripheral nervous system, the virus enters a latent stage. Although not as severe, recurrent outbreaks tend to occur.

Answer A is incorrect. Herpes simplex virus could disseminate and cause systemic illness; however, it is very unlikely in immunocompetent individuals.

Answer B is incorrect. Herpes simplex virus does not infect CD4 cells. This is characteristic of HIV, which can initially present with an acute illness somewhat resembling infectious mononucleosis. This might be followed by complete resolution followed by an asymptomatic carrier state for many years before development of full-blown AIDS.

Answer C is incorrect. Herpes simplex virus does not transport itself to the central nervous system (CNS). An example of a virus that can enter the CNS from the periphery is rabies. However, this would be a very uncommon clinical presentation for rabies. Rabies is usually acquired from animal bites (skunks, raccoons) and has a long incubation period (weeks to 3 months) followed by fatal encephalitis with seizures and hydrophobia.

Answer D is incorrect. After the primary outbreak of genital herpes, herpes simplex virus travels via retrograde, not anterograde, transport to the cell body of the peripheral nervous system. The microtubules of the cytoskeleton serve as tracks for the movement of synaptic vesicles, organelles, and other material from the neuronal cell body to the axon terminal in an anterograde direction.

4. **The correct answer is D.** The clinical picture is one of pelvic inflammatory disease (PID). Of the bacteria that cause PID, *Neisseria gonorrhoeae* is most likely to cause acute high fever and purulent discharge. The Gram's stain of the gram-negative diplococci in the vaginal discharge is diagnostic of gonococcal PID. Complications of PID include salpingitis, endometritis, hydrosalpinx, and tubo-ovarian abscess.

Answer A is incorrect. *Candida albicans* is another cause of vulvovaginitis, along with *Gardnerella* and *Trichomonas.* Pseudohyphae of this yeast can be seen on potassium hydroxide preparation.

Answer B is incorrect. Chlamydial pelvic inflammatory disease is more subacute, and the organisms are not visible on Gram's stain under a light microscope.

Answer C is incorrect. *Gardnerella vaginalis* is a cause of vulvovaginitis, and the most striking symptom is fishy vaginal odor. *Gardnerella* species are gram-variable.

Answer E is incorrect. *Trichomonas vaginalis* is a motile protozoan (seen on a wet mount) that causes yellow-green vaginal discharge upon vulvovaginal infection.

5. **The correct answer is E.** Preeclampsia usually presents with the triad of hypertension, proteinuria, and edema. Preeclampsia affects 7% of pregnant women in their third trimester. Other symptoms include headache, blurry vision, abdominal pain, edema, and hyperreflexia. Definitive treatment is delivery of the fetus. If a patient has a seizure in the setting of preeclampsia, her diagnosis changes to eclampsia, a potentially life-threatening emergency.

Answer A is incorrect. Edema of the face and extremities is one of the triad of symptoms that classify preeclampsia and would not change the initial diagnosis.

Answer B is incorrect. Hyperreflexia is a common symptom of preeclampsia and would not change the initial diagnosis.

Answer C is incorrect. Hypertension is one of the triad of symptoms that classify preeclampsia and would not change the initial diagnosis.

Answer D is incorrect. Proteinuria is one of the triad of symptoms that classify preeclampsia and would not change the initial diagnosis.

6. **The correct answer is B.** Leiomyomas, or fibroids, are common smooth muscle tumors that are most often seen in African-American women

and present with multiple masses. These tumors are benign and can be associated with menstrual pain and menorrhagia (increased bleeding). Since they are estrogen-sensitive, they tend to increase in size during pregnancy and decrease in size after menopause.

Answer A is incorrect. Leiomyomas, or fibroids, are common smooth muscle tumors that are most often seen in African-American women and present with multiple masses. These tumors are benign and are usually associated with menstrual pain and menorrhagia (increased bleeding). Since they are estrogen-sensitive, they tend to increase in size during pregnancy and decrease in size after menopause.

Answer C is incorrect. Chocolate cysts and "powder burns" are most often associated with endometriosis—non-neoplastic endometrial tissue outside the uterus. Endometriosis is often associated with severe menstrual-related pain and infertility.

Answer D is incorrect. Leiomyomas are benign tumors that are very rarely associated with malignant transformation. Malignant leiomyosarcomas most typically arise de novo with areas of necrosis and hemorrhage, not from leiomyomas.

Answer E is incorrect. Leiomyomas are benign tumors that are very rarely associated with malignant transformation, necrosis, or hemorrhage. Malignant leiomyosarcomas most typically arise de novo, not from leiomyomas.

7. **The correct answer is E.** The hypothalamus regulates prolactin release by the anterior pituitary. Thyroid-stimulating hormone stimulates prolactin release, while dopamine inhibits it. Prolactin stimulates milk production and breast development while inhibiting ovulation and spermatogenesis. Destruction of the hypothalamus would cause a reduction in dopamine secretion, increasing prolactin release.

Answer A is incorrect. ADH is released by the posterior pituitary by neurons arising from the hypothalamus. ADH increases water permeability in the late distal tubules and collecting ducts and constricts vascular smooth muscle. Destruction of the neuron bodies in the hypothalamus would reduce ADH secretion.

Answer B is incorrect. Growth hormone (GH) is released by the anterior pituitary in response to hypothalamus growth hormone releasing hormone (GHRH). GH decreases glucose uptake into cells, increases lipolysis, increases protein synthesis, and stimulates insulin-like growth factor. Destruction of the hypothalamus would reduce GHRH, thereby reducing GH.

Answer C is incorrect. Luteinizing hormone (LH) is released by the anterior pituitary in response to hypothalamic gonadotropin-releasing hormone (GnRH). LH increases testosterone synthesis by stimulating cholesterol desmolase. Destruction of the hypothalamus would reduce GnRH, thereby reducing LH.

Answer D is incorrect. Oxytocin is also released by the posterior pituitary by neurons arising from the hypothalamus. Oxytocin causes ejection of milk from the breast in response to suckling by contracting myoepithelial cells; oxytocin also contracts the uterus during labor. Destruction of the neuron bodies in the hypothalamus would reduce oxytocin secretion.

Answer F is incorrect. Testosterone is released by the testes and adrenal glands in response to luteinizing hormone from the anterior pituitary. Testosterone has many functions, including prenatal differentiation of wolffian ducts, development of male secondary sex characteristics, stimulating the pubertal growth spurt, spermatogenesis, and increasing libido. Destruction of the hypothalamus would reduce gonadotropin-releasing hormone secretion, thereby reducing luteinizing hormone and testosterone levels.

Answer G is incorrect. Thyroid-releasing hormone is released by the hypothalamus and stimulates the anterior pituitary to release thyroid-stimulating hormone; thus, prolactin levels would decrease with its destruction.

8. **The correct answer is A.** The only testicular tumor that has an elevated serum α-fetoprotein level is a yolk sac tumor, which has a peak incidence in infancy and early childhood. The yolk sac tumor is thought to be derived from endodermal cells. Symptoms include a lump or swelling in the testicle accompanied by pain.

Answer B is incorrect. This patient has a yolk sac tumor, which most often develops during infancy and early childhood rather than adolescence.

Answer C is incorrect. Embryonal carcinoma accounts for up to one third of all germ cell tumors. It tends to form glands or spaces. Typically, embryonal carcinoma presents with pain in the third decade of life.

Answer D is incorrect. Choriocarcinoma is a rare germ cell tumor that can cause an increase in serum human chorionic gonadotropin but not α-fetoprotein. It requires intensive chemotherapy and can metastasize via the bloodstream to the lungs and central nervous system. Testicular choriocarcinoma is extremely rare, or even nonexistent in prepubescent males.

Answer E is incorrect. Seminomas, which present as a painless enlargement of the testes, have a peak incidence in the fourth decade of life. Seminomas are tumors of the germ cells in the testes and are highly sensitive to radiation therapy.

9. **The correct answer is A.** This woman has Kartagener's syndrome, which is a caused by a defect in microtubule dynein, resulting in immotile cilia. Loss of cilial "sweeping" renders women infertile because eggs are not advanced through the fallopian tubes; it also results in an increased incidence of upper respiratory infections as the loss of mucociliary clearance allows debris to accumulate in the airway. Cilia have a distinct organization, with a central pair of microtubules and nine surrounding pairs, allowing them to bend and sway by differential sliding of the pairs.

Answer B is incorrect. Collagen fibrils are made up of many staggered collagen molecules, each composed of triplets of collagen α chains. A defect in collagen structure results in connective tissue diseases such as scurvy, which is characterized by easy bruising and bleeding gums and is associated with vitamin C deficiency. A defect in collagen would not cause infertility or urinary tract infections.

Answer C is incorrect. Neutrophils usually have a multilobular nucleus with granules filled with hydrolytic enzymes, lysozymes, myeloperoxidase, and lactoferrin. Neutrophils are part of the acute inflammatory response with phagocytic capabilities. A defect in neutrophils can result in conditions such as chronic granulomatous disease and Chédiak-Higashi syndrome, both of which affect immunity. However, this patient's normal WBC count suggests that this is not the case. Moreover, a defect in neutrophils would not cause infertility.

Answer D is incorrect. Zona adherens is an example of an epithelial cell junction; it consists of adjoining e-cadherin between cells and far-reaching actin filaments around the perimeter of the cells. A defect in cell junctions would not cause infertility or urinary tract infections.

Answer E is incorrect. Antibodies have two heavy chains and two light chains connected by disulfide bonds. The variable parts of the chains recognize antigens, while the constant part of the heavy chain can fix complement (e.g., IgM and IgG). A defect in antibody structure may affect immunity, but the patient's normal immunoglobulin levels suggest that this is not the case. Moreover, a defect in antibodies would not cause infertility.

10. **The correct answer is E.** During the follicular phase leading up to ovulation, estradiol levels are increasing, causing proliferation of the uterus. The estradiol levels suppress follicle-stimulating hormone and luteinizing hormone (LH) levels by negative feedback inhibition. At the end of the follicular phase, there is a burst of estradiol, resulting in positive feedback on the pituitary and a burst of LH production. This LH surge causes ovulation.

Answer A is incorrect. Estrogen is not directly responsible for ovulation. It induces a surge in luteinizing hormone that causes ovulation.

Answer B is incorrect. Follicle-stimulating hormone (FSH) is suppressed by estradiol levels during the follicular phase. Along with the luteinizing hormone surge, there is an increase in FSH production that stimulates steroid hormone synthesis by the corpus luteum. It does not affect ovulation.

Answer C is incorrect. Gonadotropin-releasing hormone (GnRH) is suppressed by the negative feedback of estradiol levels during the follicular phase. With the burst of estradiol synthesis at the end, GnRH is positively reinforced, producing a luteinizing hormone surge. It does not directly cause ovulation, however.

Answer D is incorrect. Human chorionic gonadotropin is produced by the syncytiotrophoblast after conception. It is not part of the normal menstrual cycle and has no effect on ovulation.

Answer F is incorrect. After ovulation, the corpus luteum begins to grow, secreting progesterone. Progesterone is not secreted until after ovulation and is therefore not responsible for ovulation.

11. **The correct answer is D.** The suspensory ligaments (also known as the infundibulopelvic ligaments) contain the ovarian arteries that give direct blood supply to the ovaries. The ovaries also receive collateral flow from the uterine arteries that travel in the transverse ligament within the broad ligament.

Answer A is incorrect. The cardinal ligament carries descending branches of the uterine artery. Severing the cardinal ligament should not significantly decrease blood flow to the ovary.

Answer B is incorrect. The fallopian tubes carry the ova from the ovary to the uterus during ovulation. Severing this structure would disrupt normal fertilization but would not significantly affect blood flow to the ovary.

Answer C is incorrect. The round ligament runs inferior to the ovary before attaching to the uterus. It is not a direct source of blood supply for the ovary.

Answer E is incorrect. The ureters run directly inferior to the uterine arteries before feeding into the bladder. Remember: "Water under the bridge." Severing this structure would not affect ovarian blood flow.

12. **The correct answer is A.** Androgen-binding proteins are produced in the Sertoli cells in response to follicle-stimulating hormone. These proteins play a role in sequestering testosterone near the spermatocytes, whose maturation is androgen-dependent.

Answer B is incorrect. Testosterone is transported in the blood bound to sex hormone-binding globulin or albumin, not androgen-binding globulin.

Answer C is incorrect. Inhibin is a hormone produced by the Sertoli cells in response to follicle-stimulating hormone (FSH) that functions as a negative feedback inhibitor of FSH secretion by the anterior pituitary gland. It is not bound by androgen-binding globulin.

Answer D is incorrect. Testosterone is converted into estrogen by the enzyme aromatase, not by androgen-binding globulin.

Answer E is incorrect. Androgen-binding globulin does not feed back on the Sertoli cell or the Leydig cell and does not affect androgen production.

13. **The correct answer is D.** Cervical cancer is associated with human papillomavirus (HPV) strains 16 and 18. Cervical cancers arise from disordered epithelial growth, classified as cervical intraepithelial neoplasia (CIN) 1, 2, or 3, depending on the extent of epithelial involvement from the basal layer. An important risk factor for cervical cancer includes early sexual activity and multiple sex partners, making the incidence especially high in prostitutes. Pap smears have reduced the mortality of these cancers. HPV strains 31 and 33 are also associated with malignancy.

Answer A is incorrect. Human papillomavirus strains 1 and 2 are not associated with cervical cancer. However, herpes simplex virus (HSV) can cause oral (HSV-1) and genital (HSV-2) vesicular lesions.

Answer B is incorrect. Human papillomavirus strains 6 and 11 are associated with benign warts.

Answer C is incorrect. Human papillomavirus strain 8 is not associated with cervical cancer. Human herpesvirus 8 is associated with malignant Kaposi's sarcoma, often found in HIV and immunosuppressed patients.

Answer E is incorrect. There are no human papillomavirus strains L1-3. However, *Chlamydia trachomatis* types L1–3 are associated with lymphogranuloma venereum, an acute lymphadenitis most often occurring in the inguinal area.

14. **The correct answer is C.** This female baby has masculinization of her external genitalia due to congenital adrenal hyperplasia (CAH). CAH is caused by deficiencies in enzymes required for adrenocortical steroid synthesis, such as 21-β-hydroxylase and 11-β-hydroxlyase. 21-β-hydroxylase deficiency results in a total lack of synthesis of aldosterone or cortisol so that all intermediates generate androgen synthesis, leading to elevation of androgen levels and masculinization of tissue. The lack of aldosterone leads to salt wasting, and the infant can present with hypovolemia and hypotension. Treatment includes intravenous saline and steroid hormone replacement.

Answer A is incorrect. 11-β-Hydroxylase deficiency can cause congenital adrenal hyperplasia but does not result in hypotension or hypovolemia. Instead, it can result in hypertension because one of the intermediates that is not blocked by this deficiency but is blocked by 21-β-hydroxylase deficiency acts as a mineralocorticoid to cause salt retention and hypervolemia.

Answer B is incorrect. 17-β-Hydroxylase deficiency is a cause of male pseudointersexuality, not female intersexuality. This enzyme usually converts androstenedione to testosterone. This deficiency, and the resulting lack of testosterone, causes underdevelopment of the penis and scrotum with normal male reproductive internal organs. Clinically it appears very similar to 5-α-reductase deficiency until puberty.

Answer D is incorrect. Complete androgen insensitivity is a result of a mutation in the androgen receptor gene. These 46,XY patients develop testes and female external genitalia and vagina with no internal reproductive organs. They typically present as normal-appearing females who consult their physician when they do not begin menstruation.

Answer E is incorrect. 5-α-Reductase deficiency is a cause of male pseudointersexuality, not female intersexuality, so that patients have an XY genotype. Normally, 5-α-reductase converts testosterone to dihydrotestosterone (DHT). DHT is essential in the development of the external genitalia, and a lack of DHT results in feminization of the penis and scrotum with normal internal male reproductive organs. At puberty, these patients may suddenly experience a virilization of the external organs due to the increase in testosterone.

15. **The correct answer is E.** Prolonged unopposed estrogen use is a risk factor for developing endometrial carcinoma; it stimulates endometrial gland proliferation and manifests as vaginal bleeding. Other risk factors for endometrial cancer include obesity, diabetes, and hypertension. Curiously, tobacco use is actually protective against endometrial cancer.

Answer A is incorrect. Alcoholism has little relation to endometrial cancer but is strongly associated with chronic pancreatitis and pancreatic adenocarcinoma. Smoking is also a risk factor for these conditions.

Answer B is incorrect. Early sexual activity has little relation to endometrial cancer but is a major risk factor for cervical cancer. Other risk factors for cervical cancer include early sexual activity, multiple sex partners, human papillomavirus infection, smoking, and low socioeconomic status.

Answer C is incorrect. A low-fiber diet has little relation to endometrial cancer, but it is a risk factor for colorectal cancer. Other risk factors include villous adenomas, familial adenomatous polyposis, hereditary nonpolyposis colorectal cancer, inflammatory bowel disease, and a positive personal or family history.

Answer D is incorrect. Although nulliparity is a risk factor of endometrial cancer, multiparity is protective.

16. **The correct answer is E.** Fibrocystic disease is benign and presents with diffuse breast pain and multiple bilateral masses. Fibrocystic changes can be characterized histologically and include fibrosis, cysts, sclerosis, and epithelial hyperplasia. Without the presence of atypia, these lesions are not usually associated with an increased risk of carcinoma.

Answer A is incorrect. Central necrosis is characteristic of comedocarcinoma, often resulting in a cheesy consistency. Comedocarcinomas are malignant.

Answer B is incorrect. Lymphocytic infiltration of mammary ducts and/or glands indicates medullary carcinoma. These lesions are well circumscribed, soft, and histologically cellular with scant stroma. Medullary carcinomas are malignant.

Answer C is incorrect. Lymphatic involvement of breast tissue is indicative of inflammatory carcinoma, which is malignant with a poor prognosis.

Answer D is incorrect. Paget's disease is an eczematous patch on the nipple or areola, often with underlying ductal carcinomas that are firm and fibrous on breast examination. On histology, there are large cells with surrounding halos in the epidermis, with underlying islands of tumor cells embedded in fibrosis. Paget's disease is a type of malignant breast carcinoma.

17. **The correct answer is E.** A leak into the dorsal and saphenous vein, demonstrating venous outflow, is typically due to insufficient relaxation of the smooth muscle resulting from excessive adrenergic tone or damaged parasympathetic innervation.

Answer A is incorrect. Arterial insufficiency due to atherosclerotic change or trauma can decrease blood flow to the lacunar spaces, resulting in decreased rigidity. This patient, however, has leakage into veins, not arteries.

Answer B is incorrect. Normal levels of testosterone are important for erectile function, as is demonstrated in studies showing that testosterone therapy for erectile dysfunction increases libido weeks before it has an effect on erection, but the exact role of androgens in libido is unclear.

Answer C is incorrect. Cavernosography demonstrates an organic etiology. Some common causes of psychogenic impotence are anxiety, depression, and relationship conflict.

Answer D is incorrect. Cavernosography does not test somatosensory deficits. Intact sensory nerves are required for erection because sensory nerves that originate from receptors in the penile skin travel to the S2–4 dorsal root ganglia in order to elicit the proper parasympathetic response.

18. **The correct answer is E.** A feeling of hopelessness would make one more suspicious of postpartum depression, which is a more serious disorder than postpartum blues. Women with postpartum depression present with symptoms more suggestive of a major depression, such as feelings of hopelessness and helplessness, anhedonia, and poor grooming. Without treatment, postpartum depression can last up to 1 year.

Answer A is incorrect. Women with postpartum blues may be very anxious about their infant and can worry excessively about the infant's care and health. Similarly, depression may present with anxiety symptoms, but hopelessness is a more prominent feature.

Answer B is incorrect. Fatigability is a common complaint of women with postpartum blues. Although it may be a part of postpartum depression, hopelessness is more consistent with depression.

Answer C is incorrect. Irritability is a common complaint of women with postpartum blues. Although it may be a part of postpartum depression, hopelessness is more consistent with depression.

Answer D is incorrect. Weeping is a common complaint of women with postpartum blues. A striking characteristic of postpartum blues is emotional lability. Crying and laughing can occur at the same time.

19. **The correct answer is A.** Dihydrotestosterone (DHT) is produced from the conversion of testosterone by 5-α-reductase. Prenatally, it acts to differentiate the external genitalia. Later, it is involved in secondary sexual characteristics such as hair distribution. Dihydrotestosterone also increases the size of the epididymis and prostate.

Answer B is incorrect. Estradiol does not affect prenatal differentiation of external genitalia in males.

Answer C is incorrect. Follicle-stimulating hormone acts solely to maintain spermatogenesis. It does not affect external genitalia.

Answer D is incorrect. Luteinizing hormone acts solely on the testes to produce testosterone. It does not affect prenatal differentiation of external genitalia.

Answer E is incorrect. Testosterone does not cause prenatal differentiation of the external genitalia. Its prenatal function is differentiation of the wolffian and müllerian ducts. At puberty, it causes growth of the external genitalia and increased muscle mass. It also functions to increase libido.

20. **The correct answer is C.** Without a functional sex-determining region of the Y chromosome (SRY) gene, no symptoms will be noticed, and the embryo will develop as a perfectly normal female. Normally, the SRY gene encodes the testis-determining factor (TDF), which is responsible for the differentiation of the indifferent gonads into testes. In the testes, Leydig cells produce testosterone and Sertoli cells produce mÅllerian-inhibiting substance (MIS). Testosterone causes the development of the mesonephric (wolffian) duct into male inter-

nal sex organs (remember the mnemonic **SEED: S**eminal vesicles, **E**pididymis, **E**jaculatory duct, and **D**uctus deferens), and the development of male external organs after conversion to 5-hydroxytestosterone. MIS causes regression of the paramesonephric (müllerian) duct, preventing development of female organs. In the absence of TDF, whether due to a destructive mutation of SRY or to a normal 46,XX karyotype, the wolffian duct regresses spontaneously; the mÅllerian duct develops into the fallopian tubes, uterus, and upper vagina; and the external genitalia feminize. This condition will likely be discovered incidentally if a karyotype is performed for an unrelated reason.

Answer A is incorrect. By definition, a female pseudohermaphrodite has ovaries but ambiguous genitalia. A common cause of this condition is congenital adrenal hyperplasia, often due to 21-α-hydroxylase deficiency.

Answer B is incorrect. A male pseudohermaphrodite has testes but ambiguous genitalia. Common causes of this condition include partial androgen insensitivity, 5-α-reductase deficiency, and defects in testosterone production.

Answer D is incorrect. A functional SRY gene is critical for normal male development.

Answer E is incorrect. A true hermaphrodite has both testes and ovaries with ambiguous external genitalia. This condition is quite rare but may be the product of the fertilization of a binucleated ovum by two sperm (one X and one Y).

21. **The correct answer is E.** Krukenberg's tumors are stomach cancer metastases to both ovaries that are described as mucin-secreting "signet-ring" cells. Stomach cancer is often adenocarcinoma that can spread aggressively to lymph nodes and the liver. A classic sign of metastatic stomach cancer is involvement of the supraclavicular lymph nodes, called Virchow's nodes.

Answer A is incorrect. Galactorrhea is leakage from the breasts that is not associated with normal lactation but is associated with elevated prolactin levels secondary to prolactinomas in the anterior pituitary. Prolactin stimulates breast development and milk production while also inhibiting ovulation and spermatogenesis by inhibiting the release of gonadotropin-releasing hormone and subsequently suppressing luteinizing and follicle-stimulating hormones. Galactorrhea is not associated with stomach or ovarian cancers. Prolactinomas rarely metastasize.

Answer B is incorrect. Melena is bloody stool and is often an early sign of colorectal carcinoma. Risk factors for colorectal carcinoma include villous adenomas, inflammatory bowel disease, low-fiber diet, familial adenomatous polyposis, hereditary nonpolyposis colorectal cancer, and a positive history. Melena is not associated with stomach or ovarian cancers. Colorectal carcinomas usually metastasize to the liver.

Answer C is incorrect. A palpable gallbladder (Courvoisier's sign) is associated with pancreatic duct obstruction secondary to pancreatic adenocarcinoma. Other signs and symptoms of pancreatic cancer include abdominal pain radiating to the back, weight loss, anorexia, and migratory thrombophlebitis (Trousseau's syndrome). A palpable gallbladder is not associated with stomach or ovarian cancers.

Answer D is incorrect. Basal cell carcinoma (BCC) often presents as "pearly papules" on sun-exposed areas, such as the face and arms. Papules are not associated with stomach or ovarian cancers. BCC is locally invasive but almost never metastasizes.

22. **The correct answer is A.** Ectopic pregnancies often occur in one of the fallopian tubes or occasionally in the ovary, abdominal cavity, or cervix. Ectopic pregnancies can be complicated by rupture and can develop into a life-threatening condition. Risk factors include a history of pelvic inflammatory disease, endometriosis, postoperative adhesions, and chronic salpingitis.

Answer B is incorrect. *Escherichia coli* is part of the normal flora of the vagina, along with group B streptococcus. It is also one of the

most common causes of urinary tract infection (UTI) in ambulatory young women, along with *Staphylococcus saprophyticus*. UTIs are not associated with pelvic inflammatory disease or ectopic pregnancies.

Answer C is incorrect. Herpes simplex virus (HSV) type 2 is a sexually transmitted, enveloped DNA herpes virus. Genital herpes presents with painful penile, vulvar, or cervical ulcers. HSV is also one of the ToRCHeS organisms that can cross the placenta and negatively affect the fetus. However, HSV is not associated with pelvic inflammatory disease or ectopic pregnancies.

Answer D is incorrect. Human papilloma virus is associated with cervical and anal carcinomas. It is not associated with pelvic inflammatory disease or ectopic pregnancies.

Answer E is incorrect. *Streptococcus agalactiae* is a group B streptococcus that is part of the normal flora in the vagina and would not increase the risk of developing pelvic inflammatory disease or an ectopic pregnancy.

23. **The correct answer is A.** Prolactin is a protein hormone produced by the adenohypophysis, or anterior pituitary, to prepare mammary glands for lactation. Prolactin also increases dopamine synthesis and secretion from the hypothalamus and inhibits the secretion of gonadotropin-releasing hormone, preventing ovulation. Other hormones released from the anterior pituitary include luteinizing hormone, follicle-stimulating hormone, thyroid-stimulating hormone, growth hormone, and adrenocorticotropic hormone.

Answer B is incorrect. Progesterone is secreted by the corpus luteum for the first 8 weeks of pregnancy. It acts on the endometrium to maintain the pregnancy and decrease uterine contractions. It is also used by the fetus as a precursor for steroid hormone synthesis.

Answer C is incorrect. Oxytocin is produced by the hypothalamus and stored in the posterior pituitary. It acts on the mammary glands to stimulate milk letdown, not milk production, as prolactin does. The other hormone secreted by the posterior pituitary is ADH.

Answer D is incorrect. Human placental lactogen (HPL) and progesterone are secreted by the placenta. HPL induces lipolysis, raising the level of free fatty acids and acting as a growth hormone for the fetus. Progesterone is secreted by the placenta to maintain the endometrium after week 8 of pregnancy.

Answer E is incorrect. Human chorionic gonadotropin is produced by the syncytiotrophoblast during the first trimester of pregnancy. Its action is to stimulate the production of progesterone by the corpus luteum until the 8th week of pregnancy, at which point the placenta begins secreting progesterone on its own.

24. **The correct answer is D.** The *BRCA1* and *BRCA2* genes are strongly associated with breast cancer and are found on chromosomes 17 and 13, respectively. *BRCA* is an example of a tumor suppressor gene. A mutation results in loss of function, and thus both alleles must be lost for expression of the cancer.

Answer A is incorrect. The *VHL* gene results in von Hippel–Lindau syndrome and is found on chromosome 3. Patients with this condition often present with hemangioblastomas of the retina, cerebellum, and medulla as well as renal cell carcinomas. The gene responsible for achondroplasia is also found on chromosome 3.

Answer B is incorrect. The *APC* gene, which is responsible for causing familial adenomatous polyposis, is found on chromosome 5. Adenomatous polyps form after puberty.

Answer C is incorrect. The *WT1* gene, which causes Wilms' tumor, is found on chromosome 11. Children affected with this disease present with solid, palpable renal masses.

Answer E is incorrect. The genes *DCC* and *DPC*, responsible for colon and pancreatic cancers, respectively, are both found on chromosome 18.

Answer F is incorrect. The *NF2* gene, which causes neurofibromatosis type 2, is found on

chromosome 22. These patients often have bilateral acoustic neuromas.

25. **The correct answer is E.** Androgenic steroids are used to treat hypogonadism due to failure of the hypothalamic-pituitary-gonadal axis or due to Leydig cell dysfunction. Androgens cause premature closing of the epiphyseal plates by promoting calcium deposition in the bones.

Answer A is incorrect. Some androgenic steroids increase LDL levels. The lipid profile disturbance increases the possibility of atherosclerotic change and raises the risk of coronary artery disease.

Answer B is incorrect. Androgenic steroids cause male-pattern baldness in both men and women because of increased production of dihydrotestosterone from the excess testosterone. Androgens cause growth of facial hair in women but not growth of hair on the scalp.

Answer C is incorrect. Excess androgens can cause decreased spermatogenesis by down-regulating gonadotropin-releasing hormone (GnRH). Decreased GnRH causes decreased release of luteinizing and follicle-stimulating hormones, which are necessary for spermatogenesis.

Answer D is incorrect. Nausea and vomiting are common adverse effects of estrogen therapy, not androgenic steroids.

26. **The correct answer is B.** This patient presents with pelvic inflammatory disease (PID). The vast majority of cases of PID are caused by *Chlamydia trachomatis* and/or *Neisseria gonorrhoeae*. *Chlamydia* infection is the most common STD in the United States and is usually treated with doxycycline.

Answer A is incorrect. *Candida albicans* is the causative agent in the common yeast infection, which is a fairly common cause of vulvovaginitis. Symptoms include vaginal itching and a thick, copious, cottage cheese–like vaginal discharge. *C. albicans* is not a known cause of PID and is treated with fluconazole.

Answer C is incorrect. *Gardnerella vaginalis* is the most common cause of vulvovaginitis. It is a potential etiologic agent in PID but not the most common cause.

Answer D is incorrect. *Streptococcus agalactiae* (group B strep) has been implicated as a causative agent in PID, but it is not a very common cause. It is, however, the most common cause of neonatal meningitis. Women who are pregnant and positive for group B strep must be treated with antibiotics before giving birth.

Answer E is incorrect. *Trichomonas vaginalis* can cause vaginal itching, burning, or pain (vulvovaginitis) with a foul-smelling, frothy green vaginal discharge. *T. vaginalis* infection is not a known cause of PID, but it is somewhat common as a cause of nongonococcal urethritis. Many women who carry this organism are asymptomatic.

27. **The correct answer is E.** Preeclampsia usually presents with the triad of hypertension, proteinuria, and edema. Preeclampsia affects 7% of pregnant women in their third trimester, with increased incidence in patients with pre-existing hypertension, diabetes, chronic renal disease, and autoimmune disorders such as lupus. Other symptoms include headache, blurry vision, abdominal pain, and hyperreflexia. Definitive treatment is delivery of the baby. The patient in this vignette presents with edema and hypertension; she also has lupus. A urinalysis would test for proteinuria, completing the triad for the diagnosis of preeclampsia.

Answer A is incorrect. An electroencephalogram looks at electrical brain activity and is especially useful for looking at waveforms during a seizure. Eclampsia is essentially the symptoms and signs of preeclampsia with seizures. Preeclampsia by definition does not involve seizures, and thus an electroencephalogram would not help in a definitive initial diagnosis.

Answer B is incorrect. Elevated liver enzymes are associated with the **HELLP** syndrome (Hemolysis, Elevated Liver function tests, and Low Platelets). A liver panel would reveal any elevated liver enzymes. Preeclampsia may or may not involve elevated liver enzymes, and thus a panel would not help in a definitive initial diagnosis.

Answer C is incorrect. A Pap smear allows a physician to identify dysplastic cervical koilocytes by scraping off cells from the cervix and mounting them onto a slide to be viewed under a microscope. This is useful in diagnosing disordered epithelial growth that is possibly associated with cervical carcinoma. Preeclampsia does not involve dysplastic cervical cells, and thus a Pap smear would not help in a definitive initial diagnosis.

Answer D is incorrect. Hemolysis is associated with the **HELLP** syndrome (Hemolysis, Elevated Liver function tests, and Low Platelets). A blood smear would help identify RBC fragments, indicative of hemolysis. Preeclampsia may or may not involve hemolysis, and thus a smear would not help in a definitive initial diagnosis.

28. **The correct answer is C.** This patient most likely suffers from osteoporosis, or weakened bones, as a complication of menopause. Estrogen regulates bone resorption, maintaining proper bone mass in women. Menopause, whose average age of onset is 50 years, is a cessation of estrogen production due to a decreased number of ovarian follicles, resulting in increased bone resorption. Postmenopausal women would have low estrogen levels but high levels of luteinizing hormone, follicle-stimulating hormone, and gonadotropin-releasing hormone) due to the lack of negative feedback on the anterior pituitary and hypothalamus.

Answer A is incorrect. While estrogen is indeed low in postmenopausal women, levels of luteinizing hormone (LH) and follicle-stimulating hormone (FSH) would be high due to the lack of negative feedback on the anterior pituitary. This profile suggests that the problem is in the anterior pituitary, which is receiving high gonadotropin-releasing hormone but is unable to produce enough LH and FSH to stimulate the ovaries. Menopause is a primary dysfunction of estrogen production in the ovaries.

Answer B is incorrect. While estrogen is indeed low in postmenopausal women, luteinizing hormone, follicle-stimulating hormone, and gonadotropin-releasing hormone (GnRH) levels would be high due to the lack of negative feedback on the anterior pituitary and hypothalamus. This profile suggests that the problem is in the hypothalamus, releasing low GnRH and suboptimally stimulating the anterior pituitary and ovaries. Menopause is a primary dysfunction of estrogen production in the ovaries.

Answer D is incorrect. Menopause is a primary dysfunction of estrogen production in the ovaries. Thus, estrogen levels would be low.

Answer E is incorrect. Menopause is a primary dysfunction of estrogen production in the ovaries. Thus, estrogen levels would be low.

29. **The correct answer is D.** Ketoconazole is an antifungal drug used to treat mucocutaneous candidiasis that acts by blocking formation of fungal membrane sterols. It also has an endocrine effect because it blocks enzymes necessary for testosterone and cortisol synthesis. Other endocrine effects include decreased libido, impotence, and gynecomastia in men.

Answer A is incorrect. Amphotericin B is an antifungal drug used to treat systemic mycoses. It acts by disrupting fungal wall synthesis by binding to ergosterol (a component of the cell wall). Adverse effects include fever and chills, decreased creatinine clearance, hypotension, and anemia.

Answer B is incorrect. Fluconazole is an antifungal drug with the same mechanism of action as ketoconazole, but without the endocrine side effects. It has good penetration into the cerebrospinal fluid and is used to treat *Cryptococcus neoformans*. Adverse effects include nausea and vomiting.

Answer C is incorrect. Flucytosine is an antifungal drug used solely in combination with amphotericin B to treat systemic *Cryptococcus neoformans* and systemic *Candida*. Adverse effects include pancytopenia, elevated liver function tests, and nausea and vomiting.

Answer E is incorrect. Itraconazole is an antifungal that lacks the endocrine effects of ketoconazole. It is used to treat blastomycosis and AIDS-associated histoplasmosis. Adverse effects include nausea and vomiting, as well as rash in immunocompromised patients.

30. **The correct answer is A.** The history of a past inguinal repair strongly suggests an obstructive abnormality of the vas deferens, leading to disordered sperm transport. The vas deferens can be accidentally ligated, or scar tissue can make passage through the vas deferens impossible. In the case of vas deferens obstruction, the semen volume will be low with decreased or absent sperm. In these cases, testicular biopsy can confirm normal sperm production, and sperm can be collected for intracytoplasmic sperm injection in vitro fertilization.

Answer B is incorrect. Primary gonadal deficiency is unlikely given the husband's normal testosterone level. Typically, gonadal deficiency results in low testosterone with high luteinizing hormone and follicle-stimulating hormone levels.

Answer C is incorrect. Secondary hypogonadism is unlikely given the husband's normal testosterone level. A low testosterone level in association with low luteinizing hormone and low follicle-stimulating hormone levels would suggest pituitary or hypothalamic dysfunction.

Answer D is incorrect. The results from the testicular biopsy demonstrate sperm within normal parameters. Normal fertility is associated with sperm motility exceeding 63% and more than 12% of sperm exhibiting normal morphology.

Answer E is incorrect. A Y-chromosome deletion has been associated with azoospermia (no sperm) or oligospermia (low sperm count). In this case, the husband has normal sperm on testicular biopsy, making it unlikely that he has a Y-chromosome abnormality.

31. **The correct answer is F.** This patient presents with symptoms of a urinary tract infection, most likely caused by prolonged urethral

catheterization. Nosocomial urinary tract infection is most often associated with *Escherichia coli*, *Proteus mirabilis*, *Pseudomonas aeruginosa*, *Klebsiella pneumoniae*, *Serratia marcescens*, staphylococci, enterococci, and Candida albicans. Although the patient's symptoms are not specific for any of these organisms, the urine culture tells us that (1) the organism is a gram-negative rod, and (2) the organism produces a red pigment. *S. marcescens* is a gram-negative rod that produces a red pigment called prodigiosin.

Answer A is incorrect. The presence of *Candida albicans* in an otherwise normal female usually represents colonization rather than infection. Urinary tract infection with *Candida* usually can be attributed to structural abnormalities, metabolic or hormonal abnormalities, or impaired host defenses. *C. albicans* is a yeast.

Answer B is incorrect. *Escherichia coli* is the most common cause of urinary tract infection. Although it is a gram-negative rod, it does not produce any pigments.

Answer C is incorrect. *Klebsiella pneumoniae* is a gram-negative rod and is responsible for approximately 8% of nosocomial infections. It is a significant cause of urinary tract infection and pneumonia in hospitalized and ambulatory patients. *K. pneumoniae* does not produce any pigments.

Answer D is incorrect. *Proteus mirabilis* is a gram-negative bacillus and is a frequent cause of nosocomial urinary tract infection. It produces the enzyme urease, which serves to create a more alkaline environment for itself (urea → ammonia + carbon dioxide) but does not produce any pigments.

Answer E is incorrect. *Pseudomonas aeruginosa* has been known to cause catheter-associated urinary tract infection. Although it is a gram-negative rod, it produces a blue-green pigment called pyocyanin.

Answer G is incorrect. *Staphylococcus saprophyticus* is the second most common cause of urinary tract infection in young women. It is a gram-positive coccus and does not produce any pigments.

32. **The correct answer is C.** A blood-filled chocolate cyst is characteristic of endometriosis, a condition that results in non-neoplastic endometrial glands/stroma abnormally located outside the uterus. The ovary is one of the most common sites, and the cysts are formed from cyclic bleeding from the tissue, mimicking menstruation. Severe menstrual-related pain and infertility are possible complications of endometriosis.

Answer A is incorrect. Abnormal vaginal bleeding in a nonpregnant woman can be associated with endometrial hyperplasia, hormonal imbalances, and malnutrition, among many other things. Endometriosis does not commonly present with abnormal vaginal bleeding, since the ectopic glands are often outside the uterus and are stimulated by hormonal changes during menstruation (i.e., bleeding would occur during regular menstruation).

Answer B is incorrect. Common cancers in the reproductive tract include endometrial carcinoma, which can arise from endometrial hyperplasia caused by excess estrogen stimulation, and cervical carcinoma, associated with human papillomavirus infection. Endometriosis does not progress to cancer.

Answer D is incorrect. Polycystic ovarian syndrome (Stein-Leventhal syndrome) manifests with amenorrhea, infertility, obesity, and hirsutism due to increased androgen production from theca cells secondary to increased luteinizing hormone levels. Endometriosis is not associated with masculinization.

Answer E is incorrect. Polycystic ovarian syndrome (Stein-Leventhal syndrome) manifests with amenorrhea, infertility, obesity, and hirsutism due to increased androgen production from theca cells secondary to increased LH levels. Endometriosis is not associated with obesity.

33. **The correct answer is C.** Milk letdown is a reflex that causes milk ejection from the breast.

Typically, milk letdown is induced by infant suckling. Oxytocin is produced by the posterior pituitary in response to suckling and, when produced synthetically, is used to induce labor or promote milk letdown in nursing mothers. It causes milk letdown by stimulating contraction of the myoepithelial cells around the mammary alveoli, causing ejection of the milk.

Answer A is incorrect. ADH is also produced by the posterior pituitary. Its action is mainly within the kidney to cause water resorption in the collecting tubules. It is largely used to treat patients with diabetes insipidus.

Answer B is incorrect. Human chorionic gonadotropin (hCG) is a placental hormone that stimulates progesterone production during pregnancy. In men, hCG can be used to treat hypogonadism because it promotes sexual maturation.

Answer D is incorrect. Somatostatin is a growth hormone (GH) inhibitor. It is used to treat acromegaly, a syndrome of excess GH characterized by periosteal bone growth, organomegaly, and glucose intolerance.

Answer E is incorrect. Somatotropin, or growth hormone (GH), is released by the anterior pituitary. It is used for its anabolic properties in GH-deficient children.

34. **The correct answer is B.** The spermatic cord is a thick cord containing the structures that run to and from the testes. It is covered by three layers: external spermatic fascia derived from the external oblique muscle, cremasteric muscle and fascia derived from the internal oblique muscle, and internal spermatic fascia derived from the transversalis fascia. The ilioinguinal nerve arises from L1, passes through the inguinal ligament on top of the spermatic cord, and supplies cutaneous sensation to the scrotum/labia and medial aspect of the thigh. It is not a part of the spermatic cord and must be isolated separately from the cord during hernia surgeries to ensure that there is no loss of sensation to these areas.

Answer A is incorrect. The ductus deferens is the tube that carries sperm from the testes to the ejaculatory duct. It is at the center of the spermatic cord.

Answer C is incorrect. The pampiniform plexus, or testicular venous plexus, drains blood from the testes and is a part of the spermatic cord.

Answer D is incorrect. The testicular artery supplies blood to the testes and epididymis and runs in the spermatic cord. Remember that anything running to or from the testes will be a part of the spermatic cord. Even if you don't know the layers of the cord, you can eliminate structures that you know have something to do with testicular function.

Answer E is incorrect. The testes, as vascular organs, do produce lymph that needs to be drained by lymphatic vessels. Since the spermatic cord contains structures that run away from the testes, the testicular lymph vessels are a part of the spermatic cord.

35. **The correct answer is D.** Cancer is 35–48 times more likely in cryptorchidism than in the normally descended testis. About 5% of full term babies and one third of premature babies have one undescended testis at birth, but descent is typically complete by the end of the first few weeks of life.

Answer A is incorrect. Hypogonadotropic hypogonadism is due to congenital or acquired causes, not cryptorchidism. Impaired secretion of luteinizing hormone (LH) and follicle-stimulating hormone (FSH) due to congenital gonadotropin-releasing hormone deficiency results in secondary hypogonadism, characterized by low testosterone in the setting of low LH and FSH.

Answer B is incorrect. An indirect inguinal hernia is a protrusion of bowel through the deep inguinal ring that is unrelated to cryptorchidism. The bowel may descend all the way into the scrotum. Clinical signs include a tender mass in the inguinal region that cannot be reduced with pressure.

Answer C is incorrect. Retractile testes are a physiologic retraction of the testes into the abdominal cavity in response to cold, a benign condition requiring no treatment.

Answer E is incorrect. Torsion of the spermatic cord is rarely seen in cryptorchidism. The incidence of testicular torsion is increased, however, in males in whom the tunica vaginalis is attached high on the spermatic cord.

36. **The correct answer is E.** Sildenafil acts by increasing levels of cGMP phosphodiesterase, leading to smooth muscle relaxation of the corpus cavernosum. The muscle relaxation allows increased blood flow. Some of the adverse effects include headache, flushing, and disturbances in color vision.

Answer A is incorrect. Testosterone cannot be given orally due to issues of hepatotoxicity. It can be administered intramuscularly, topically, or buccally but is rarely effective in the setting of normal testosterone levels and is discouraged because of the adverse effects of decreased spermatogenesis, gynecomastia, and possible impotence.

Answer B is incorrect. Clomiphene is an antiestrogen that interferes with estrogen's binding site on the hypothalamus and the pituitary, thus increasing the secretion of gonadotropin-releasing hormone. It is used to treat women with infertility associated with anovulatory cycles.

Answer C is incorrect. Alprostadil is an intraurethral prostaglandin pellet that increases arterial inflow and decreases venous outflow, thereby increasing erection by binding G proteins and stimulating adenylyl cyclase. It is also available as an intracavernosal injection, but this form is associated with a higher risk of priapism.

Answer D is incorrect. Sildenafil works via inhibition of cyclic cGMP phosphodiesterase because cGMP causes increased smooth muscle relaxation; cAMP phosphodiesterase does not.

37. **The correct answer is A.** A Tzanck test is a smear of an opened skin lesion to detect multinucleated giant cells and assay for the herpes simplex virus (HSV). The Tzanck test can detect HSV-1 and -2 and the varicella-zoster virus.

Answer B is incorrect. Auer rods are rod-shaped bodies in myeloid cells. They are found in acute myelogenous leukemia.

Answer C is incorrect. Call-Exner bodies are spaces between granulosa cells in ovarian follicles and in granulosa cell tumors.

Answer D is incorrect. Cowdry A inclusions are intranuclear eosinophilic inclusions surrounded by a clear halo. They are seen in pathology preparations of herpes zoster skin rashes but are not seen in the histology image.

Answer E is incorrect. Mallory bodies are eosinophilic intracytoplasmic inclusions found in hepatic cells and seen in a variety of diseases, including alcoholic liver disease.

38. **The correct answer is D.** Placenta previa occurs when the placenta overlies the cervical os. This can be asymptomatic, or it may present with vaginal bleeding. Classically, the bleeding is painless; however, it may be associated with contractions. If a digital vaginal examination is performed and the placenta is disrupted, it can result in massive vaginal bleeding. Prior to pelvic examination, a sonogram should be performed to verify placental location in all pregnant patients with vaginal bleeding in the second or third trimesters.

Answer A is incorrect. Abruptio placentae is the premature separation of the placenta from the uterine wall, usually during the third trimester of pregnancy. It is usually associated with painful vaginal bleeding. Severe abruption may result in fetal death and disseminated intravascular coagulation.

Answer B is incorrect. Eclampsia is characterized by a seizure in the second or third trimester in a patient who has not been previously diagnosed with a seizure disorder. Eclampsia is not usually associated with independent painless vaginal bleeding.

Answer C is incorrect. A hydatidiform mole is a pathologic ovum that causes swelling of chorionic villi and proliferation of chorionic epithelium, resulting in a "honeycombed uterus" or "cluster of grapes." This is associated with extremely elevated β-hCG. Complete moles would present earlier in pregnancy and would not have fetal heart tones.

Answer E is incorrect. Preeclampsia is characterized by hypertension, edema, and proteinuria, which this patient does not display. There is an increased incidence in patients with pre-existing hypertension, diabetes, chronic renal disease, and autoimmune diseases. Preeclampsia is not usually associated with independent painless vaginal bleeding.

39. **The correct answer is D.** This infant has a hypospadia, in which the penile urethra opens on the ventral surface of the penis rather than the tip. Hypospadias are caused by incomplete closure of the urethral folds. In the male, the urethral folds give rise to the ventral shaft of the penis; in the female, they give rise to the labia minora.

Answer A is incorrect. The glans clitoris arises from the genital tubercle, which produces the glans penis in the male.

Answer B is incorrect. The glands of Bartholin are derived from the urogenital sinus. The urogenital sinus produces the corpus spongiosum, the bulbourethral glands, and the prostate gland in the male.

Answer C is incorrect. The labia majora are derived from the labioscrotal swelling, which gives rise to the scrotum in the male.

Answer E is incorrect. The urethral and paraurethral glands of Skene are derived from the urogenital sinus. The urogenital sinus produces the corpus spongiosum, the bulbourethral glands, and the prostate gland in the male.

Answer F is incorrect. The urogenital sinus produces the vestibular bulbs, the glands of Bartholin, and the glands of Skene in the female. It produces the corpus spongiosum, the bulbourethral glands, and the prostate gland in the male.

40. **The correct answer is E.** Oral contraceptive pills (OCPs) act by suppressing ovulation, thickening the cervical mucus, and thinning the endometrial lining. Three different formulations exist: fixed-dose estrogen-progesterone combination, phasic estrogen-progesterone combination, and progesterone alone. The combination pills have a theoretical effectiveness of 99.9%, while the progesterone-only pills have a theoretical effectiveness of 99.5%. Absolute contraindications for OCP use include a previous thromboembolic event, a history of an estrogen-dependant tumor, pregnancy, abnormal uterine bleeding, and hypertriglyceridemia.

Answer A is incorrect. Anticonvulsant drug therapy is a relative contraindication for oral contraceptive pill use. A relative contraindication means that the therapy should be provided only if it is absolutely necessary. The woman should receive more medical supervision than would other women using anticonvulsant medications.

Answer B is incorrect. There is an increased risk of cervical cancer in woman who uses oral contraceptive pills. It is not a contraindication for usage.

Answer C is incorrect. There is an increased risk of coronary heart disease in women over the age of 35 who smoke and use oral contraceptive pills (OCPs). It is not a contraindication for OCP use.

Answer D is incorrect. Hypertension is a relative contraindication to oral contraceptive pill use. A relative contraindication means that the therapy should be provided only if it is absolutely necessary. A woman with hypertension should receive more medical supervision than a woman without hypertension.

41. **The correct answer is E.** The ureters are muscular ducts with narrow lumina that carry urine from the kidneys to the urinary bladder. These retroperitoneal structures cross the external iliac artery just beyond the common iliac bifurcation and pass under the ductus deferens and testicular vessels.

Answer A is incorrect. Efferent ductules transport sperm from the rete testis to the epididymis, where it is stored. The tail of the epididymis is continuous with the ductus deferens, the next sperm destination. Efferent ductules are located inferior to the ductus rather than posterior.

Answer B is incorrect. The spermatic cord contains the ductus deferens, the testicular artery, the pampiniform plexus, and the lymphatic vessels. It does not cross posterior to ductus deferens.

Answer C is incorrect. Sympathetic nerve fibers are constituents of the spermatic cord that run on arteries. They run parallel to the ductus deferens but do not cross posteriorly.

Answer D is incorrect. The testicular artery arises from the aorta and supplies the testis and epididymis. It runs parallel to, but does not cross, the ductus deferens to enter the spermatic cord.

42. **The correct answer is B.** Paget's disease is an eczematous patch on the nipple or areola, often with underlying ductal carcinomas that are firm and fibrous on breast examination. On histologic examination, there are large cells with surrounding halos in the epidermis, with underlying islands of tumor cells embedded in fibrosis. Risk factors for breast cancer include nulliparity, early menarche, late menopause, obesity, high-fat diet, and a positive family history.

Answer A is incorrect. Paget's disease is almost always associated with intraductal carcinoma, not intralobular. Infiltrating lobular carcinomas are often bilateral, made up of cells in clusters or in "Indian file" within ductules.

Answer C is incorrect. Medullary carcinoma involves lymphocytic infiltration and scant stroma. The tumors are often soft and fleshy, not firm. Medullary carcinomas are not associated with Paget's disease.

Answer D is incorrect. Comedocarcinoma is a tumor with a "cheesy" consistency and central necrosis. While this is also an intraductal carcinoma in situ, it is not associated with Paget's disease.

Answer E is incorrect. Mucinous (colloid) carcinomas have a gelatinous consistency and show pools of extracellular mucous surrounding clusters of tumor cells. These are not associated with Paget's disease.

Answer F is incorrect. Proliferation of normal-looking epithelial cells describes epithelial hyperplasia; it poses no increased risk of carcinoma. This is an example of a fibrocystic change that often occurs in women older than 30 years. These tumors are benign and are not associated with Paget's disease or malignancy.

Answer G is incorrect. Proliferation of normal-looking glands and ducts suggests intraductal papilloma, which can often present with nipple discharge. These tumors are benign and are not associated with Paget's disease or malignancy.

43. **The correct answer is D.** Tamoxifen as a chemotherapeutic agent is useful only in estrogen receptor-positive breast cancer. It is an estrogen antagonist whose mechanism of action relies on binding estrogen receptors to impede the production of estrogen-responsive genes. Thus, the growth effects of the hormone are reduced. Tamoxifen is not useful in a breast cancer that is estrogen receptor-negative. In this case, the patient's breast cancer is Her-2/neu-positive, which may have a better response to the chemotherapeutic agent trastuzumab (Herceptin).

Answer A is incorrect. Tamoxifen does not cause hypersensitivity reactions. Its major adverse reactions include hot flashes, nausea, and vomiting. Hypersensitivity is an adverse reaction of paclitaxel, a chemotherapeutic agent used to treat metastatic breast cancer.

Answer B is incorrect. First, osteoporosis is uncommon in women under the age of 65 years. Second, tamoxifen does not exacerbate osteoporosis. In fact, because tamoxifen increases bone mineralization, it may have a protective effect in osteoporosis.

Answer C is incorrect. Tamoxifen actually decreases LDL cholesterol, thus decreasing the risk of atherosclerotic heart disease.

Answer E is incorrect. Tamoxifen is effective as an oral medication. It is metabolized by the liver and excreted into the bile.

44. **The correct answer is A.** The prostate produces prostate-specific antigen (PSA), a serine protease that liquefies semen after ejaculation. PSA is specific to the prostate, not to prostatic cancer. Elevated PSA can be caused by prostatitis and sometimes benign prostatic hypertrophy.

    Answer B is incorrect. Although the prostate does produce some seminal fluid, the seminal vesicle is the main organ that performs this function. Seminal fluid contains fructose and choline, and nourishes the sperm.

    Answer C is incorrect. The testes are the site of spermatogenesis, not the prostate. The testes require the cooler temperature of the scrotal sac in order to produce sperm. This is why cryptorchidism often results in sterility; the temperature within the body is too warm for spermatogenesis to take place.

    Answer D is incorrect. The prostate has no role in erectile function. Erection is controlled by parasympathetic nervous system activation of the muscles in the penis.

    Answer E is incorrect. The epididymis is a coiled duct continuous with the efferent ductules at the head and with the ductus deferens at the tail. Sperm maturation and storage take place in the first two thirds of the epididymis.

45. **The correct answer is A.** 5-α-Reductase is the enzyme that is required to convert testosterone to dihydrotestosterone (DHT). DHT is required for the masculinization of the external genitalia before birth. The infant has testes and normal levels of testosterone, estrogen, and luteinizing hormone. At puberty, the dramatic increase in testosterone levels causes the genitalia to be masculinized.

Answer B is incorrect. Males with the genotype XYY are phenotypically normal, so their genitalia are unambiguous.

Answer C is incorrect. Female pseudohermaphroditism occurs when ovaries are present (not testes) and the external genitalia are ambiguous. This condition is usually due to exposure to androgens early in gestation.

Answer D is incorrect. Testicular feminization syndrome is a defect in the dihydrotestosterone receptor resulting in feminine-appearing external genitalia. Testes are present, as the individual is XY, and levels of testosterone, estrogen, and luteinizing hormone are all high. Genitalia do not masculinize at puberty, and gender identity is female.

Answer E is incorrect. True hermaphroditism occurs only when both ovary and testicular tissue is present.

46. **The correct answer is C.** The right gonadal vein drains directly into the inferior vena cava (IVC). The left gonadal vein would have to cross the aorta to drain into the IVC; instead, it courses superiorly in the retroperitoneum to the left renal vein. The left renal vein crosses the aorta anteriorly and drains into the IVC.

    Answer A is incorrect. The inferior mesenteric vein becomes part of the portal circulation that carries blood from the digestive tract to the liver. The gonadal venous drainage does not need to be directly sent to the liver and drains into the systemic circulation. Make the distinction between portal and systemic circulation, and you should be able to logically eliminate this choice.

    Answer B is incorrect. Do not confuse the gonadal arteries with the veins. Both gonadal arteries arise from the aorta; the right gonadal artery crosses the inferior vena cava to supply the right testis/ovary. The veins, on the other hand, never cross the aorta.

    Answer D is incorrect. Keep in mind the relationship between the inferior vena cava (on the right) and the aorta (on the left). If you re-member that the veins never cross the aorta, you can figure out which one (the left) must drain into the renal vein.

Answer E is incorrect. Remember that the go-nadal veins drain to different locations. Then remember the relationship of the inferior vena cava (IVC) to the aorta. The IVC is on the right, so it logically makes sense that the right gonadal vein drains to the IVC, as the left would have to cross the aorta to drain into the IVC.

47. **The correct answer is D.** The disorder de-scribed is Stein-Leventhal syndrome, or poly-cystic ovarian syndrome. Although there is a great deal of variation in clinical presentation in this syndrome, a subset of patients have ele-vated serum luteinizing hormone (LH) levels and elevated LH:follicle-stimulating hormone (FSH) ratios. Consistently high levels of LH can lead to anovulation due to downregulation of the LH receptors at the ovaries. Elevated LH also stimulates the thecal cells of the ovaries to secrete excess androstenedione, which can be converted into testosterone by most peripheral tissues, leading to hirsutism, acne, or male-patterned alopecia.

Answer A is incorrect. The majority of pa-tients with polycystic ovarian syndrome have elevated or normal estrone and estradiol levels.

Answer B is incorrect. Serum androgen lev-els, including testosterone, androstenedione, and dehydroepiandrosterone sulfate, are in-creased in the majority of patients with poly-cystic ovarian syndrome.

Answer C is incorrect. Follicle-stimulating hormone (FSH) levels may be normal or low in polycystic ovarian syndrome, contributing to the elevated luteinizing hormone/FSH ratio seen in many patients.

Answer E is incorrect. Elevated luteinizing hormone levels and reduced ovulation leads to deficient ovarian progesterone secretion. Pa-tients with polycystic ovarian syndrome are at an increased risk for endometrial hyperplasia

and carcinoma due to the unopposed estrogen stimulation of the endometrium.

48. **The correct answer is B.** A hydatidiform mole is a pathologic ovum with no DNA that causes cystic swelling of chorionic villi and prolifera-tion of the trophoblast, resulting in a mass that can look like a "cluster of grapes," as seen in the image. The genotype of a complete mole is 46,XX, completely consisting of paternal DNA. There is no associated fetus with this entity de-spite the elevated hCG.

Answer A is incorrect. Maternally derived 46,XX would not cause a hydatidiform mole. Moles are derived from "empty" ova that are then fertilized by sperm.

Answer C is incorrect. 46,XX describes the genotype of a normal fetus, receiving one set of chromosomes from each parent.

Answer D is incorrect. Paternally derived 69,XXX describes another possible DNA make-up of a partial mole. A partial mole contains more than two sets of chromosomes that usu-ally consist of two paternal and one maternal set of chromosomes, resulting in triploidy or tetraploidy. Partial moles may present with a similar grapelike mass but are also associated with fetal parts.

Answer E is incorrect. Maternally and pater-nally derived 69,XXY describes one possible DNA make-up of a partial mole. A partial mole contains more than two sets of chromo-somes that usually consist of both paternal and maternal sets, resulting in triploidy or tet-raploidy. Partial moles may present with a simi-lar grapelike mass but are associated with fetal parts.

49. **The correct answer is D.** Human chorionic gonadotropin (hCG) is produced by the pla-centa immediately following fertilization. hCG acts on the corpus luteum to rescue it from regression. The corpus luteum then goes on to produce estriol and progesterone to maintain the pregnancy until the placenta takes over this role in the second and third

trimesters. hCG levels peak at week 9 and then start to decline until reaching a steady state around week 25.

Answer A is incorrect. Progesterone raises the threshold for uterine contraction, not human chorionic gonadotropin. This helps prevent spontaneous abortion of the fetus.

Answer B is incorrect. Human chorionic gonadotropin does not initiate parturition at the end of pregnancy. The actual initiating event is unknown.

Answer C is incorrect. Lactation is stimulated by oxytocin and prolactin secretion, not human chorionic gonadotropin. Estrogen stimulates prolactin secretion from the anterior pituitary so that prolactin levels increase during the pregnancy. Prolactin secretion is maintained after birth by the infant's suckling action, which also causes prolactin to be released from the pituitary gland.

Answer E is incorrect. Estrogen and progesterone, produced by the corpus luteum in the first trimester and by the placenta in the second and third trimesters, stimulate the growth of breasts during pregnancy, not human chorionic gonadotropin.

50. **The correct answer is E.** *Candida albicans* infection can cause thrush in immunocompromised patients. It can also cause vulvovaginitis, disseminated candidiasis (to any organ), and chronic mucocutaneous candidiasis. Diagnosis is made through cultures and tissue biopsy for invasive systemic disease.

Answer A is incorrect. Coccidioidomycosis is the second most common fungal infection en-

countered in the United States. About 60% of these infections cause no symptoms, and in the remaining 40% of cases, the symptoms can range from mild to severe. Severe forms of the infection can present with blood-tinged sputum, loss of appetite, weight loss, a painful red rash on the legs, and change in mental status.

Answer B is incorrect. Histoplasmosis does not typically lead to any symptomatic presentation. When symptoms are present, they usually present as a flu-like illness with fever, cough, headaches, and myalgias. Histoplasmosis can result in lung disease resembling tuberculosis and widespread disseminated infection affecting the liver, spleen, adrenal glands, mucosal surfaces, and meninges. Histoplasmosis occurs most commonly in the Mississippi and Ohio River valleys.

Answer C is incorrect. *Aspergillus fumigatus* infection can present with bronchopulmonary aspergillosis, lung cavity aspergillomas ("fungus balls"), and invasive aspergillosis. A. *fumigatus* is a mold with septate hyphae that branch at a V-shaped 45-degree angle. A. *fumigatus* is not dimorphic.

Answer D is incorrect. *Cryptococcus neoformans* infection does not often present with any symptoms in an immunocompetent host. However, in an immunocompromised individual, it can present with meningoencephalitis. *Cryptococcus* is a heavily encapsulated yeast that is not dimorphic. The fungus is found in soil and pigeon droppings.

CHAPTER 14

Respiratory

QUESTIONS

1. A 25-year-old woman with asthma presents to the emergency department in severe cardiovascular distress after taking a theophylline overdose in an attempt to commit suicide. At presentation, she is convulsing, her blood pressure is 80/40 mm Hg, and she has developed a cardiac arrhythmia. Considering the mechanism of action of theophylline, which of the following drugs may be used to counteract its effects?

   (A) Albuterol
   (B) β-Blockers
   (C) Digoxin
   (D) Epinephrine
   (E) Furosemide

2. A 70-year-old woman who smokes comes in with complaints of shortness of breath and chronic cough, sometimes producing blood. Suspecting the worst, she is worked up for lung carcinoma. Tests come back in favor of the proposed diagnosis and the patient is told that she has lung carcinoma. When the patient comes back in for her appointment, one of her eyelids is droopy and the pupil on the same side is smaller than the contralateral pupil. Upon questioning, she reveals that the side of her body with the droopy lid doesn't sweat. Which of the following is the most likely etiology of the patient's symptoms?

   (A) Apical lung tumor
   (B) Paraneoplastic endocrine hormone production
   (C) Pleural effusion
   (D) Recurrent laryngeal nerve paralysis
   (E) Superior vena cava obstruction

3. A 50-year-old man is treated for septic shock with multiple antibiotics. Seven days later, the patient is alert and oriented, and his tissue perfusion has returned to normal. However, he describes a terrible feeling that "the world is spinning." Which of the following therapeutic agents is most likely responsible for this patient's symptom?

   (A) Ciprofloxacin
   (B) Erythromycin
   (C) Gentamicin
   (D) Imipenem
   (E) Piperacillin-tazobactam

4. Oxygen binds to hemoglobin in RBCs while in the lungs to be circulated throughout the blood to oxygenate peripheral tissues. Many factors determine hemoglobin's affinity for O_2. Which of the following factors is associated with an increased hemoglobin affinity for O_2?

   (A) Acidotic blood pH
   (B) High altitude
   (C) High levels of 2,3-diphosphoglycerate
   (D) Hypermetabolic state
   (E) Increased body temperature
   (F) Presence of fetal hemoglobin

5. A 65-year-old obese woman underwent bilateral total knee replacement. The patient has been receiving low-molecular-weight heparin postoperatively. The patient has not been able to ambulate at all, and she presents on postoperative day 7 with a fever of 38.5° C (101.3° F) without infection. The patient complains of acute shortness of breath, chest pain, and that she has a tender left lower extremity. On examination she is tachycardic, tachypneic, hypotensive, and has a right ventricular gallop rhythm to auscultation with widely split S_2. Which of the following is a risk factor for this patient's likely condition?

   (A) Healthy heart
   (B) Immobility
   (C) Low-molecular-weight heparin use
   (D) Slender body habitus
   (E) Warfarin use

6. A 25-year-old medical student presents with a nonproductive cough, low-grade fever, and malaise of 3 weeks' duration. He says that a few of the people he studies with have been feeling the same way. Sputum cultures come

back negative. The patient denies exposure to farm animals, travel, or HIV. The physician decides to treat for an atypical pneumonia. Which of the following is the most likely cause of this patient's ailment?

(A) *Coxiella burnetii*
(B) *Klebsiella pneumoniae*
(C) *Mycoplasma pneumoniae*
(D) *Pneumocystis carinii pneumonia*
(E) *Staphylococcus aureus*
(F) *Streptococcus pneumoniae*

7. A 50-year-old man complains of shortness of breath on exertion of a few months' duration. On inspection there is an increased anteroposterior diameter of the chest, pursed lips, and dyspnea with no scleral icterus or jaundice. On physical examination, the patient is noted to be tachycardic, have hyperresonant lungs with decreased breath sounds, and no hepatomegaly or liver nodules on palpation. Which of the following is the most likely diagnosis?

(A) α_1-Antitrypsin deficiency
(B) Asthma
(C) Bronchiectasis
(D) Centriacinar emphysema
(E) Chronic bronchitis
(F) Panacinar emphysema

8. A 13-year-old white girl with a past medical history of nasal polyps develops severe bronchoconstriction and wheezing after taking a large dose of aspirin, having mistaken it for a cold medication. After presenting to the emergency department, she is found to have a past history of aspirin allergy. Which of the following medications can be used effectively to stop the bronchoconstriction resulting from her aspirin allergy?

(A) Cromolyn
(B) Dopamine
(C) Methylxanthines
(D) Prednisone
(E) Zileuton

9. A 60-year-old white man presents with a productive cough of a few months' duration. The patient reports that the cough lasts 4 months and that he has had three of these episodes over the past 2 years. On examination, the patient is cyanotic, wheezing, and has crackles in the lungs upon auscultation. Lung biopsy reveals hypertrophy of mucus-secreting glands in the bronchioles giving a Reid index of > 50%. A diagnosis of chronic bronchitis is given. Which of the following is clearly linked with chronic bronchitis?

(A) Alcohol intake
(B) Cigarette smoking
(C) Cold climate
(D) Hypertension
(E) Intravenous drug abuse
(F) Seasonal allergies

10. During dental procedures, it is possible that small fragments may be aspirated into the trachea and cause aspiration pneumonia. If the patient is sitting upright during the procedure, which of the following is the most common site of aspiration pneumonia?

(A) Left lower lobe
(B) Left upper lobe
(C) Lingula
(D) Right lower lobe
(E) Right upper lobe

11. A 57-year-old man with a 40-year history of smoking has chronic obstructive lung disease. He presents to the physician with a blood pressure of 150/95 mm Hg. Which of the following antihypertensive agent is contraindicated in this patient?

(A) Acebutolol
(B) Atenolol
(C) Esmolol
(D) Metoprolol
(E) Nadolol

12. Gas exchange in the lungs occurs in the alveoli. There are two components to this exchange, diffusion and perfusion. Either of these components can limit the exchange of oxygen from the air into the bloodstream. Which of the following describes perfusion-limited exchange?

(A) It is illustrated by CO and O_2 concentrations during strenuous exercise

(B) It is illustrated by gas equilibrating early along the length of the pulmonary capillary

(C) It is illustrated by gases other than N_2O and CO_2 under healthy, resting conditions

(D) It is illustrated by the gas partial pressure difference being maintained between alveolar air and pulmonary capillary blood

(E) It is illustrated in disease states such as fibrosis and emphysema

(F) It is not affected by change in blood flow

13. While examining a patient, the physician notices decreased breath sounds at the right lower lobe, dullness on percussion, and decreased tactile fremitus without tracheal deviation. These findings most likely represent which of the following?

(A) Bronchial obstruction

(B) Intestinal infiltration

(C) Lobar pneumonia

(D) Pleural effusion

(E) Pneumothorax

14. A 65-year-old man with an 80-pack-year history of smoking presents with a cough and increasing dyspnea over the past 6 weeks. A 2-cm diameter mass is seen in the left lower lobe in an x-ray film of the chest. A sample of non-neoplastic tissue from a bronchial biopsy is shown in the image. Which of the following types of epithelium not normally present in the lung is seen this image (denoted by *E*)?

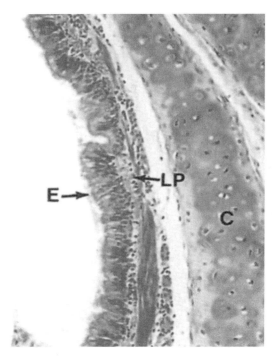

Reproduced, with permission, from Berman I. *Color Atlas of Basic Histology*, 3rd ed. New York, McGraw-Hill, 2003: 214, Fig. 14-3.

(A) Pseudostratified columnar

(B) Simple squamous

(C) Stratified columnar

(D) Stratified squamous

(E) Transitional

15. The oxygen-hemoglobin dissociation curve represents the percent saturation of hemoglobin with oxygen as a function of the partial pressure of oxygen in the blood. This curve is sigmoidal in shape due to the change in affinity of heme groups for oxygen as each successive oxygen molecule binds. Which of the following causes a shift in this curve to the left?

(A) High altitude

(B) Increased 2,3-diphosphoglycerate

(C) Increased partial pressure of carbon dioxide in the blood

(D) Increased pH

(E) Increased temperature

16. A 69-year-old man is hospitalized for an exacerbation of asthma. He is placed on albuterol and an inhaled corticosteroid, but due to low oxygen saturation, he is intubated. After 3 days in the hospital, he has a temperature of 39.4° C (103.1° F), a blood pressure of 104/63 mm Hg, a pulse of 108/min, and a respiratory rate of 35/min. On physical examination, the patient is found to have coarse rhonchi at the base of the lung fields bilaterally. The patient is producing purulent, foul-smelling sputum that shows *Pseudomonas aeruginosa* on culture analysis. Which of the following agents could be used to treat *Pseudomonas aeruginosa* infection?

(A) Cefoperazone
(B) Cefotaxime
(C) Cefotetan
(D) Ceftriaxone
(E) Cefuroxime

17. A 7-year-old boy is brought to the pediatrician because of a chronic cough, fatty diarrhea, and failure to thrive. *Pseudomonas aeruginosa* is cultured from his respiratory tract. The physician informs the patient's parents that their son has a disease that is caused by a mutation in a specific ion transporter. This patient has a mutation in the ion transporter of which of the following electrolytes?

(A) Ca^{2+}
(B) Cl^-
(C) HCO_3^-
(D) K^+
(E) Na^+

18. An 18-year-old man comes to the physician complaining of a runny nose, sneezing, and difficulty breathing for the past 2 days. On questioning, the patient says that his younger sister received a baby kitten as a birthday present 2 days ago. The response seen in this patient is mediated by which of the following?

(A) Antigen cross-linking IgE on presensitized mast cells and basophils
(B) Antigen-antibody complexes activating complement
(C) IgM and IgG binding to antigens on enemy cells

(D) Sensitized T lymphocytes releasing lymphokines
(E) Serum sickness

19. A 24-year-old medical student was studying one night for the boards and decided to take a break to eat. While eating quickly, he was reading something that made him laugh. A piece of food got stuck and he started having trouble breathing. At the emergency department, an x-ray film showed a piece of chicken stuck in his trachea. This meant that there was no air getting to the alveoli, but blood was still flowing. Which of the following best describes the relationship between ventilation and perfusion in the lungs?

(A) Compared to the apex, the ventilation/perfusion ratio in the base is much greater
(B) During exercise, the ventilation/perfusion ratio in the apex does not change
(C) In a complete airway obstruction (shunt), the ventilation/perfusion ratio approaches infinity
(D) In hypoxic vasoconstricted areas, the ventilation/perfusion ratio approaches zero
(E) Relative to the base, the apex arterial partial oxygen pressure is less and arterial partial carbon dioxide pressure is greater
(F) The ventilation/perfusion ratio in the apex of the lung indicates wasted perfusion
(G) Ventilation is greatest at the base of the lungs

20. A 5-year-old girl is brought to the emergency department by her aunt because of a sore throat. The patient is visiting from Nicaragua and has had very few immunizations. Physical examination reveals a grayish-white membrane on the pharynx with marked cervical lymphadenopathy and edema of the throat and neck area. The girl is, however, afebrile. Definitive diagnosis is made by gram-positive rods growing on which of the following media?

(A) Bordet-Gengou agar
(B) Chocolate agar with factors V and X
(C) Sabouraud's agar
(D) Tellurite agar
(E) Thayer-Martin agar

21. A 57-year-old man from Colombia presents to the emergency department with fever, night sweats, and a productive cough. A sputum smear shows acid-fast bacilli, and the patient is started on several antituberculosis medications. Three months later, the patient returns to the emergency department with reduced visual acuity and an inability to see the color green. Which of the following is the most likely cause of this patient's change in visual acuity?

    (A) Ethambutol toxicity
    (B) Isoniazid toxicity
    (C) Pyrazinamide toxicity
    (D) Rifampin toxicity
    (E) Tuberculous eye infection

22. A 76-year-old man comes to the physician in the early fall with a high fever, dry cough, and shortness of breath. Rales are heard on auscultation, and he has mild cyanosis. X-ray film of his chest shows diffuse interstitial infiltrates; a sputum culture is negative. Which of the following reflects how the standard treatment of this disease will affect the prognosis of this patient?

    (A) Although the fever will abate, the dry cough and shortness of breath will be prolonged
    (B) Immunity to future infection is bolstered
    (C) Symptom duration is reduced by 1–1.5 days
    (D) Symptom duration is reduced by half
    (E) Symptoms will initially get worse, then better

23. A 21-year-old man underwent emergent surgery for a strangulated inguinal hernia. After removal of 6 in of ileum, the patient was admitted to his postoperative room. The following day, the patient spiked a fever and had difficulty breathing. The doctor notes that the most common cause for fever 1–2 days postoperatively is atelectasis. Which of the following is most characteristic of alveoli?

    (A) Compliance in small alveoli is increased relative to large alveoli
    (B) Large alveoli have an increased tendency to collapse

    (C) Large surfactant-lined alveoli have the highest chance of collapsing
    (D) Small alveoli have a decreased pressure required to keep open
    (E) Surfactant-lined alveoli have increased compliance

24. A 7-year-old girl is brought to the pediatrician because of a fever of 39.7° C (103.5° F), trouble swallowing, and drooling. Within a few minutes of arriving at the office, she develops inspiratory stridor and respiratory distress. An x-ray film of her neck is shown. Which of the following organisms is most likely responsible for this patient's condition?

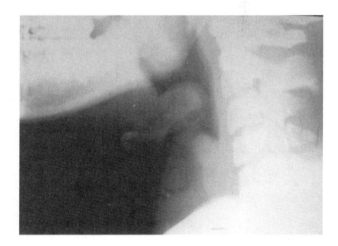

Reproduced, with permission, from Stone CK, Humphries RL. *Current Emergency Diagnosis & Treatment*. New York, McGraw-Hill, 2004: Fig. 48-4.

    (A) *Haemophilus influenzae*
    (B) *Mycoplasma pneumoniae*
    (C) Parainfluenza virus
    (D) Respiratory syncytial virus
    (E) *Streptococcus pyogenes*

25. An 8-year-old boy comes to the physician with his mother, who wants to discuss respiratory problems that have arisen since an upper respiratory infection 4 months ago. The mother says that the patient has attacks characterized by wheezing and shortness of breath that usually resolve after an hour. On one occasion, an

attack required a visit to the emergency department, and the mother remembers the treating physician saying something about an abnormally high level of eosinophils in the patient's blood. Which of the following is the most likely diagnosis for this patient?

(A) Asbestosis
(B) Asthma
(C) Coronavirus infection
(D) Croup
(E) Cystic fibrosis

26. A 46-year-old woman presents to the emergency department with a 4-week history of worsening nausea and lethargy. While she is waiting to see the doctor, the patient experiences a seizure. Her past medical history is significant for hypertension and tuberculosis. Laboratory values are as follows:

Serum Na$^+$: 125 mEq/L
Serum osmolality: 255 mOsm/kg
Urine osmolality: 1550 mOsm/kg
Hematocrit: 27%

Which of the following is the most likely diagnosis?

(A) Central diabetes insipidus
(B) Epilepsy
(C) Nephrogenic diabetes insipidus
(D) Psychogenic polydipsia
(E) Syndrome of inappropriate ADH secretion

27. Which of the following occurs during inspiration?

(A) Air passively moves into the lungs against a pressure gradient
(B) Alveolar pressure increases to more than atmospheric pressure
(C) At peak inspiration the lung volume equals functional residual capacity minus one tidal volume
(D) Inspiratory muscles relax causing thoracic volume to decrease
(E) Intrapleural pressure becomes more negative

(F) The diaphragm relaxes, increasing thoracic cavity volume

28. An HIV-positive 24-year-old man from Southern California comes in to his physician's office with a dry cough, headache, mild wheezing, and slight fever. A complete blood count shows elevated eosinophils, and a potassium hydroxide sputum smear is positive for microorganisms. The infectious form of the organism shown in the image possesses which of the following key components?

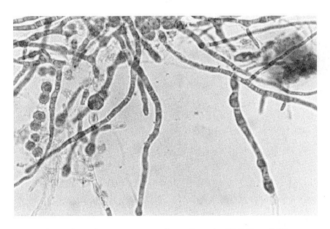

Reproduced, with permission, from Brooks GF, Butel JS, Morse SA. *Jawetz, Melnick, & Adelberg's Medical Microbiology*, 23rd ed. New York, McGraw-Hill, 2004: Fig. 45-15.

(A) Dipicolinic acid
(B) Hemagglutinin
(C) Lipopolysaccharide
(D) Polysaccharide
(E) Teichoic acid

29. A 74-year-old patient with increased shortness of breath presents because his respiratory problem is causing him distress. A sputum sample reveals golden-brown beaded fibers, which results from iron- and protein-coated fibers. On CT scan, dense hyalinized fibrocalcific plaques of the parietal pleura are seen. A particular pneumoconiosis is suspected. Which of the following is the likely etiology of the patient's condition?

(A) Autoimmune attack of lung parenchyma
(B) Chronic inhalation of asbestos fibers
(C) Idiopathic (unknown) etiology
(D) Living in a polluted city for years
(E) Long-term complication of steroid abuse
(F) Reactivation of a contained primary disease
(G) Working in a coal mine for 40 years

30. A 158.8-kg (350-lb) man with a body mass index of 40 comes to the physician complaining of frequent fatigue, shortness of breath, general sleepiness, and an inability to concentrate. Physical examination shows an extremely obese, tired-looking man with hypertension and an elongated uvula. Which of the following metabolic findings is most likely?

(A) Decreased serum glucose
(B) Increased HDL cholesterol
(C) Increased renal H^+ reabsorption
(D) Increased renal HCO_3^- reabsorption
(E) Renal HCO_3^- secretion

31. A 55-year-old woman presents with a painless mass at the angle of the mandible 1 week after undergoing a dental procedure. On physical examination, her physician notes that the mass is draining pus and yellowish granules. A stained sample from the abscess shows branching gram-positive rods. She is treated with penicillin. What was the most likely causative organism?

(A) *Actinomyces israeli*
(B) *Candida albicans*
(C) *Clostridium perfringens*
(D) *Nocardia asteroides*
(E) *Staphylococcus epidermidis*

32. Respiratory rate changes dynamically with input from many different sources. There are central control, chemoreceptors, and other receptors responsible for respiration. What is one mechanism by which the body exerts control over respiration?

(A) Aortic and carotid bodies are considered to be central chemoreceptors
(B) Central chemoreceptors affect breathing by directly detecting the H^+ blood levels
(C) Central control of breathing is located in the hypothalamus and amygdala
(D) Peripheral chemoreceptors stimulate breathing at partial oxygen pressure levels less than 60 mm Hg
(E) Stretch, irritant, and J receptors all function outside of the lung to regulate breathing

33. A 21-year-old college student presents to his student health center with complaints of malaise, headaches, fever up to 38.3° C (101° F), chills, and a nonproductive cough of 1 week's duration. On physical examination the patient appears fatigued and his vital signs are as follows: temperature 38.1° C (100.6° F), heart rate 90/min, respiratory rate 20/min, and blood pressure 118/75 mm Hg. Auscultation of lungs reveals bilateral diffuse wheezes and rales. X-ray of the chest reveals bilateral infiltrates. The doctor prescribed ceftriaxone, but the patient failed to show any improvement over the next week. What antibiotic should be added to the patient's regimen?

(A) Ampicillin
(B) Azithromycin
(C) Cefotaxime
(D) Clindamycin
(E) Penicillin

34. A tall, thin 23-year-old man comes to the emergency department (ED) complaining of sudden pleuritic chest pain and shortness of breath. On physical examination, the trachea is displaced to the left and there is right-sided hyperresonance to percussion, decreased breath sounds, and decreased tactile fremitus. X-ray film of the

chest that was made in the ED is shown in the image. A subpleural bleb is noted at lung decompression surgery. Which of the following is the most likely diagnosis?

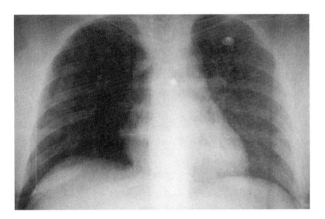

Reproduced, with permission, from Stone CK, Humphries RL. *Current Emergency Diagnosis & Treatment.* New York, McGraw-Hill, 2004: Fig. 11-3.

(A) Asbestosis
(B) Asthma
(C) Bronchiectasis
(D) Bronchitis
(E) Emphysema
(F) Oat cell carcinoma
(G) Pneumothorax

35. A 40-year-old patient with AIDS presents to the clinic with fatigue and weakness. An x-ray film of the chest shows a diffuse, patchy infiltrate. A methenamine silver stain of a bronchoalveolar lavage specimen is positive. Treatment with trimethoprim-sulfamethoxazole is contraindicated because the patient has a sulfa allergy. Which of the following agents should be used to treat this patient's infection?

(A) Ivermectin
(B) Metronidazole
(C) Penicillin
(D) Pentamidine
(E) Protamine

36. A 71-year-old man is brought to the emergency department (ED) by ambulance after he was found by his neighbor walking around his garden confused and unable to answer questions. In the ED, the patient is confused and oriented only to person. His vital signs are a temperature of 37.6° C (99.7° F), heart rate is 110/min, respiratory rate is 20/min, and blood pressure is 130/92 mm Hg. While in the ED the patient has a seizure. Laboratory testing shows a serum Na^+ of 115 mEq/L, a serum K^+ level of 3.8 mEq/L, a serum glucose level of 100 g/dL, and a serum osmolality of 250 mOsmol/kg. Urine electrolyte testing show a urine osmolality of 500 mOsmol/kg. X-ray of the chest shows a mass in the lung. Which of the following is the most likely etiology of the mass?

(A) Metastatic brain cancer
(B) Pneumonia
(C) Small cell carcinoma
(D) Squamous cell carcinoma
(E) Tuberculosis

37. Several cases of severe pneumonia occur in a community. Patients present with a high fever; sputum specimens show very few small, gram-negative rods on Gram's stain. The outbreak is traced back to a water mist machine used in the produce section of a supermarket. Which of the following is the most likely causative organism in this outbreak?

(A) *Bordetella pertussis*
(B) *Haemophilus influenzae* type B
(C) *Legionella pneumophila*
(D) *Mycobacterium tuberculosis*
(E) *Streptococcus pneumoniae*

38. Medium-sized bronchi are the major site of airway resistance in the lungs. Bronchial smooth muscle can change bronchial diameter by contracting or relaxing. Which of the following conditions is associated with dilation of airways?

(A) Asthma
(B) Atelectasis
(C) Bronchiectasis
(D) Idiopathic pulmonary fibrosis
(E) Neonatal respiratory distress syndrome

39. A 69-year-old woman with a history of intractable pain presents to the emergency department unconscious and in respiratory arrest. Her husband says that she recently visited a pain clinic, where she was given a new medication. On physical examination, she is noted to have a greatly distended abdomen. Which of the following is the most appropriate treatment for this patient?

(A) Aminocaproic acid
(B) Flumazenil
(C) Naltrexone
(D) Physostigmine
(E) Protamine

40. At a checkup during her 22nd week of pregnancy, a woman tells her doctor that she feels like she is "abnormally large" considering how long she has been pregnant. Her doctor agrees, and performs an ultrasound, which reveals an excess of fluid in the uterus. In addition, the stomach, spleen, and a portion of the small intestine are visible in the fetus's thorax. What structure(s) most likely failed to form completely in the fetal thorax?

(A) Dorsal mesentery of the esophagus
(B) Foregut
(C) Lateral body wall
(D) Pleuroperitoneal folds
(E) Septum transversum

41. Which of the following letter choices represents the residual volume?

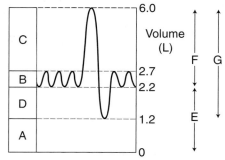

Reproduced, with permission, from USMLERx.com.

(A) A
(B) B

(C) C
(D) D
(E) E
(F) F
(G) G

42. A call at 3 A.M. reveals a pregnant patient who is in labor. While rushing to get to the hospital to assist with the delivery, the doctor realizes that the patient is only 29 weeks pregnant. The patient had no signs of preeclampsia (hypertension, edema, or proteinuria), but the patient was dealing with maternal diabetes mellitus. Upon arrival at the hospital, the doctors decide that she will have to have a cesarean section. Knowing the risk this baby faces, it is suggested that maternal steroids be started immediately and that surfactant is ready to administer to the infant immediately after birth. This course of treatment is intended to prevent which of the following?

(A) Diffuse alveolar damage
(B) Hyaline membrane disease
(C) Hypersensitivity pneumonitis
(D) Intra-alveolar exudative consolidation
(E) Localized proliferation of histiocytes
(F) Noncaseating granulomatous disease
(G) Panacinar emphysema

43. A 37-year-old man is brought to the emergency department after he is stabbed immediately superior the right nipple with an unknown object. On physical examination, the patient's blood pressure is 100/60 mm Hg, his heart rate is 126/min, his respiratory rate is 26/min, and his oxygen saturation is 94% on 100% oxygen face mask. The wound is small but is bubbling, and the skin immediately around the wound is moving in and out with respirations. Which of the following will likely be found on x-ray of this patient's chest?

(A) Right hemothorax
(B) Right ninth and tenth rib fractures
(C) Right pleural effusion
(D) Right pneumothorax
(E) Right upper lobe consolidation

44. A 67-year-old homeless man reports to the physician with a 1-week history of a productive cough, shortness of breath, and high fever. He denies alcohol, drug, or tobacco use. The patient says that the onset of symptoms was sudden. A chest x-ray taken in the emergency department shows a large left lower lobe opacity. Which of the following antibiotics would best initially treat this patient's infection?

(A) Azithromycin
(B) Ceftriaxone
(C) Doxycycline
(D) Erythromycin
(E) Levofloxacin

45. A 26-year-old recent immigrant from China presents to the emergency department with a 3-week history of fevers accompanied by night sweats and chills, weight loss of 2.3 kg (5 lb), and cough that is often productive of blood-tinged sputum. Results of an acid-fast sputum stain are shown in the image. Which of the following should be included in the treatment regimen of this patient?

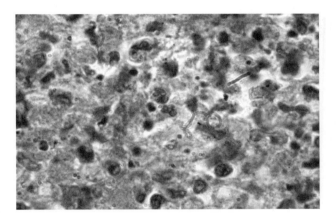

Image courtesy of PEIR Digital Library (http://peir.net).

(A) Vitamin B$_1$
(B) Vitamin B$_6$
(C) Vitamin B$_{12}$
(D) Vitamin C
(E) Vitamin E

46. A 15-year-old white boy with a history of severe asthma presents to the emergency department in obvious respiratory distress. After admission and multiple nebulizer treatments, he develops nausea, vomiting, and weakness. Studies reveal a potassium level of 2.6 mEq/L and U waves on ECG. Which of the following medications may have elicited these symptoms?

(A) Albuterol
(B) Ipratropium
(C) Prednisone
(D) Theophylline
(E) Zileuton

47. A 32-year-old woman presents to her physician complaining of "swollen lymph nodes" under her chin. Further questioning reveals that she has had a cough for the past 2 months and some increased shortness of breath. After completing a full physical examination, her physician orders an x-ray of the chest, which shows an abnormality. A lung biopsy is ordered, and a micrograph of the biopsy is shown. What is her most likely diagnosis?

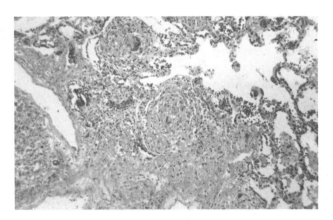

Image courtesy of PEIR Digital Library (http://peir.net).

(A) Goodpasture's syndrome
(B) Sarcoidosis
(C) Small-cell lung cancer
(D) Systemic lupus erythematosus
(E) Tuberculosis

48. A farmer presents to the physician with a dry cough and pressure in his chest. He quickly develops bloody pleural effusions, hemorrhagic mediastinitis, and septic shock. Which of the following organisms is most likely responsible for this patient's symptoms?

   (A) *Bacillus anthracis*
   (B) *Legionella pneumophila*
   (C) *Mycoplasma pneumoniae*
   (D) *Nocardia asteroides*
   (E) *Streptococcus pneumoniae*

49. A 44-year-old man comes into the office for "personal reasons." Upon meeting the doctor, the patient is nervous but not unstable. He explains that his father died of a myocardial infarction at the age of 45, and his birthday is coming up in a month. History reveals that he was diagnosed with type 2 diabetes mellitus, has high cholesterol, and smokes a pack of cigarettes per day. The patient does not take any vitamins or aspirin. After having an ECG that comes back suspicious, the patient is sent for an exercise stress test. With regard to CO_2 during exercise, which of the following physiologic processes is taking place?

   (A) All of the dissolved CO_2 becomes converted to bicarbonate, which binds to hemoglobin
   (B) Bicarbonate travels in the RBCs until it reaches the lung, where it gets exhaled as CO_2

   (C) Carbaminohemoglobin (CO_2 bound to hemoglobin) becomes the primary CO_2 transport carrier
   (D) In the lungs, the acidic environment shifts the hemoglobin-O_2 curve to the right and causes the release CO_2 from hemoglobin
   (E) More chloride is entering the RBCs peripherally to compensate for increased carbonic anhydrase activity

50. A 65-year-old patient comes in for an insurance physical that requires pulmonary function tests to ensure his lungs are working normally before the insurance company will cover him. The patient has been a chronic smoker for most of his life. Laboratory testing reveals an arterial blood partial carbon dioxide pressure (P_{CO_2}) of 40 mm Hg and his expired air P_{CO_2} is 30 mm Hg. His physiologic dead space is determined to be 0.125 L (125 mL). What is the value of the patient's tidal volume?

   (A) 0.01 L
   (B) 0.05 L
   (C) 0.1 L
   (D) 0.5 L
   (E) 1 L
   (F) 5 L

1. **The correct answer is B.** An overdose of theophylline will cause a decrease in the hydrolysis of cyclic adenosine monophosphate (cAMP) to adenosine monophosphate, resulting in an increasing and potentially toxic level of cAMP. In order to decrease cAMP in the patient, β-blockers may be given to stop the conversion of ATP to cAMP via adenylate cyclase.

Answer A is incorrect. Albuterol would potentiate the effects of theophylline.

Answer C is incorrect. Digoxin, a medication for congestive heart failure, is unrelated to theophylline overdose.

Answer D is incorrect. Epinephrine would potentiate the effects of theophylline.

Answer E is incorrect. Furosemide, a diuretic, is unrelated to theophylline overdose. It is used for edematous states.

2. **The correct answer is A.** A tumor at the apex of the lung, or superior sulcus, is known as a Pancoast's tumor. This can affect the cervical sympathetic plexus, resulting in Horner's syndrome (ptosis, miosis, enophthalmos, and anhidrosis).

Answer B is incorrect. A paraneoplastic endocrine syndrome would be a lung carcinoma that secretes products similar to ACTH, antidiuretic hormone, or parathyroid hormone. These would cause Cushing's syndrome, the syndrome of inappropriate secretion of antidiuretic hormone, or hypercalcemia, respectively.

Answer C is incorrect. Pleural effusion would present with dyspnea, and on physical examination one would hear crackles, most likely at the bases of the lungs.

Answer D is incorrect. Recurrent laryngeal nerve paralysis would cause a patient to present with hoarseness of the voice, not the other symptoms mentioned.

Answer E is incorrect. Superior vena cava (SVC) syndrome results when a tumor compresses the SVC. Clinically, one would see facial swelling, cyanosis, and dilation of the veins of the head, neck, and upper extremities, not eyelid droop and hemianhidrosis.

3. **The correct answer is C.** Gentamicin is an aminoglycoside antibiotic used in the treatment of gram-negative rod infections. It is often combined with β-lactam antibiotics because it acts synergistically. Aminoglycosides can cause nephrotoxicity and nonoliguric acute tubular necrosis, or ototoxicity, which can present as either vestibular or cochlear damage. Vestibular toxicity may result in vertigo, nausea, vomiting, or ataxia, whereas cochlear damage causes tinnitus or hearing loss. The patient in this question is experiencing vertigo.

Answer A is incorrect. Ciprofloxacin is a fluoroquinolone antibiotic used to treat urinary tract infection and severe gram-negative infections as well as a variety of other infections. Toxicity may cause gastrointestinal upset, rash, dizziness, and tendonitis.

Answer B is incorrect. Erythromycin is a macrolide antibiotic used to treat atypical pneumonias and upper respiratory infections caused by *Legionella, Chlamydia, Mycoplasma,* and *Neisseria* species. Erythromycin toxicity causes gastrointestinal discomfort, acute cholestatic hepatitis, eosinophilia, and skin rash.

Answer D is incorrect. Imipenem is a β-lactamase-resistant agent that has a wide spectrum of activity. It is not effective for treating methicillin-resistant *Staphylococcus aureus*, vancomycin-resistant enterococcus, or some strains of *Pseudomonas* species infections. Adverse effects of imipenem include gastrointestinal distress and seizures.

Answer E is incorrect. Piperacillin-tazobactam is used to treat *Pseudomonas* species infections, resistant *Staphylococcus aureus* infections, and many gram-negative infections. Adverse reactions include hypersensitivity reactions and diarrhea.

4. The correct answer is F. A left shift of the hemoglobin-O_2 dissociation curve occurs in the presence of fetal hemoglobin.

Answer A is incorrect. Acidotic blood pH has an increased amount of H^+ ions, which decreases O_2 affinity and displaces O_2 from hemoglobin.

Answer B is incorrect. High altitude is associated with hypoxemia, shifting the curve to the right.

Answer C is incorrect. A right shift of the hemoglobin-O_2 dissociation curve occurs when the levels of 2,3-diphosphoglycerate are high.

Answer D is incorrect. Increased metabolic needs require increased levels of O_2 delivery to the tissue. For this to happen, hemoglobin affinity for O_2 has to decrease.

Answer E is incorrect. Increased body temperature shifts the curve to the right.

5. The correct answer is B. The patient most likely has a pulmonary embolism (PE), which can be a life-threatening situation. Malignancy (cancer), multiple fractures, use of oral contraceptive pills, prolonged bed rest (immobility), and congestive heart failure are clinical settings in which a PE can occur.

Answer A is incorrect. Congestive heart failure and previous myocardial infarction are risk factors for pulmonary embolism.

Answer C is incorrect. Low-molecular-weight heparin would affect the prothrombin time, inhibiting the coagulation cascade and the formation of a deep venous thrombosis.

Answer D is incorrect. Obesity is a risk factor for pulmonary embolism.

Answer E is incorrect. Warfarin would "thin" the blood and is used in the treatment of thromboembolic disease.

6. The correct answer is C. *Mycoplasma pneumoniae* is the most common cause of interstitial (atypical) pneumonia, along with viruses. It cannot be cultured and is diagnosed by the cold agglutinin test.

Answer A is incorrect. *Coxiella burnetii* (Q fever) is associated with infected cattle or sheep, or drinking unpasteurized products, none of which were among this patient's exposures.

Answer B is incorrect. *Klebsiella pneumoniae* is associated with alcoholics and hospitalized patients, neither of which is likely the case here.

Answer D is incorrect. *Pneumocystis carinii* pneumonia is a very common opportunistic infection in patients diagnosed with HIV that have $CD4^+$ counts of $< 200/\mu L$.

Answer E is incorrect. *Staphylococcus aureus* pneumonia is often a complication of influenza or viral pneumonias.

Answer F is incorrect. *Streptococcus pneumoniae* (pneumococcus) is the most common cause of lobar pneumonia, and presents with classic symptoms such as acute fever, productive cough, and shortness of breath.

7. The correct answer is D. Although the vignette did not give information about smoking, smoking is the most likely cause of centriacinar emphysema. The stem mentions an absence of jaundice and liver problems, making α_1-antitrypsin deficiency unlikely.

Answer A is incorrect. α_1-Antitrypsin deficiency usually presents with emphysema and liver cirrhosis (jaundice).

Answer B is incorrect. Asthma would present with wheezing after exposure to a trigger. However, asthma is reversible most of the time, and would not produce a barrel chest or pursed lips.

Answer C is incorrect. Bronchiectasis is permanent abnormal bronchial dilation caused by chronic infection. This is characterized by copious purulent sputum.

Answer E is incorrect. Chronic bronchitis patients are given the classic name "bluebloaters." This patient does not have a history of productive cough, thus he is unlikely to have chronic bronchitis.

Answer F is incorrect. Panacinar emphysema is a result of α_1-antitrypsin deficiency.

8. **The correct answer is E.** Aspirin serves to inhibit the cyclooxygenase enzymes. An allergy to aspirin is thought to result from the diversion of arachidonic acid to the leukotriene pathway when the cyclooxygenase-catalyzed prostaglandin pathway is blocked. The resulting increase in leukotriene synthesis leads to the bronchoconstriction that is typical of an aspirin allergy. Zileuton is an effective inhibitor of the 5-lipoxygenase pathway and thus blocks the conversion of arachidonic acid to leukotrienes. Because of this, zileuton can be used in the treatment of aspirin allergy.

Answer A is incorrect. Cromolyn may be used as prophylactic treatment for aspirin allergy because it inhibits the release of inflammatory mediators from mast cells. However, it cannot be used to treat active aspirin allergy because the mast cell mediators have already been released.

Answer B is incorrect. Dopamine, which is used in shock and heart failure, is not used for aspirin allergy.

Answer C is incorrect. Methylxanthines such as theophylline are not effective in treating aspirin allergy because they affect the phosphodiesterase pathway rather than the leukotriene pathway.

Answer D is incorrect. Prednisone is not effective in treating aspirin allergy.

9. **The correct answer is B.** Cigarette smoking is the leading cause of chronic bronchitis.

Answer A is incorrect. Alcohol intake is not directly associated with chronic bronchitis.

Answer C is incorrect. Air pollution is associated with chronic bronchitis, not cold climate.

Answer D is incorrect. Hypertension is not associated with chronic bronchitis.

Answer E is incorrect. Intravenous drug abuse is not associated with chronic bronchitis.

Answer F is incorrect. Seasonal allergies are not related to chronic bronchitis.

10. **The correct answer is D.** The right main bronchus is more vertical and wider than the left, and aspirated particles are more likely to lodge at the junction of the right inferior and right middle bronchi. Because of this, aspiration pneumonia contracted when an individual is in an upright position is most common in the right lower and middle lobes.

Answer A is incorrect. The left main bronchus is narrower and less vertical than the right main bronchus. The right main bronchus is more vertical and wider than the left, and aspirated particles are more likely to lodge at the junction of the right inferior and right middle bronchi.

Answer B is incorrect. The left main bronchus is narrower and less vertical than the right main bronchus. The right main bronchus is more vertical and wider than the left, and aspirated particles are more likely to lodge at the junction of the right inferior and right middle bronchi.

Answer C is incorrect. The lingula is in the left lung, and the left main bronchus is narrower and less vertical than the right main bronchus. The right main bronchus is more vertical and wider than the left, and aspirated particles are more likely to lodge at the junction of the right inferior and right middle bronchi.

Answer E is incorrect. When a person is supine, aspiration pneumonia may affect the upper lobes and posterior segments of the lungs, since they become the gravity-dependent regions when a person lies flat.

11. **The correct answer is E.** Nonselective β-blockers are contraindicated in patients with lung disease because they can cause bronchoconstriction by blocking the β_2 receptors responsible for relaxation of bronchial smooth muscle. β_2 Agonists are a mainstay of asthma therapy. Acebutolol, atenolol, esmolol, metoprolol, and betaxolol are all cardioselective β_1-blockers that could be used in a patient with

lung/airway disease. Nadolol is a nonselective β-blocker and should **not** be used in a patient with lung disease.

Answer A is incorrect. Acebutolol is not cardio-selective and could cause asthma exacerbation.

Answer B is incorrect. Atenolol is not cardio-selective and could exacerbate obstructive lung disease.

Answer C is incorrect. Esmolol is not cardio-selective and could exacerbate obstructive lung disease.

Answer D is incorrect. Metoprolol is not cardioselective and could exacerbate obstructive lung disease.

12. **The correct answer is B.** In perfusion-limited exchange, gas equilibrates early along the length of the pulmonary capillary, because it is not a problem with gas diffusion.

Answer A is incorrect. Diffusion-limited exchange is illustrated by CO and O_2 during strenuous exercise.

Answer C is incorrect. Perfusion-limited exchange is illustrated by N_2O and CO_2 under normal conditions, along with O_2 under normal conditions.

Answer D is incorrect. The partial pressure of the gas in the pulmonary capillary blood becomes equal to the partial pressure in the alveolar air. It is maintained in diffusion-limited exchange.

Answer E is incorrect. Diffusion-limited exchange is illustrated in disease states such as fibrosis and emphysema, because it's the gas, not the blood flow, that is the problem.

Answer F is incorrect. Perfusion-limited exchange is increased only if blood flow increases, and it decreases when blood flow decreases.

13. **The correct answer is D.** Small to moderate pleural effusions can present without tracheal deviation, decreased breath sounds over the effusion, dullness to resonance, and decreased tactile fremitus.

Answer A is incorrect. Bronchial obstruction would present with absent breath sounds over the area, decreased resonance, decreased tactile fremitus, and tracheal deviation toward the side of the lesion.

Answer B is incorrect. Intestines can appear in the thoracic cavity if there is a diaphragmatic hernia. There would be no breath sounds at all, and the patient could have tracheal deviation.

Answer C is incorrect. Lobar pneumonia may have bronchial breath sounds over the lesion, dullness to percussion, increased tactile fremitus, and no tracheal deviation.

Answer E is incorrect. Pneumothorax presents with decreased breath sounds, hyperresonant lungs to percussion, absent tactile fremitus, and tracheal deviation away from the side of the lesion.

14. **The correct answer is D.** The letter E in the image points to pseudostratified ciliated columnar epithelium; LP refers to the lamina propria and C refers to hyaline cartilage. In smokers, pseudostratified ciliated columnar epithelium can undergo metaplasia and transform into stratified squamous epithelium. Stratified epithelium is defined as epithelial membrane composed of more than one cell layer. Stratified epithelium is defined as epithelial membrane composed of more than one cell layer. Stratified squamous epithelium is classified by the flattened shape of the cells in the surface layer. Examples of tissues with stratified squamous epithelium include the skin, mouth, anus, vagina, and esophagus.

Answer A is incorrect. Pseudostratified columnar epithelium is the normal respiratory epithelium. This type of epithelium only appears stratified; however, all cells are in contact with basal lamina and only some cells reach the surface of epithelium.

Answer B is incorrect. Simple squamous epithelium lines alveoli, loops of Henle, and endothelial linings of blood vessels. Simple epithelium indicates that the epithelial membrane is composed of a single layer of cells. Under the microscope, simple squamous epithelium is characterized by a single sheet of flattened cells lying on a basal lamina. It does not play a role in this case.

Answer C is incorrect. Stratified columnar epithelium is found in only a few places in the body—namely, the conjunctivae of the eye and regions of the male urethra. It is composed of a low polyhedral to cuboidal deeper layer in contact with the basal lamina along with a superficial layer of columnar cells.

Answer E is incorrect. The bladder, not the lung, is lined by transitional epithelium. Transitional epithelium is characterized by several layers of cuboidal cells, with the surface layer being large and dome-shaped.

15. **The correct answer is D.** A shift in the curve to the left indicates an increased affinity of the hemoglobin for oxygen. This is caused by increased pH and by decreased temperature, 2,3-diphosphoglycerate levels, and P_{CO_2}, as well as fetal hemoglobin.

    Answer A is incorrect. This will cause a shift in the curve to the right, indicating a decreased affinity for oxygen.

    Answer B is incorrect. This will cause a shift in the curve to the right, indicating a decreased affinity for oxygen.

    Answer C is incorrect. This will cause a shift in the curve to the right, indicating a decreased affinity for oxygen.

    Answer E is incorrect. This will cause a shift in the curve to the right, indicating a decreased affinity for oxygen.

16. **The correct answer is A.** Cephalosporins are β-lactam antibiotics that inhibit bacterial cell wall synthesis. They are generally well tolerated and easy to administer; however, adverse effects include anaphylaxis and nephrotoxicity when combined with aminoglycosides. Three cephalosporins may be used to treat *Pseudomonas aeruginosa* infection (and should be memorized): cefoperazone, ceftazidime, and cefepime. Cefoperazone and ceftazidime, third-generation cephalosporins, are similar except

that ceftazidime has better activity against the Enterobacteriaceae family and is more commonly used. Cefepime is a fourth-generation cephalosporin with activity against both gram-positive and gram-negative organisms, including *Pseudomonas aeruginosa*.

Answer B is incorrect. Cefotaxime is similar to ceftriaxone but has a shorter half-life, which limits its usage.

Answer C is incorrect. Cefotetan is a second-generation cephalosporin with a spectrum of activity similar to that of the first-generation cephalosporins. The major advantage of cefotetan is its activity against *Bacteroides* species, making it an ideal prophylactic agent in abdominal surgeries.

Answer D is incorrect. Ceftriaxone is a third-generation cephalosporin that is particularly useful for penicillin-resistant gonorrhea, Lyme disease, and meningitis. Along with cefotetan and the cephalosporins with *Pseudomonas* species activity, this is a popular USMLE subject.

Answer E is incorrect. Cefuroxime is a second-generation cephalosporin with effectiveness against *Haemophilus influenzae* as well as strains of *Enterobacter* and *Proteus* species. It was previously used to treat *H. influenzae* meningitis but has been supplanted by the third-generation agents.

17. **The correct answer is B.** Cystic fibrosis (CF) is an autosomal recessive disease that most commonly occurs in the white population. It is usually caused by a mutation in the CF transmembrane conductance regulator (CFTR) protein, a protein that functions as a Cl⁻ channel and is regulated by cyclic adenosine monophosphate (cAMP). The delta F508 mutation is the most common gene abnormality associated with the disease; it involves the deletion of three base pairs from the gene and the consequent loss of a phenylalanine from the protein. Because three base pairs are deleted, there is no frameshift. Dysfunction of this channel causes abnormal Cl⁻ conductance with associated water transport abnormalities, leading to viscous secretions in exocrine glands. Failure to clear secretions in the respi-

ratory tract, pancreas, sweat glands, and other exocrine tissues results in recurrent pneumonias, exocrine pancreatic insufficiency, abnormal sweat gland function, urogenital dysfunction, and, ultimately, failure to thrive.

Answer A is incorrect. Ca^{2+} transporters are not affected in cystic fibrosis.

Answer C is incorrect. HCO_3^- transporters are not affected in cystic fibrosis.

Answer D is incorrect. K^+ transporters are not affected in cystic fibrosis.

Answer E is incorrect. Na^+ transporters are not affected in cystic fibrosis.

18. **The correct answer is A.** This response is an example of a type I hypersensitivity reaction. In these reactions, an allergen cross-links antigen-specific IgE on the surface of mast cells and basophils. Subsequently, the mast cells and basophils release vasoactive amines. Since antibodies are preformed in this type of hypersensitivity, the reaction develops quite rapidly.

Answer B is incorrect. Antigen-antibody complexes activate complement in a type III hypersensitivity reaction. This reaction would not present with sneezing and a runny nose but rather with local inflammation.

Answer C is incorrect. IgM and IgG binding occurs in a type II hypersensitivity reaction, which leads to a cytotoxic response to the allergen in the serum. This reaction would not present with sneezing and a runny nose, but rather with local inflammation.

Answer D is incorrect. In type IV hypersensitivity, or delayed-type hypersensitivity, one sees sensitized T lymphocytes releasing cytokines. This reaction would not present with sneezing and a runny nose but rather with local inflammation such as that associated with contact dermatitis from poison ivy. In addition, the clinical response occurs several days after antigen exposure.

Answer E is incorrect. Serum sickness is a type II hypersensitivity reaction in which antibodies to foreign proteins are formed. It presents a few days after an immunologic insult with urticaria, fever, arthralgia, and proteinuria.

19. **The correct answer is G.** Going from the apex to the base, both the ventilation and perfusion increase. Their rates of increase are different, but they both do increase.

Answer A is incorrect. From apex to base, the perfusion and ventilation both increase. However, because the blood flow increases at a higher rate, the ventilation/perfusion ratio decreases from apex to base.

Answer B is incorrect. During exercise, apical capillaries vasodilate and the ventilation/perfusion ratio approaches 1 (originally it is about 3).

Answer C is incorrect. As in the vignette about the piece of chicken occluding the trachea, no air is getting to the alveoli (there is no ventilation). Thus, the ventilation/perfusion ratio approaches zero.

Answer D is incorrect. Hypoxic vasoconstriction (physiologic dead space) indicates a lack of perfusion, thus the ventilation/perfusion ratio approaches infinity.

Answer E is incorrect. Apex arterial partial oxygen pressure is higher (wasted ventilation) and arterial partial carbon dioxide pressure is less (less perfusion).

Answer F is incorrect. In the apex, the blood flow is the lowest. Thus, there is more ventilation than perfusion, and the ventilation/perfusion ratio is high.

20. **The correct answer is D.** The disease described in this vignette is diphtheria, which is caused by the gram-positive rod *Corynebacterium diphtheriae*. Diphtheria classically presents with a grayish-white pseudomembrane on the pharynx or tonsils. Underlying tissue of the throat and neck becomes edematous, and lymphadenopathy develops. Fever is usually mild or absent. It is seen very rarely in vaccinated populations but is endemic to certain parts of the world. Culture of *C. diphtheriae* requires tellurite to prevent growth of normal upper respiratory tract flora.

Answer A is incorrect. Bordet-Gengou agar is used to culture *Bordetella pertussis*. Pertussis presents with paroxysmal coughing spells and whooping sounds on inspiration.

Answer B is incorrect. Chocolate agar is used to grow *Haemophilus influenzae*. Encapsulated strains of *H. influenzae* cause invasive diseases such as septicemia, meningitis, cellulitis, septic arthritis, epiglottitis, and pneumonia. Nonencapsulated strains are likely to cause otitis media, conjunctivitis, bronchitis, and sinusitis.

Answer C is incorrect. Sabouraud's agar is used to grow fungi.

Answer E is incorrect. Thayer-Martin agar is a chocolate agar plate which has VCN antibiotics (vancomycin, colistin, and nystatin) that suppress the growth of endogenous flora while supporting *Neisseria gonorrhoeae* growth. This patient does not have symptoms of gonorrhea.

21. **The correct answer is A.** Ethambutol is active only against *Mycobacterium tuberculosis*. The mechanism of action appears to be inhibition of polymerization of cell wall precursors. Although the drug is generally well tolerated, its most common adverse effects involve ocular toxicity, which usually appears several months after the initiation of treatment. Ethambutol is usually used with rifampin for patients who either cannot tolerate isoniazid or are infected with isoniazid-resistant *M. tuberculosis*.

Answer B is incorrect. Although rifampin is considered the best antituberculous agent, isoniazid is used for prophylaxis in asymptomatic patients with a positive PPD. A 6-month course of isoniazid prevents active tuberculosis in 90% of patients for at least 20 years. Isoniazid blocks mycolic acid cell wall synthesis and is bactericidal for rapidly multiplying organisms. Major adverse effects include hepatotoxicity and peripheral neuropathy, but many other adverse effects occur, such as lupuslike syndrome and optic atrophy.

Answer C is incorrect. Like isoniazid, the spectrum of action of pyrazinamide is limited to *Mycobacterium tuberculosis*. The site of activity for pyrazinamide is thought to be a fatty

acid synthase gene. The major adverse effect of pyrazinamide therapy is hepatotoxicity, but it is rare at recommended dosages. Another major adverse effect is hyperuricemia and gout.

Answer D is incorrect. Rifampin is the most potent antituberculous agent available. Rifampin blocks DNA-dependent RNA polymerase, preventing RNA synthesis. Although it is a better agent than isoniazid for preventing active tuberculosis infection, it has a significant risk of liver toxicity that outweighs its benefits in this population.

Answer E is incorrect. *Mycobacterium tuberculosis* can have extrapulmonary manifestations, but the eye is not commonly involved. Miliary tuberculosis infection can affect the eye and cause chorioretinitis, uveitis, and conjunctivitis, but these manifestations are rare. Color blindness would not be associated with such an infection.

22. **The correct answer is C.** Rimantadine, amantadine, oseltamivir, and zanamivir are the four drugs most commonly used to treat influenza virus infection. They have been proven to reduce the duration of symptoms by 1–1.5 days if given within 48 hours of onset of symptoms. The disease presents with the symptoms outlined in the stem and can be very severe if the patient is young, old, or immunocompromised.

Answer A is incorrect. The duration of all of his symptoms will be reduced by 1–1.5 days.

Answer B is incorrect. No future immune protection is conferred by the use of antiviral treatment.

Answer D is incorrect. The duration of symptoms will be reduced by 1–1.5 days, not reduced by half.

Answer E is incorrect. The severity of flu symptoms is reduced with use of rimantadine, amantadine, oseltamivir, and zanamivir therapies.

23. **The correct answer is E.** Surfactant decreases surface tension, preventing small alveoli from collapsing and thus increasing compliance.

Answer A is incorrect. Compliance in small alveoli is decreased relative to large alveoli, because smaller alveoli are more likely to collapse.

Answer B is incorrect. Large alveoli are less likely to collapse because they have increased radii.

Answer C is incorrect. Small alveoli without surfactant have the most chance of collapsing.

Answer D is incorrect. Small alveoli have smaller radii, causing an increased collapsing pressure, requiring increased pressure to keep them open.

24. **The correct answer is A.** High fever, dysphagia, drooling, inspiratory stridor, and respiratory distress are all consistent with the diagnosis of epiglottitis. The x-ray film shows thickening of the epiglottic (thumbprint sign) and aryepiglottic folds. The most common etiologic agent associated with epiglottitis is *Haemophilus influenzae*.

Answer B is incorrect. *Mycoplasma pneumoniae* causes atypical pneumonia that presents with cough and shortness of breath, and bilateral diffuse infiltrates are visible on an x-ray film. This patient's symptoms and x-ray findings are not consistent with this disease.

Answer C is incorrect. Parainfluenza virus is associated with croup. This disease can present with inspiratory stridor, seal-like barking cough, retractions, and coryza. The x-ray film shows a characteristic steeple sign and not the thumbprint sign.

Answer D is incorrect. Respiratory syncytial virus is an etiologic agent of bronchiolitis that is characterized by gradually developing respiratory distress and paroxysmal wheezing.

Answer E is incorrect. *Streptococcus pyogenes* (group A) can cause pharyngitis. Patients with this illness present with headache, abdominal pain, and vomiting. The patient's symptoms are not consistent with this diagnosis.

25. **The correct answer is B.** This boy suffers from asthma, which is characterized by airway hyperresponsiveness and airflow obstruction. This condition can be precipitated by several factors, including allergens, upper respiratory infections, drugs, and stress. Clinically, asthmatics experience episodes of wheezing, coughing, and dyspnea. Sputum samples may demonstrate Curschmann's spirals and Charcot-Leyden crystals. Blood tests will typically reveal eosinophilia. Other causes of eosinophilia include neoplasms, parasites, collagen vascular diseases, and allergic processes.

Answer A is incorrect. Asbestosis is characterized by diffuse interstitial fibrosis and an increased risk of mesothelioma and bronchogenic carcinoma. Intermittent obstructive episodes are not associated with asbestosis. Ferruginous bodies in the lungs are necessary for this diagnosis.

Answer C is incorrect. Coronavirus is an RNA virus that causes the common cold.

Answer D is incorrect. Croup is laryngotracheobronchitis due to infection with the RNA virus parainfluenza. Croup is characterized by a seal-like barking cough, not intermittent obstructive episodes.

Answer E is incorrect. Cystic fibrosis is an autosomal recessive disease resulting from ineffective chloride transport due to a defective *CFTR* gene. This condition is characterized by pulmonary infections, chronic bronchitis, and pancreatic insufficiency. High concentrations of chloride in a sweat test would confirm this diagnosis, not high levels of eosinophils.

26. **The correct answer is E.** The patient is suffering from syndrome of inappropriate antidiuretic hormone secretion (SIADH), a condition in which excessive ADH is secreted independent of serum osmolality; this can be seen in pulmonary diseases such as tuberculosis. SIADH is caused by central nervous system disturbances, such as strokes; certain drugs, such as cyclophosphamide; and ectopic secretion by certain carcinomas, such as small-cell lung carcinoma, as a part of a paraneoplastic syndrome. Excessive ADH secretion can lead to nausea, lethargy, seizures, and even coma. The patient's laboratory values are typical of someone with SIADH, showing hyponatremia,

serum hypo-osmolality, urine hyperosmolarity, and decreased hematocrit secondary to dilution.

Answer A is incorrect. In central diabetes insipidus, there is deficient secretion of ADH by the posterior pituitary, resulting in a clinical picture opposite from SIADH. Patients with central diabetes insipidus present with large quantities of dilute urine, serum hyperosmolality, and hypernatremia, and will report polydipsia and polyuria. Central diabetes insipidus can be caused by posterior pituitary tumors, meningitis, sarcoid and skull-based trauma or surgery, and can be corrected with administration of exogenous ADH.

Answer B is incorrect. Hyponatremia and glucose abnormalities can be found following epileptic seizures; however, the presence of serum hypoosmolality, urine hyperosmolality, and decreased hematocrit secondary to dilution would be unlikely if epilepsy were the diagnosis.

Answer C is incorrect. The signs and symptoms of nephrogenic diabetes insipidus (DI) are similar to those of central DI; however, unlike central DI, nephrogenic DI cannot be corrected with exogenous ADH because it results from ADH receptor dysfunction at the kidneys. Nephrogenic DI is a potential adverse effect of demeclocycline and lithium.

Answer D is incorrect. Although patients with psychogenic polydipsia drink excessive amounts of fluid and may present with decreased serum osmolality, they will have appropriate ADH suppression and will thus have a large volume of hypotonic, not hypertonic urine, as seen in this patient.

27. **The correct answer is E.** Lung volume increases during inspiration, increasing the elastic recoil strength of the lungs. Thus, intrapleural pressure becomes more negative than at rest.

Answer A is incorrect. Inspiration under normal conditions is active, while expiration is usually passive. Air moves with the pressure gradient.

Answer B is incorrect. During inspiration, alveolar pressure decreases to less than atmospheric pressure, allowing air to enter the alveoli.

Answer C is incorrect. At peak inspiration, the lung volume is functional residual capacity plus one tidal volume, as air is brought into the lung.

Answer D is incorrect. Inspiratory muscles contract during inspiration, causing an increase in the volume of the thorax.

Answer F is incorrect. The diaphragm is the most important inspiratory muscle. During inspiration it contracts, pushing abdominal contents downward and ribs upward and outward. This expands the thoracic cavity.

28. **The correct answer is A.** The description is a typical presentation and appearance of coccidioidomycosis, which is endemic to the southwestern United States. This infection causes disseminated disease in immunocompromised patients and forms spherules in tissue. Infection is caused by inhalation of spores of the fungus, *Coccidioides immitis*. Dipicolinic acid is a key component of fungal spores, which provide the fungus with resistance to dehydration, heat, and chemicals.

Answer B is incorrect. Hemagglutinin is an influenza virus antigen.

Answer C is incorrect. Lipopolysaccharide is an antigen located in the cell wall of most gram-negative bacteria.

Answer D is incorrect. Encapsulated bacteria and yeast have capsules made of polysaccharide; one exception is *Bacillus anthracis*, whose capsule contains D-glutamate.

Answer E is incorrect. Teichoic acid is a bacterial surface antigen that induces tumor necrosis factor-α and interleukin-1.

29. **The correct answer is B.** Asbestosis is caused by inhalation of asbestos fibers and histologically is marked by ferruginous bodies.

Answer A is incorrect. Asbestos is not related to an autoimmune phenomenon.

HIGH-YIELD SYSTEMS

Respiratory

Answer C is incorrect. The cause of asbestos is the inhalation of asbestos fibers into the lungs.

Answer D is incorrect. Living in a city for years causes anthracosis, which causes no harm.

Answer E is incorrect. Ferruginous bodies and ivory-white pleural plaques are not long-term sequelae of steroid abuse.

Answer F is incorrect. Tuberculosis has a Ghon's complex in the primary infection and cavitary lesions are present in the secondary re-activation.

Answer G is incorrect. Working in a coal mine can cause "coal workers' pneumoconio-sis" or silicosis.

30. **The correct answer is D.** This man is likely suffering from obstructive sleep apnea (OSA) secondary to extreme obesity (pickwickian syn-drome). During the night he has intermittent cessation of airflow at the nose and mouth. During this progressive asphyxia, he has a brief arousal, restores airway patency, and returns to sleep. This patient's obesity and elongated uvula are very good indicators of OSA, as are his daytime sleepiness, inability to concentrate, and hypertension. Periodic, recurrent asphyxia has the effect of causing a respiratory acidosis that, when present chronically, is compensated for by renal retention of HCO_3^-.

Answer A is incorrect. If anything, this pa-tient's glucose is likely elevated.

Answer B is incorrect. This patient likely has a decreased HDL level.

Answer C is incorrect. Increased reabsorption of H^+ would worsen acidosis.

Answer E is incorrect. Renal secretion of HCO_3^- would worsen acidosis.

31. **The correct answer is A.** *Actinomyces israeli* is a microaerophilic organism that causes oral and facial abscesses, with characteristic "sulfur granules" that may drain through sinus tracts in skin.

Answer B is incorrect. *Actinomyces*'s long branched filaments can resemble fungi, such as *Candida albicans*. The oral lesions caused by *Candida*, known as thrush, usually occur on the mucous membranes such as the throat and tongue in immunocompromised patients and appear white. It would be an unlikely cause of an oral abscess in a patient with a healthy immune system.

Answer C is incorrect. *Clostridium perfrin-gens* is also a gram-positive anaerobic rod; how-ever, it typically causes food poisoning from meat dishes or myonecrosis (gas gangrene), not dental abscesses.

Answer D is incorrect. Like *Actinomyces*, *No-cardia* is also an obligate anaerobe that is part of the normal gastrointestinal flora, but causes pulmonary infections in immunocompromised patients.

Answer E is incorrect. *Staphylococcus epider-midis* is a gram-positive clustering coccus, not a rod. It is part of the normal skin flora and usually pathologic only in immunocompro-mised patients.

32. **The correct answer is D.** Peripheral, not cen-tral, chemoreceptors stimulate breathing in re-sponse to O_2 levels that are below 60 mm Hg.

Answer A is incorrect. Aortic and carotid bod-ies are not central chemoreceptors. They are the peripheral chemoreceptors that are able to respond to decreased partial oxygen pressure levels in the arterial blood.

Answer B is incorrect. Central chemorecep-tors do affect breathing with varying levels of H^+ in the blood, but it is indirect. The H^+ in blood cannot cross the blood-brain barrier. Thus, CO_2 in the blood crosses the cere-brospinal fluid and combines with H_2O to form H^+ and HCO_3^-. The resulting H^+ acts di-rectly on the receptors.

Answer C is incorrect. Central control is lo-cated in the brainstem and cerebral cortex. Particularly important are the medullary respi-ratory center located in the reticular forma-tion, the apneustic center in the lower pons, the pneumotaxic center in the upper pons, and the cerebral cortex.

Answer E is incorrect. Stretch, irritant, and J receptors all function within the lung to regulate breathing. Stretch receptors are located in the smooth muscle, irritant receptors are located in the airway epithelial cells, and the J (juxtacapillary) receptors are located in the alveolar walls close to the capillaries.

33. **The correct answer is B.** The patient's presentation is most consistent with an atypical pneumonia likely caused by *Mycoplasma pneumoniae*. Macrolide antibiotics such as azithromycin are effective in treating this disease. Mycoplasma is not sensitive to cephalosporins, which are used to treat pneumococcal pneumonia.

    Answer A is incorrect. Mycoplasma is not sensitive to ampicillin. Some cases of pneumococcal pneumonia are sensitive to and can be treated effectively with ampicillin.

    Answer C is incorrect. Cefotaxime is a cephalosporin that can be used to treat pneumococcal pneumonia, but will be ineffective against *Mycoplasma*. Given the lack of response of the patient to ceftriaxone, cefotaxime is not an appropriate choice.

    Answer D is incorrect. Clindamycin is used in the treatment of anaerobic bacterial infections, not mycoplasma infections.

    Answer E is incorrect. Mycoplasma is not sensitive to penicillins. Some cases of pneumococcal pneumonia are sensitive to penicillin and can be treated effectively with this drug.

34. **The correct answer is G.** Patients with pneumothorax typically present this way. In this case, an apparent mass at the left hilum completely collapsed the left lung.

    Answer A is incorrect. Asbestosis presents with dyspnea and is associated with a history of exposure to asbestos, persistent bibasilar crackles, reduced lung volumes, and fibrosis on the radiograph.

    Answer B is incorrect. Asthma is characterized by hyperreactivity of the airways and ob-

struction, and not with the symptoms in the stem of this question.

Answer C is incorrect. Bronchiectasis is dilation of the bronchial tree. It does not present with tracheal shift or pleuritic chest pain.

Answer D is incorrect. Bronchitis presents with productive cough and an increased Reid index, not with pleuritic chest pain and tracheal deviation.

Answer E is incorrect. Emphysema typically is found in an older smoker who is barrel-chested. Also, there is no tracheal deviation.

Answer F is incorrect. Oat cell carcinoma would present in an older person with cough, hemoptysis, and possibly with a paraneoplastic endocrine syndrome.

35. **The correct answer is D.** Diffuse, patchy infiltrate is consistent with *Pneumocystis jiroveci* (formerly *carinii*) pneumonia, which is confirmed by methenamine silver stain of lavage or biopsy sample. The first-line treatment of this condition is trimethoprim-sulfamethoxazole for patients with no contraindications to sulfa drugs. In the case of a patient with a sulfa allergy, the first-line treatment is pentamidine.

    Answer A is incorrect. Ivermectin is used to treat onchocerciasis (river blindness). It is thought to block the release of microfilariae from gravid female worms. One dose reduces microfilarial counts by up to 95%.

    Answer B is incorrect. Metronidazole is used to treat a wide variety of anaerobic bacterial infections. It is also effective against parasitic infections such as *Giardia lamblia*, *Entamoeba histolytica*, *Gardnerella vaginalis*, and *Trichomonas vaginalis*.

    Answer C is incorrect. Penicillin is used to treat a variety of bacterial infections but is not effective in the treatment of *Pneumocystis jiroveci* (formerly *carinii*) pneumonia.

    Answer E is incorrect. Protamine is used to treat heparin overdose. It binds to heparin to form a stable complex that has no anticoagulant activity. Used alone, protamine has anticoagulant properties.

36. **The correct answer is C.** The patient's presentation is consistent with syndrome of inappropriate ADH secretion (low serum osmolality and Na^+, with high urine osmolarity), which can be caused by the secretion of ADH from small-cell carcinomas of the lung. This type of carcinoma is clearly associated with cigarette smoking.

    Answer A is incorrect. Brain cancer could cause the altered mental status, but would not be associated with the observed electrolyte abnormalities.

    Answer B is incorrect. Pneumonia would not cause the electrolyte abnormality noted in this patient.

    Answer D is incorrect. Squamous cell carcinoma is associated with the secretion of parathyroid hormone and causes hypercalcemia.

    Answer E is incorrect. Tuberculosis would not cause the electrolyte abnormality seen in this patient.

37. **The correct answer is C.** *Legionella pneumophila* is a gram-negative rod that causes Legionnaires' disease, a condition in which patients develop a severe pneumonia and a high fever. Other signs and symptoms include hyponatremia and central nervous system changes. The organism is present only in water sources (e.g., air-conditioning systems, whirlpools, mist sprayers) and can cause infection when aerosolized water droplets are inhaled. The organism is not transmitted by person-to-person contact.

    Answer A is incorrect. *Bordetella pertussis* is a gram-negative rod, but it causes an upper respiratory infection or whooping cough. It is transmitted by person-to-person contact, not through infected water sources.

    Answer B is incorrect. *Haemophilus influenzae* type B is a gram-negative rod, but it is more likely to be associated with acute epiglottitis or meningitis. The Hib vaccine has rendered these infections far less common.

    Answer D is incorrect. *Mycobacterium tuberculosis* is an acid-fast mycobacterium that causes tuberculosis. It would not present this

acutely, and the organism is not transmitted via water sources.

Answer E is incorrect. *Streptococcus pneumoniae* is a significant cause of bacterial pneumonia, but it is a gram-positive rod. It is transmitted by person-to-person contact.

38. **The correct answer is C.** Bronchiectasis can be caused by a chronic necrotizing infection of the bronchi leading to dilated airways.

    Answer A is incorrect. Asthma is a condition associated with airway constriction, marked by wheezing.

    Answer B is incorrect. Atelectasis is alveolar collapse, not associated with airway dilation.

    Answer D is incorrect. Idiopathic pulmonary fibrosis causes restrictive lung disease and does not involve the major airways.

    Answer E is incorrect. Neonatal respiratory distress syndrome is related to surfactant deficiency, causing alveolar collapse. Dilated airways are not a feature of the syndrome.

39. **The correct answer is C.** This patient has been receiving an opioid analgesic and has overdosed. Morphine use can lead to constipation, the cause of the patient's distention, and overdose can present with coma, miosis, and respiratory depression. Both naloxone and naltrexone competitively inhibit opioids at the opioid receptor, reversing their effects.

    Answer A is incorrect. Aminocaproic acid is used to treat overdose of thrombolytics.

    Answer B is incorrect. Flumazenil is used to treat overdose of benzodiazepines.

    Answer D is incorrect. Physostigmine is used to treat overdose of anticholinergics.

    Answer E is incorrect. Protamine is used to treat overdose of heparin.

40. **The correct answer is D.** The ultrasound reveals a congenital diaphragmatic hernia (CDH) in the fetus. The diaphragm is derived from four embryological structures: the septum transversum, the pleuroperitoneal folds, the dorsal mesentery of the esophagus, and a muscular

outgrowth of the lateral body wall. The pleuroperitoneal folds form a large portion of the fetal diaphragm; if they fail to form completely, the thorax and the abdomen are incompletely separated posterolaterally and the abdominal contents often herniate into the thorax. Pressure from abdominal organs results in lung hypoplasia, which in turn can lead to polyhydramnios. Typical newborns with CDH have a flat stomach and a heart displaced to the right.

Answer A is incorrect. The dorsal mesentery of the esophagus forms the central part of the fetal diaphragm. Post-embryonically, this structure becomes the crura of the diaphragm. It is not normally defective in congenital diaphragmatic hernia.

Answer B is incorrect. Although the foregut is displaced from the abdomen into the thorax in the presence of a congenital diaphragmatic hernia, its formation is normal.

Answer C is incorrect. Muscular outgrowths of the lateral body wall form the lateral edge of the diaphragm, bordering the left and right costodiaphragmatic recesses. These structures are not commonly defective in congenital diaphragmatic hernia.

Answer E is incorrect. The septum transversum grows out from the ventrolateral body wall and separates the heart from the liver in the embryo. Ultimately, it gives rise to the central tendon of the diaphragm. However, defects in the septum transversum are rarely the cause of congenital diaphragmatic hernia.

41. **The correct answer is A.** Choice A represents the residual volume, which is the volume that remains in the lungs after a maximal expiration.

Answer B is incorrect. Choice B represents the total volume, which is the volume inspired or expired with each normal breath.

Answer C is incorrect. Choice C represents the inspiratory reserve volume, which is the volume that can be inspired over and above the tidal volume.

Answer D is incorrect. Choice D represents the expiratory reserve volume, which is the volume that can be expired after the expiration of the tidal volume.

Answer E is incorrect. Choice E represents the functional reserve capacity. It is the sum of expiratory residual volume and residual volume, and is the volume that remains in the lungs after a tidal volume is expired.

Answer F is incorrect. Choice F represents the inspiratory capacity, which is the sum of tidal volume and inspiratory reserve volume.

Answer G is incorrect. Choice G represents vital capacity, which is the sum of tidal volume, inspiratory reserve volume, and expiratory reserve volume. Vital capacity (also called forced vital capacity) is the volume of air that can be forcibly expired after a maximal inspiration.

42. **The correct answer is B.** Hyaline membrane disease (neonatal respiratory distress syndrome) is the most common cause of death in premature infants. It is associated with prematurity, maternal diabetes mellitus, and cesarean section delivery.

Answer A is incorrect. Diffuse alveolar damage is caused by a wide variety of mechanisms and toxic agents. The formation of intra-alveolar hyaline membranes leads to impaired gas exchange.

Answer C is incorrect. Hypersensitivity pneumonitis is an immunologically-induced non–IgE-mediated inflammatory lung disease resulting from the sensitization and subsequent recurrent exposure to any of a wide variety of inhaled organic dusts.

Answer D is incorrect. Intra-alveolar exudative consolidation is typically seen in lobar pneumonia caused most frequently by *Streptococcus pneumoniae* (pneumococcus).

Answer E is incorrect. Localized proliferation of histiocytes is characteristic of eosinophilic granuloma, which has associated Birbeck's granules.

Answer F is incorrect. Multiple noncaseating granulomas are seen in sarcoidosis, a disease of unknown etiology (i.e., it is not caused by early delivery) that affects multiple organ systems.

Answer G is incorrect. Panacinar emphysema is caused by α_1-antitrypsin deficiency, which is a genetically inherited condition affecting the lungs and liver.

43. **The correct answer is D.** The medical student should be very familiar with both the anatomy and the physiology of the sucking chest wound, as described in this patient. A penetrating wound to the chest can puncture the pleura, making an opening for air to be sucked into the pleural space. With inspiration, the diaphragm descends, lowering the intrapleural pressure. If there is a communication directly between the pleural space and the outside world, air is sucked into this negative pressure space and collapses the lung. Air in the pleural space is known as a pneumothorax and is seen on chest x-ray as a collapsed lung.

Answer A is incorrect. It is possible to have a hemopneumothorax, but this vignette describes a pneumothorax injury. You may also see blood in the dependent portions of the thorax, but a hemothorax may not be present in this case, while a pneumothorax definitely will be present.

Answer B is incorrect. There may be rib fractures on chest x-ray, but the stab wound is above the nipple, which is about the level of the fourth and fifth ribs, superior to the ninth and tenth ribs.

Answer C is incorrect. A pleural effusion is seen on x-ray as a fluid collection in the dependent portions of the thorax. The injury above describes the chest wall around the wound moving with respirations. This is from air moving in and out of the pleural space. Fluid would fill the gravity-dependent portions of the lung and not move with respirations.

Answer E is incorrect. Right upper lobe consolidation would be consistent with right upper lobe pneumonia, which is not described in this vignette.

44. **The correct answer is B.** The patient described in the question stem has a case of typical pneumonia that is characterized by high-grade fever, productive cough, and acute onset. Common bacteria include *Streptococcus pneumoniae*, *Staphylococcus aureus*, and *Haemo-philus influenzae*, which could be covered with ceftriaxone.

Answer A is incorrect. Azithromycin is a macrolide antibiotic that has a mechanism and spectrum of activity similar to erythromycin but with less severe adverse effects. It should not be taken with milk or antacids because they can cause problems with absorption. It is commonly used in the empiric treatment of community-acquired pneumonia.

Answer C is incorrect. Doxycycline is a tetracycline analog that can be used in patients with renal failure. Its mechanism of action is binding to the 30S subunit and preventing attachment of aminoacyl-tRNAs. It can be used to treat causes of atypical pneumonia such as *Chlamydia* and *Mycoplasma* species infection. Side effects include gastrointestinal distress, photosensitivity, and rash.

Answer D is incorrect. Erythromycin is a macrolide antibiotic used to treat *Legionella*, *Chlamydia*, *Mycoplasma*, and *Neisseria* species infection. It is typically used to treat atypical pneumonias and upper respiratory infections. Erythromycin toxicity causes gastrointestinal discomfort, acute cholestatic hepatitis, eosinophilia, and skin rash.

Answer E is incorrect. Levofloxacin is a fluoroquinolone antibiotic used to treat infection with gram-negative rods and some gram-positive organisms. Fluoroquinolones such as levofloxacin are used to treat upper respiratory infections and urinary tract infections.

45. **The correct answer is B.** The patient is suffering from tuberculosis, and his treatment regimen will include isoniazid. One of the adverse effects of isoniazid therapy is peripheral neuropathy, which can be prevented by coadministration of vitamin B_6.

Answer A is incorrect. There is no role for the administration of vitamin B_1 in the treatment of tuberculosis. Vitamin B_1 is used to treat alcoholics to prevent Wernicke-Korsakoff syndrome.

Answer C is incorrect. There is no role for the administration of vitamin B$_{12}$ in the treatment of tuberculosis. Vitamin B$_{12}$ is used to treat patients with vitamin B$_{12}$ deficiency who are showing neurological symptoms and macrocytic anemia.

Answer D is incorrect. There is no role for the administration of vitamin C in the treatment of tuberculosis. Vitamin C is used to treat scurvy.

Answer E is incorrect. There is no role for the administration of vitamin E in the treatment of tuberculosis.

46. **The correct answer is A.** β-Agonists such as albuterol may cause potassium to shift into cells, resulting in hypokalemia. This may lead to ECG abnormalities due to destabilization of cardiac cell membranes, the classic examples of which are U waves. Short-acting β-agonists such as albuterol are used in the treatment of acute asthma exacerbations because of their relaxing effects on bronchial smooth muscle. Long-acting β-agonists such as salmeterol are used for prophylaxis of bronchospasm.

Answer B is incorrect. Ipratropium is used for both asthma and chronic obstructive pulmonary disease.

Answer C is incorrect. Prednisone, an oral steroid, is an excellent treatment for asthma, but it does not cause hypokalemia.

Answer D is incorrect. Theophylline may also cause cardiotoxicity but does not result in hypokalemia.

Answer E is incorrect. Zileuton is an asthma medication that blocks the production of leukotrienes.

47. **The correct answer is B.** This histology shows noncaseating granulomas, characteristic of sarcoidosis. Sarcoidosis is a multiorgan inflammatory disorder of unknown etiology. It is thought to be immune mediated and is characterized by noncaseating granulomas. The lung is the most frequently involved organ, but other commonly affected organs are lymph nodes, skin, eyes, kidneys, the heart, and the central nervous system. Findings that might be expected

in a patient with sarcoidosis would include **G**amma-globulinemia, **R**heumatoid arthritis, elevated **A**ngiotensin-converting enzyme levels, **I**nterstitial fibrosis, and **N**oncaseating granulomas (remember the mnemonic **GRAIN**).

Answer A is incorrect. Goodpasture's syndrome is caused by anti-basement membrane antibodies. It is not associated with noncaseating granulomas.

Answer C is incorrect. Small-cell lung cancer is not associated with granulomas and is recognized by numerous small blue neoplastic cells.

Answer D is incorrect. Systemic lupus erythematosus can be associated with pleuritis, but it is not associated with noncaseating granulomas.

Answer E is incorrect. Tuberculosis is characterized by caseating granulomas, which can be recognized by the necrotic, cheeselike center in the granuloma.

48. **The correct answer is A.** *Bacillus anthracis* can cause cutaneous anthrax, inhalation anthrax, and gastrointestinal anthrax. Bloody pleural effusions, hemorrhagic mediastinitis, dry cough, and substernal pressure are consistent with inhalation anthrax, also known as wool-sorter's disease.

Answer B is incorrect. *Legionella* is a cause of severe pneumonia, particularly in cigarette smokers and immunocompromised individuals. It is associated with environmental water sources. It does not cause mediastinitis or hemorrhagic pleural effusions.

Answer C is incorrect. *Mycoplasma pneumoniae* causes atypical pneumonia with cough, shortness of breath, and bilateral infiltrates that are visible on an x-ray film of the chest. The symptoms described in this patient are not consistent with this disease.

Answer D is incorrect. *Nocardia asteroides* is an acid-fast aerobe also found in soil. This organism causes pulmonary infections primarily in immunocompromised individuals.

Answer E is incorrect. *Streptococcus pneumoniae* causes typical pneumonia that is characterized by sudden onset of chills, fever, cough, and pleuritic pain. It is not associated with bloody pleural effusions or hemorrhagic mediastinitis.

49. **The correct answer is E.** In the tissues, more CO_2 is being produced and entering the RBCs. It is combined with H_2O by carbonic anhydrase to form H_2CO_3, which then becomes H^+ and HCO_3^-. The HCO_3^- leaves the RBCs while Cl^- enters.

Answer A is incorrect. Dissolved CO_2 that remains in the plasma accounts for about 5% of transport. In addition, bicarbonate does not bind to hemoglobin, H^+ does.

Answer B is incorrect. Bicarbonate travels in the plasma, not the RBCs. When it gets to the lung, it goes into the RBCs, gets transformed back to H_2O and CO_2, and the CO_2 is exhaled.

Answer C is incorrect. The primary transport of CO_2 in the blood is via HCO_3^- (90%). Carbaminohemoglobin only accounts for about 5%.

Answer D is incorrect. The lungs do not have an acidic environment, the peripheral tissues do. The oxygenation of hemoglobin in the lungs promotes the dissociation of CO_2 (the Haldane effect).

50. **The correct answer is D.** If one applies the equation $V_d = V_t \times ((\text{Pa}CO_2 - \text{Pe}CO_2)/\text{Pa}CO_2)$, where $\text{Pa}CO_2$ is partial carbon dioxide pressure and $\text{Pe}CO_2$ is partial expired carbon dioxide pressure, and plugs in the numbers given in the stem, the answer is 0.5 L.

Answer A is incorrect. See calculation.

Answer B is incorrect. See calculation.

Answer C is incorrect. See calculation.

Answer E is incorrect. See calculation.

Answer F is incorrect. See calculation.

Full-Length Examinations

Test Block 1

1. A new patient presents to a clinic in Denver, Colorado, with complaints of dyspnea and fatigue on exertion. On history, the patient informs the doctor that she just moved from the California coastline less than 1 week ago, and has been attempting to do her 3-mile run every morning. The patient is told to limit her running until her body adjusts to the new altitude. Which of the following will occur in this woman's body in response to the high altitude?

(A) An increased partial oxygen pressure at 50% saturation on the hemoglobin-O_2 curve
(B) Decreased pulmonary vascular resistance
(C) Decreased RBC 2,3-diphosphoglycerate concentration
(D) Increased arterial partial oxygen pressure
(E) Right ventricular atrophy

2. A 13-year-old girl suffers from seizures that last for approximately 10 seconds. During a seizure, she cannot respond to questions but has no loss of postural tone; afterward, she immediately returns to a normal level of consciousness. Which of the following results would you expect to find on an EEG obtained during this patient's seizures?

(A) Centrotemporal spike pattern
(B) Diffuse slowing with generalized spike-and-wave complexes
(C) Polyspike or slow spike-and-wave complexes
(D) Posterior asymmetric slowing of background
(E) Regular and symmetric bursts of 3-Hz spike-and-wave complexes

3. A 35-year-old man with no significant past medical history presents to his primary care physician complaining of shortness of breath on exertion. The patient acknowledges recent heart palpitations, but denies chest pain, cough, lower extremity edema, paroxysmal nocturnal dyspnea, or weakness. He further denies any recent illness, and he states that he does not smoke. Cardiac examination shows an irregularly irregular rhythm, a widely split fixed S_2, and a systolic ejection murmur over the left upper sternal border. The patient's ECG is shown. Based on these findings, the physician concludes that these symptoms are due to pathology of which of the following fetal structures?

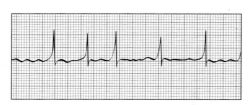

Reproduced, with permission, from USMLERx.com.

(A) Aorticopulmonary septum
(B) Ductus arteriosus
(C) Ductus venosus
(D) Foramen ovale
(E) Interventricular septum

4. A 10-year-old boy is referred to the neurologist with intellectual deterioration, personality changes, generalized seizures, and visual disturbances that have worsened over the last few months. The patient's cerebrospinal fluid culture shows no bacterial growth. Further analysis shows normal glucose levels and normal protein. The patient is afebrile and reports no headache. The child's parents say that he has not received any vaccinations since arriving in the United States last year. They also say that he has had only one major illness prior to this. The child was approximately 2 years old when he developed a high fever, cough, and runny nose. Soon after the onset of these symptoms, he developed a red maculopapular rash that spread downward from his head. Antibodies against which of the following are likely to be found in this patient's cerebrospinal fluid?

(A) Herpes simplex virus type 2
(B) Measles virus
(C) Mumps virus
(D) *Neisseria meningitidis*
(E) *Treponema pallidum*

5. A 34-year-old man comes to the clinic because his gums have become swollen and have exhibited a tendency to bleed. He states that he has been brushing his teeth at least twice a day. On examination, he is found to have several bruises on his legs in different stages of healing. The patient adds that his bruises have been taking longer than usual to heal. His complete blood cell count and coagulation panel are within normal limits. What is the likely cause of this patient's symptoms?

(A) Decreased platelet count
(B) Defect in hydroxylation of collagen residues
(C) Decreased von Willebrand factor
(D) Mutation of dystrophin gene
(E) Mutation of spectrin

6. A 21-year-old woman with no family or personal history of breast cancer presents with a small, firm mass in the lower inner quadrant of her right breast that seems mobile when palpated. It is nontender. There are no overlying skin changes or nipple discharge. Which of the following would most likely be found on biopsy of this mass?

(A) Blue dome cysts and some atypical epithelial hyperplasia
(B) Cells in a single-file formation
(C) Fibrosing stroma around normal-looking glands
(D) Large cells with clear "halos"
(E) Multicentric lobes with lymphocytic infiltrate

7. A 50-year-old woman who works as a secretary comes to the physician because of numbness and tingling in her hands. On examination, the patient is found to have decreased sensation in all of her fingers except her fifth digit. Which of the following muscles is most commonly weakened in patients with this condition?

(A) Adductor pollicis
(B) Dorsal interossei
(C) Lumbricals (3 and 4)
(D) Opponens digiti minimi
(E) Opponens pollicis

8. A 19-year-old man presents to the emergency department complaining of fatigue, lethargy, and a history of a recent upper respiratory infection. His temperature is 37° C (98.6° F) and his physical examination shows jaundice and prominent splenomegaly. Blood counts show low hemoglobin (9 g/dL), elevated mean cell hemoglobin concentration, and increased reticulocyte count. A peripheral blood smear for this patient is shown. Which of the following treatments is most appropriate in severe cases of this disease?

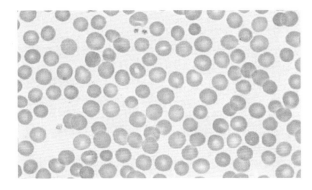

Reproduced, with permission, from Lichtman MA, Beutler E, Kipps TJ, Seligsohn U, Kaushansky K, Prchal JF. *Williams Hematology*, 7th ed. New York, McGraw-Hill, 2006: Color Plate III-7.

(A) Blood transfusion
(B) Chemotherapy
(C) Folic acid supplementation
(D) Iron chelation therapy
(E) Iron supplementation
(F) Splenectomy

9. A 33-year-old man patient presents with a headache. His symptoms are consistent with tension headaches that he has had sporadically in the past, which were alleviated with ibuprofen. He read on the Internet that severe headaches can be a sign of subarachnoid hemorrhage and feels that this may be "the worst headache of his life." He rates it as a 9 out of 10, with 10 being the worst pain he has ever experienced. The physician is ready to send him home, but the patient would like a CT scan of his head. What is the appropriate next step?

(A) Avoid his concern and send him home
(B) Call in a neurology consult
(C) Discuss why he would like the CT scan
(D) Send him for a CT scan
(E) Send him for a less costly x-ray film of the head
(F) Tell him ibuprofen will cure subarachnoid hemorrhage

10. A 34-year-old man presents to the emergency department complaining of a 2-day history of fatigue and double vision. Physical examination shows a right nystagmus. A detailed history reveals that he recently began treatment for recurrent tonic-clonic seizures. Routine laboratory studies show the following results:

Na^+: 143 mEq/L
K^+: 4.5 mEq/L
Cl^-: 103 mEq/L
HCO_3^-: 26 mEq/L
Blood urea nitrogen: 45 mg/dL
Creatinine: 4.3 mg/dL

Which of the following agents is most likely responsible for this patient's condition?

(A) Acetaminophen
(B) Clozapine
(C) Imipramine
(D) Lithium
(E) Phenytoin
(F) Sumatriptan

11. A 4-year-old boy has a sublingual mass. A scan using ^{99m}Tc pertechnetate, which behaves as iodine and approximates iodine uptake, shows significant uptake in this region with little activity lower in the neck. Which of the following is the embryologic explanation for this mass?

(A) The third and fourth branchial (pharyngeal) arches have hypertrophied
(B) The thymus has developed ectopically
(C) The thyroid has failed to migrate caudally
(D) The thymus has hypertrophied
(E) The thyroid has migrated too far rostrally

12. A 27-year-old healthy man presents because he and his wife have been repeatedly unsuccessful getting pregnant. The wife has been tested and determined to be fertile. On history, the patient denies coronary or lipid abnormalities but admits to having multiple sinus infections and a chronic productive cough. On physical examination, the apical impulse is felt on the right fifth intercostal space and the liver is palpated on the left side. The prostate is not enlarged on examination. Which of the following is the most likely etiology for the patient's infertility?

(A) Age-related increase in estradiol with possible prostate dihydrotestosterone sensitization
(B) Autosomal recessive dysfunction of a chloride ion channel
(C) Failure of testicles to descend into the scrotum
(D) Familial disease causing early atherosclerosis leading to erectile dysfunction
(E) Lack of dynein ATPase arms in microtubules of cilia

13. An anxious young woman presents to the emergency department with an acute onset of severe abdominal pain. She states that she "partied a little bit last night" and consumed approximately 8 or 9 alcoholic drinks. Her stool is guaiac-negative, but she has periumbilical tenderness to palpation. An arterial blood gas study shows that her pH is 7.5 and her HCO_3^- is 19 mEq/L, with a P_{CO_2} of 25 mm Hg. Her serum shows normal NaCl levels. Which of the following is the origin of her acid-base disturbance?

(A) A buildup of unmeasured anions due to hepatic metabolism of alcohol
(B) Chronic diuretic use
(C) Hyperventilation secondary to pain
(D) Hypoventilation due to the respiratory depression caused by alcohol ingestion
(E) Vomiting

14. A 38-year-old white woman presents to the physician with a 2-week history of aching pain in her left calf that is made worse by dorsiflexion of her foot. On physical examination, her left calf is found to be erythematous, warm, and swollen. Which of the following measures should she take to decrease similar problems in the future?

(A) Begin taking a bile acid resin
(B) Begin taking a statin
(C) Begin taking low-dose oral contraceptives
(D) Exercise 30 minutes three times per week
(E) Quit smoking
(F) Reduce alcohol consumption to one or two glasses of red wine per week

15. An 18-year-old woman presents to her physician's office with jaundice after recently beginning birth control medication. She denies drug use and reports consistent condom use. On physical examination, the patient shows no hepatomegaly or right upper quadrant tenderness. Laboratory studies show a total bilirubin level of 4 mg/dL, a direct bilirubin level of 1 mg/dL, and an indirect bilirubin level of 3 mg/dL. Which of the following is the most likely diagnosis?

(A) Crigler-Najjar syndrome type I
(B) Dubin-Johnson syndrome
(C) Gilbert's disease
(D) Hepatitis C
(E) Oral contraceptive–associated cholestasis

16. A 44-year-old man is brought to the emergency department after he became combative and was screaming that "the little people" were after him. The emergency department staff is unable to obtain a history or physical examination because of his agitation, although the triage nurse is able to obtain his vital signs, which are significant for a temperature of 40° C (104° F) and a blood pressure of 90/50 mm Hg. His family reports that he was fine earlier in the day and that he has never had any psychiatric issues before. By the time the psychiatrist arrives, the patient is somnolent and somewhat confused. Which of the following is this patient's most likely diagnosis?

(A) Brief psychosis
(B) Delirium
(C) Delusion
(D) Mania
(E) Schizophrenia

17. A 34-year-old woman who is at 26 weeks of gestation and who has a history of multiple spontaneous abortions presents with severe abdominal pain, jaundice, ascites, and mental status change. Ultrasonography reveals an obscure hepatic venous connection to the inferior vena cava and absence of any waveform in the hepatic veins. She has a positive serum antiphospholipid antibody titer with a history of childhood seizures. Which of the following is this patient's most likely diagnosis?

(A) Budd-Chiari syndrome
(B) Congestive heart failure
(C) Polymyalgia rheumatica
(D) Portal vein thrombosis
(E) Veno-occlusive disease

18. A 5-year-old girl is brought to the pediatrician by her mother for evaluation of readiness to enter school. The mother is worried because the child had to be withdrawn from preschool last year because of an inability to cope with the other children. She reports that the child becomes very upset if her daily routine is interrupted. The child's birth history and past medical history are unremarkable. She reached all of her neurodevelopmental milestones on schedule. Which of the following is the most likely diagnosis in this child?

(A) Autistic disorder
(B) Asperger's syndrome
(C) Childhood disintegrative disorder
(D) Expressive language disorder
(E) Rett's disorder

19. A 4-year-old boy with a history of mental retardation and seizures is brought to the physician with a 3-month history of worsening shortness of breath. During physical examination, the physician notices numerous acnelike papules on the patient's face. Echocardiography shows significant left ventricular outflow obstruction. Which of the following is the most likely diagnosis for this patient's heart condition?

(A) Coronary artery disease
(B) Dilated cardiomyopathy
(C) Myxoma
(D) Rhabdomyoma
(E) Transposition of the great vessels

20. The association between autoimmune diseases and the expression of certain cytokines has prompted several advances in pharmacotherapy. Which of the following is an accurate statement regarding drug therapy, cytokines, and autoimmune disease?

(A) Adalimumab, a synthetic TNF-α analog, is not indicated for rheumatoid arthritis, a disease associated with an overexpression of TNF-α
(B) Anakinra, a synthetic interleukin-1-receptor antagonist, is not indicated for rheumatoid arthritis, a disease associated with an overexpression of endogenous interleukin-1-receptor antagonist
(C) Etanercept, a fusion protein of a TNF-α receptor and IgG₁, is indicated for rheumatoid arthritis, a disease associated with an overexpression of TNF-α
(D) Infliximab, a monoclonal antibody against TNF-α, is indicated for systemic lupus erythematosus, a disease associated with an underexpression of TNF-α
(E) Infliximab, a synthetic TNF-α analog, is not indicated for rheumatoid arthritis, a disease associated with an overexpression of TNF-α

21. A 45-year-old man visited his primary care physician 1 month ago because of chest pain that he had experienced four times in the past 4 months. The onset of the pain is sudden and radiates to his left jaw. He usually feels the pain when he is sitting in front of the television but has never felt it during exertion. During last month's visit, the physician prescribed sublingual nitroglycerin, and the patient reports that this has shortened the duration of his episodes. Last month's ECG is shown. Which of the following is the most likely cause of this patient's chest pain?

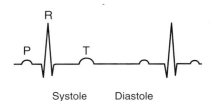

Systole   Diastole

Reproduced, with permission, from USMLERx.com.

(A) Myocardial infarction
(B) Pericarditis
(C) Prinzmetal's angina
(D) Stable angina
(E) Unstable angina

22. A clinical study at a research facility based in Utah is performed with young male subjects who have deafness, ocular abnormalities, and a nephritic syndrome. Kidney biopsies of these subjects show no pathology under immunofluorescence or light microscopy. Which of the following is the most common pathological characteristic likely to be seen under electron microscopy?

(A) Diffuse epithelial foot process fusion
(B) Immune complex deposits
(C) Split basement membrane
(D) Subendothelial spike and dome pattern
(E) Wire-loop appearance

23. A researcher is designing an in vitro experimental system to study the kinetics of GLUT4-mediated glucose transport into mammalian cells. The system will measure radiolabeled glucose concentrations in cell culture media both before and at intervals following the addition of insulin. Which of the following cell types is the best choice for use in this experimental system?

(A) Adipocytes
(B) Cortical neurons
(C) Erythrocytes
(D) Hepatocytes
(E) Pancreatic β cells

24. Myasthenia gravis is a disorder that affects nearly 3 in 100,000 people, with a 3:2 female-to-male predominance. Affected people classically present with complaints of muscle weakness and fatigue secondary to the formation of autoantibodies to the acetylcholine receptors at the neuromuscular junctions, with subsequent loss of the receptors. The most accurate method of diagnosis involves the detection of autoantibodies against the acetylcholine receptor. This test possesses an approximately 80% sensitivity and 90% specificity. If an individual has a positive test for autoantibodies against the acetylcholine receptor, what is the approximate posttest probability of having this disease, assuming a pretest probability of disease contraction of 50%?

(A) 75%
(B) 80%
(C) 85%
(D) 90%
(E) 95%
(F) 99%

[handwritten: 80% sens   20% not picked up]
[handwritten: 90% spec.   10% false pos]

25. An 85-year-old man is rushed to the emergency department from his primary care physician's office after his physician palpates a pulsating mass in his abdomen. The patient is diagnosed with an abdominal aortic aneurysm. Instead of repairing the aneurysm by surgically opening the abdomen, the surgeon decides to perform endovascular stenting and grafting. The stent is inserted into the femoral artery and threaded up toward the aortic defect. To access the femoral artery the surgeon must open the femoral sheath and expose its contents. Which of the following structures is enclosed inside the femoral sheath?

(A) Cooper's ligament
(B) Femoral canal
(C) Femoral nerve
(D) Obturator nerve
(E) Tunica vaginalis

26. A 6-year-old girl is found to be nearsighted during a vision screening at school, and the school nurse tells the parents the child should be fitted for corrective lenses. Her mother is upset because her daughter is already much taller than her classmates, has an awkward gait, and was recently diagnosed with scoliosis. She is afraid that the glasses will only add to her daughter's problems at school, where her classmates frequently tease her. When the ophthalmologist observes that the patient's right lens is dislocated, he suspects that her symptoms are in fact related to an enzyme deficiency. As a result of this deficiency, which of the following amino acids is essential in this patient's diet?

(A) Cysteine
(B) Lysine
(C) Methionine
(D) Tryptophan
(E) Tyrosine

27. A 57-year-old man presents to his primary care physician with complaints of fatigue and nausea over the past month. On physical examination, the patient is found to have a low-grade fever, scattered lymphadenopathy including two firm 2-cm lymph nodes in the left axilla, and an enlarged spleen. Biopsy of the lymph nodes yields a diagnosis of diffuse large cell lymphoma. Upon consultation with an oncologist, the patient begins a multidrug regimen that includes cyclophosphamide. Although generally safe, cyclophosphamide treatment can produce severe adverse effects in some patients. Which of the following drug-symptom combinations correctly states the treatment strategy for a common adverse event associated with this medication?

(A) Acrolein for hemorrhagic cystitis
(B) Acrolein for myelosuppression
(C) Acrolein for nausea and vomiting
(D) N-acetylcysteine for hemorrhagic cystitis
(E) N-acetylcysteine for myelosuppression
(F) N-acetylcysteine for nausea and vomiting

28. An obese 46-year-old, multiparous woman presents to the physician with nonradiating right upper quadrant pain and fever that was preceded by nausea and vomiting. Ultrasonography shows hyperechogenic structures in the right upper quadrant. Laboratory testing reveals a WBC count of 14,500/mm³, an erythrocyte sedimentation rate of 40 mm/hr, and a serum amylase level of 70 U/L. Which of the following is the most likely diagnosis in this patient?

(A) Acute acalculous cholecystitis
(B) Acute calculous cholecystitis
(C) Acute pancreatitis
(D) Carcinoma of the pancreas
(E) Cholesterolosis

29. A 60-year-old woman with a history of chronic renal insufficiency presents with pruritus, diffuse bone pain, and proximal muscle weakness. Laboratory studies show a serum Ca^{2+} level of 6.5 mg/dL, a serum phosphate level of 6.0 mg/dL, a serum creatinine level of 4.5 mg/dL, and an intact parathyroid hormone level of 300 pg/mL. The laboratory findings in this patient are most likely due to which of the following conditions?

(A) Parathyroid adenoma
(B) Parathyroid insufficiency
(C) Renal failure
(D) Underlying malignancy
(E) Vitamin D intoxication

30. A 73-year-old man who has atrial fibrillation has been treated pharmacologically for 10 years. He presents to his primary care physician complaining of generalized dyspnea. Pulmonary function tests show forced expiratory volume in 1 second (FEV_1) and forced vital capacity (FVC) are both less than 70% of the predicted value, with a ratio of FEV_1 to FVC of 81%. The flow-volume curve is shown. Which of the following is a possible etiology of this presentation?

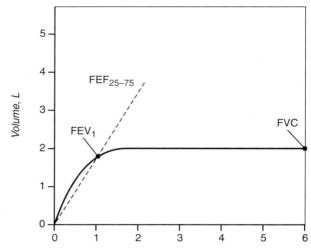

Reproduced, with permission, from USMLERx.com.

(A) Adult-onset asthma
(B) Amiodarone
(C) Diltiazem
(D) Sotalol
(E) Tobacco

31. A 23-year-old man comes to the emergency department complaining of bloody diarrhea and a fever. Laboratory tests of blood and stool cultures show an oxidase-negative, motile, gram-negative bacillus that does not grow on MacConkey agar. Which of the following is the most likely causative organism?

(A) *Escherichia coli*
(B) *Pseudomonas aeruginosa*
(C) *Salmonella* spp.
(D) *Shigella* spp.
(E) *Vibrio cholerae*

32. A 35-year-old man is brought to the emergency department by ambulance after having a tonic-clonic seizure at work. The patient reports that he has always been healthy and has never had a seizure before. On further questioning, the patient reports that he has been having intermittent bloody stools for the past 4 months. A CT scan of the head reveals an irregular 3 × 4-

cm mass extending from the right to the left hemisphere. CT of the abdomen shows multiple polypoid masses in the sigmoid colon. Which of the following is the most likely diagnosis?

(A) Familial adenomatous polyposis
(B) Gardner's syndrome
(C) Hereditary nonpolyposis colorectal carcinoma
(D) Tuberous sclerosis
(E) Turcot syndrome

33. A patient's serum is placed on a plate that is precoated with a specific antigen. The plate is then washed free of non–antigen-binding antibodies. Anti-immunoglobulin antibodies coupled to an enzyme are then added to the mixture. Excess anti-immunoglobulin antibodies are washed free, and a substrate that changes color when cleaved by the enzyme is added to the plate. Which of the following laboratory techniques does this describe?

(A) Allele-specific oligonucleotide probe
(B) Enzyme-linked immunosorbent assay
(C) Northern blot
(D) Polymerase chain reaction
(E) Sequencing
(F) Southern blot
(G) Western blot

34. A 3-year-old boy comes to the physician because of fever and erythema in his conjunctivae, oral mucosa, palms, and soles for the past week. Physical examination is significant for fever, enlarged cervical lymph nodes, and edema of the hands and feet. Although the precise cause of the patient's disease is unknown, it is speculated that autoantibodies may play a role. Based on the known structure that is primarily affected in the patient's disease, what autoantibodies are suspected to be associated with this condition?

(A) Anticentromere antibodies
(B) Anti–endothelial cell antibodies
(C) Antihistone antibodies
(D) Anti-IgG antibodies
(E) Antinuclear antibodies

35. A 6-year-old boy arrives at the emergency department breathing rapidly and complaining of tinnitus and nausea. His parents explain that he swallowed half a bottle of aspirin that they had accidentally left out. The emergency department physician decides to administer a medication that alters the pH of the boy's urine in order to improve excretion of the drug. How does altering the pH of the urine improve the excretion of aspirin?

(A) Acidification of the urine traps ionized molecules in the urine
(B) Acidification of the urine traps nonionized molecules in the urine
(C) Acidification of urine will increase the glomerular filtration rate
(D) Alkalinization of the urine traps ionized molecules in the urine
(E) Alkalinization of the urine traps nonionized molecules in the urine
(F) Alkalinization of urine will increase the glomerular filtration rate

36. A 61-year-old man with a past medical history of cancer presents with a 2-week history of constant and severe headaches. He also notes changes in his vision associated with the headaches. Physical examination shows a healing ecchymotic lesion on the right forearm, papilledema in the left eye, a right-sided pronator drift, and weakness of the right arm. The diagnosis of an intracranial hemorrhage is confirmed with a head CT scan. Which of the following cancers is most likely to have resulted in this patient's presentation?

(A) Angiosarcoma
(B) Basal cell carcinoma
(C) Colorectal carcinoma
(D) Melanoma
(E) Prostate cancer

37. A 7-year-old boy presents to the physician with acute-onset edema and facial swelling. Dipstick urinalysis reveals 4+ proteinuria. Renal biopsy shows no appreciable changes under light and fluorescence microscopy, but electron microscopy demonstrates glomerular epithelial cell foot process effacement. A diagnosis of minimal change disease is made. How does this disease affect the pressures governing the flow of fluid across the glomeruli?

(A) Bowman's space hydrostatic pressure will be decreased
(B) Bowman's space hydrostatic pressure will be increased
(C) Bowman's space oncotic pressure will be decreased
(D) Glomerular capillary hydrostatic pressure will be increased
(E) Glomerular capillary oncotic pressure will be decreased

38. A 15-year-old boy is riding his skateboard down a rail when the board slips and he falls, straddling the rail. He comes to the emergency department in extreme pain. On physical examination, he is found to be febrile and tachycardic. His genital examination is notable for ecchymosis and swelling of the scrotum and perineal region due to urinary leakage. Which of the following is the source of this urinary leakage?

(A) Anterior bladder wall rupture
(B) Penile urethra rupture
(C) Superior bladder wall rupture
(D) Urethral rupture above the urogenital diaphragm
(E) Urethral rupture below the urogenital diaphragm

39. A gram-positive organism is isolated and cultured. Analyses show the organism is catalase-negative with no hemolysis, and is resistant to optochin and penicillin. The organism is able to grow in 40% bile salts and in 6.5% sodium chloride solution. Which of the following organisms has been isolated?

(A) *Enterococcus faecalis*
(B) *Streptococcus agalactiae*
(C) *Staphylococcus epidermidis*
(D) *Streptococcus pneumoniae*
(E) *Streptococcus sanguis*

40. The mother of a 16-month-old girl is concerned because she noticed that her daughter became lethargic and irritable 2 days after an ear infection. The mother recalls periodically noticing sweet-smelling urine in her child's diaper but that otherwise her development has been normal. An inability to metabolize which amino acid(s) would explain these symptoms?

(A) Histidine
(B) Phenylalanine
(C) Phenylalanine and tyrosine
(D) Tyrosine and histidine
(E) Valine and isoleucine
(F) Valine, isoleucine, and leucine

41. A 35-year-old man presents to the physician with a 2-month history of nonbloody, nonmucoid, nonoily watery diarrhea. He has a diastolic murmur that gets louder with inspiration and is best heard over the left lower sternal border. His face is warm and appears to be engorged with blood for several minutes during the examination. His laboratory studies show the following:

Vanillylmandelic acid: 5 mg/day (normal 0–7 mg/day)
Metanephrine, urine: 250 μg/g of creatinine (normal 0–300 μg/g)
Homovanillic acid, urine: 14 mg/day (normal 0–15 mg/day)
5-HIAA: 28 mg/day (normal 0–9 mg/day)

A lower gastrointestinal endoscopy is most likely to show a lesion located near which of the following?

(A) Appendiceal cecal orifice
(B) Gastroesophageal junction
(C) Pancreaticoduodenal junction
(D) Rectosigmoid junction
(E) Splenic flexure

42. A 57-year-old woman presents with violet discoloration of her upper eyelids, periorbital edema, and erythematous patches over her knuckles, elbows, and knees for the past several months. She also complains of bilateral muscle weakness that causes difficulty swallowing and trouble getting up from a chair. Which of the following secondary disease processes is this patient most likely to have?

(A) Cancer of a visceral organ
(B) Osteoarthritis
(C) Psoriasis
(D) Secondary syphilis
(E) Zenker's diverticulum

43. A 20-year-old man presents to the emergency department with a 3-day history of worsening fever and swelling and redness over his left leg. On physical examination, the patient has erythema and edema of his left leg that is exquisitely tender. The patient is admitted to the hospital and given intravenous antibiotics. The erythema and swelling decrease over the next 3 weeks. During the fourth week, the patient develops new onset of weakness, fatigue, fever, and a maculopapular rash. Significant laboratory findings include a BUN level of 45 mg/dL and creatinine level of 2.8 mg/dL. Blood studies show increased WBCs and eosinophils, and urinalysis shows hematuria, mild proteinuria, and increased WBCs, including a high number of eosinophils. Which of the following is the most likely cause of this patient's new onset of symptoms?

(A) Poststreptococcal glomerulonephritis
(B) IgA nephropathy
(C) Interstitial nephritis due to medications
(D) Rapidly progressive glomerulonephritis
(E) Systemic lupus erythematosus

44. A 10-year-old boy is brought to the emergency department after becoming less responsive following several bouts of nausea and vomiting. The patient is tachycardic and is breathing deeply and slowly. Laboratory studies are re-markable for a serum pH of 7.21, a serum glucose level of 700 mg/dL, a serum HCO_3^+ level of 16 mEq/L, and a serum anion gap of 22 (normal 7–16). Intravenous fluids and insulin are administered. Management of which of the following electrolytes is most critical in this patient?

(A) Ca^{2+}
(B) Cl^-
(C) HCO_3^-
(D) K^+
(E) Na^+

45. A 34-year-old woman presents to her primary care physician with a lump on the front of her neck, at the midline. A fine needle biopsy reveals papillary thyroid cancer. The patient elects to have a total thyroidectomy. The surgery is uneventful, but the patient finds that after surgery her voice has changed, and is now hoarse and raspy. Which of the following structures has most likely been damaged?

(A) Accessory nerve
(B) External laryngeal nerve
(C) Phrenic nerve
(D) Recurrent laryngeal nerve
(E) Suprascapular nerve

46. A 3-year-old girl is brought to the emergency department because she is feeling sick and has had a temperature of 38.9° C (102° F) for 3 days. The intern notices a shallow, healing laceration on the girl's right calf with an erythematous papule in the same area. On questioning, her brother states that a cat may have scratched the toddler because he "saw her playing with a stray." Which of the following organisms is the most likely cause of this illness?

(A) *Bartonella henselae*
(B) *Borrelia burgdorferi*
(C) *Eikenella corrodens*
(D) *Francisella tularensis*
(E) *Pasteurella multocida*

47. A 35-year-old man presents comes to his primary care physician with a chief complaint of palpitations and occasional chest pain. Further questioning reveals a recent history of weight loss, diarrhea, and heat intolerance. Laboratory evaluation shows anti–thyroid-stimulating hormone (TSH) receptor antibodies in the patient's serum. Which of the following best describes this patient's TSH and thyroid hormone levels relative to normal baseline values?

Choice	Thyroid-Stimulating Hormone	Total Thyroxine	Free Thyroxine
A	↑	↑	↑
B	↑	↓	↑
C	↑	↓	↓
D	↓	↑	↑
E	↓	↓	↓

(A) A
(B) B
(C) C
(D) D
(E) E

48. A 35-year-old woman presents to her primary care physician with a fever of 38.3° C (101° F), night sweats, and fatigue. The patient says that she has lost about 6.7 kg (15 lb) over the past year. A CT scan demonstrates mediastinal lymphadenopathy. Biopsy of the nodes shows a small number of large cells with "owl-eye" nucleoli, multiple nuclei, and an abundance of pale cytoplasm on a background of many reactive lymphocytes, macrophages, and granulocytes. Which of the following drugs could be used to treat this condition?

(A) Azathioprine
(B) Cisplatin
(C) Doxorubicin
(D) β-Interferon
(E) Paclitaxel

49. The blood-brain barrier (BBB) is made up of three structures: choroid plexus epithelium, intracerebral capillary endothelium, and arachnoid. Which of the following statements about the BBB is correct?

(A) Amino acids cross the BBB by active transport
(B) Carbon dioxide cannot cross the BBB
(C) Dopamine cannot cross the BBB
(D) Glucose crosses the BBB by passive diffusion
(E) Polar molecules cross the BBB more readily than nonpolar molecules

50. A 22-year-old woman presents to her family physician because of increasing fatigue and because she looks "pale" despite spending many hours outside as a camp counselor. She also states that her urine looks "cola-colored" when she first goes to the bathroom in the morning. The patient feels well otherwise. Blood analysis shows a low platelet count, a low RBC count, and a low WBC count. The patient's RBCs are mixed with acidified normal serum and compared to normal RBCs at room temperature and at 37° C (98.6° F); both temperatures cause the patient's, but not the normal, RBCs to lyse. Based on this clinical picture and the laboratory tests, this patient most likely has which of the following disorders?

(A) Alkaptonuria
(B) Cystinuria
(C) Hemophilia A
(D) Maple syrup urine disease
(E) Paroxysmal nocturnal hemoglobinuria

1. **The correct answer is A.** In response to high altitude, the hemoglobin-O_2 curve shifts right (to release O_2 more easily at the tissues). The P_{50} (the P_{O_2} at 50% saturation of hemoglobin) will increase.

Answer B is incorrect. Pulmonary vasoconstriction (hypoxic vasoconstriction) is a result of hypoxemia (decreased arterial partial oxygen pressure), thus increasing pulmonary arterial pressure (i.e., pulmonary vascular resistance).

Answer C is incorrect. 2,3-Diphosphoglycerate (2,3-DPG) binds to the β chains of deoxyhemoglobin, decreasing the affinity of hemoglobin for O_2. An increase in 2,3-DPG shifts the hemoglobin-O_2 dissociation curve to the right, which is what happens in response to high altitudes.

Answer D is incorrect. At increased altitudes, barometric pressure decreases, which decreases alveolar partial oxygen pressure. As a result, arterial partial oxygen pressure is decreased (hypoxemia).

Answer E is incorrect. As a result of increased pulmonary vascular resistance, there is increased work on the right side of the heart, resulting in hypertrophy of the right ventricle to counteract the increased afterload.

2. **The correct answer is E.** This patient is suffering from absence seizures, which have a higher incidence in children aged 3–13 years. The seizures typically involve episodes of persistent staring that can involve stereotyped activity followed by an abrupt return to consciousness. Also known as petit mal seizures, these seizures can be inherited as an autosomal recessive trait.

Answer A is incorrect. A centrotemporal spike pattern on EEG is characteristic of benign rolandic epilepsy, an epileptic disorder that usually begins in childhood. It is characterized by focal partial seizures that involve the face and may subsequently spread to be generalized and involve the entire side of the body initially affected.

Answer B is incorrect. Diffuse slowing with generalized spike-and-wave complexes is characteristic of grand mal seizures.

Answer C is incorrect. Polyspike or slow spike-and-wave complexes are consistent with the EEG pattern evident in myoclonic seizures.

Answer D is incorrect. Posterior asymmetric slowing of background on EEG is consistent with febrile seizures. Such seizures typically affect children between 3 months and 5 years of age, are precipitated by a high temperature, and are without an organic cause.

3. **The correct answer is D.** The clinical picture is consistent with a patent foramen ovale. Excessive resorption of the septum primum or septum secundum (the two components of the atrial septum) will prevent the foramen ovale from fully closing at birth as it normally does. If small, a patent foramen ovale may go undetected well into adulthood, and it is the most common congenital heart disease in adults. The clinical presentation is as described in the question. Note that the ECG pattern shows atrial fibrillation (which also explains the irregularly irregular pulse), an arrhythmia commonly seen with patent foramen ovale.

Answer A is incorrect. The aorticopulmonary (AP) septum forms the division between the pulmonary trunk and the aorta, which are both derived from the truncus arteriosus. Pathology of the AP septum is associated with transposition of the great vessels and tetralogy of Fallot. Both of these conditions cause early cyanosis and thus are not consistent with this clinical presentation.

Answer B is incorrect. The ductus arteriosus may fail to close at birth, producing a patent ductus arteriosus (PDA). While this can cause exertional dyspnea, it is typically discovered much earlier in life and produces a continuous "machinelike" murmur, not a purely systolic murmur. PDA is associated with maternal rubella infection during pregnancy and with premature birth, but is not associated with atrial fibrillation.

Answer C is incorrect. The ductus venosus shunts blood from the portal vein to the inferior vena cava and thus is not associated with cardiac pathology.

Answer E is incorrect. The interventricular septum divides the fetal primitive ventricle into right and left ventricles. Pathology of this structure produces a membranous ventricular septal defect (VSD). A VSD produces exertional dyspnea but is obvious in an infant and would never remain occult until the age of 35. A smaller distinction to note is that the harsh pansystolic murmur of a VSD is best heard over the left lower sternal border.

4. **The correct answer is B.** This patient is most likely suffering from subacute sclerosing panencephalitis. This is a rare progressive demyelinating disease associated with chronic central nervous system infection with measles virus. There is often a history of primary measles infection at an early age (approximately 2 years) followed by a latent interval of 6–8 years. Initial manifestations include poor school performance and mood and personality changes. Fever and headache do not occur. As the disease progresses, patients develop progressive intellectual deterioration, focal and/or generalized seizures, myoclonus, ataxia, and visual disturbances. The cerebrospinal fluid (CSF) is acellular with normal or mildly elevated protein and markedly elevated gamma globulin (> 20% of total CSF protein). CSF antimeasles antibodies are elevated. CT and MRI show evidence of multifocal white matter lesions, cortical atrophy, and ventricular enlargement.

Answer A is incorrect. Herpes simplex virus 2 (HSV-2) can cause a recurrent meningitis. As with the other examples, one would expect to see signs of meningeal irritation as well as an increase in lymphocytes. Infection with HSV-2 is often associated with genital lesions.

Answer C is incorrect. The patient has no evidence of current mumps infection. Mumps virus can cause acute viral meningitis, but one would expect to see classic signs of meningitis as well as an increase in lymphocytes in the cerebrospinal fluid.

Answer D is incorrect. *Neisseria meningitidis* can cause bacterial meningitis. These organisms would likely be discovered on culture of the cerebrospinal fluid (CSF). Bacterial meningitis would also manifest in a high fever with meningeal signs (headache, nuchal rigidity) as well as decreased CSF glucose, increased CSF protein, and mononuclear and/or polymorphonuclear cells.

Answer E is incorrect. Infection with *Treponema pallidum* can eventually lead to neurosyphilis, which can include some of the symptoms described in this case. The patient has neither elevated cerebrospinal fluid protein nor the presence of mononuclear cells. There is also little evidence in the history of prior or current infection with *T. pallidum*.

5. **The correct answer is B.** A defect in the hydroxylation of proline and lysine residues of collagen is a result of vitamin C deficiency and is associated with scurvy. Patients with scurvy can present with swollen gums and poor wound healing.

Answer A is incorrect. Thrombocytopenia, or decreased platelet counts, may account for easy bleeding. Thrombocytopenia may be a result of many factors, including decreased platelet production (secondary to viral infections or to chemotherapy or radiation), increased platelet destruction (which may be idiopathic or secondary to disseminated intravascular coagulation, thrombotic thrombocytopenic purpura, or hemolytic uremic syndrome), or distribution (splenomegaly). The characteristic symptom of thrombocytopenia is mucosal or cutaneous bleeding. However, this diagnosis is ruled out by a normal platelet count.

Answer C is incorrect. von Willebrand's factor (vWF) plays an important role in primary hemostasis by binding to both platelets and endothelial components, forming an adhesive bridge between platelets and vascular subendothelial structures as well as between adjacent platelets at sites of endothelial injury. It also contributes to fibrin clot formation by acting as a carrier protein for factor VIII, which has a greatly shortened half-life and abnormally low concentration unless it is bound to vWF. Von Willebrand's disease is characterized by mutations that lead to impairment in the synthesis or function of vWF. Patients with von Willebrand's disease have a tendency to bleed, as the disease is associated with an increased partial thromboplastin time and bleeding time, both of which are normal in this patient.

Answer D is incorrect. Dystrophin is a protein that is located on the cytoplasmic face of the plasma membrane of muscle fibers. It functions as a component of a large, tightly associated glycoprotein complex and shields the complex from degradation. Mutations in the dystrophin gene lead to digestion of the glycoprotein complex by proteases. Loss of these membrane proteins may initiate the degradation of muscle fibers, resulting in muscle weakness characteristic of Duchenne's muscular dystrophy.

Answer E is incorrect. Spectrin is a protein that ties the skeleton of a red blood cell to its outer lipid bilayer. Mutations of spectrin can lead to a disease called hereditary spherocytosis. Patients with this red blood cell membrane defect typically present with hemolytic anemia, jaundice, and splenomegaly.

6. **The correct answer is C.** Fibroadenomas are the most common tumor in young women, presenting as small, firm, mobile masses. They are not associated with malignancy. On histology, fibrosing stroma is seen around normal duct and gland structures.

Answer A is incorrect. Blue dome cysts are seen in fibrocystic diseases of the breast. These lesions have associated risks of carcinoma with the presence of atypia.

Answer B is incorrect. Paget's disease presents with eczematous skin findings with underlying ductal carcinomas. Paget's cells are large cells with halolike clearings.

Answer D is incorrect. Infiltrating lobular carcinomas are often multilocular and bilateral.

These cells are found in clusters or in a linear formation.

Answer E is incorrect. Any lymphocytic infiltrate suggests inflammatory carcinoma with a poor prognosis.

7. **The correct answer is E.** This woman has carpal tunnel syndrome, which occurs in individuals whose work involves repetitive hand motions. The median nerve is compressed in the carpal tunnel, leading to decreased sensation on the first three and one-half digits and loss of strength of the thumb due to weakness of the abductor pollicis brevis and opponens pollicis. The opponens pollicis is supplied by the median nerve and functions to aid in opposition.

Answer A is incorrect. The adductor pollicis is innervated by a branch of the ulnar nerve and thus would not be affected by carpal tunnel syndrome. It functions to adduct the thumb toward the middle digits.

Answer B is incorrect. Dorsal interossei muscles are innervated by a branch of the ulnar nerve, which functions to abduct the digits.

Answer C is incorrect. The third and fourth lumbricals are innervated by a branch of the ulnar nerve.

Answer D is incorrect. The opponens digiti minimi muscle is innervated by a branch of the ulnar nerve and brings the pinky in opposition with the thumb.

8. **The correct answer is F.** The most likely diagnosis in this patient is hereditary spherocytosis (HS) caused by a defect in cytoskeletal proteins in RBCs, such as spectrin and ankyrin. HS is most commonly inherited as an autosomal dominant disorder and presents with a triad of anemia, jaundice, and splenomegaly. Anemia may be intermittent and can be aggravated by infection or bone marrow suppression. Laboratory indices that are supportive of HS include evidence of hemolytic anemia (elevated reticulocyte count and low hemoglobin), elevated mean cell hemoglobin concentration due to loss of membrane stability, and

increased osmotic fragility. HS is most characteristically defined on peripheral blood smear by the presence of spherocytic RBCs. Spherocytes are formed by the activity of splenic reticuloendothelial cells, which remove portions of abnormal membrane from the cytoskeletal defects found on these RBCs. Symptomatic treatment for anemic crises includes folic acid and blood transfusions. In more severe cases, the only treatment for HS anemia is splenectomy. Even following splenectomy, however, spherocytes will still be observed due to the underlying defect in the RBC membrane.

Answer A is incorrect. Both folic acid supplements and blood transfusion are important in treating the symptoms of anemia in hereditary spherocytosis, but they are not curative measures.

Answer B is incorrect. Chemotherapy is not appropriate and would induce a state of aplastic anemia.

Answer C is incorrect. Both folic acid supplements and blood transfusion are important in treating the symptoms of anemia in hereditary spherocytosis, but they are not curative measures.

Answer D is incorrect. Iron chelation therapy would be appropriate in iron-overloaded states, such as in thalassemic patients requiring many transfusions or in hemochromatosis.

Answer E is incorrect. Iron supplementation would be appropriate in iron deficiency anemia.

9. **The correct answer is C.** It is appropriate to discuss the patient's concerns. Explanation of the symptoms and the disease process may alleviate the patient's fears, especially because the patient appears to want a more active role in his care.

Answer A is incorrect. Avoiding a patient's concerns ultimately results in more work than addressing them directly. This choice would also be incorrect because it would leave the patient anxious and feeling unresolved.

Answer B is incorrect. This type of answer is almost always incorrect on Step 1. One must deal with worried patients constantly on the wards. It is important to be compassionate and not pass the responsibility on to someone else.

Answer D is incorrect. It is unfortunate that physicians may feel they need to send this patient for a CT scan of the head to "cover their own back." While this may ultimately be the course of action, it is more appropriate to discuss care with patients first.

Answer E is incorrect. This would essentially be performing a fake test. Some would argue of the power of peace of mind, but this would be a waste of medical resources, unethical, and even potentially harmful.

Answer F is incorrect. It is never appropriate to lie to a patient. It is also never appropriate to pick such an answer on a boards-type examination.

10. **The correct answer is E.** Phenytoin toxicity, as with many of the antiepileptic medications, can lead to nystagmus, diplopia, lethargy, and ataxia. It can also lead to tubulointerstitial nephritis, which can cause a sharp increase in creatinine levels.

Answer A is incorrect. Acetaminophen overdose can cause hepatic toxicity.

Answer B is incorrect. Clozapine is an antipsychotic that possesses extrapyramidal and anticholinergic adverse effects.

Answer C is incorrect. Imipramine is a tricyclic antidepressant that can lead to the "3 C's": Convulsion, Coma, and Cardiotoxicity.

Answer D is incorrect. Lithium toxicity presents with tremor, polyuria, slurred speech, and poor coordination.

Answer F is incorrect. Sumatriptan is a 5-HT_1 agonist used to treat migraines. Sumatriptan toxicity can present with chest discomfort and tingling.

11. **The correct answer is C.** The uptake of ^{99m}Tc pertechnetate (which is captured by thyroid tissue just as iodine is) in this mass and its sublingual position strongly suggest that it is composed of ectopic thyroid tissue. Normally,

the thyroid diverticulum develops from the floor of the primitive pharynx and descends from there into the neck. Therefore, finding thyroid tissue still attached to the tongue implies that it has failed to migrate caudally. The tongue is the most common site of ectopic thyroid tissue for this reason.

Answer A is incorrect. The third and fourth branchial (pharyngeal) arches form the posterior third of the tongue. However, the ^{99m}Tc pertechnetate uptake in this mass indicates that it is composed of thyroid, and not lingual, tissue.

Answer B is incorrect. The thymus is located in the anterior mediastinum, deep to the sternum. There would be no embryologic explanation for finding thymic tissue in the upper neck. Furthermore, the uptake of ^{99m}Tc pertechnetate implies that this mass is composed of thyroid, and not thymus, tissue.

Answer D is incorrect. The thymus is not normally found in the neck; it is instead located in the anterior mediastinum. Thymic hypertrophy would not explain this location. Furthermore, the uptake of ^{99m}Tc pertechnetate indicates that this mass is composed of thyroid, and not thymus, tissue.

Answer E is incorrect. The thyroid does not migrate rostrally during development. Instead, it develops near the tongue and migrates caudally (descends) to its normal position in the lower neck.

12. **The correct answer is E.** This patient has Kartagener's syndrome, which is caused by a lack of dynein arms in microtubules in cilia, rendering them immotile.

Answer A is incorrect. Benign prostatic hypertrophy could cause impairment of ejaculation by not allowing semen to be expelled from the body. Because the patient is without an enlarged prostate and is 27 years old, this diagnosis is highly unlikely.

Answer B is incorrect. Cystic fibrosis does cause infertility, but is associated with gastrointestinal problems and not associated with situs inversus.

Answer C is incorrect. Hypogonadism is associated with infertility and an increased risk of testicular cancer. It is usually found at a very young age and resolves by itself or is surgically corrected before serious complications occur.

Answer D is incorrect. Familial hypercholesterolemia can cause atherosclerosis of the vessels of the male genitalia, causing erectile dysfunction. Without a history of erectile dysfunction or a lipid history, this diagnosis is highly unlikely.

13. **The correct answer is C.** According to her pH, P_{CO_2}, and HCO_3^-, this young woman has a respiratory alkalosis. Respiratory alkalosis is caused by a loss of CO_2, which is balanced by an increased excretion of HCO_3^-. Hence, a low CO_2 and low HCO_3^- level indicate respiratory alkalosis. The key to this question is to recognize that respiratory alkalosis can be caused only by an increase in ventilation, which can be caused by low oxygen (in high altitudes) or by sympathetic stimulation such as anxiety, panic attack, or pain.

Answer A is incorrect. An increase in anions would be consistent with anion-gap metabolic acidosis. Metabolic acidosis is indicated by the presence of a low pH with a low plasma HCO_3^- and a low CO_2, and an increased anion gap, measured by ($[Na^+] - [Cl^-] - [HCO_3^-]$), which is normally between 10 and 16 mEq/L.

Answer B is incorrect. Diuretic use can cause metabolic alkalosis by volume contraction. This causes the kidney to compensate by reabsorbing sodium and excreting hydrogen ions. A metabolic alkalosis would present with elevated pH, elevated CO_2, and elevated HCO_3^-.

Answer D is incorrect. Hypoventilation causes a reduction in pH due to CO_2 retention. This will lead to a respiratory acidosis with a low pH, a high CO_2, and a high HCO_3^-. The compensatory mechanism for respiratory acidosis is an increase in HCO_3^- retention by the kidneys to normalize the pH.

Answer E is incorrect. Vomiting causes a metabolic alkalosis secondary to the loss of acid and chloride from the stomach. If this were the cause, this patient's lab results would show a high pH, a high HCO_3^-, and (with respiratory compensation) a high CO_2. The causes of metabolic alkalosis include vomiting, diuretic therapy, and chloride restriction. The compensation for metabolic alkalosis is hypoventilation.

14. **The correct answer is E.** This patient presents with deep venous thrombosis (DVT). Erythematous, warm, and tender unilateral calf swelling is classic for DVT. Risk factors for DVT and subsequent pulmonary thromboembolism include Virchow's triad, which consists of stasis (e.g., immobility, obesity, congestive heart failure), endothelial injury (e.g., trauma, surgery, previous DVT), and hypercoagulable state (e.g., pregnancy, oral contraceptive use, coagulation disorders, malignancies, smoking). This patient also has a positive Homans' sign (calf pain on forced dorsiflexion), which further supports the diagnosis. Not only should this patient be anticoagulated with heparin or warfarin on presentation, but she should quit smoking to decrease her clotting tendencies.

Answer A is incorrect. Bile acid resins such as cholestyramine and colestipol decrease serum triglycerides and cholesterol, which may indirectly, although not directly, improve vascular health.

Answer B is incorrect. Statins decrease LDL cholesterol but do not affect the rate of deep venous thrombosis formation.

Answer C is incorrect. Oral contraceptives are associated with hypercoagulable state, so they would make deep venous thrombosis more likely.

Answer D is incorrect. Moderate exercise has been linked to improved cardiovascular health and a decreased incidence of acute coronary syndromes, although it is not specifically linked to deep venous thrombosis. Stasis, however, can make deep venous thrombosis more likely.

Answer F is incorrect. Modest alcohol consumption has been associated with improved cardiovascular health, although no specific link to deep venous thrombosis has been proven.

15. **The correct answer is E.** This patient has an increase in both direct and indirect bilirubin levels. Oral contraceptives can cause jaundice, which is very similar to intrahepatic cholestasis. This condition would lead to increased direct and indirect bilirubin levels. This condition is reversible when the medication is discontinued.

Answer A is incorrect. Crigler-Najjar syndrome type I is an indirect bilirubinemia that is caused by a complete absence of glucuronosyltransferase. It presents in infancy with high unconjugated bilirubin.

Answer B is incorrect. Dubin-Johnson syndrome is a direct bilirubinemia that presents with elevations in both direct and indirect bilirubin due to a defect in excretion of bilirubin. The liver in these patients is typically black. Jaundice is exacerbated by illness, pregnancy, and oral contraceptive use. These patients typically have an enlarged liver and mild right upper quadrant tenderness.

Answer C is incorrect. Gilbert's disease is an indirect bilirubinemia that typically presents in the second decade of life in response to a stressor (infection, surgery, excessive alcohol consumption, exertion, or fasting). These patients typically present with normal liver function tests, high serum bilirubin, and low/normal direct bilirubin levels.

Answer D is incorrect. Patients with hepatitis typically present with increased levels of both indirect and direct bilirubin. This patient also denies two of the common risk factors for hepatitis, unprotected intercourse and drug use.

16. **The correct answer is B.** Delirium is characterized by a decreased attention span and level of arousal, disorganized thinking, hallucinations, illusions, misperceptions, disturbance in sleep-wake cycle, and cognitive dysfunction. In addition to a high temperature, a low blood pressure, and a rapidly developing course of illness, this patient is exhibiting rapidly fluctuat-

ing levels of consciousness. Delirium is the most common psychiatric diagnosis on medical and surgical floors and can commonly be seen in patients with high temperatures as well as in patients who are in a shocklike state. A Mini-Mental State Examination will reveal associated deficits.

Answer A is incorrect. Brief psychotic disorder lasts for more than 1 day but less than 1 month. Patients do not meet the criteria for schizophrenia.

Answer C is incorrect. Delusions are disorders in the content of thought. The patient holds onto them despite all evidence to the contrary.

Answer D is incorrect. Mania is a distinct period of abnormally elevated or irritable mood that lasts at least 1 week. This patient has had symptoms only for the past few hours.

Answer E is incorrect. Schizophrenia is characterized by psychotic symptoms lasting for at least 6 months.

17. **The correct answer is A.** Budd-Chiari syndrome (BCS) is a nearly complete obstruction to blood flow by an acute clot in the hepatic veins or in the inferior vena cava. This sudden event is followed by the onset of hepatomegaly, pain, ascites, and jaundice. The patient has classical hypercoagulable risk factors for developing BCS, including pregnancy and antiphospholipid antibody syndrome (positive antiphospholipid antibody titer, seizures, and multiple abortions). In addition to the clinical presentation and risk factors, imaging study further supports the diagnosis by suggesting hepatic venous occlusion.

Answer B is incorrect. Although pregnancy increases the patient's risk for congestive heart failure (CHF), this patient's clinical presentation, combined with the ultrasound findings, is unlikely to result from CHF.

Answer C is incorrect. Polymyalgia rheumatica is a rheumatologic disorder characterized by pain in several muscle groups with an increased erythrocyte sedimentation rate. It does not involve the liver or related vasculature.

Answer D is incorrect. Unlike Budd-Chiari syndrome (BCS), the presenting symptom of portal vein thrombosis is almost always variceal hemorrhage with melena. In contrast to BCS, ultrasound testing reveals an echogenic thrombus in the portal vein.

Answer E is incorrect. Veno-occlusive disease (VOD) is characterized by occlusion of terminal hepatic venules and hepatic sinusoids. It can clinically resemble Budd-Chiari syndrome; however, the risk factors for developing this disorder are different. They include bone marrow transplantation, chemotherapy, hepatic irradiation, and Jamaican bush tea. Hypercoagulable states such as pregnancy and antiphospholipid syndrome are not risk factors for the disorder. Hence, the most likely diagnosis is not VOD.

18. **The correct answer is B.** Asperger's syndrome is now considered to be a milder form of autism. These children have normal intelligence and language skills but are unable to show emotion or attachment to other people. They exhibit some characteristics of autism, including repetitive behaviors and relationship problems. This condition is associated with poor visuospatial skills, gauche social behavior, and clumsiness. Many of the difficulties evident in patients with Asperger's syndrome are closely associated with right hemisphere dysfunction.

Answer A is incorrect. Children with autistic disorder exhibit pervasive cognitive and behavioral deficits. Their intelligence is generally below normal. This child does not exhibit severe disability.

Answer C is incorrect. Children with childhood disintegrative disorder develop normally and reach developmental milestones until about 2 years of age, after which they show loss of abilities. Eventually, these children become severely mentally retarded.

Answer D is incorrect. Expressive language disorder is a disorder of communication. These children are not mentally retarded and exhibit no difficulties other than with speech.

Answer E is incorrect. Rett's disorder is an X-linked condition that is seen only in girls (affected boys die at birth). Most of the classic signs and symptoms, including neurodevelopmental regression and mental retardation, are first noticed after the age of 4.

19. **The correct answer is D.** Tuberous sclerosis is a genetic condition (autosomal dominant) characterized by nodular proliferation of multinucleated atypical astrocytes. These form tubers, which are found throughout the cerebral cortex and periventricular areas. The classic triad, which is manifest in only the most severe of cases, consists of seizures, mental retardation, and facial angiofibromas (also known as adenoma sebaceum). Half of patients with tuberous sclerosis develop rhabdomyomas, primary tumors of cardiac muscle that, although benign, may compromise cardiac function, especially of the atrioventricular valves. Tuberous sclerosis is also notable for a link to angiomyolipomas of the kidney.

Answer A is incorrect. Coronary artery disease (CAD) can cause progressive shortness of breath, but in conjunction with the facial lesions, the outflow obstruction on echo, and the patient's age, CAD is an unlikely diagnosis.

Answer B is incorrect. Dilated cardiomyopathy is often idiopathic. It involves four-chamber hypertrophy and dilation, and eventually heart failure. This condition is not associated with tuberous sclerosis. Note that hypertrophic cardiomyopathy also causes ventricular outflow obstruction and is often responsible for sudden death in young athletes.

Answer C is incorrect. Myxomas, like rhabdomyomas, are capable of obstruction. However, these are seen in adults and are often located in the atria.

Answer E is incorrect. Transposition of the great vessels is a situation in which the pulmonary trunk arises from the left ventricle and the aorta arises from the right ventricle. This arrangement is incompatible with life, and a compensatory anomaly such as a patent ductus arteriosus is necessary.

20. **The correct answer is C.** All of the facts in this statement are correct. Tumor necrosis factor-α (TNF)-α is a potent inflammatory cytokine found in increased amounts in the serum and synovial fluid of people with rheumatoid arthritis. TNF-α also promotes the release of other proinflammatory cytokines. Furthermore, it makes logical sense that you would treat rheumatoid arthritis with etanercept, a drug that can bind the excess TNF-α and remove it via an IgG-mediated immune response.

Answer A is incorrect. Adalimumab binds and inhibits tumor necrosis factor-α (TNF)-α; it is sometimes prescribed for moderate to severe cases of rheumatoid arthritis. It is not a synthetic TNF-α analog.

Answer B is incorrect. Rheumatoid arthritis is associated with an underexpression of endogenous interleukin-1-receptor antagonist (i.e., it causes an excess of available interleukin-1 receptors), and thus some cases can be treated with anakinra, a synthetic interleukin-1-receptor antagonist.

Answer D is incorrect. Systemic lupus erythematosus is associated with an underexpression of tumor necrosis factor-α (TNF)-α. This answer can be ruled out, however, by (1) knowing that infliximab is a monoclonal antibody against TNF-α, and (2) realizing that one would not treat an underexpression of TNF-α with an antibody against TNF-α.

Answer E is incorrect. Infliximab is a monoclonal antibody against tumor necrosis factor-α (TNF)-α, not a synthetic TNF-α analog.

21. **The correct answer is C.** This patient has classic symptoms of cardiac ischemia: chest pain with sudden onset that radiates to his left shoulder or jaw and is relieved by sublingual nitroglycerin. However, the patient is young, and the pain is not prompted by activity but occurs at rest. Additionally, his ECG is normal, showing no evidence of infarct or ischemia. As a result, he probably suffers from vasospasm or Prinzmetal's angina.

Answer A is incorrect. If myocardial infarctions were the etiology of the four episodes of chest pain in the past 4 months, his ECG would show evidence of infarct (T-wave inversion, pathologic Q waves, etc.).

Answer B is incorrect. Pericarditis can cause sudden onset of chest pain without exertion, but the pain would be not relieved with nitroglycerin. Typically, an ECG would also show diffuse ST-segment elevations.

Answer D is incorrect. Although the patient's clinical symptoms are of cardiac ischemia, they are not induced by a specific amount of exercise, which is the classic definition of stable angina.

Answer E is incorrect. Because the patient's symptoms are not prompted by a light amount of exercise or strain, it is unlikely that they are due to unstable angina.

22. **The correct answer is C.** Alport's syndrome is a heterogeneous (although most commonly X-linked) genetic disorder with absent or mutated collagen IV. It is characterized by renal disease, nerve disorders (deafness), and ocular disorders. There is no evidence of disease under low-power microscopy or immunofluorescence, as it is not an immune-mediated disease. However, under electron microscopy, there is evidence of a split basement membrane due to the collagen IV mutation.

Answer A is incorrect. Minimal change disease, the most common cause of nephrotic syndrome in children, includes a histopathologic finding of diffuse epithelial foot process fusion on electron microscopy.

Answer B is incorrect. Alport's syndrome is genetic, not immune-mediated. Therefore, there will be no immune complex deposits visible under electron microscopy.

Answer D is incorrect. A diagnosis of membranoproliferative glomerulonephritis is based on a histologic presentation that includes mesangial proliferation, thickening of the peripheral capillary walls by subendothelial spike-and-dome immune deposits, and mesangial interposition into the capillary wall, giving

rise to a tram-track appearance that is visible on light microscopy.

Answer E is incorrect. A wire-loop appearance under electron microscopy is peculiar to systemic lupus erythematosus (SLE), which is accompanied by subendothelial basement membrane deposits. SLE is a chronic autoimmune disease that affects multiple organ systems, including the kidney. SLE affects young adults (women more than men) and usually presents with a combined nephritic and nephrotic picture.

23. **The correct answer is A.** Adipocytes are the cells that comprise adipose tissue. GLUT4-mediated glucose transport occurs in only two tissue types: adipose (fat) and skeletal muscle. This is the only choice among those listed that could be used in the hypothetical experimental system described.

Answer B is incorrect. Cortical neurons are derived from the brain, where glucose transport occurs independent of insulin stimulation. Thus, these cells could not be used in this hypothetical system.

Answer C is incorrect. Insulin has no effect on glucose uptake in erythrocytes, so this cell type could not be used in this hypothetical system.

Answer D is incorrect. Insulin has no effect on glucose uptake in hepatocytes, so this cell type could not be used in this hypothetical system.

Answer E is incorrect. Pancreatic β cells express GLUT2 transporters, which serve as glucose sensors. These cells do not express GLUT4 transporters and would not be appropriate for use in this hypothetical system.

24. **The correct answer is D.** In this scenario, we are given the sensitivity and specificity of the test for autoantibodies against the acetylcholine receptor and the pretest probability of having myasthenia gravis. We are being asked to calculate the positive predictive value (PPV) of the test, which can be calculated with the following formula, where TP is true-positive re-

sults and FP is false-positive results: TP/(TP + FP). To get these values we need to set up any hypothetical 2 × 2 table in which the number of subjects with the disease is equal to the number not having the disease. This satisfies the pretest probability of 50%. If we set that number as 10, then TP = 8 and FP =1, given the sensitivity of 80% and specificity of 90%. Therefore, the PPV would be calculated as 8/(8 + 1) = 89% ≈ 90%. The same answer can also be obtained by converting the pretest probability to an odds ratio (1:1) and multiplying it by the test's positive likelihood ratio (LR+), which can be calculated using the formula LR+ = sensitivity/(1 − specificity) = 0.80/(1 − 0.90) = 8. Therefore, the posttest odds of having the disease is 8:1 or 8/9 = 89% ≈ 90% once the figure is converted back into a probability.

Answer A is incorrect. This value is too low to be the correct answer.

Answer B is incorrect. This value is too low to be the correct answer.

Answer C is incorrect. This value is too low to be the correct answer.

Answer E is incorrect. This answer is too high to be the correct answer.

Answer F is incorrect. This answer is too high to be the correct answer.

25. **The correct answer is B.** The femoral canal contains the deep inguinal lymph nodes and is enclosed inside the femoral sheath with the femoral artery and vein. In a femoral hernia, this is the potential space into which abdominal contents herniate. A mnemonic for the contents of the femoral triangle is **N(AVEL)** (laterally to medially) for **N**erve, **A**rtery, **V**ein, **E**mpty space, **L**ymphatics.

Answer A is incorrect. Cooper's ligament (lacunar ligament) is an extension of the inguinal ligament and forms the medial border of the femoral ring.

Answer C is incorrect. The femoral nerve is found outside of the femoral sheath.

Answer D is incorrect. The obturator nerve runs along the medial edge of the psoas muscle and is posterior to the femoral triangle.

Answer E is incorrect. The tunica vaginalis is the reflection of the peritoneal membrane that invests the testis and spermatic cord. It is formed when the testis descends from the abdomen into the outpouching of peritoneum known as the processus vaginalis. The processus vaginalis normally closes but can remain patent in up to 20% of men. A patent processus vaginalis can lead to hydroceles or indirect hernias, but this structure is not found in the femoral triangle.

26. **The correct answer is A.** Homocystinuria is an inborn error of metabolism caused by a defect in cystathionine synthase, the enzyme that converts homocysteine to cystathionine. Cystathionine is later converted to cysteine, so patients with this enzyme deficiency are required to supplement their diets with exogenous cysteine. In addition to marfanlike features and subluxation of the lens, these patients are at increased risk of a variety of cardiovascular derangements, including premature vascular disease and early death.

Answer B is incorrect. Lysine is another of the essential amino acids (recall the mnemonic **PVT TIM HALL** used to remember the 10 essential amino acids: Phenylalanine, Valine, Tryptophan, Threonine, Isoleucine, Methionine, Histidine, Arginine, Lysine, and Leucine). It is not related to homocystinuria.

Answer C is incorrect. Homocystinuria is a disorder of methionine metabolism; this patient would actually have an excess of methionine as opposed to a deficiency.

Answer D is incorrect. Tryptophan is an amino acid often confused with tyrosine. It is already an essential amino acid and does not have any relationship to homocystinuria.

Answer E is incorrect. Tyrosine is the amino acid affected in phenylketonuria (PKU), a deficiency of phenylalanine hydroxylase. This enzyme deficiency results in an inability to convert phenylalanine to tyrosine, making the latter an essential amino acid in patients with PKU. However, it has no role in homocystinuria.

27. **The correct answer is D.** The adverse effects of cyclophosphamide include nausea, vomiting, myelosuppression, and hemorrhagic cystitis. During its metabolism, cyclophosphamide is converted to its active form by the hepatic cytochrome P-450 enzymes. The final step in the production of the active form is nonenzymatic and produces phosphoramide mustard, the desired cytotoxic agent, and acrolein, an unwanted cytotoxic compound that is directly responsible for hemorrhagic cystitis. This dreaded adverse effect is ameliorated by increasing fluid intake and administering N-acetylcysteine, a sulfhydryl donor. N-acetylcysteine has little impact on the other adverse effects. Mesna is another thiol compound commonly used to prevent cyclophosphamide-induced hemorrhagic cystitis.

Answer A is incorrect. Acrolein is an unwanted cytotoxic compound and is not a treatment.

Answer B is incorrect. Acrolein is an unwanted cytotoxic compound and is not a treatment.

Answer C is incorrect. Acrolein is an unwanted cytotoxic compound and is not a treatment.

Answer E is incorrect. N-acetylcysteine has little impact on myelosuppression.

Answer F is incorrect. N-acetylcysteine has little impact on nausea and vomiting.

28. **The correct answer is B.** Right upper quadrant pain in an obese, middle-aged, multiparous woman with ultrasonographic findings consistent with gallstones is a classic sign and symptom of acute calculous cholecystitis. Acute calculous cholecystitis is an acute inflammation of the gallbladder commonly resulting from a gallbladder stone obstructing the gallbladder neck or cystic duct. Risk factors

are the "4F's": Female, "Fat," Fertile, and Forty. Definitive treatment is cholecystectomy.

Answer A is incorrect. Acute acalculous cholecystitis, in contrast to acute calculous cholecystitis, occurs in the absence of gallstones, generally in a severely ill patient.

Answer C is incorrect. Acute pancreatitis usually presents with radiating epigastric pain and increased serum amylase levels. This is in contrast to the nonradiating right upper quadrant abdominal pain and normal amylase levels seen in this patient.

Answer D is incorrect. Carcinoma of the pancreas often presents with jaundice and abdominal pain radiating to the back. It may also present with migratory thrombophlebitis (Trousseau's sign). This presentation differs significantly from the one described in the question.

Answer E is incorrect. Cholesterolosis, or strawberry gallbladder, is characterized by yellow cholesterol-containing flecks in the mucosal surface. In contrast to this patient's diagnosis, it is not associated with inflammatory changes (normal erythrocyte sedimentation rate and WBC count) and has no special association with cholelithiasis.

29. **The correct answer is C.** This vignette describes a patient with secondary hyperparathyroidism due to chronic renal insufficiency or renal osteodystrophy. The central problems in this disorder are impaired Ca^{2+} reabsorption and phosphate excretion from the kidneys due to nephron loss. The resulting hypocalcemia stimulates increased secretion of parathyroid hormone (secondary hyperparathyroidism), causing increased bone turnover and contributing to the hyperphosphatemia. Moreover, nephron loss results in impaired conversion of 25-OH vitamin D to 1,25-dihydroxy vitamin D, reducing Ca^{2+} absorption in the intestines and thus exacerbating hypocalcemia in this syndrome.

Answer A is incorrect. Parathyroid adenoma would cause increased secretion of parathyroid hormone, resulting in hypercalcemia rather than hypocalcemia, in tandem with hypophosphatemia rather than hyperphosphatemia.

Answer B is incorrect. Parathyroid insufficiency would result in hypocalcemia but cannot account for the hyperphosphatemia presented in this case.

Answer D is incorrect. Malignancy usually results in hypercalcemia due to lytic metastases to bone (with increased serum alkaline phosphatase activity and hyperphosphatemia) or production of parathyroid hormone–related peptide (with hypophosphatemia).

Answer E is incorrect. Vitamin D intoxication results in hypercalcemia and hyperphosphatemia and thus would be consistent with the laboratory findings presented in the vignette, but this patient's symptoms are more consistent with hyperparathyroidism. Given the history of renal insufficiency, renal osteodystrophy is more likely to be the cause of the findings in this case.

30. **The correct answer is B.** This is a clinical picture of restrictive lung disease; the FEV_1:FVC ratio is approximately normal, but both are dramatically reduced. Amiodarone is an antiarrhythmic that can cause pulmonary fibrosis, a restrictive lung disease.

Answer A is incorrect. Asthma is a cause of chronic obstructive pulmonary disease.

Answer C is incorrect. Diltiazem is an antiarrhythmic that is sometimes used in intravenous form to treat atrial fibrillation. It infrequently causes hypotension or bradyarrhythmias, but is not known to cause pulmonary fibrosis.

Answer D is incorrect. Sotalol has both β-blocking and action potential–prolonging activity. It is used for treatment of ventricular and supraventricular arrhythmias in children and for life-threatening ventricular arrhythmias in adults. It can sometimes cause torsades de pointes when taken at higher doses. However, sotalol does not cause pulmonary fibrosis.

Answer E is incorrect. Tobacco is a known risk factor for chronic obstructive pulmonary

disease (COPD). COPD presents with an FEV_1:FVC ratio of < 80% and a sloping flow-volume curve.

31. **The correct answer is C.** Bloody diarrhea and fever can have a number of bacterial causes, including *Escherichia coli* (O157:H7), *Salmonella*, and *Shigella* species. Other bacterial causes include *Campylobacter jejuni* and *Yersinia enterocolitica*. Both *Salmonella* and *Shigella* species are gram-negative rods that do not ferment lactose and are oxidase-negative. *Salmonella*, however, is motile, while *Shigella* is not. When a bacterium that ferments lactose is plated on MacConkey agar, the colonies are pink/red. If the plated bacteria do not ferment lactose, the colonies are clear.

Answer A is incorrect. Certain strains of *Escherichia coli* (O157:H7) can cause bloody diarrhea. However, *E. coli* does ferment lactose.

Answer B is incorrect. *Pseudomonas aeruginosa* is a frequent cause of nosocomial pulmonary infection in intubated patients and those with cystic fibrosis. It does not cause bloody diarrhea, and although it is a non–lactose-fermenting, gram-negative bacillus, it is oxidase-positive.

Answer D is incorrect. Enteric shigellosis can present similarly to *Salmonella* species infection. They also are oxidase-negative, non–lactose-fermenting, gram-negative rods. However, *Shigella* species are nonmotile, while *Salmonella* species are motile.

Answer E is incorrect. *Vibrio* species are curved, motile, gram-negative rods. However, *Vibrio cholerae* causes rice-water stools, not bloody diarrhea.

32. **The correct answer is E.** This patient has Turcot syndrome, an autosomal dominant disease characterized by colorectal polyposis and central nervous system tumors, particularly gliomas. All familial polyposis syndromes, with the exception of Peutz-Jeghers syndrome, predispose to colorectal cancer. Turcot syndrome has also been reported in association with both familial adenomatous polyposis (FAP) and

hereditary nonpolyposis colorectal carcinoma, but FAP is the more classic association.

Answer A is incorrect. Familial adenomatous polyposis is associated with hundreds of colorectal polyps, and nearly all affected patients will develop colorectal cancer.

Answer B is incorrect. Gardner's syndrome is characterized by colorectal polyposis and osteomas or other bone and soft tissue tumors.

Answer C is incorrect. Hereditary nonpolyposis colorectal carcinoma is associated with dozens of colorectal polyps, and a majority of affected patients will develop colorectal cancer.

Answer D is incorrect. Tuberous sclerosis is an autosomal dominant condition characterized by mental retardation, seizures, tuberous central nervous system tumors, angiomyolipomas of the kidneys, leptomeningeal tumors, and skin lesions such as ash-leaf spots and sha-green patches.

33. **The correct answer is B.** This question describes enzyme-linked immunosorbent assay (ELISA). ELISA is an immunologic technique used in laboratories to determine whether a particular antibody is present in a patient's blood. Labeled antibodies are used to detect whether the serum contains antibodies against a specific antigen precoated on an ELISA plate. The patient's serum can also be challenged with a specific antibody to determine whether the corresponding antigen is present in the patient's blood.

Answer A is incorrect. Allele-specific oligonucleotide probes are short-labeled DNA sequences complementary to an allele of interest. These probes can be used to detect the presence of disease-causing mutations.

Answer C is incorrect. Northern blots are similar to Southern blots except that in Northern blotting, mRNA is separated by electrophoresis instead of DNA. This is not the technique described above.

Answer D is incorrect. Polymerase chain reaction is a laboratory technique used to produce many copies of a segment of DNA. In the procedure, DNA is mixed with two specific primers, deoxynucleotides and a heat-stable polymerase. The solution is heated to denature the DNA and is then cooled to allow synthesis. Twenty cycles of heating and cooling amplify the DNA over a million times. This is not the procedure described above.

Answer E is incorrect. Sequencing is a laboratory technique that utilizes dideoxynucleotides to randomly terminate growing strands of DNA. Gel electrophoresis is used to separate the varying lengths of DNA. The DNA sequence can then be read based on the position of the bands on the gel. This is not the technique described above.

Answer F is incorrect. In a Southern blot procedure, DNA is separated with electrophoresis, denatured, transferred to a filter, and hybridized with a labeled DNA probe. Regions on the filter that base-pair with the labeled DNA probes can be identified when the filter is exposed to film that is sensitive to the radiolabeled probe. This is not the technique described above.

Answer G is incorrect. In a Western blot procedure, protein is separated by electrophoresis and labeled antibodies are used as a probe. This technique can be used to detect the existence of an antibody to a particular protein.

34. **The correct answer is B.** To answer this question, one must know that Kawasaki's syndrome (also referred to as mucocutaneous lymph node syndrome) is an arteritis that primarily affects medium- and small-sized arteries. Hence, it makes sense that there is evidence suggesting the formation of anti–endothelial cell (and anti–smooth muscle cell) autoantibodies in patients with this disease. The clinical manifestations of this disease include fever for more than 5 days, cervical lymphadenopathy, a skin rash (which often has desquamation, or shedding of the skin), and erythema of the conjunctivae, oral mucosa, palms, and soles. Eighty percent of patients are under the age of 4. Twenty percent of patients develop cardiovascular disease, including coronary artery vasculitis and coronary artery aneurysm.

Answer A is incorrect. Anticentromere antibodies, which are found in 90% of patients with the CREST variant of scleroderma, are not particularly associated with Kawasaki's syndrome.

Answer C is incorrect. Antihistone antibodies, which are found in over 95% of patients with drug-induced lupus erythematosus, are not particularly associated with Kawasaki's syndrome.

Answer D is incorrect. Anti-IgG (rheumatoid factor) is not particularly associated with Kawasaki's syndrome. Elevated levels of serum rheumatoid factor are present in 80% of patients with rheumatoid arthritis.

Answer E is incorrect. Antinuclear antibodies, which are present in over 95% of patients with systemic lupus erythematosus, are not particularly associated with Kawasaki's syndrome.

35. **The correct answer is D.** Aspirin is a weak acid with a pK_a near 3.5. Thus, it can interconvert between neutral and negatively charged forms depending on the pH. Alkalinizing the tubular fluid shifts the equilibrium toward the deprotonated charged state, which cannot diffuse across the cell membrane into the tubular cells and bloodstream. Thus, neutral molecules diffusing into the lumen will become ionized and trapped, and the clearance of aspirin will greatly increase.

Answer A is incorrect. Acidification of the urine would lower the pH and shift the equilibrium toward the protonated neutral form of aspirin. These nonionized molecules could then move back into the bloodstream and clearance of aspirin would be decreased.

Answer B is incorrect. Acidification of the urine would lower the pH and shift the equilibrium toward the protonated neutral form of aspirin, but these molecules can diffuse across cell membranes back into the bloodstream and would not be trapped.

Answer C is incorrect. Acidification of the urine has no effect on the glomerular filtration rate, which is affected by the difference in pressures across the glomerulus and glomerular permeability.

Answer E is incorrect. Alkalinization of urine promotes ionization of aspirin in the urine; the concentration of nonionized molecules of aspirin would decrease as the urine is alkalinized.

Answer F is incorrect. Alkalinization of the urine has no effect on the glomerular filtration rate, which is affected by the difference in pressures across the glomerulus and glomerular permeability.

36. **The correct answer is D.** Intracranial metastases represent nearly half of all brain tumors, yet only 15% of tumors metastasize to the brain. Intracranial hemorrhages are a recognized but relatively uncommon complication of brain tumors and can result in intraparenchymal, subarachnoid, subdural, and epidural hematomas. Focal neurologic signs are frequently evident and are due to pressure exerted on the brain parenchyma. To answer the question, first determine the most likely source of intracranial metastases and then select which of those cancers demonstrate a propensity to bleed. Lung, breast, colon, and renal carcinomas as well as melanomas are all common sources of intracranial metastases. However, only renal cell carcinomas, choriocarcinomas, melanomas, retinoblastomas, and lung and breast cancers can result in hemorrhagic brain metastases. Since melanoma is a relatively frequent source of metastatic lesions to the brain (although less common than breast or lung carcinoma) and demonstrates a tendency to hemorrhage, melanoma is the correct answer in this case.

Answer A is incorrect. Angiosarcomas are malignant endothelial neoplasms that resemble hemangiomas. Although these tumors may bleed, angiosarcomas rarely metastasize, and only a few case reports exist of hemorrhage of cerebral metastasis from angiosarcoma.

Answer B is incorrect. Some cancers rarely metastasize to the brain; these include carcinomas of the oropharynx, esophagus, and prostate as well as nonmelanoma skin cancers.

Answer C is incorrect. Colorectal carcinoma does metastasize to the brain (although less frequently than melanoma) but does not typically result in intracranial hemorrhage. Since colorectal carcinoma is less likely than melanoma to result in brain metastases and is less likely to hemorrhage, it is a less likely option.

Answer E is incorrect. Carcinoma of the prostate almost never results in metastatic brain disease and therefore represents an extremely unlikely etiology for this patient's disease.

37. **The correct answer is E.** Minimal change disease results in nephrotic syndrome, which is primarily manifested in the loss of significant protein in the urine. As a result of this protein loss, the plasma protein concentration will go down, thus decreasing the oncotic pressure in the glomerular capillary. According to the Starling equation ($GFR = K_f [(P_{GC} - P_{BS}) - (\pi_{GC} - \pi_{BS})]$), this change will lead to a higher glomerular filtration rate by decreasing the oncotic forces that normally oppose ultrafiltration.

Answer A is incorrect. Tubular hydrostatic pressures are not affected by nephrotic syndrome. The Bowman's space hydrostatic pressure generally does not decrease.

Answer B is incorrect. Tubular hydrostatic pressures are not affected by nephrotic syndrome. The Bowman's space hydrostatic pressure could be increased in a patient with an obstruction to urine flow.

Answer C is incorrect. Bowman's space oncotic pressure will increase, not decrease, as protein is filtered into Bowman's space and thus increases the protein concentration there.

Answer D is incorrect. Hydrostatic pressures are not affected in minimal change disease. The glomerular capillary hydrostatic pressure could be increased with constriction of the efferent arteriole, for example.

38. **The correct answer is E.** The male urethra is made up of three parts. The prostatic urethra runs through the prostate. The membranous urethra runs through the urogenital diaphragm, and the penile urethra runs through the penis. Rupture of the urethra below the urogenital diaphragm (at the junction between the membranous and the penile urethra) from a so-called "straddle injury" causes urine to flow into the scrotum and the perineal region.

Answer A is incorrect. Anterior bladder wall rupture is caused by a fractured pelvis. In this kind of injury, urine will flow into the retropubic space.

Answer B is incorrect. Penile urethra rupture occurs following a crush injury. Urine will flow into the deep fascia of Buck within the penis.

Answer C is incorrect. Superior bladder wall rupture, also called dome rupture, is caused by forceful compression of a full bladder. This form of bladder rupture causes urine to flow into the peritoneal cavity.

Answer D is incorrect. Urethral rupture above the urogenital diaphragm (at the junction of the prostatic and membranous urethra) due to a fractured pelvis or improper catheter insertion causes urine to flow into the retropubic space.

39. **The correct answer is A.** *Enterococcus faecalis* and *E. faecium* (Lancefield group D streptococci) are normal flora of the intestine and can cause both urinary tract infection and infectious endocarditis. They are very hardy organisms that are able to grow in salt and bile solutions. They can be α- or β-hemolytic and are optochin- and penicillin-resistant. Recently, strains of enterococcus have become resistant to vancomycin. Vancomycin-resistant enterococci can cause a life-threatening nosocomial infection.

Answer B is incorrect. *Streptococcus agalactiae* is a bacitracin-resistant, β-hemolytic group B streptococcus. It is the leading cause of neonatal meningitis but does not usually cause symptomatic infection in adults. *S. agalactiae* is usually penicillin-sensitive.

Answer C is incorrect. *Staphylococcus epidermidis* is a catalase-positive, coagulase-negative, novobiocin-sensitive organism. It is the cause of infection in many patients with artificial prosthetic devices such as catheters, heart valves, and vascular shunts.

Answer D is incorrect. *Streptococcus pneumoniae* is a significant cause of many different types of infections, including pneumonia. *S. pneumoniae* is an α-hemolytic, optochin-sensitive organism. The majority of *S. pneumoniae* strains are still sensitive to penicillin and do not grow in bile.

Answer E is incorrect. *Streptococcus sanguis* is similar to *Enterococcus faecalis* in that it is optochin-resistant and bile-tolerant. Although resistance to penicillin among the viridans group of streptococci (which includes *S. sanguis*) is increasing, most strains are still susceptible. The viridans streptococci are α-hemolytic, while the enterococci can be either α- or β-hemolytic.

40. **The correct answer is F.** This child has intermittent maple syrup urine disease (MSUD). MSUD is caused by an inability to degrade the carbon skeleton of the three branched-chain amino acids leucine, valine, and isoleucine. MSUD has many subtypes; the two most common are classical and intermittent. Classical MSUD presents with ketonuria 48 hours to 1 week after birth. The intermittent form presents during times of catabolism such as after infections. If left untreated, MSUD can lead to seizure, coma, and death. Dietary restriction of branched-chained amino acids is the mainstay of treatment.

Answer A is incorrect. Histidine breakdown is impaired in histidase, an enzyme deficiency that results in histidinemia. Mental retardation is common but not always present in this disease. It is 20 times more common than maple syrup urine disease.

Answer B is incorrect. Phenylalanine degradation deficiencies are characteristic of phenylke-

tonuria. This is screened for at birth and the main symptom is mental retardation.

Answer C is incorrect. Phenylalanine is converted to tyrosine, which is degraded by homogentisate oxidase. Deficiency of this enzyme causes alkaptonuria, which causes black-appearing urine when left untreated.

Answer D is incorrect. No disease involves tyrosine alone and histidine.

Answer E is incorrect. Valine and isoleucine share a common degradation pathway; however, leucine is also initially degraded by α-ketoacid dehydrogenase and thus its degradation is affected in MSUD.

41. **The correct answer is A.** This patient presents with chronic diarrhea, intermittent facial flushing, and a murmur consistent with tricuspid stenosis—a triad of findings classic for carcinoid tumor. Carcinoid tumors are most often benign bowel neoplasms that classically occur on or near the appendix, which is located near the ileocecal valve. Carcinoid tumors secrete serotonin, causing vasoactive responses such as those mentioned. Electron microscopy reveals "salt and pepper" granulation of cells, consistent with their neuroendocrine origin. Elevated urinary 5-HIAA is diagnostic.

Answer B is incorrect. The gastroesophageal junction is affected by gastroesophageal reflux disease, not carcinoid tumors.

Answer C is incorrect. The pancreaticoduodenal junction is the site where pancreatic endocrine and exocrine secretions empty into the small bowel to aid in digestion.

Answer D is incorrect. The rectosigmoid junction is not a common location for carcinoid tumors.

Answer E is incorrect. The splenic flexure is a watershed area that is susceptible to ischemic damage if cardiac output becomes low. It is not, however, a common site for carcinoid tumors.

42. **The correct answer is A.** The clinical vignette gives a description of dermatomyositis, an im-

mune-mediated disorder that involves the skin and skeletal muscles. The distinctive rash of this disease is characterized by a violet discoloration of the upper eyelids together with periorbital edema. Patients often develop a gradual symmetric muscle weakness of the proximal muscles, which may manifest as difficulty getting up from chairs; one-third of patients develop muscle weakness that causes dysphagia. The disease often also presents with Gottron's lesions, which are erythematous patches over the knuckles, elbows, and knees. Between 6% and 45% of patients with dermatomyositis have an underlying visceral cancer.

Answer B is incorrect. Osteoarthritis is a degenerative joint disease characterized by joint inflammation and destruction secondary to wear and tear. It is not notably associated with dermatomyositis.

Answer C is incorrect. The diagnosis of psoriasis is characterized by nonpruritic scaly/silvery erythematous plaques with well-defined borders. Nevertheless, psoriasis is not notably associated with dermatomyositis.

Answer D is incorrect. Secondary syphilis often develops 6 weeks after an untreated primary chancre of syphilis has healed. It is characterized by fever, lymphadenopathy, skin rashes (widespread small, flat lesions that particularly involve the palms, soles, and oral mucosa), and condylomata lata (painless wartlike lesions that present in the vulva, the scrotum, or other warm, moist areas of the body). This disease is not notably associated with dermatomyositis.

Answer E is incorrect. Zenker's diverticulum, also known as pharyngoesophageal diverticulum, is an outpouching of the esophageal wall above the level of the upper esophageal sphincter that results from herniation of mucosa through a defective muscular layer. While this disease may cause dysphagia, it is not notably associated with dermatomyositis.

43. **The correct answer is C.** Allergic interstitial nephritis is an intrarenal cause of acute renal failure. The pathologic process includes edema and infiltration with polymorphonu-

clear leukocytes and lymphocytes in the interstitium of the kidney. In severe cases, there may be tubule cell necrosis. The cause of interstitial nephritis is usually medications, but infections and immunologic disorders occasionally precipitate the disorder. Medications that cause interstitial nephritis include penicillins (particularly methicillin and nafcillin), cephalosporins, sulfonamides, and nonsteroidal anti-inflammatory drugs. Clinical findings include fever, rash, and peripheral eosinophilia. Urinalysis commonly reveals RBCs and proteinuria. Also, eosinophils are often seen on urinalysis in patients with interstitial nephritis due to medications.

Answer A is incorrect. Poststreptococcal glomerulonephritis is a type of immune complex glomerulonephritis that causes enlargement of glomeruli with infiltration of neutrophils and mesangial cell proliferation. This condition usually presents about 10 days after pharyngitis or 2 weeks after skin infection and is usually seen in children. Most patients have antistreptolysin O, which can be helpful in making the diagnosis. The classic presentation is oliguric renal failure with nephritic syndrome. It is not associated with eosinophilia.

Answer B is incorrect. IgA nephropathy (Berger's disease) is a primary renal disease with deposition of IgA in the glomerulus. It is associated with hepatic cirrhosis, celiac disease, HIV, and cytomegalovirus. Patients present with gross hematuria and can have upper respiratory infection, gastrointestinal symptoms, or a flulike illness. Unlike postinfectious glomerulonephritis, no latent period exists between pharyngitis and renal symptoms. Eosinophilia is not present.

Answer D is incorrect. In rapidly progressive glomerulonephritis (RPGN), patients develop renal failure over a period of weeks to months. They present with renal failure and nephritic syndrome. Pathologically, RPGN is characterized by crescent formation involving most glomeruli. There are many etiologies for nephritic syndrome/RPGN. One would not expect to see eosinophils.

Answer E is incorrect. Systemic lupus erythematosus (SLE) is an inflammatory autoimmune disorder that affects multiple organ systems. SLE frequently causes renal damage that can present as either nephrotic or nephritic syndrome or be asymptomatic. Urinalysis typically shows microscopic hematuria and proteinuria but not eosinophilia. End-stage renal disease is a common cause of death in SLE.

44. **The correct answer is D.** This patient is in diabetic ketoacidosis (DKA), which is often the presenting syndrome in type 1 diabetes. The initial management of this condition requires aggressive fluid resuscitation and correction of hyperglycemia with insulin. Insulin stimulates the shift of K^+ from the extracellular compartment to the intracellular compartment, causing a decrease in serum K^+ levels and possible cardiac conduction abnormalities. In addition, the increase in serum pH will cause H^+ ions to come out of the cells, and their positive charge will be replaced by K^+ ions moving intracellularly, leading to further hypokalemia. Hence, following the administration of insulin, judicious administration of K^+ is the most important step in the treatment of DKA. In addition, Ca^{2+} gluconate should be administered to protect cardiac myocytes and prevent arrhythmias.

Answer A is incorrect. Ca^{2+} does not undergo insulin-mediated transcellular shifts, as is the case with K^+; hence, serum levels of Ca^{2+} do not fluctuate to the same extent with diabetic ketoacidosis and insulin administration. Calcium gluconate is generally administered to protect cardiomyocytes against arrhythmias that may result from abnormal serum K^+ levels; serum Ca^{2+} levels per se are usually not the concern in patients with diabetic ketoacidosis.

Answer B is incorrect. Cl^- does not undergo insulin-mediated transcellular shifts, as is the case with K^+; hence, serum levels of Cl^- do not fluctuate to the same extent with diabetic ketoacidosis and insulin administration. Appropriate fluid resuscitation is generally sufficient to manage serum Cl^- levels in patients who may be dehydrated.

Answer C is incorrect. HCO_3^- does not undergo insulin-mediated transcellular shifts as is the case with K^+. HCO_3^- levels often normalize with the correction of hyperglycemia and fluid administration with diuresis of serum ketoacids. HCO_3^- should be administered only when serum HCO_3^- levels are less than 15 mEq/L.

Answer E is incorrect. Na^+ does not undergo insulin-mediated transcellular shifts, as is the case with K^+. Serum levels of Na^+ therefore do not fluctuate to the same extent with diabetic ketoacidosis and insulin administration. Fluid resuscitation is generally sufficient to manage serum Na^+ levels in patients who may be dehydrated.

45. **The correct answer is D.** Damage to one or both of the recurrent laryngeal nerves is a complication of thyroid, lung, or heart surgery. Injury can also occur during placement of an endotracheal tube or by masses or swollen lymph nodes in the mediastinum. The most common symptoms of recurrent laryngeal nerve damage are hoarseness, difficulty speaking, and dysphagia. When bilateral damage occurs, bilateral vocal cord paralysis leads to obstruction of the upper airway, and intubation is contraindicated. A tracheostomy, the creation of a surgical opening into the trachea, must be performed to restore the airway.

Answer A is incorrect. The accessory nerve passes posteroinferiorly through the posterior triangle of the neck before traveling deep to the anterior border of the trapezius. It has cranial and spinal roots that supply the soft palate and pharynx (cranial root) and sternocleidomastoid and trapezius muscles (spinal root) but does not innervate the larynx. Damage to the spinal root of this nerve results in winging of the scapula and impaired neck rotation.

Answer B is incorrect. The external laryngeal nerve is a terminal branch of the superior laryngeal nerve (itself a branch of the vagus). This nerve supplies the cricothyroid muscle, which varies the length and tension of the vocal cord, and so injury to this nerve results in a monotone voice.

Answer C is incorrect. The phrenic nerve arises from C3–5 and contains motor, sensory, and sympathetic nerve fibers. It supplies the diaphragm, mediastinal pleura, and pericardium. Injury to this nerve results in paralysis of half of the diaphragm. Remember the mnemonic "**C3, 4, 5** keeps the **diaphragm** alive."

Answer E is incorrect. The suprascapular nerve passes laterally through the posterior triangle of the neck and innervates the supraspinatus and infraspinatus muscles and the glenohumeral joint. Injury to this nerve results in the "waiter's tip position" due to loss of lateral rotation of the humerus at the shoulder.

46. **The correct answer is A.** *Bartonella henselae* is a gram-negative bacillus that is the cause of cat-scratch disease. Typically (in 60% of cases), a child is scratched by a bacteremic young cat, and a papule or pustule develops in the area 3–5 days later. Tender regional lymphadenopathy develops in 1–2 weeks. Most patients present with systemic symptoms such as anorexia, fever, and malaise.

Answer B is incorrect. The spirochete *Borrelia burgdorferi* is the cause of Lyme disease. The spirochete is carried by the *Ixodes* tick, which is most common in the northeastern United States. It initially presents with an expanding ring-shaped lesion known as erythema migrans, which begins at the site of the tick bite.

Answer C is incorrect. *Eikenella corrodens* is a gram-negative organism that is part of the normal flora of the mouth and nasopharynx. It is associated with infections resulting from human bites.

Answer D is incorrect. *Francisella tularensis* is the cause of tularemia. This disease is carried by wild rabbits and ticks in the southeastern United States. It often presents with lymphadenopathy and an ulcer at the site of entry as well as with fever.

Answer E is incorrect. *Pasteurella multocida* is caused by cat bites and dog bites. This infection causes a rapid inflammation (often within hours) and is accompanied by purulent drainage.

47. **The correct answer is D.** The vignette describes a classic history of an autoimmune hyperthyroidism, Graves' disease. In this disorder, thyroid follicular cells are stimulated to synthesize and secrete thyroid hormone by anti-TSH receptor antibodies, leading to increased levels of thyroxine (T_4) and triiodothyronine (T_3) in the blood, which results in negative feedback on the anterior pituitary and suppression of TSH secretion. Thus, both free T_4 and total T_4, which includes free T_4 and T_4 bound to proteins in the blood (e.g., albumin and thyroxine-binding globulin) will be increased, while blood TSH levels will be low relative to the normal baseline.

Answer A is incorrect. An elevated TSH level is not characteristic of Graves' disease, and elevated T_4 levels should result in a lower TSH level due to negative feedback on the anterior pituitary.

Answer B is incorrect. An elevated TSH level is not characteristic of Graves' disease, and an elevated free thyroxine (T_4) level should result in a lower TSH level due to negative feedback on the anterior pituitary. Furthermore, thyroid hormone binding to proteins in the blood should not be decreased but instead should be increased in the setting of increased free T_4. Therefore, the total T_4 level should be elevated rather than low.

Answer C is incorrect. Graves' disease is characterized by a low TSH due to the circulating thyroid-stimulating immunoglobulins which elevate the triiodothyronine (T_3) and thyroxine (T_4) levels and, via negative feedback, down-regulate the level of TSH. In this answer choice, the level of TSH is elevated with would lead to elevated, not diminished, levels of T_3 and T_4.

Answer E is incorrect. Total and free thyroxine (T_4) levels are expected to be low in the setting of low TSH levels. However, in Graves' disease, stimulation of TSH receptors on the thyroid follicular cells by anti-TSH receptor antibodies stimulates the secretion of thyroid hormones and results in increased total and free T_4 levels in the setting of normal or even low TSH levels. The resulting negative feedback loop to the anterior pituitary leads to reduced TSH levels.

48. **The correct answer is C.** The classic symptoms of Hodgkin's disease include nonspecific constitutional symptoms such as night sweats, fatigue, fever, and weight loss. Additionally, mediastinal lymphadenopathy is common, and biopsy of affected nodes will show Reed-Sternberg cells on a background of reactive inflammatory cells, just as described in the question stem. A variety of chemotherapeutic agents can be used for treatment of Hodgkin's disease, including doxorubicin.

Answer A is incorrect. Azathioprine is used as an immunosuppressant in kidney transplant patients and those with autoimmune disorders.

Answer B is incorrect. Cisplatin (as well as other platinum-based chemotherapeutics) is used in the treatment of testicular, ovarian, and lung cancers.

Answer D is incorrect. β-Interferon is used in treatment of multiple sclerosis.

Answer E is incorrect. Paclitaxel (Taxol) is used for treatment of ovarian and breast cancers.

49. **The correct answer is C.** The main function of the BBB is to limit entry of certain macromolecules and allow others through. L-dopa, not dopamine, crosses the BBB. In Parkinson's disease, L-dopa crosses the BBB and is converted to dopamine within the brain to produce its desired effect.

Answer A is incorrect. Amino acids cross by a carrier-mediated transport mechanism, not active transport.

Answer B is incorrect. Substances such as carbon dioxide, oxygen, and water easily penetrate the BBB.

Answer D is incorrect. Glucose crosses by a carrier-mediated transport mechanism, not passive diffusion.

Answer E is incorrect. Nonpolar/lipid-soluble molecules cross more readily than do polar/water-soluble ones.

50. **The correct answer is E.** Paroxysmal nocturnal hemoglobinuria (PNH) is caused by a defect in synthesis of the cellular anchor used to hold surface proteins to the cell membranes of RBCs, WBCs, and platelets. This defect leads to the clinical manifestations of the disorder: anemia caused by intravascular hemolysis (leading to hemoglobinuria and the darkened urine), thromboses in unusual veins, and hematopoietic deficiencies leading to pancytopenia. The hemolysis occurs all day, but the concentrated urine formed overnight shows an obvious color change. The Ham test (mixing the patient's RBCs with acidified serum) is used to diagnose PNH. Lysis of the patient's RBCs indicates PNH.

Answer A is incorrect. Alkaptonuria presents with urine that darkens after exposure to air as a result of alkapton bodies (accumulations of homogentisic acid), as well as darkening of connective tissues. Patients may also have arthralgias.

Answer B is incorrect. Cystinuria is due to a defect in the tubular amino acid transporter in the kidneys. Patients can form cystine kidney stones due to excess cystine in the urine.

Answer C is incorrect. Hemophilia A is an X-linked disease characterized (in moderate to severe deficiency) by spontaneous bleeding, easy bruising into soft tissues, and hemarthrosis into weight-bearing joints (hip, knee, and ankle).

Answer D is incorrect. Maple syrup urine disease is caused by a deficiency of α-ketoacid dehydrogenase. Patients present with lethargy, seizures, failure to thrive, mental retardation, and urine that smells like maple syrup.

Test Block 2

1. A new patient presents to a clinic in Denver, Colorado, with complaints of dyspnea and fatigue on exertion. On history, the patient informs the doctor that she just moved from the California coastline less than 1 week ago, and has been attempting to do her 3-mile run every morning. The patient is told to limit her running until her body adjusts to the new altitude. Which of the following will occur in this woman's body in response to the high altitude?

(A) 10.0%
(B) 37.5%
(C) 60.0%
(D) 88.8%
(E) 90.0%
(F) 95.2%

2. A 27-year-old woman who is pregnant at 32 weeks' gestation presents to the emergency department following a motor vehicle accident. Radiologic studies demonstrate a fractured femur. Fetal heart monitoring is reassuring, and there is no evidence of rupture of membranes. The patient is admitted to the hospital for observation. The patient is placed on strict bed rest in expectation of induction of labor at 37 weeks' gestation. Which of the following medications would be most appropriate for this patient?

(A) Heparin
(B) Indomethacin
(C) Prostaglandin E_2
(D) Streptokinase
(E) Warfarin

3. A 38-year-old woman with a history of type 2 diabetes mellitus gives birth to a term male infant. Immediately after birth, the infant is noted to be cyanotic and tachypneic. His hypoxemia quickly worsens over minutes, and he is taken to cardiac catheterization, where a balloon is guided to perforate the atrial septum. He is also given an infusion of prostaglandin E_1. The infant's hypoxia stabilizes, and he is later taken for definitive, corrective surgery.

Which of the following is the underlying pathophysiology of this infant's hypoxemia?

(A) Coarctation of the aorta
(B) Concomitant ventricular septal defect
(C) Delayed closure of the ductus arteriosus
(D) Failure of the aorticopulmonary to spiral
(E) Overriding aorta

4. A 34-year-old man presents to his primary care physician with night sweats, a fever of 38° C (100.2° F), and weight loss of 5 kg (12 lb) over the last 3 months. A CT scan demonstrates mediastinal lymphadenopathy, and results of a biopsy of the node are shown in the image. Which of the following drug therapies could be used to manage this disease?

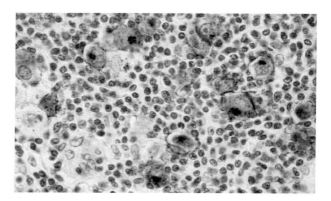

Reproduced, with permission, from Lichtman MA, Beutler E, Kipps TJ, Seligsohn U, Kaushansky K, Prchal JF. *Williams Hematology*, 7th ed. New York, McGraw-Hill, 2006: Color Plate XXII-34.

(A) Colchicine
(B) Cyclosporine
(C) Hydroxyurea
(D) Metformin
(E) Prednisone

5. A 14-year-old high school freshman presents to her family doctor for a sports physical. She has not played organized sports in the past but is in good physical shape. She mentions that she experienced severe leg cramps after trying out for

the soccer team last week. The night after the tryouts, she noticed that her urine had a reddish tinge. She has no other medical complaints. Her physician orders an ischemic forearm exercise test, which reveals no increase in venous lactate. Which of the following enzymes is most likely deficient in this patient?

(A) Acid maltase
(B) Cystathionine synthase
(C) Glucose-6-phosphatase
(D) α-1,6-Glucosidase
(E) Glycogen phosphorylase

6. A 35-year-old man comes to the physician because he has been experiencing bone pain, in addition to confusion, lethargy, recurrent renal stones, duodenal ulcer, and a small nodule on the anterior neck. His laboratory values are as follows:

Serum Ca^{2+}: 17 mg/dL
Serum phosphate: 1.0 mg/dL
Alkaline phosphatase: 500 U/L
Serum parathyroid hormone: 900 pg/mL

Which of the following conditions is most likely to be seen in this patient's bones?

(A) Hypertrophic osteoarthropathy
(B) Osteitis fibrosa cystica
(C) Osteopetrosis
(D) Osteoporosis
(E) Paget's disease of the bone

7. A 45-year-old man comes to the physician with a 3-day history of a temperature of 39° C (102.2° F). He also complains of headache, neck stiffness, and a maculopapular rash on his trunk. A diagnosis of meningitis is made, and a smear and culture of his cerebrospinal fluid identify *Neisseria meningitides* as the causative agent. In the most severe form of meningococcemia, which of the following symptoms can develop?

(A) Acute renal failure and thrombocytopenia with hemolytic anemia
(B) Fever, migratory polyarthritis, and carditis

(C) Fever, new murmur, small erythematous lesions on the palms, and splinter hemorrhages on the nail bed
(D) Shock, widespread purpura, disseminated intravascular coagulation, and adrenal insufficiency
(E) Symmetric ascending muscle weakness beginning in the distal lower extremities

8. The relationship between coxibs (cyclooxygenase-2 inhibitors) and cardiovascular events is now under question. Which of the following proposals might explain why coxibs cause more cardiovascular events than does aspirin?

	CHOICE	PGI_2	TxA_2
A	COX-2 inhibitor	↑	—
	Aspirin	↓	↓
B	COX-2 inhibitor	—	↑
	Aspirin	↓	↓
C	COX-2 inhibitor	↓	↓
	Aspirin	↓	↓
D	COX-2 inhibitor	↓	—
	Aspirin	↑	↑
E	COX-2 inhibitor	↓	—
	Aspirin	↓	↓

(A) A
(B) B
(C) C
(D) D
(E) E

9. A 30-year-old woman with systemic lupus erythematosus treated with high-dose prednisone comes to her physician with symptoms of anemia. The patient's blood studies show a low hemoglobin level (10 g/dL), a low serum iron level, an elevated ferritin level, and a low total iron-binding capacity with normocytic RBCs on blood smear. Which of the following is the most appropriate treatment for this patient's anemia?

(A) Erythropoietin
(B) Ferrous sulfate
(C) Folate
(D) Parenteral vitamin B_{12}
(E) Phlebotomy

10. A laboratory discovers a heat-sensitive strain of *Escherichia coli*. When incubated above 37° C (98.6° F), the bacteria die. It is determined that the heat-sensitive strain of *E. coli* is no longer able to form continuous strands of DNA from Okazaki fragments above 37° C (98.6° F). These findings are most likely due to a mutation in which of the following proteins?

(A) Helicase
(B) Ligase
(C) Polymerase
(D) Primase
(E) RNase H

11. An obese 56-year-old African-American man with a history of smoking experiences chest pain associated with an apparent heart attack. The pain radiates to the man's left shoulder and down his left arm. What is the reason for referred pain to this region?

(A) Common origin of sensory neurons in the anterior horn of the spinal cord
(B) Common origin of sensory neurons in the posterior horn of the spinal cord
(C) Lymphatic drainage of mediators of inflammation and pain
(D) Shared parasympathetic pathways
(E) Shared sympathetic pathways

12. A 5-year-old girl is brought to the emergency department with acute onset of projectile vomiting and severe headache. Her parents report that over the past couple of months her gait has become increasingly shaky. Her medical history is negative for seizures and signs of meningitis. Physical examination is notable for truncal ataxia and papilledema. A CT scan reveals a mass at the cerebellar vermis. Which of the following is most likely to be seen on a histological examination of tissue from this mass?

(A) Fried egg cells
(B) Psammoma bodies
(C) Pseudopalisading tumor cells with necrosis
(D) Rod-shaped blepharoblasts near nuclei
(E) Small blue cells in perivascular rosettes

13. A 63-year-old man who is an alcoholic is brought into the emergency department by his daughter. She claims that her father "has not been himself" lately. She further states that the patient's memory has been very poor, and he constantly creates elaborate yet untrue stories. On physical examination, the patient is noted to have ataxia as well as a bilateral horizontal nystagmus. Wernicke-Korsakoff syndrome is suspected. Which of the following is the result of another water-soluble vitamin deficiency?

(A) Increased erythrocyte hemolysis
(B) Neonatal hemorrhage
(C) Night blindness
(D) Osteomalacia
(E) Pellagra

14. A woman with a 2-year-old son comes to her physician because she has been unable to conceive a second child for more than a year. The woman is currently breast-feeding her son. Which of the following explains how lactation suppresses ovulation?

(A) Lactation antagonizes estrogen action
(B) Lactation decreases secretion of prolactin
(C) Lactation increases secretion of follicle-stimulating hormone
(D) Lactation increases secretion of sterility hormones
(E) Lactation inhibits secretion of gonadotropin-releasing hormone

15. A 5-day-old normally developed boy presents to the emergency department with vomiting

and constipation. The mother states that the child has not passed stool since birth but only recently began vomiting. The vomitus has a greenish coloration. On examination, it is noted that the abdomen is markedly distended and is tympanic to percussion. Digital rectal examination shows an empty rectum, but stool is passed explosively following the examination. A sweat chloride test is negative. The disorder in this infant arises from cells derived from which of the following embryologic germ cell layers?

(A) Endoderm
(B) Neural crest
(C) Neuroectoderm
(D) Mesoderm
(E) Surface ectoderm

16. A woman strikes her head in a car crash and is admitted to the hospital, where she begins urinating up to 1 L every few hours and complaining of constant thirst. The most appropriate agent to treat her problem is which of those listed?

(A) Demeclocycline
(B) Desmopressin
(C) Furosemide
(D) Insulin
(E) Mannitol

17. A 65-year-old man presents to his family doctor for a regularly scheduled check-up. He is recently widowed and appears unkempt at this visit. His past medical history is significant for alcoholism, hypertension, and type 2 diabetes mellitus. His current medications are hydrochlorothiazide, metformin, and clonidine. On physical examination, his blood pressure is found to be poorly controlled at 158/90 mm Hg. He is obese with a body mass index (BMI) of 33 kg/m^2, although this is decreased from his previous visit 3 months ago (BMI = 36 kg/m^2). On further questioning, the patient ad-

mits to owning a gun and states that he has thought repeatedly of shooting himself in the head. Which of the following actions is most appropriate in the care of this patient?

(A) Hospitalize voluntarily or involuntarily
(B) Prescribe an antidepressant
(C) Refer to a psychiatrist
(D) Schedule for a regular visit
(E) Tell the patient's children

18. A 57-year-old man who is HIV-positive presents to his physician with headache, nausea and vomiting, and a change in mental status. No nuchal rigidity is noted. A lumbar puncture is performed and shows a high opening pressure. A preparation of his cerebrospinal fluid with India ink stain is shown. Antimicrobial treatment is started. Which of the following adverse effects might occur with this patient's initial treatment?

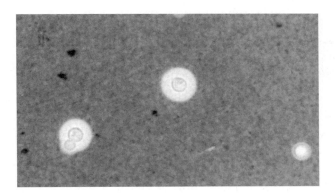

Reproduced, with permission, from Brooks GF, Butel JS, Morse SA. *Jawetz, Melnick, & Adelberg's Medical Microbiology*, 23rd ed. New York, McGraw-Hill, 2004: 648.

(A) Arrhythmia
(B) Bone marrow suppression
(C) Flushing
(D) Gynecomastia
(E) Nausea and vomiting

19. A patient presents to the emergency department with a crushing injury to her right ankle. A medical student working in the emergency department is told to evaluate the vascular integrity of the patient's right lower extremity. She feels for femoral, dorsalis pedis, and posterior tibial pulses and finds that they are intact and symmetric bilaterally. In which of the following locations did the student palpate the posterior tibial pulse?

(A) Between the two heads of the gastrocnemius muscle
(B) Deep in the popliteal fossa
(C) Immediately anterior to the medial malleolus
(D) Immediately posterior to the lateral malleolus
(E) Immediately posterior to the medial malleolus

20. A 53-year-old man with a long-standing history of allergic rhinitis and asthma presents with uveitis, mild hearing loss, numbness and tingling in his right hand, and diffuse joint pain for the past 10 days. Physical examination shows weak to absent left knee patellar reflexes (right knee reflex strong and intact). Laboratory studies show a markedly elevated eosinophil count. A diagnosis is made, and the patient is treated with cyclophosphamide. Further laboratory studies show elevated serum levels of the most common autoantibody associated with this condition. What structure is primarily targeted by the autoantibodies that are most likely elevated in this patient's serum?

(A) Acetylcholine receptors
(B) Neutrophils
(C) Oligodendrocytes
(D) RBCs
(E) Thyroid-stimulating hormone receptors

21. A 23-year-old woman comes to the physician with severe abdominal cramping and lower back pain correlating with her menstrual cycle. On pelvic examination, the physician palpates a nodular, enlarged ovary. A laparoscopy is performed and multiple lesions are found over the ovary. One of the lesions is biopsied, and the pathology report indicates ectopic en-

dometrium. Which of the following is the medication class of the drug used to treat this patient's condition?

(A) Androgen
(B) Antiestrogen
(C) Estrogen
(D) Mineralocorticoids
(E) Progesterone

22. A 59-year-old man with a long history of untreated gastroesophageal reflux undergoes endoscopic study of the esophagus. A biopsy is taken from a red, irregular lesion in the distal esophagus. The pathologist finds that the tissue stains abnormally for colonic-type mucin. This patient most likely has which of the following conditions?

(A) Barrett's esophagus
(B) *Candida* esophagitis
(C) Chagas' disease
(D) Esophageal varices
(E) Laceration

23. A mutation in the elongation factor EF1-α causes it to have a higher affinity for guanosine diphosphate than normal. This decreases the growth rate of the cells due to a decrease in protein synthesis. A secondary mutation in the cells increases the growth rate back toward normal. Which of the following is the secondary mutation?

(A) Decreased affinity of elongation factor EF1-α for guanosine triphosphate
(B) Decreased affinity of elongation factor EF1-β for guanosine triphosphate
(C) Elimination of EF1-α
(D) Elimination of EF1-β
(E) Increased affinity of elongation factor EF1-β for the mutant EF1-α

24. A 55-year-old woman presents to her primary care physician with complaints of nausea, fatigue, early satiety, and abdominal distension. Physical examination reveals the presence of ascites as well as significant pelvic discomfort. CT scanning reveals the presence of multiple masses spread diffusely throughout the abdomen. The patient is subsequently taken to

surgery to reduce her tumor burden and to confirm a diagnosis of metastatic ovarian cancer. Her oncologist then places her on a treatment regimen that includes paclitaxel. Which of the following characterizes the mechanism of this chemotherapy agent?

(A) Alkylating agent that covalently links DNA
(B) Binds tubulin and hyperstabilizes polymerized microtubules
(C) Depolymerizes microtubules
(D) Inhibits DNA polymerase
(E) Inhibits topoisomerase II

25. A 7-year-old girl has numerous vesicles on her face, particularly around her mouth. Over a few days, the vesicles turn into pustules and crust over, becoming flaky and light yellow in color. Which of the following statements about the organism most likely responsible for this girl's infection is correct?

(A) Sabouraud's agar is required to culture this bacterium
(B) The bacterium is bacitracin-sensitive
(C) The bacterium is a facultative intracellular organism
(D) The bacterium is a group B β-hemolytic organism
(E) The bacterium is protected from host defenses by protein M

26. Patients with von Hippel-Lindau disease have hemangioblastomas, or cavernous hemangiomas of the retina, cerebellum, and medulla. They can also present with adenomas and cysts of the liver, kidneys, and pancreas. Which of the following tumors are patients with von Hippel-Lindau disease at an increased risk of developing?

(A) Acute lymphocytic leukemia
(B) Colon cancer
(C) Pheochromocytoma
(D) Renal cell carcinoma
(E) Testicular seminoma

27. A 42-year-old woman comes to the physician with severe itching for the past 4 days. Her physical examination is significant for hepatomegaly and three xanthomas on her right

lower extremity. Laboratory studies reveal a normal total bilirubin level and elevated serum cholesterol and alkaline phosphatase levels. A liver biopsy shows granulomatous destruction of medium-sized intrahepatic bile ducts. Which of the following autoantibodies is most likely to be significantly elevated in this patient?

(A) Anticentromere antibodies
(B) Antihistone antibodies
(C) Antimitochondrial antibodies
(D) Antinuclear antibodies
(E) Rheumatoid factor

28. A 25-year-old woman comes to her family physician for a routine check-up. Her physical examination shows a mildly overweight woman but is otherwise unremarkable. A fasting lipid panel, however, shows an LDL cholesterol level of 310 mg/dL, an HDL level of 42 mg/dL, a triglyceride level of 150 mg/dL, and a total cholesterol level of 382 mg/dL. She is diagnosed with familial hypercholesterolemia. In addition to modification of diet and regular exercise, which of the following treatment options will the physician most likely recommend?

(A) B complex vitamins
(B) Hormone replacement therapy
(C) LDL apheresis
(D) Liver transplant
(E) Statin medications

29. Informed consent is the legal demonstration of a patient's understanding of risks, benefits, and outcomes of treatments and alternatives. Which of the following circumstances represents an exception for obtaining informed consent?

(A) A competent patient whose son wishes to waive his father's right
(B) A fellow physician agrees that informing the patient will be detrimental to the patient's health
(C) A mentally retarded patient who is legally competent
(D) A nursing volunteer has already obtained informed consent
(E) A paralyzed patient who cannot speak but can nod his head for consent

30. A 43-year-old man presents to the emergency department with the sudden onset of a headache, sweating, and palpitations. On physical examination, he appears anxious and his face is flushed. His blood pressure is 150/95 mm Hg. Urinalysis reveals high levels of vanillylmandelic acid. Which of the following is the most appropriate pharmacologic treatment for this patient's condition?

(A) Phenelzine
(B) Phenoxybenzamine
(C) Phenylephrine
(D) Prazosin
(E) Propranolol

31. A 78-year-old man comes to the physician for evaluation after falling five times in 2 months. An x-ray skeletal survey reveals no fractures, but the patient admits to worsening urinary incontinence over the previous 4 months. His wife states that his memory and concentration have deteriorated recently. The patient's vital signs are normal, and his physical examination is notable for a wide-based gait with short steps. A Mini-Mental State Examination results in a score of 26/30. His funduscopic examination is normal, and his neurologic examination is notable for slight bradykinesia without tremor. Laboratory tests, including serum vitamin B_{12}, folate, and thyroid-stimulating hormone, are normal. What is the most likely etiology of this patient's recent decline?

(A) Alzheimer's disease
(B) Hypothyroidism
(C) Multi-infarct dementia
(D) Normal pressure hydrocephalus
(E) Parkinson's disease

32. An 8-month-old girl is brought into the emergency department by her parents because they have noted she appears swollen. The parents weaned the child from formula 3 weeks ago. They wanted to give the child soy milk instead, but have accidentally been giving her rice milk for 1 month. The child is diffusely edematous on examination with 2+ pitting edema in her wrists and shins. This type of malnutrition is caused by a deficiency of which class of nutrients?

(A) Fat and calories
(B) Fat only
(C) Protein and calories
(D) Protein only
(E) Vitamins

33. A 19-year-old man who recently immigrated from Asia comes to the emergency department because of blood in his sputum. On history, the patient mentions he has had weight loss and night sweats. On examination, the patient has a fever and bronchial breath sounds with crepitant rales. Laboratory tests show lymphocytosis and an increased erythrocyte sedimentation rate. X-ray film of the chest shows a calcified lung lesion and hilar lymphadenopathy. A sputum sample is obtained from the patient, and it shows acid-fast bacilli. Which of the following is the stain used to identify the most likely infectious organism?

(A) Congo red
(B) Giemsa's
(C) India ink
(D) Periodic acid-Schiff
(E) Ziehl-Neelsen

34. A 65-year-old postmenopausal woman presents with progressive constipation and frequent, excessive urination. On history, she mentions she has been smoking a pack per day since she was 19 years old. On review of systems, she mentions that she feels like she is having palpitations constantly. On physical examination, there are respiratory findings, which prompts an x-ray film of the chest. A circular lesion in the lung is found. Laboratory testing shows a normal phosphorus level. Which of the following is the most likely cause of this patient's symptoms?

(A) Central bronchogenic carcinoma
(B) Cervical sympathetic chain compression
(C) Chronic silica exposure
(D) Congenital chloride channel dysfunction
(E) Dynein arm defect in cilia
(F) Ectopic antidiuretic hormone production
(G) Solitary parathyroid adenoma

35. The illustration demonstrates a specialized epithelium that overlies a type of peripheral lymphoid tissue. What is the main class of antibodies associated with this lymphoid tissue?

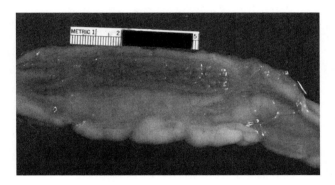

Image courtesy of PEIR Digital Library (http://peir.net).

(A) IgA
(B) IgD
(C) IgE
(D) IgG
(E) IgM

36. A 45-year-old man with essential hypertension presents to the emergency department with light-headedness. Peaked T waves and prolonged PR intervals are noted on ECG. Which of the following medications could be the underlying cause of the changes noted on this patient's ECG?

(A) Acetazolamide
(B) Furosemide
(C) Hydrochlorothiazide
(D) Mannitol
(E) Spironolactone

37. A 45-year-old woman presents with a history of generalized muscles weakness and bone pain. Her history reveals that she is not yet postmenopausal; however, she eats poorly, rarely drinks milk, and does not get outside much. A carpal spasm is noted after the cuff is inflated while the patient's blood pressure is measured. Laboratory tests show a total calcium level of 6.0 mg/dL and a phosphate level of 2.0 mg/dL.

Radiographs demonstrate a diffuse radiolucency and reduced bone density. Osteomalacia is suspected. Which of the following increases the activity of 1-α-hydroxylase in the kidney?

(A) Elevated 1,25-dihydroxycholecalciferol
(B) Elevated parathyroid hormone
(C) Elevated serum calcium
(D) Elevated serum phosphate
(E) Increased sun exposure

38. A 64-year-old woman presents to her primary care physician with fatigue, weakness, and a weight loss of 4.5 kg (10 lb) in the past 4 months. Additionally, she notes that her vision has deteriorated over that time, and has had several severe nosebleeds. Physical examination demonstrates hepatosplenomegaly, and laboratory tests show an increased total protein. Serum protein electrophoresis reveals a monoclonal M spike. Which of the following is the most likely diagnosis?

(A) Chronic lymphocytic leukemia
(B) Diabetes mellitus
(C) Hodgkin's disease
(D) Multiple myeloma
(E) Waldenström's macroglobulinemia

39. A pharmaceutical company has created a new drug that, when taken daily, is thought to be highly effective at preventing the onset of migraines. The company would like to market the drug and is conducting a study to look at its benefits and possible risks. In coordination with a physician at a local hospital, it enrolls 800 people for the study. The physician places 100 patients with the worst and most frequent migraines in the medication group, as he thinks that they are in most need of the drug's benefit. Which of the following best explains why the drug may not perform up to expectations?

(A) Differences in group size
(B) Late-look bias
(C) Recall bias
(D) Sampling bias
(E) Selection bias

40. The human papillomavirus promotes neoplasia through production of the viral proteins E6 and E7, which interfere with the normal function of *Rb* and *p53*. What general function is common to both *Rb* and *p53*?

    (A) Cell cycle regulation
    (B) Cellular adhesion
    (C) Direct transcriptional control
    (D) DNA repair
    (E) Inhibition of signal transduction

41. A 95-year-old woman is transferred to the intensive care unit after a 3-day history of cough and declining mental status. Her blood pressure is 85/50 mm Hg, pulse is 124/min, temperature is 39.8° C (103.6° F), and respiratory rate is 27/min. Crackles are heard at the left lower lung base, and the patient is suffering from rigors intermittently. Blood and sputum cultures drawn at the onset of symptoms grow strains of *Klebsiella pneumoniae* resistant to all antibiotics except polymyxin B. Which of the following is a serious adverse reaction of polymyxin B?

    (A) Granulocytopenia
    (B) Hearing loss
    (C) Hemolysis in patients with glucose
        6-phosphate dehydrogenase deficiency
    (D) Numbness of the extremities
    (E) Severe vomiting

42. A 20-year-old woman presents to the physician with a history of bloody diarrhea and abdominal pain. She states that she has not traveled recently or changed her eating habits. A stool culture is negative for any known infectious cause of diarrhea. A flexible sigmoidoscopy is performed and shows numerous lesions in the descending colon interrupted by normal-appearing mucosa. Which of the following features would most likely be present on a tissue biopsy of the affected region?

    (A) Cells with loss of mucin and hyperchromatic nuclei
    (B) Hyperplastic goblet cells
    (C) Mucus-filled cells in crypts
    (D) Noncaseating granulomas
    (E) Ulcerated mucosa only

43. A 38-year-old man dies in the emergency department due to heart failure. On autopsy, an enlarged and flaccid heart is observed. Microscopy of a blood sample taken in the emergency department earlier that day shows flagellated parasites. A histologic section of the heart shows nonmotile amastigotes. Which of the following parasites did this man most likely harbor?

    (A) *Cryptosporidium* spp.
    (B) *Entamoeba histolytica*
    (C) *Giardia lamblia*
    (D) *Toxoplasma gondii*
    (E) *Trypanosoma cruzi*

44. A 59-year-old health care worker is taking a course of isoniazid for tuberculosis prophylaxis. After 4 months of treatment, she presents to the emergency department with confusion and slurred speech. A detailed history and review of her medication shows that this patient has been taking four times the recommended dose. She says that she had a seizure the previous day. Administration of which of the following drugs is most appropriate at this time?

    (A) Diazepam
    (B) Phenobarbital
    (C) Pyridoxine
    (D) Rifampin
    (E) Thiamine

45. A 10-month-old infant is taken to the doctor for persistent jaundice and easy fatigability. Laboratory studies are ordered and a peripheral smear is obtained. Which of the following characteristics would be seen in hereditary spherocytosis?

   (A) Hypersegmented polymorphonuclear cells
   (B) Increased mean corpuscular hemoglobin concentration
   (C) Increased total iron-binding capacity
   (D) Positive direct Coombs' test
   (E) Rouleaux formation of red blood cells

46. Albinism is an autosomal recessive disorder in which a deficiency in tyrosinase activity leads to a lack of pigmentation in the hair, skin, and eyes. The cells most involved in this condition are derived from which of the following germ cell layers?

   (A) Ectoderm
   (B) Endoderm
   (C) Mesoderm
   (D) Neuroectoderm, neural crest cells
   (E) Neuroectoderm, non-neural crest cells

47. A 24-year-old woman patient presents to the physician with fatigue. Physical examination reveals splenomegaly and signs of anemia. A peripheral blood smear demonstrates the presence of spherocytes. The patient says that she recently finished a course of penicillin for treatment of otitis media. In the etiology of drug-induced hemolytic anemia, penicillin is believed to act as which of the following?

   (A) Adjuvant
   (B) Antibody
   (C) CD4+ helper epitopes
   (D) Hapten
   (E) Soluble antigen

48. A 53-year-old man presents to his physician with complaints of chest pain that is worse on exertion and at times of stress. An angiogram reveals fibrous plaques in the intima of the proximal portions of his coronary arteries. Fibrous plaques are indicative of which of the following disorders?

   (A) Arteriosclerosis
   (B) Atherosclerosis
   (C) Medial calcific sclerosis
   (D) Mönckeberg's arteriosclerosis
   (E) Takayasu's arteritis

49. A 14-year-old boy presents to the physician with severe lower extremity pain. His past medical history is significant for a gallstone diagnosed 1 year ago. His hemoglobin level is found to be 9 g/dL. If, in the future, this patient develops fever, chills, cough, and pleuritic chest pain, which of the following organisms is most likely infecting him?

   (A) *Mycoplasma pneumoniae*
   (B) *Pseudomonas aeruginosa*
   (C) Respiratory syncytial virus
   (D) *Salmonella* spp.
   (E) *Streptococcus pneumoniae*

50. A 7-year-old girl is brought to the emergency department by her parents because of concerns that she is not growing and not developing appropriately. The parents say that the patient has cold intolerance, easy fatigability, and polyuria. A physical examination is notable for short stature and bilateral papilledema. Thyroid function tests are notable for low levels of triiodothyronine, thyroxine, and thyroid-stimulating hormone. An MRI shows an enhancing multilobulated suprasellar mass with ring calcification in the region of the sella turcica. If the lesion represents a primary intracranial neoplasm, which of the following is the most likely diagnosis?

   (A) Craniopharyngioma
   (B) Ependymoma
   (C) Hemangioblastoma
   (D) Prolactinoma
   (E) Thyrotropinoma

1. **The correct answer is C.** It is important to understand that the question is asking for the sensitivity. It is calculated by TP/(TP + FN), where TP means true-positive and FN means false-negative. The true-positives in the vignette represent those with the cancer who correctly tested positive with this new test (60). False-negatives are those with the cancer who tested negative with the new test (40); thus, 60/(60 + 40) = 60%. Screening tests theoretically would aim to identify all those with the disease, and therefore high sensitivities are desired. In this case, 60% represents a low number, and the ca-1panc blood test would not be a good screening test for the cancer.

   Answer A is incorrect. The 10.0% figure represents the prevalence of the disease, calculated as total cancer/total people (100/1,000).

   Answer B is incorrect. The 37.5% figure is the positive predictive value, or the probability that someone with a positive test (ca-1panc) truly does have the cancer. The predictive values vary with how prevalent a disease is in the population. It is calculated as TP/(TP + FP) (where TP means true-positive and FP means false-positive) or 60/(60 + 100) = 37.5%.

   Answer D is incorrect. The 88.8% figure represents the specificity of the blood test, which measures how well the test detects those without the disease. It is important to correctly detect those without the disease in order to prevent them from undergoing unnecessary treatment or studies that could be painful or harmful to the patient. It is calculated as TN/(TN + FP) (where TN means true-negative and FP means false-positive), or 800/(800 + 100) = 88.8%

   Answer E is incorrect. The 90.0% figure simply represents the percentage of people without the cancer, 900/1000.

   Answer F is incorrect. The 95.2% figure is the negative predictive value, or the probability that the person with a negative test really does not have the cancer. It is calculated as TN/(TN + FN) (where TN means true-negative and FN means false-negative), or 800/(800 + 40) = 95.2%.

2. **The correct answer is A.** Pregnancy is considered to be a state of hypercoagulability with an increased risk for deep venous thrombosis and pulmonary embolus. A major concern is that a deep venous thrombus can lodge within the pulmonary arterial system. This, in turn, can result in pulmonary hypertension, hypoxia, and, in the worst case, right-sided heart failure and death. Pregnant women who have an indication for anticoagulation therapy (in this case, both stasis and endothelial injury secondary to her trauma) should be treated with an anticoagulant. Heparin is the preferred anticoagulant because it does not cross the placenta.

   Answer B is incorrect. Indomethacin is a nonsteroidal anti-inflammatory agent and is contraindicated in the third trimester of pregnancy because it will close the ductus arteriosus prematurely.

   Answer C is incorrect. Prostaglandin E_2 can be applied topically to ripen the cervix and promote induction of labor; however, in this patient, immediate induction of labor is not desired.

   Answer D is incorrect. Streptokinase is a thrombolytic agent used in the treatment of early myocardial infarction.

   Answer E is incorrect. Warfarin cannot be used because it can cross the placenta and has been implicated in nasal hypoplasia and skeletal abnormalities in the fetus in the first trimester. It also causes diffuse central nervous system abnormalities, particularly optic atrophy during pregnancy.

3. **The correct answer is D.** The neonate suffers from transposition of the great vessels, in which the aorta rises from the right ventricle and the pulmonary artery from the left ventricle. It is a common congenital heart defect in

the children of mothers with diabetes. Without a shunt, transposition is incompatible with life. If the infant is born without the shunt, an artificial shunt can be created by balloon atrial septostomy, and prostaglandin E_1 can be given to salvage whatever patent ductus arteriosus might remain. Once stabilized, the infant can then be taken for corrective surgery.

Answer A is incorrect. Coarctation of the aorta would not cause early cyanosis and is not associated with transposition of the great vessels.

Answer B is incorrect. A concomitant ventricular septal defect (VSD), while sometimes present in patients with transposition of the great vessels, is not the underlying pathophysiology of this infant's cyanosis. Additionally, if this patient had a VSD, there probably would have been little reason to create an additional shunt in the atria.

Answer C is incorrect. A prostaglandin E_1 infusion delays the closure of the PDA; however, this confers a protective advantage in patients with transposition of the great vessels, as it allows for mixing of blood. It is not the underlying pathophysiology of transposition of the great vessels.

Answer E is incorrect. An overriding aorta is one component of tetralogy of Fallot. Although tetralogy of Fallot is a cause of early cyanosis, an isolated overriding aorta would not cause the emergent hypoxia seen in this infant.

4. **The correct answer is E.** The patient presents with the classic signs of Hodgkin's disease, and the biopsy demonstrates the presence of Reed-Sternberg cells with reactive lymphocytes. Prednisone is a part of many of the multidrug treatment regimens for treating Hodgkin's disease.

Answer A is incorrect. Colchicine is used for acute gout.

Answer B is incorrect. Cyclosporine is an immunosuppressant used in transplant patients and autoimmune disorders.

Answer C is incorrect. Hydroxyurea is used for treatment of sickle cell anemia and to suppress high WBC counts in acute leukemia and chronic myelogenous leukemia.

Answer D is incorrect. Metformin is a drug used in diabetes treatment.

5. **The correct answer is E.** This patient suffers from McArdle's disease, a glycogen storage disorder in which glycogen phosphorylase is deficient in muscle. The enzyme is responsible for liberating individual units of glucose-1-phosphate from branches of a glycogen molecule. Onset of the disease typically occurs in adolescence or early adulthood and is characterized by muscle cramping, rapid fatigue, and poor endurance during exertion. Severe myoglobinuria is also observed in some patients.

Answer A is incorrect. Acid maltase is the defective enzyme in Pompe's disease, another glycogen storage disorder. The findings in Pompe's disease typically manifest in early childhood and include respiratory difficulties (due to diaphragmatic weakness) and progressive loss of muscle tone.

Answer B is incorrect. Homocystinuria is an inborn error of metabolism caused by a defect in cystathionine synthase, the enzyme that converts homocysteine to cystathionine. In addition to marfanlike features, these patients are at increased risk of a variety of cardiovascular derangements, including premature vascular disease and early death.

Answer C is incorrect. Glucose-6-phosphatase is the enzyme responsible for converting glucose-6-phosphate to glucose. It is a component of gluconeogenesis. A deficiency of this enzyme could cause a mild hypoglycemia in some individuals but would not be expected to produce the symptoms observed in this patient.

Answer D is incorrect. α-1,6-Glucosidase is the enzyme responsible for the debranching of glycogen. It is implicated in Cori's disease but is not implicated in McArdle's disease.

FULL-LENGTH EXAM

Test Block 2

6. **The correct answer is B.** This patient is likely suffering from hyperparathyroidism due to a parathyroid adenoma. Primary hyperparathyroidism causes hypercalcemia, hypophosphatemia, increased alkaline phosphatase activity, and an increase in serum parathyroid hormone (PTH). Hypercalcemia can cause metastatic calcification, including nephrocalcinosis, and development of renal stones and peptic duodenal ulcer disease. Furthermore, PTH elevation can lead to a variety of bone abnormalities, including osteitis fibrosa cystica, a condition that results from excessive bone resorption and fibrous replacement of the marrow, leading to cystic spaces and areas of hemorrhage, or "brown tumors." Clinically, patients may present with bone pain and fractures.

Answer A is incorrect. Hypertrophic osteoarthropathy is seen in patients with a variety of illnesses, including lung cancer, sepsis, endocarditis, and inflammatory bowel disease. Patients frequently present with digital clubbing and painful swelling of wrists, fingers, elbows, and other joints. New bone formation is present at the ends of these bones.

Answer C is incorrect. Osteopetrosis is characterized by brittle, dense, thickened bones that fracture easily. The disease has an autosomal dominant and recessive mode of inheritance.

Answer D is incorrect. Osteoporosis, which is characterized by decreased bone mass, pain, and fractures, is most commonly seen in postmenopausal women and the elderly. Osteoporosis is associated with normal Ca^{2+} and phosphorus levels, and increased alkaline phosphatase activity.

Answer E is incorrect. Paget's disease of the bone, like osteitis fibrosa cystica, is a result of excessive bone resorption. In Paget's disease, the resorbed bone is replaced by a soft, disorganized bone matrix with a mosaic, rather than trabecular, pattern. Alkaline phosphatase activity is increased. Patients can present with bone pain, fractures, deformity, and sensory deficits due to nerve impingement.

7. **The correct answer is D.** Waterhouse-Friderichsen syndrome is a possible complication of meningococcemia. In this disorder, bilateral hemorrhage into the adrenal gland causes adrenal insufficiency. This results in hypotension, tachycardia, a rapidly enlarging petechial skin lesion, disseminated intravascular coagulation, and coma.

Answer A is incorrect. Hemolytic-uremic syndrome (HUS) is characterized by acute renal failure and thrombocytopenia with hemolytic anemia. HUS can be a complication of infection caused by *E. coli* O157:H7 and not *Neisseria meningitidis*.

Answer B is incorrect. Rheumatic fever is characterized by fever, migratory polyarthritis, and carditis. It may follow group A streptococcal pharyngitis.

Answer C is incorrect. Fever, a new murmur, Janeway lesions, and nail-bed hemorrhages are all signs of bacterial endocarditis. Acute endocarditis is caused by *Staphylococcus aureus* and subacute infection can be caused by *Streptococcus viridans*.

Answer E is incorrect. Guillain-Barré syndrome is characterized by rapidly progressing ascending paralysis. It is thought to follow a variety of infectious diseases, such as cytomegalovirus, Epstein-Barr virus, HIV, and gastroenteritis caused by *Campylobacter jejuni*.

8. **The correct answer is E.** Prostaglandin (PG) I_2 inhibits platelet aggregation and therefore is an antithrombotic agent. On the other hand, thromboxane (Tx) A_2 increases platelet aggregation and is a prothrombotic agent. COX-2 inhibitors selectively decrease PGI_2 leaving the action of TxA_2 unopposed. This could well result in increased cerebrovascular and cardiovascular events due to the tonic, unopposed prothrombotic action of TxA_2.

Answer A is incorrect. Coxibs do not increase prostaglandin (PG) I_2. Coxibs are thought to spare the gastric mucosa because they selectively block the synthesis of other prostaglandins, not because they increase the production of PGI_2.

Answer B is incorrect. Coxibs do not increase the activity of thromoboxane (Tx) A_2. They lead to a prothrombotic state by decreasing the activity of the antithrombotic prostaglandin I_2, which normally opposes TxA_2 and keeps it in check.

Answer C is incorrect. Coxibs do not decrease thromboxane A_2, they leave its prothrombotic action unopposed.

Answer D is incorrect. Aspirin is a COX-1 and COX-2 inhibitor that nonselectively decreases all prostaglandins.

9. **The correct answer is A.** This patient's clinical presentation is consistent with anemia of chronic disease (ACD) in the setting of systemic lupus erythematosus. ACD presents with low serum iron levels, elevated ferritin levels, decreased total iron-binding capacity, and microcytic/normocytic RBCs on blood smear. ACD resolves if the underlying condition is corrected, but in the absence of a successful primary treatment, erythropoietin can be effective in treating the anemia. Iron therapy is not effective in treating this disorder.

Answer B is incorrect. Iron therapy is inappropriate in treating anemia of chronic disease, since iron stores are not low.

Answer C is incorrect. Folate supplementation would be appropriate in macrocytic anemia caused by folate deficiency.

Answer D is incorrect. Parenteral vitamin B_{12} therapy is appropriate for pernicious anemia caused by lack of intrinsic factor, which is necessary for vitamin B_{12} absorption.

Answer E is incorrect. Phlebotomy is appropriate in treating cases of iron overload, as seen in patients with chronic transfusion therapy and hemochromatosis.

10. **The correct answer is B.** DNA ligase is an enzyme that binds two polynucleotide chains together. It joins Okazaki fragments together to form a continuous section of DNA on the lagging strand.

Answer A is incorrect. Helicase is a eukaryotic enzyme that unwinds double-stranded DNA.

Answer C is incorrect. Polymerases synthesize new DNA strands.

Answer D is incorrect. Primase is an RNA polymerase that makes RNA primers.

Answer E is incorrect. RNase H is an enzyme that digests RNA primers.

11. **The correct answer is B.** Afferent pain fibers of the heart enter the posterior horn of the spinal cord at the same level as the brachial plexus, thus leading to pain that is perceived as being located in the neck and shoulder region.

Answer A is incorrect. Sensory neurons have their origin in the posterior horn of the spinal cord, not the anterior horn, where efferent neurons arise.

Answer C is incorrect. Lymphatic drainage does occur in the left upper quadrant, but it plays no role in the model of referred myocardial pain.

Answer D is incorrect. The heart and the neck and shoulder region do not share similar parasympathetic innervation patterns.

Answer E is incorrect. The heart and the neck and shoulder region do not share similar sympathetic innervation patterns.

12. **The correct answer is E.** Gait disturbances and ataxia are results of the tumor impinging on the cerebellar vermis. Some of the symptoms arise from obstructive hydrocephalus. Medulloblastomas, ependymomas, and hemangioblastomas are childhood primary brain tumors that can result in hydrocephalus by obstruction of the fourth ventricle. However, the patient's gait disturbances and truncal ataxia indicate medulloblastoma as the most likely cause. Medulloblastomas are a form of primitive neuroectodermal tumor (PNET) and ap-

pear as small blue cells arranged in perivascular rosettes. They are most often found at the cerebellar vermis.

Answer A is incorrect. Fried egg cells are typical of oligodendrogliomas, which are more common in adults.

Answer B is incorrect. Psammoma bodies are typical of meningiomas, which are not likely to cause the symptoms listed. In addition, meningiomas are more common in adults.

Answer C is incorrect. Pseudopalisading tumor cells with necrosis indicate glioblastoma multiforme, which is more common in adults.

Answer D is incorrect. Rod-shaped blepharoblasts (basal ciliary bodies) are typical of ependymomas.

13. **The correct answer is E.** Pellagra is caused by vitamin B_3 (niacin) deficiency. Patients classically present with diarrhea, dermatitis, and dementia (and beefy glossitis). Other water-soluble vitamins include B_2 (riboflavin), niacin (B_3), biotin, folate, and cobalamin (B_{12}).

Answer A is incorrect. Increased erythrocyte hemolysis is the result of vitamin E deficiency, which results in increased fragility of erythrocytes. Vitamin E is an antioxidant that protects erythrocytes from hemolysis. It is fat-soluble.

Answer B is incorrect. Osteomalacia is due to vitamin D deficiency. Vitamin D is a fat-soluble vitamin.

Answer C is incorrect. Night blindness is a consequence of vitamin A (retinol) deficiency. Vitamin A is a constituent of visual pigments and is a fat-soluble vitamin.

Answer D is incorrect. Osteomalacia is due to vitamin D deficiency. Vitamin D is a fat-soluble vitamin.

14. **The correct answer is E.** Lactation is maintained by prolactin secretion from the anterior pituitary. Prolactin prevents ovulation by several mechanisms. It inhibits the secretion of gonadotropin-releasing hormone (GnRH) from the hypothalamus and inhibits the action of GnRH at the anterior pituitary, thus de-

creasing the secretion of luteinizing hormone (LH) and follicle-stimulating hormone (FSH). Finally, it inhibits the actions of LH and FSH on the ovaries. Before this woman can become pregnant, she will have to stop nursing her son.

Answer A is incorrect. Lactation and the resulting high levels of prolactin do not affect estrogen's action on the ovary.

Answer B is incorrect. Lactation is maintained by prolactin. It does not decrease its secretion.

Answer C is incorrect. Lactation results in decreased secretion of follicle-stimulating hormone.

Answer D is incorrect. Lactation does not cause sterility.

15. **The correct answer is B.** The disorder described in the question is Hirschsprung's disease, a disorder of neural crest cells. Specifically, neural crest cells fail to migrate to distal portions of the colon, leading to a congenital lack of parasympathetic ganglion cells. This produces a functional obstruction of the colon, as peristalsis cannot take place. As a result, the abdomen becomes distended, eventually causing bilious vomiting. Pathology will reveal a lack of ganglia in Meissner's and Auerbach's plexuses and nerve fiber hypertrophy in Meissner's plexus.

Answer A is incorrect. The endoderm gives rise to the epithelial lining of much of the gastrointestinal tract, but this is not a disorder of the epithelium.

Answer C is incorrect. The neuroectoderm gives rise to most components of the nervous system but not to the ganglia.

Answer D is incorrect. The mesoderm gives rise to smooth muscle, but this patient has Hirschsprung's disease, a disorder of colonic ganglion cells, not smooth muscle.

Answer E is incorrect. The surface ectoderm gives rise to the epithelial lining of the lower anal canal, but this patient has Hirschsprung's disease, which is not a disorder of the epithelium.

16. **The correct answer is B.** Desmopressin (dDAVP) is 1-deamino-8-D-arginine vasopressin, an analog of ADH. This woman has central diabetes insipidus caused by trauma to the posterior pituitary. This inhibits secretion of ADH. Repleting her ADH is the most appropriate therapy of the options given. If dDAVP is chosen, the patient's sodium and fluid status should be carefully monitored, because acute trauma to the posterior pituitary can lead to a triphasic response. In phase 1, the injured pituitary ceases secretion of ADH, resulting in the clinical picture presented in the question stem. In phase 2, the death of pituitary tissue causes the release of ADH stores, leading to fluid retention and hyponatremia consistent with the syndrome of inappropriate ADH secretion. Phase 3 arises from permanent damage to the posterior pituitary, resulting in persistent central diabetes insipidus.

Answer A is incorrect. Demeclocycline is used to treat the syndrome of inappropriate ADH secretion. This compound acts to inhibit ADH action and would exacerbate her condition.

Answer C is incorrect. Furosemide is a loop diuretic and is likely to exacerbate her condition.

Answer D is incorrect. Insulin is an inappropriate treatment. Central diabetes insipidus shares only the symptoms of polydipsia and polyuria with diabetes mellitus. The treatments and causes are completely different.

Answer E is incorrect. Mannitol is an osmotic diuretic that would exacerbate her condition.

17. **The correct answer is A.** This patient has a number of risk factors for suicide completion, including an organized plan, male gender, older age, depression, ethanol abuse, and no spouse (other risk factors include loss of rational thinking, lack of social support, and chronic illness). Suicide completers tend to have major depressive disorder or alcoholism, carefully laid-out plans, and effective suicidal means (e.g., guns or hanging). In addition, they often hide their plans from friends and family. Asking patients about suicide does not put ideas in their heads. If a patient has suicidal ideation and lacks family support, a hospital is the best place to manage them acutely.

Answer B is incorrect. This patient may be given an antidepressant while in the hospital, but a prescription alone is insufficient care for this patient. Also, antidepressants can take up to 3–4 weeks to take effect.

Answer C is incorrect. The patient does need to speak with a psychiatrist, but an inpatient setting is more appropriate than an outpatient setting.

Answer D is incorrect. Ignoring this patient's major depressive disorder with suicidal ideation is a serious breach of standard of care.

Answer E is incorrect. The patient has not been declared incompetent. You cannot tell his children against his wishes.

18. **The correct answer is A.** Patients with AIDS are susceptible to a variety of infections that are unusual in the immunocompetent population. Among diseases that cause fever and headache in these patients are *Cryptococcus*, toxoplasmosis, and central nervous system lymphoma. An encapsulated yeast that stains with India ink is a pathognomonic description of *Cryptococcus neoformans*, which is a yeast found in pigeon droppings. Infection occurs when patients inhale fungus particles, which can lead to pneumonia. Initial treatment of *C. neoformans* is IV amphotericin B, followed by fluconazole once the patient's condition is stable. Amphotericin toxicity can cause fever and chills, hypotension, nephrotoxicity, and arrhythmias. The arrhythmias are due to QT prolongation, which is exacerbated by changes in potassium and magnesium levels.

Answer B is incorrect. Bone marrow suppression is seen with a number of drugs, including flucytosine.

Answer C is incorrect. Flushing can be caused by caspofungin, an antifungal medication used to treat aspergillosis infection. Caspofungin inhibits synthesis of an essential component of the fungal cell wall. Other adverse effects include gastrointestinal upset.

Answer D is incorrect. Gynecomastia is an adverse effect of fluconazole treatment. The -azole antifungals inhibit ergosterol synthesis. They are used to treat systemic mycoses but are less effective than amphotericin B. Other adverse effects include liver dysfunction and fever.

Answer E is incorrect. Nausea and vomiting are seen with flucytosine, which is used to treat systemic fungal infections. Flucytosine inhibits DNA synthesis because it is converted to fluorouracil in vivo.

19. **The correct answer is E.** Recall that blood supply to the entire leg comes from the femoral artery. The femoral artery runs anteriorly on the thigh until reaching the adductor hiatus, where it dives deep and becomes the popliteal artery. The posterior tibial artery branches from the popliteal artery and runs deep in the calf until the ankle, where it lies in the superficial fossa immediately posterior to the medial malleolus. When there is a penetrating or crushing injury to the leg, it is important to palpate this artery and assess for symmetry.

Answer A is incorrect. The posterior tibial artery does run between the heads of the gastrocnemius muscle, but it is deep in the leg and is nonpalpable. You should remember from anatomy that the palpable pulses in the leg are the femoral artery in the groin, the popliteal artery in the popliteal fossa on the posterior aspect of the knee, the posterior tibial posterior to the medial malleolus, and the dorsalis pedis in the first interosseous space on the dorsum of the foot.

Answer B is incorrect. The popliteal artery is found in the popliteal fossa on the posterior aspect of the knee.

Answer C is incorrect. There is no palpable artery anterior to the medial malleolus.

Answer D is incorrect. The dorsalis pedis artery runs along the dorsal surface of the foot and is a continuation of the anterior tibial artery.

20. **The correct answer is B.** This patient has Churg-Strauss syndrome (also known as allergic granulomatosis and angiitis), which is one of a trio of diseases (Wegener's granulomatosis and microscopic polyangiitis being the others) that are commonly referred to as the ANCA (antineutrophil cytoplasmic antibody)–associated vasculitides (ie, diseases causing inflammation of blood or lymphatic vessels). Fifty to seventy percent of patients have elevated levels of ANCA, usually the perinuclear pattern of staining type. Patients often have preexisting asthma and allergic rhinitis, and they often present with markedly elevated eosinophil counts and mononeuritis multiplex (simultaneous deficits of two or several peripheral nerves in different areas of the body). Other symptoms include uveitis, conductive hearing loss, and muscle/joint pain. An eosinophilic gastroenteritis may precede the onset of the other symptoms.

Answer A is incorrect. Autoantibodies to acetylcholine receptors are not particularly associated with Churg-Strauss syndrome. Myasthenia gravis is characterized by an autoimmune attack on the acetylcholine receptors of the neuromuscular junction between motor neurons and skeletal muscle fibers.

Answer C is incorrect. Autoantibodies to oligodendrocytes are not particularly associated with Churg-Strauss syndrome. There is evidence suggesting that multiple sclerosis may be partially caused by autoimmune antibody attack on central nervous system myelin-secreting oligodendrocytes.

Answer D is incorrect. Autoantibodies to RBCs, which may be found in certain cases of immune hemolytic anemia, are not particularly associated with Churg-Strauss syndrome.

Answer E is incorrect. Autoantibodies to thyroid-stimulating hormone (TSH) receptors are not particularly associated with Churg-Strauss syndrome. Graves' disease is a disorder resulting from IgG-type autoantibodies to the TSH receptor.

21. **The correct answer is C.** Danazol is an androgen that is commonly used to treat en-

dometriosis. The excess testosterone decreases gonadotropin-releasing hormone secretion from the hypothalamus, lessening the release of luteinizing and follicle-stimulating hormones, which are necessary to the growth of the endometrium during the menstrual cycle. Adverse effects include menstrual irregularities, weight gain, and acne.

Answer A is incorrect. The antiestrogens clomiphene and tamoxifen are used for infertility and breast cancer treatment, respectively. Tamoxifen has an adverse effect on the endometrium, predisposing patients to uterine cancer.

Answer B is incorrect. Estrogen supplementation would exacerbate the endometriosis, not alleviate the symptoms. Endometriosis is an ectopic endometrium that continues to respond to the hormonal fluctuations of the menstrual cycle, including estrogen.

Answer D is incorrect. Mineralocorticoids such as aldosterone help maintain body water control and electrolyte balance. Aldosterone has no effect on the endometrium.

Answer E is incorrect. Progesterone promotes the development of the endometrium. Giving exogenous progesterone would only exacerbate endometriosis.

22. **The correct answer is A.** The key word here is *colonic*. Barrett's esophagus is the term used to describe benign intestinal metaplasia of the distal esophagus. Normally, this epithelium should be squamous. A long history of gastroesophageal reflux leads to Barrett's esophagus through repetitive injury of the mucosa. Metaplastic cells are often goblet cells, normally present in the colon. These goblet cells stain for mucin, which can be used as a marker for intestinal metaplasia in the biopsy specimen. Barrett's esophagus may be a harbinger of adenocarcinoma of the esophagus.

Answer B is incorrect. *Candida* esophagitis is associated with immunosuppression, antibiotic therapy, and a few other conditions, but not gastroesophageal reflux. On endoscopy, the lesion would appear patchy white on the mucosa.

Answer C is incorrect. Chagas' disease is caused by *Trypanosoma cruzi*, a protozoan parasite prevalent in South America. These organisms invade and impinge on striated muscle, including cardiac muscle. The esophageal sphincter may be affected, leading to achalasia (persistent contraction of the lower esophageal sphincter and aperistalsis). Mucin-positive cells are not involved.

Answer D is incorrect. Esophageal varices are dilated submucosal veins seen in portal hypertension. This condition may lead to severe bleeding and death. The varices can be seen on endoscopy and do not involve mucin-positive cells.

Answer E is incorrect. Longitudinal lacerations are typically irregular longitudinal tears along the gastroesophageal junction. Such lacerations resulting from trauma or severe vomiting put the patient at risk for Mallory-Weiss syndrome: bleeding from the gastroesophageal junction as a result of severe retching. Esophageal varices also may lead to such bleeding.

23. **The correct answer is E.** Before binding mRNA, aminoacyl-tRNA first binds guanosine triphosphate (GTP) and elongation factor EF1-α. When tRNA binds to the A site of the ribosome, GTP is hydrolyzed to guanosine diphosphate (GDP). The GDP-EF1-α complex then binds elongation factor EF-β, allowing GDP to be released. Next, GTP binds the complex and EF-β disassociates, leaving GTP-EF1-α regenerated for another cycle. Therefore, increased affinity of EF1-β for the mutant EF1-α counteracts the increased affinity of EF1-α for GDP.

Answer A is incorrect. Decreased affinity of elongation factor EF1-α for guanosine triphosphate would decrease protein synthesis even further.

Answer B is incorrect. Decreased affinity of elongation factor EF1-β for guanosine triphosphate would decrease protein synthesis.

Answer C is incorrect. Elimination of elongation factor EF1-α would completely halt protein synthesis.

Answer D is incorrect. Elimination of elongation factor EF1-β would completely halt protein synthesis.

24. **The correct answer is B.** Paclitaxel (Taxol) binds tubulin and hyperstabilizes polymerized microtubules, thus preventing anaphase. It is derived from the pacific yew tree (*Taxus brevifolia*), and is currently used with carboplatin as first-line therapy for metastatic ovarian carcinoma. It is also used to treat metastatic adenocarcinoma of the breast.

Answer A is incorrect. Cyclophosphamide and ifosfamide are alkylating agents that covalently link DNA and are useful in the treatment of non-Hodgkin's lymphoma and breast and ovarian carcinomas. Cisplatin and carboplatin are platinum-derived compounds that are also thought to act like alkylating agents—they are used with paclitaxel for primary chemotherapy for ovarian cancer, and are also effective for treatment of testicular, bladder, and lung carcinomas.

Answer C is incorrect. Colchicine depolymerizes microtubules and is derived from the autumn crocus (*Colchicum autumnale*). It is used in the treatment of acute gout attacks.

Answer D is incorrect. Cytarabine inhibits DNA polymerase and is useful in the treatment of acute myelogenous leukemia.

Answer E is incorrect. Etopoadverse inhibits topoisomerase II and is derived from a springtime herb (*Podophyllum peltatum*). It is used in the treatment of oat cell and testicular carcinomas.

25. **The correct answer is B.** This girl has impetigo, caused by *Streptococcus pyogenes*, a gram-positive group A β-hemolytic organism that is bacitracin-sensitive. This infection is characterized by an eruption of vesicles on the face. These vesicles later turn into pustules with a characteristic honey-colored crust. A distinctly *bullous* form of impetigo is caused by S. *aureus*.

Answer A is incorrect. Sabouraud's agar is required to culture fungi, not *Streptococcus pyogenes*.

Answer C is incorrect. *Mycobacterium, Brucella, Francisella, Listeria, Yersinia, Legionella,* and *Salmonella* are facultative intracellular organisms, but *Streptococcus pyogenes* is not.

Answer D is incorrect. The bacterium is a group A β-hemolytic organism. *Streptococcus agalactiae* is a group B β-hemolytic organism.

Answer E is incorrect. Protein M protects the bacterium from phagocytosis, but it makes the bacterium more sensitive to host defenses due to antibody production against protein M.

26. **The correct answer is D.** Patients with von Hippel–Lindau disease are at increased risk of developing renal cell carcinoma.

Answer A is incorrect. Patients with Down's syndrome, or trisomy 21, are at increased risk of developing acute lymphocytic leukemia.

Answer B is incorrect. Patients with familial adenomatous polyposis develop colon cancer if the polyps are not resected.

Answer C is incorrect. Patients with neurofibromatosis type 1 are at increased risk of developing malignancies.

Answer E is incorrect. Patients with androgen insensitivity are normal-appearing females but can have undescended (inguinal) testicles. If these are not excised, the risk of malignancy, including testicular seminoma, is greatly increased.

27. **The correct answer is C.** This patient most likely has primary biliary cirrhosis, which is a chronic autoimmune liver disorder that may initially present with severe itching, hepatomegaly, and xanthomas (yellow nodules/plaques filled with lipid-laden histiocytes, often a sign of hypercholesterolemia). Jaundice develops later in the disease, as hyperbilirubinemia does not occur until there is marked liver damage. The pathologic hallmark is described by the liver biopsy results in the question stem. Over 90% of patients have elevated levels of antimitochondrial antibodies.

Answer A is incorrect. While patients with primary biliary cirrhosis may also have other autoimmune disorders, the association with anticentromere antibodies is not as strong as the association with antimitochondrial antibodies. It is worth noting that the presence of elevated levels of anticentromere antibodies is often associated with the CREST variant of scleroderma.

Answer B is incorrect. While patients with primary biliary cirrhosis may also have other autoimmune disorders, the association with antihistone antibodies is not as strong as the association with antimitochondrial antibodies. It is worth noting that the presence of antihistone antibodies is often associated with drug-induced lupuslike syndromes.

Answer D is incorrect. While patients with primary biliary cirrhosis may also have other autoimmune disorders, the association with antinuclear antibodies is not as strong as the association with antimitochondrial antibodies.

Answer E is incorrect. While patients with primary biliary cirrhosis may also have other autoimmune disorders, the association with rheumatoid factor is not as strong as the association with antimitochondrial antibodies. It is worth noting that the presence of elevated levels of rheumatoid factor is often associated with rheumatoid arthritis.

28. **The correct answer is E.** Dietary modification (drastically limiting saturated and trans fats and cholesterol), weight loss, and aerobic exercise are the first-line treatment options for any patient with elevated cholesterol levels, and these lifestyle modifications should be attempted by this patient. Even though these efforts potentiate the effects of drug therapy in lowering LDL levels, they will likely have only a minimal effect in a patient with familial hypercholesterolemia. Statin medications are 3-hydroxy-3-methylglutaryl coenzyme A reductase inhibitors. By blocking the rate-limiting step in cholesterol synthesis, they can lower cholesterol levels, and are the most readily available pharmacologic agents used to treat elevated cholesterol. High-dose therapy with a statin such as atorvastatin, or combined therapy with one of the fibrate drugs, is usually initiated.

Answer A is incorrect. Niacin (vitamin B_3) can lower LDL and increase HDL levels. However, statin medications are first-line therapy for this disorder. Niacin can be added to the regimen as a third drug (with a fibrate) or can be used in patients who are refractory to statin treatment. Its use is often limited by tolerability (it causes flushing in the majority of patients).

Answer B is incorrect. Hormone replacement therapy is contraindicated in patients with high cholesterol due to the increased risk of heart attack and stroke. Also, hormone replacement therapy is not necessary for a woman in her 20s.

Answer C is incorrect. LDL apheresis is a method for selectively removing LDL molecules from the blood using immunoadsorption columns. This process takes at least 3 hours and is done every 1–2 weeks. It is very expensive and not readily available.

Answer D is incorrect. Liver transplantation can dramatically lower LDL levels in patients with familial hypercholesterolemia by providing them with normal LDL receptors. However, the risks associated with transplantation make this option a last resort.

29. **The correct answer is B.** The therapeutic privilege is a rare case of an appropriate exception to informed consent. The principle is that informing the patient will not be medically sound for the patient. In general, a physician should consult another physician not involved in the patient's care, a psychiatrist, and/or an ethics committee when invoking this principle. It does not refer to withholding information a physician believes will make a patient less likely to have a procedure performed.

Answer A is incorrect. Only a patient can waive their own right to informed consent.

Answer C is incorrect. Any competent adult can make informed consent.

Answer D is incorrect. Usually, physicians must obtain informed consent. In some instances, a qualified nurse or other medical professional may obtain informed consent; however a nursing volunteer can certainly not.

Answer E is incorrect. A competent patient may acknowledge informed consent by any means.

30. **The correct answer is B.** This patient has the classic presentation of pheochromocytoma, a tumor of the adrenal medulla that causes hypersecretion of catecholamines. Patients tend to experience sudden "spells" of elevated blood pressure, palpitations, headache, diaphoresis, and anxiety. Diagnosis of this disorder is made by demonstration of elevated urinary excretion of catecholamines or their metabolites, metanephrines and vanillylmandelic acid. Pharmacologically, this disorder is managed with nonselective α antagonists (phenoxybenzamine and phentolamine).

Answer A is incorrect. Phenelzine, a monoamine oxidase inhibitor, is used to treat depression and would have no effect in treating this disorder.

Answer C is incorrect. Phenylephrine, an α agonist, would not be appropriate for the treatment of pheochromocytoma because it would worsen the patient's hypertension via its vasoconstrictive effect at α_1 receptors.

Answer D is incorrect. Prazosin, a selective competitive blocker of α_1 receptors, is useful in the treatment of hypertension, but it is not routinely used in the treatment of pheochromocytoma.

Answer E is incorrect. Propranolol, a nonselective β-blocker, is not indicated for the treatment of pheochromocytoma because its actions are limited to β receptors. Thus, it would have little effect in antagonizing the α_1-agonist actions of norepinephrine that are of concern in these tumors.

31. **The correct answer is D.** This patient has a potentially reversible case of dementia caused by normal pressure hydrocephalus (NPH), with the classic triad of incontinence, mental decline, and gait difficulty. Patients with NPH often demonstrate mild bradykinesia, and their gait has been described as "magnetic" because their feet seemingly cling to the floor. The score of 26/30 on the Mini-Mental State Examination (MMSE) is not indicative of serious cognitive impairment but indicates that an abnormality is present. Regardless, the patient should be imaged with magnetic resonance imaging to rule out a mass lesion that could cause similar symptoms. The pathophysiology of NPH is not well understood, but it is thought to be due to disruption of the neurons because of stretching secondary to dilation of the ventricles due to excessive cerebrospinal fluid production, decreased absorption, or both. It is imperative to identify these patients because timely intervention with a ventriculoperitoneal shunt can reverse the dementia and decline. The Miller Fisher test can help determine the potential success of shunting; after removal of approximately 30 mL of cerebrospinal fluid, the gait is reassessed for improvement.

Answer A is incorrect. Alzheimer's disease can present with some of the symptoms in this case. However, significant physical impairment tends to occur later in the Alzheimer's disease process and would thus correlate with a much lower score on the Mini-Mental State Examination. The time course and the relatively rapid progression in symptoms are not consistent with the diagnosis.

Answer B is incorrect. Hypothyroidism, another potential cause of reversible dementia in the elderly, should be ruled out early in the workup. This patient's thyroid-stimulating hormone level is normal, indicating euthyroidism.

Answer C is incorrect. Multi-infarct dementia is the most common cause of cognitive decline with a stepwise drop in function in the setting of prior cerebrovascular disease and stroke. In this case, the decline has been steadily progressive in a patient with no history of vascular disease.

Answer E is incorrect. Parkinson's disease classically presents with bradykinesia, masklike facies, shuffling gait, tremor, and rigidity. This patient has mild bradykinesia and no rigidity or tremor, so this diagnosis is a less likely possibility.

32. **The correct answer is D.** Protein malnutrition, or kwashiorkor, is characterized by an inadequate intake of protein but adequate intake of calories. Edema is the most common presenting symptom, but depigmented hair, anorexia, fatty liver changes, and skin lesions are also seen. Edema is caused by low levels of protein that decrease the plasma oncotic pressure and results in a loss of fluid into interstitial spaces. This patient's history and presentation are consistent with a low-protein, normal-calorie diet.

Answer A is incorrect. If this child was getting rice milk only and developed a fat deficiency, then she would likely have fat and calorie malnutrition but would not present with edema.

Answer B is incorrect. Fat malnutrition would be unlikely in this child based on the presentation. Rice milk has about one-fourth the amount of fat in cow's milk or soy milk. Fats, especially the essential fatty acids linoleic and linolenic acid, are largely obtained in the diet. They are required for the development of cell membranes and nerve cell sheaths. Deficiency in fat causes developmental delays but not edema. In addition, with adequate calories, the body can generate most fatty acids.

Answer C is incorrect. Marasmus describes protein and calorie malnutrition. The deficiency of calories, however, is the real problem, and marasmus can occur even with an adequate protein intake. Like kwashiorkor, marasmus is seen in infants at times of diet change such as weaning from breast milk in areas of the world where food can be scarce. The symptoms, however, are muscle wasting, weakness, arrested growth, and anemia.

Answer E is incorrect. Vitamin deficiencies have various effects. Prolonged thiamine deficiency in children can cause edema, but edema in the setting of low protein intake is more likely caused by the protein deficiency.

33. **The correct answer is E.** Ziehl-Neelsen stain is used to reveal acid-fast bacteria. This patient most likely has tuberculosis, which is an acid-fast, gram-positive aerobic bacillus.

Answer A is incorrect. Congo red is used to visualize amyloid, showing apple-green birefringence in polarized light.

Answer B is incorrect. Giemsa's stain is useful for *Borrelia, Plasmodium,* trypanosomes, and *Chlamydia.*

Answer C is incorrect. India ink is the stain of choice for *Cryptococcus neoformans.*

Answer D is incorrect. Periodic acid-Schiff stains glycogen, and thus it can be used to visualize mucopolysaccharides. In addition, is used to diagnose Whipple's disease.

34. **The correct answer is A.** The patient has symptoms of hypercalcemia, which because of a normal phosphorus level is unlikely to be due to an overactive parathyroid gland. With a history of smoking and "coin" lesion in the lung, you should suspect a lung tumor that produces parathyroid hormone–related peptide. Squamous cell carcinoma is a centrally located bronchogenic carcinoma.

Answer B is incorrect. Horner's syndrome is characterized by ptosis, miosis, and anhidrosis. It is a complication of lung cancer at the apex, referred to as a Pancoast tumor.

Answer C is incorrect. Chronic silica exposure is associated with increased tuberculosis susceptibility. Tuberculosis usually presents with chronic cough, hemoptysis, fevers, chills, and weight loss.

Answer D is incorrect. Cystic fibrosis causes respiratory, reproductive, and gastrointestinal symptoms.

Answer E is incorrect. Kartagener's syndrome is associated with sinusitis, bronchiectasis, and infertility.

Answer F is incorrect. Ectopic antidiuretic hormone production, which you could see with small-cell carcinoma, would cause water retention (oliguria) and fatigue.

Answer G is incorrect. Solitary parathyroid adenoma can present with hypercalcemia, but would have low serum phosphorus, not normal levels.

35. **The correct answer is A.** The gut-associated lymphoid tissue is a vital collection of peripheral lymphoid tissue. The image depicts the epithelium that lies above the Peyer's patches. Note that this epithelium is quite distinctive; several M cells can be seen (they are specialized for endocytosis and phagocytosis of gut luminal particles). Secretory polymeric (often dimerized) IgA is the main antibody present within the mucosal lining of the gut. It is synthesized by plasma cells that reside within the lamina propria. Of note is the fact that several gut pathogens, called IgA protease, express a virulence factor that cleaves the dimeric IgA antibodies.

Answer B is incorrect. IgD is found only on the surface of B lymphocytes; its function is not known.

Answer C is incorrect. IgE orchestrates the type I hypersensitivity response.

Answer D is incorrect. IgG is the main antibody produced during a secondary immune response and also the most abundant.

Answer E is incorrect. While IgM can be found within the gut lumen, IgA predominates.

36. **The correct answer is E.** Peaked T waves and prolonged PR intervals are evident on ECG in cases of hyperkalemia. Spironolactone is a potassium-sparing diuretic that inhibits K^+ secretion at the cortical collecting duct; therefore, an important side effect of spironolactone use is hyperkalemia.

Answer A is incorrect. Acetazolamide inhibits carbonic anhydrase at the proximal convoluted tubule to cause increased excretion of HCO_3^-. It has no effect on potassium concentrations and thus would not result in hyperkalemia.

Answer B is incorrect. As a loop diuretic, furosemide inhibits the cotransport ions (Na^+, K^+, and $2Cl^-$) in the thick ascending loop of Henle and causes secretion of potassium from the kidney. Hypokalemia can result.

Answer C is incorrect. Hydrochlorothiazide inhibits the reabsorption of NaCl at the distal tubule, and the resulting decrease in plasma volume will activate the renin-angiotensin-aldosterone system, leading to increased secretion of K^+ from the cortical collecting duct. Thus, hypokalemia is a side effect of excess hydrochlorothiazide.

Answer D is incorrect. Mannitol is an osmotic diuretic that increases urine output by increasing the osmolarity of fluid in the nephron. It has no effect on ion transport proteins and thus does not change potassium excretion.

37. **The correct answer is B.** This patient is suffering from vitamin D deficiency and osteomalacia. Osteomalacia can present with bone pain and muscles weakness with reduced bone density on radiographic exam. Vitamin D can be consumed in milk (ergocalciferol) or formed in sun-exposed skin (cholecalciferol). The active form of vitamin D is 1,25-dihydroxycholecalciferol (calcitriol), which is produced in the kidney, and its production is catalyzed by the enzyme 1-α-hydroxylase. The activity of 1-α-hydroxylase is increased by an elevated parathyroid hormone level, decreased serum calcium concentration, or decreased serum phosphate concentration.

Answer A is incorrect. With the help of 1-α-hydroxylase, 1,25-dihydroxycholecalciferol levels increase. Elevated levels do not increase the activity of this enzyme.

Answer C is incorrect. A decreased, rather than increased, serum Ca^{2+} will increase the enzyme's activity.

Answer D is incorrect. A decreased, rather than increased, serum phosphate will increase the enzyme's activity.

Answer E is incorrect. Increased sun exposure results in an increase of vitamin D_3 (cholecalciferol), which is formed in sun-exposed skin.

38. **The correct answer is E.** The disease that is described is Waldenström's macroglobuline-

mia, which is characterized by weakness, weight loss, a monoclonal M spike on serum protein electrophoresis, and a hyperviscosity syndrome. The hyperviscosity syndrome is caused by a large amount of IgM protein in the blood produced by a B-neoplasm. The IgMs are large proteins that interfere with microvascular and cellular processes, causing blood vessel damage, headaches due to impaired cranial blood flow, and disturbances in vision due to poor ocular blood flow. The circulating IgM proteins can bind to clotting factors and inhibit them, causing increased bleeding. Additionally, cryoglobulinemia can result.

Answer A is incorrect. Chronic lymphocytic leukemia (CLL) typically presents with lymphadenopathy, hepatosplenomegaly, a warm antibody autoimmune hemolytic anemia, and smudge cells in the peripheral blood. The hyperviscosity syndrome is not present in CLL.

Answer B is incorrect. Diabetes presents with nocturia, polyuria, and polydipsia. Blood tests would demonstrate increased glucose. Superficial resemblances between the hyperviscosity syndromes and diabetic retinopathy, and diabetic kidney disease with the renal insufficiency of multiple myeloma, may be misleading. However, bleeding complications due to diabetes alone would be rare.

Answer C is incorrect. Hodgkin's disease presents with constitutional symptoms and mediastinal lymphadenopathy. A monoclonal M spike is not a characteristic of this disease.

Answer D is incorrect. Multiple myeloma is similar to the condition described with abnormal plasma cells overproducing immunoglobulin, and an M spike is critical for diagnosis. However, instead of a hyperviscosity syndrome, multiple myeloma typically presents with lytic bone lesions, hypercalcemia, and renal insufficiency.

39. **The correct answer is E.** Selection bias is being displayed in this scenario. The physician is selecting his more serious cases for the treatment group (ie, those who are in most need of the benefit). The placebo group contains pa-

tients who are healthier, less symptomatic, and more likely to have a better outcome. Therefore, when it comes time for collecting data, the drug's beneficial effect compared to placebo may be blunted.

Answer A is incorrect. Studies can still be valid if there are differences in group size. There is no evidence that there is a difference in group size in this scenario.

Answer B is incorrect. Late-look bias occurs when information or results are gathered at an inappropriate time. Late-look bias is not displayed in this scenario.

Answer C is incorrect. Recall bias occurs when knowledge of the presence of a disorder alters the way a subject remembers his or her history. For example, a patient may over- or underestimate his or her consumption of a certain drug upon learning of its detrimental effect to the body. Recall bias is not displayed in this scenario.

Answer D is incorrect. Sampling bias occurs when those in the trial are not truly representative of the general population. Therefore, the results (both positive and negative) of the study cannot be truly applied to the general population. There is no evidence of sampling bias in this scenario.

40. **The correct answer is A.** This question addresses mechanisms of neoplastic transformation via loss of tumor suppressors. Each of the choices is a valid tumor suppressor function which, if lost, promotes malignancy. *Rb* and *p53* act as red flags that halt the cell cycle if, for example, DNA is damaged.

Answer B is incorrect. E-cadherin is a tumor suppressor that is involved in cellular adhesion. Some breast and stomach cancers are associated with mutations in e-cadherin.

Answer C is incorrect. WT-1, a nuclear transcription factor, is mutated in Wilms' tumor. *p53* is a transcription factor, but *Rb* interacts only with transcription factors, thereby indirectly affecting gene expression.

Answer D is incorrect. The breast cancer-associated genes *BRCA1* and *BRCA2* are involved in DNA repair.

Answer E is incorrect. Tumor suppressors such as *APC* (gastrointestinal cancers and melanoma) and *NF1* (neurofibromatosis type 1) inhibit signal transduction.

41. **The correct answer is D.** Polymyxins bind to gram-negative bacterial cell membrane phospholipids and destroy the membrane by acting like a detergent. They have no activity against gram-positive organisms or fungi. Polymyxins are predominantly used to treat severe gram-negative infections that are resistant to less toxic antimicrobials. Polymyxins are rarely used owing to their association with nephrotoxicity and neurotoxicity. Numbness of the extremities is one manifestation of neurotoxicity, but dizziness, drowsiness, confusion, nystagmus, and blurred vision are also possible.

Answer A is incorrect. Granulocytopenia refers to a low number of granulocytes (neutrophils, eosinophils, and basophils). Certain medications can cause granulocytopenia, most commonly clozapine, ticlopidine, sulfasalazine, and antithyroid drugs. Among antibiotics, trimethoprim and dapsone are most commonly implicated.

Answer B is incorrect. Ototoxicity is a common adverse effect of aminoglycosides and vancomycin, particularly when the two agents are used in combination. It is not an adverse effect of polymyxins.

Answer C is incorrect. T Patients with glucose-6-phosphate dehydrogenase deficiency are predisposed to hemolysis, and drugs with a high redox potential can precipitate rapid destruction of RBCs. In particular, primaquine and sulfonamides can precipitate a severe anemia characterized by sudden onset of jaundice, pallor, and dark urine with back pain.

Answer E is incorrect. Vomiting is an adverse effect of many antibiotics, but it is not an adverse effect of polymyxins.

42. **The correct answer is D.** Inflammatory bowel disease (IBD) typically presents during late adolescence to early adulthood with symptoms of abdominal pain and frequent bouts of diarrhea. Types of IBD are differentiated and diagnosed on the basis of their clinical picture, their appearance on endoscopy and biopsy, and the exclusion of other intestinal infectious etiologies. In this patient, the areas of normal-appearing mucosa should immediately point to the diagnosis of Crohn's disease as opposed to ulcerative colitis. Ulcerative colitis is characterized by mucosal inflammation that is limited to the colon and frequently involves the rectum. Crypt abscesses and ulceration of the mucosa are classically seen on biopsy. Crohn's disease, however, shows transmural inflammation interspersed with normal mucosa (skip lesions), as seen in this patient. It can affect any part of the gastrointestinal tract but usually spares the rectum. Noncaseating granulomas may be found in Crohn's disease but are not found in ulcerative colitis.

Answer A is incorrect. Cells with loss of mucin and hyperchromatic nuclei are present in colon cancer, which is more commonly associated with ulcerative colitis.

Answer B is incorrect. Hyperplasia of goblet cells is the central feature of hyperplastic polyps, the most common type of non-neoplastic polyp. Although usually asymptomatic, they may cause bleeding, abdominal pain, and, rarely, obstruction.

Answer C is incorrect. Mucus-filled cells in crypts are part of normal colonic mucosa.

Answer E is incorrect. Ulceration limited to the mucosa is a feature of ulcerative colitis. In Crohn's disease, the inflammation is often transmural and interspersed with areas of normal-appearing tissue, as described in this vignette.

43. **The correct answer is E.** *Trypanosoma cruzi* infection can cause aganglionic megacolon and Chagas' disease, a condition in which the heart is enlarged and flaccid. *T. cruzi* is transmitted via the reduviid bug. Microscopic examination reveals flagellated trypomastigotes in the blood and nonmotile amastigotes in tissue culture. *T. cruzi* infection is treated with nifurtimox.

Answer A is incorrect. *Cryptosporidium* species infection presents with severe diarrhea in HIV-positive patients and mild watery diarrhea in HIV-negative patients. *Cryptosporidium* is transmitted via cysts in water (fecal-oral transmission). Microscopically, acid-fast staining cysts are found. Unfortunately, there is no treatment available for *Cryptosporidium* infection; however, in healthy patients, cryptosporidiosis is self-resolving.

Answer B is incorrect. *Entamoeba histolytica* infection presents with bloody diarrhea (dysentery), abdominal cramps with tenesmus, and pus in the stool. It can also cause right upper quadrant pain and liver abscesses. *E. histolytica* is transmitted via cysts in water (fecal-oral transmission). On microscopy, one observes amebas with ingested RBCs. Treatment for *E. histolytica* infection includes metronidazole and iodoquinol.

Answer C is incorrect. *Giardia lamblia* infection presents with bloating, flatulence, foul-smelling diarrhea, and light-colored fatty stools. *G. lamblia* is transmitted via cysts in water (fecal-oral transmission). On microscopy, one observes teardrop-shaped trophozoites with a ventral sucking disc or cysts. Metronidazole is used to treat *G. lamblia* infection.

Answer D is incorrect. *Toxoplasma gondii* infection presents with brain abscesses in HIV-positive patients and with birth defects if infection occurs during pregnancy (toxoplasmosis is one of the TORCH organisms). *T. gondii* is transmitted via cysts in raw meat or cat feces. The definitive stage (sexual stage) occurs in cats. Microscopically, acid-fast staining cysts are found. Sulfadiazine and pyrimethamine are used to treat toxoplasmosis.

44. **The correct answer is C.** Isoniazid works by inhibiting mycolic acid synthesis and also acts as a competitive antagonist to pyridoxine (vitamin B_6), which is used in the biosynthesis of γ-aminobutyric acid (GABA); the reduced levels of GABA, an inhibitory neurotransmitter, can therefore promote seizures. Peripheral neuropathy and hepatitis can also result. Adminis-

tration of pyridoxine can both prevent and reverse these effects.

Answer A is incorrect. Diazepam would be an appropriate treatment if the patient were actively seizing but is not indicated for isoniazid overdose.

Answer B is incorrect. Phenobarbital, like diazepam, is GABAergic and would be indicated for active seizures.

Answer D is incorrect. Rifampin is an antimycobacterial agent that inhibits DNA-dependent RNA polymerase but would have no effect on the vitamin B_6 deficiency produced in isoniazid overdose.

Answer E is incorrect. Thiamine is indicated for treatment of Wernicke-Korsakoff syndrome and beriberi, conditions of thiamine deficiency.

45. **The correct answer is B.** Hereditary spherocytosis is an autosomal dominant, inherited membrane disorder caused by a defect in the spectrin protein of erythrocyte membranes. An intrinsic anemia, it is characterized by an increase in mean corpuscular hemoglobin concentration. Morphologically, it presents as large round red cells with no central pallor.

Answer A is incorrect. Vitamin B_{12} and folate deficiencies lead to megaloblastic anemia, which is characterized on peripheral blood smear by enlarged, oval-shaped erythrocytes and hypersegmented polymorphonuclear cells.

Answer C is incorrect. Iron deficiency is common in children of all ages. Iron-deficiency anemia is characterized by an elevated total iron-binding capacity (TIBC). In anemia of chronic disease, the TIBC will be decreased.

Answer D is incorrect. Autoimmune hemolytic anemia has a clinical presentation similar to that of hereditary spherocytosis, but it is distinguished by having a positive direct Coombs' test.

Answer E is incorrect. Rouleaux formation, which is described as red blood cells lined up like "stacks of coins," is seen on a peripheral blood smear in patients with increased serum protein. It can be seen in association with hyperfibrinogenemia or in hypergammaglobulinemic states such as that which occurs with multiple myeloma.

46. **The correct answer is D.** The lack of pigmentation in the hair, skin, and eyes that is seen in albinism results from a lack of tyrosinase activity in melanocytes. Without tyrosinase, these cells are unable to convert tyrosine to melanin, putting the affected person at an increased risk of squamous and basal cell carcinoma and malignant melanoma. Melanocytes, odontoblasts, pia and arachnoid mater, Schwann cells, cells of the ganglia, parafollicular C cells of the thyroid, chromaffin cells, the aorticopulmonary septum, pharyngeal arch skeletal components, and the neurocranium are all derived from neural crest cells, a specific portion of the neuroectoderm.

    Answer A is incorrect. Although the ectoderm does give rise to the epidermis and the hair (as well as many other structures), it does not produce melanocytes.

    Answer B is incorrect. The endoderm is responsible for the epithelial lining of many internal organs as well as other structures, but plays no role in albinism.

    Answer C is incorrect. The mesoderm produces many structures, including the dermis, but does not produce melanocytes.

    Answer E is incorrect. The neuroectoderm cells outside of the neural crest are the source of the iris (as well as several other optic and nonoptic structures) but do not give rise to melanocytes.

47. **The correct answer is D.** This is a case of penicillin-induced autoimmune hemolytic anemia. Penicillin is believed to act as a hapten, a molecule that on its own, cannot elicit an immune response. However, when a hapten molecule binds to a protein, the hapten-protein conjugate is capable of eliciting an immune response. In this case, penicillin binds to proteins on the surface of RBCs, eliciting an immune response and autoimmune destruction of the RBCs. It also explains the patient's anemia.

    Answer A is incorrect. Penicillin is not acting as an adjuvant (nonspecific immune activator), but rather as a hapten.

    Answer B is incorrect. Penicillin is not an antibody.

    Answer C is incorrect. Penicillin does not contribute CD4+ helper epitopes.

    Answer E is incorrect. Penicillin acts as a hapten, not a soluble antigen.

48. **The correct answer is B.** Atherosclerosis is caused by the formation of a central core of cholesterol and cholesterol esters, lipid-laden macrophages (foam cells), calcium, and necrotic debris in the intima of the coronary arteries as well as in the circle of Willis, lower extremity arteries, and renal and mesenteric arteries.

    Answer A is incorrect. *Arteriosclerosis* is a general term for vascular disease characterized by rigidity and often thickening of blood vessels.

    Answer C is incorrect. Medial calcific sclerosis, also known as Mönckeberg's arteriosclerosis, involves the media of medium-sized muscular arteries.

    Answer D is incorrect. Mönckeberg's arteriosclerosis is characterized by ringlike calcifications that do not cause obstruction to arterial flow because the intima is not involved.

    Answer E is incorrect. Takayasu's arteritis is also known as "pulseless disease" because of thickening of the aortic arch or proximal great vessels, which leads to weak pulses in the upper extremities and ocular disturbances.

49. **The correct answer is E.** A hemoglobin level of 9 g/dL, acute episodes of pain, and a history of gallstones in children and teenagers are all consistent with a diagnosis of sickle cell disease. Patients with this disease are more susceptible to infection by encapsulated organisms. Fever, chills, cough, and pleuritic pain are symptoms consistent with pneumonia. The

most likely organism causing pneumonia in patients with sickle cell disease is *Streptococcus pneumoniae.*

Answer A is incorrect. *Mycoplasma pneumoniae* causes atypical pneumonia. It is not thought to be particularly associated with sickle cell disease.

Answer B is incorrect. *Pseudomonas aeruginosa* causes pneumonia in patients with cystic fibrosis.

Answer C is incorrect. Respiratory syncytial virus (RSV) is a major cause of pneumonia and bronchiolitis in infants and young children; older children do not usually develop serious RSV infections. It is not particularly associated with sickle cell disease.

Answer D is incorrect. *Salmonella* species infection is also commonly found in patients with sickle cell disease but is more likely to cause osteomyelitis.

50. **The correct answer is A.** Craniopharyngiomas account for 80–90% of neoplasms arising in the pituitary region and are the most common supratentorial tumor of childhood. They originate from squamous rest cells in the remnant of Rathke's pouch between the adenohypophysis and neurohypophysis. Eighty percent of patients have evidence of endocrine dysfunction at diagnosis; growth hormone deficiency is the most common (75%), followed by gonadotropin deficiency (40%), and ACTH or thyroid-stimulating hormone deficiency (25%).

Even though these masses are frequently large at presentation, it is rare for the pituitary stalk to be disrupted; only 20% of patients have prolactinemia, and 10–15% have diabetes insipidus secondary to pituitary stalk dysfunction.

Answer B is incorrect. Ependymomas are most commonly found in the fourth ventricle and can result in hydrocephalus; however, it is very rare for ependymomas to cause the hormonal changes evident in this patient.

Answer C is incorrect. Hemangioblastomas are the most common cerebellar tumors in children and are associated with von Hippel–Lindau syndrome when found with retinoblastomas. Such a tumor would not affect hormonal release.

Answer D is incorrect. While a prolactinoma can cause many of the same symptoms (pubertal delay/failure) and may present with symptoms similar to those of a craniopharyngioma, it represents a far less likely diagnosis (accounting for 2.7% of childhood tumors) than craniopharyngioma.

Answer E is incorrect. Thyrotropinomas present with hyperthyroidism without thyroid-stimulating hormone suppression, goiter, visual symptoms, and headache. It would be uncommon for them to suppress growth hormone release, and they are very rare in childhood.

FULL-LENGTH EXAM

Test Block 2

Test Block 3

1. A patient with major depression that is resistant to treatment with selective serotonin receptor inhibitors and therapy is given a monoamine oxidase inhibitor by a physician who has been treating him for 3 years. The patient develops the serotonin syndrome and subsequently dies. Considering the defining characteristics of malpractice, which of the following best describes the actions of the physician?

(A) Not malpractice because no harm was caused directly from the treatment
(B) Not malpractice because the patient was not harmed at all by this physician
(C) Not malpractice because the physician did not neglect her duties
(D) Not malpractice because the physician had no obligation to treat this patient
(E) This is an instance of malpractice

2. A 64-year-old man with a history of coronary artery disease and high cholesterol presents to the physician with increasing lower extremity edema. His blood pressure is 190/110 mm Hg, and laboratory studies show hypernatremia and hypokalemia. Imaging shows no abnormalities except an area of right renal artery vessel constriction. Which of the following are the likely aldosterone and renin levels in this patient?

(A) Decreased/decreased
(B) Decreased/elevated
(C) Elevated/decreased
(D) Elevated/elevated
(E) No change/no change

3. A 41-year-old man is admitted to the hospital for the subacute onset of herpes encephalitis. On admission, the patient's serum sodium level is 114 mEq/L and the patient is significantly obtunded. Treatment is initiated, and 7 hours later the patient's serum sodium level is 134 mEq/L. Over the next 4 days, the patient's condition worsens with the development of dysarthria, dysphagia, and paraparesis in the setting of treatment with appropriate antiviral agents. Which of the following is the most serious complication that may result from the aggressive treatment of this patient's condition?

(A) Cerebral edema
(B) Diffuse axonal injury
(C) Intracerebral hemorrhage
(D) Osmotic demyelination
(E) Uncal herniation

4. When a particular ligand binds to its receptor, there is an increase in the cleavage of phosphatidylinositol biphosphate into inositol triphosphate and diacylglycerol. Both of these substances have actions within the cell. Which of the following would be an example of a receptor that functions in this manner?

(A) γ-Aminobutyric acid receptor
(B) Dopamine receptor
(C) Insulin receptor
(D) Muscarinic acetylcholine receptor
(E) Serotonin receptor

5. A 59-year-old man presents to his primary care physician with a 2-year history of increasing lethargy, weakness, bone pain, a pathologic hip fracture 1 year ago, and polyuria. X-rays show lytic bone lesions in the hip and spine. Total serum protein is elevated, and serum protein electrophoresis shows an M spike in the gamma immunoglobulin region. Bence Jones proteins are seen in the urine. If a kidney biopsy were taken, which of the following would most likely be found in this patient?

(A) Destruction of glomeruli with crescents of proliferating cells adherent to Bowman's capsule
(B) Fibrillary deposits in the mesangium and subendothelium that stain positive with Congo red
(C) Focal lesions involving collapse of the basement membrane, increase in matrix, and deposition of hyaline masses with detachment of the epithelial cells from the basement membrane

(D) Normal appearance under light microscopy but with foot process effacement observed under electron microscopy

(E) Ovoid hyaline masses located in the periphery of the glomerulus, with prominent wire looping

6. A 34-year-old nonsmoker presents to the physician with progressive shortness of breath. Physical examination shows an increase in the anteroposterior diameter of the chest and hyper-resonance to percussion. Laboratory studies reveal elevated liver enzymes. Which of the following parts of the respiratory pathway is affected by α_1-antitrypsin deficiency?

(A) Bronchi
(B) Larynx
(C) Respiratory bronchioles
(D) Terminal bronchiole
(E) Trachea

7. A 70-year-old man is brought to the emergency department by his wife because of a 2-day history of altered mental status. His past medical history is significant for alcoholism with hepatic cirrhosis. He does not have a history of dementia. His current medications are hydrochlorothiazide, ranitidine, metoprolol, metformin, and testosterone. Which of his medications is most likely to have caused his delirium?

(A) Hydrochlorothiazide
(B) Metformin
(C) Metoprolol
(D) Ranitidine
(E) Testosterone

8. An 8-year-old boy comes to the physician with a fever of 39.4° C (103° F), cough, chills, and dyspnea. His mother reports that he has had numerous respiratory infections over the past 3 years and has a history of foul-smelling, fatty stools. The physical examination is significant for crackles, decreased breath sounds, and dullness to percussion in the lower left lung. The patient also has clubbing of his digits. Which of the following organisms is most likely responsible for this patient's current illness?

(A) *Chlamydia pneumoniae*
(B) *Haemophilus influenzae*

(C) *Klebsiella pneumoniae*
(D) *Mycoplasma pneumoniae*
(E) *Pseudomonas aeruginosa*
(F) Respiratory syncytial virus
(G) *Streptococcus pneumoniae*

9. During a motor vehicle crash, a 45-year-old man is thrown from his car and suffers severe lacerations with profound hemorrhage. Sensing a rapid loss in intravascular volume, baroreceptors trigger the renin-angiotensin-aldosterone system as well as the production of renal prostaglandins in order to modulate renal blood flow and glomerular filtration rate. Referring to the image (where A is the afferent arteriole and B is the efferent arteriole), which of the following most accurately reflects the actions of angiotensin II and prostaglandins in this patient?

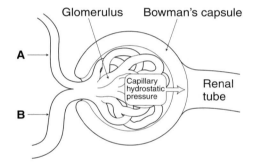

Reproduced, with permission, from USMLERx.com.

(A) Angiotensin II vasoconstricts both A and B; prostaglandins vasodilate A and vasoconstrict B; there is an overall reduction in glomerular filtration rate

(B) Angiotensin II vasoconstricts both A and B; prostaglandins vasodilate both A and B; there is an overall reduction in glomerular filtration rate

(C) Angiotensin II vasoconstricts B with minimal effects on A; prostaglandins vasodilate both A and B; there is an overall increase in glomerular filtration rate

(D) Angiotensin II vasodilates B and vasoconstricts A; prostaglandins have minimal effects on A and B; overall glomerular filtration rate is reduced

(E) Angiotensin II vasodilates both A and B; prostaglandins vasodilate A and vasoconstrict B; overall glomerular filtration rate is unchanged

10. A 24-year-old man presents to the emergency department with hypertension, tachycardia, an elevated body temperature, diaphoresis, mydriasis, and severe agitation. When asked, his mother states that her son and his friends "probably used some drugs they got in the neighborhood." Which of the following agents is the most appropriate therapy for this patient?

(A) Atropine
(B) Flumazenil
(C) Fluoxetine
(D) Labetalol
(E) Physostigmine
(F) Sumatriptan

11. A 39-year-old woman presents to the physician with complaints of itchy skin and diarrhea. On examination, the patient appears slightly confused and is having trouble remembering what she did earlier in the day. A physical examination shows that the patient has a large, deeply pigmented tongue with thickened papillae. On further questioning, it is discovered that the patient has been taking isoniazid for suspected tuberculosis infection. Which of the following supplements should this patient take?

(A) Ascorbic acid
(B) Biotin
(C) Folic acid
(D) Niacin
(E) Riboflavin
(F) Thiamine
(G) Vitamin D

12. Acute allograft rejection is mediated by cytotoxic T lymphocytes that recognize and are activated by the major histocompatibility complex proteins expressed by the donated organ. A depleting monoclonal antibody to which of the following cell surface molecules would be most useful in reducing this immune-mediated graft rejection?

(A) CD3
(B) CD4
(C) CD14
(D) CD16
(E) CD19

13. Routine blood studies for a 73-year-old man show an elevated serum alkaline phosphatase level. All other values, including liver function tests, are within normal limits. The physician subsequently checks the patient's prostate-specific antigen level, which is elevated. A fine-needle biopsy of the prostate is done, revealing adenocarcinoma. Which of the following situations best explains this patient's laboratory results?

(A) Hepatitis
(B) Metastasis to bone
(C) Paraneoplastic syndrome
(D) Severe anaplasia
(E) Urethral obstruction

14. A 28-year-old woman with a past medical history significant for pelvic inflammatory disease presents to the emergency department with right lower quadrant abdominal pain. The pain began 2 hours ago, has been consistently localized to the right lower quadrant without migration, and has been associated with nausea and vomiting. Although her periods are usually regular, her last menstruation was approximately 6 weeks ago. On examination, she is found to be afebrile with a blood pressure of 90/60 mm Hg, a pulse of 110/min, and a respiratory rate of 26/min. Abdominal examination shows localized tenderness with guarding in the right lower quadrant. Pelvic examination is deferred due to excessive pain, but vaginal bleeding is noted. Laboratory studies show a hematocrit of 29.8% and an elevated human chorionic gonadotropin (hCG). Which of the following is the most likely etiology of this patient's disorder?

(A) A blastocyst has implanted in the ampulla, leading to rupture of the uterine tube
(B) A blastocyst has implanted in the posterior superior uterine wall, leading to rupture of the uterine wall
(C) A fecalith has obstructed the appendiceal lumen, leading to rupture of the appendix
(D) Ectopic endometrial tissue has implanted on the ovary
(E) Two spermatozoa have fertilized a single ovum

15. In one afternoon, a pediatrician sees two children with a hereditary defect in fructose metabolism for regular visits. The physician reminds the parents of the first child to maintain the child on a low-fructose, low-sucrose diet. The physician tells the parents of the second child, in response to their concerns about fructose in their girl's blood and urine, that the child is unlikely ever to experience any symptoms of the disorder. Which of the following actions describes the function of the enzyme deficient in the second child?

(A) Converts fructose-1-phosphate to dihydroxyacetone-phosphate
(B) Converts fructose-1-phosphate to glyceraldehydes
(C) Converts fructose to fructose-1-phosphate
(D) Converts glyceraldehyde-3-phosphate to 1,3-bisphosphoglycerate
(E) Converts glyceraldehyde to glyceraldehyde-3-phosphate

16. Calcium channel blockers are commonly used cardiovascular drugs that are effective antihypertensives, antianginals, and antiarrhythmics. Diltiazem is more effective than nifedipine for cardiac indications because diltiazem slows the recovery of the slow calcium channel while also reducing the influx of calcium into the myocyte. Which of the following is an effect of diltiazem?

(A) Increase in cardiac chronotropy
(B) Increase in cardiac inotropy
(C) Increase in conduction velocity
(D) Increase vascular smooth muscle tone
(E) Prolongation of the PR interval

17. A 42-year-old man comes to his physician complaining of erectile dysfunction. He has been having this problem for several months and is now presenting because of the strain it is having on his marriage. On reviewing the patient's chart, the physician notes that the patient has a history of back injury and begins to work him up for a neurologic problem. Which of the following is the spinal location of the nerves that induce erection?

(A) C2–4
(B) T8–12
(C) T12–L2
(D) L1–5
(E) S2–4

18. A 69-year-old smoker presents with "double vision" and lower extremity muscle weakness with exertion. After a full neurologic, cardiovascular, and ophthalmologic workup comes back negative, he has an x-ray film of the chest made. A small circular lesion in the right lung hilum is seen. Suspecting cancer, a full cancer workup is done, which reveals metastases throughout the body. Biopsy report from the pathologist gives the diagnosis of oat cell carcinoma. Which of the following is the most likely cause for this man's diplopia and weakness?

(A) Antibodies against presynaptic Ca^{2+} channels at the neuromuscular junction
(B) Autoimmune disease with anti–double-stranded DNA, anti-DNA, and anti-Smith antibodies
(C) Autoantibodies to acetylcholine receptors at the neuromuscular junction
(D) Inflammatory disorder of synovial joints with pannus formation
(E) Reactivation of a peripheral subpleural parenchymal lesion and hilar lymph nodes

19. A 33-year-old man from Connecticut comes to his physician because he began experiencing flulike symptoms and an expanding rash on his leg following a camping trip 1 week ago. The physician diagnoses him with Lyme disease and prescribes tetracycline. The man finds some tetracycline in his bathroom from about 6 years ago and decides to use this instead of buying a new bottle. One week later, the man presents to the emergency department and is diagnosed with which of the following renal conditions?

(A) Diffuse cortical necrosis
(B) Glomerulonephritis
(C) Kidney stones
(D) Renal papillary necrosis
(E) Renal tubular dysfunction

20. A 26-year-old woman presents to her primary care physician because of difficulty swallowing for the past 2 weeks. Her physical examination is unremarkable. For the past 4 years, this patient has presented to her doctor with complaints of episodic nausea, vomiting, and diarrhea as well as dyspareunia, low back pain, and menorrhagia. She had a negative ultrasound of the gallbladder after complaining of severe right upper quadrant pain. She also had a normal colonoscopy with biopsies after complaining of rectal pain and the passage of blood and mucus in her stool. In the absence of organic pathology, what is this patient's most likely diagnosis?

    (A) Body dysmorphic disorder
    (B) Conversion disorder
    (C) Hypochondriasis
    (D) Pain disorder
    (E) Somatization disorder

21. Which of the following skin cells is chiefly responsible for immunogenic antigen presentation?

    (A) Clear cells
    (B) Dark cells
    (C) Langerhans cells
    (D) Melanocytes
    (E) Merkel's cells

22. Niemann-Pick disease is one of the lysosomal storage diseases. It is caused by a deficiency of sphingomyelinase. Patients with this disease show only 1–10% sphingomyelinase enzyme activity compared to normal individuals. Affected individuals display hepatosplenomegaly, failure to thrive, and progressive central nervous system deterioration; they usually die by 3 years of age. Which of the following is the function of sphingomyelinase in normal individuals?

    (A) Converts ceramide trihexoside to lactosyl cerebroside
    (B) Converts galactocerebroside to cerebroside
    (C) Converts ganglioside M_2 to ganglioside M_3
    (D) Converts glucocerebroside to cerebroside
    (E) Converts sphingomyelin to cerebroside

23. A 46-year-old woman had been taking paroxetine for depression, but her physician switches her medication to an agent effective against anxiety. A few hours after beginning the anxiolytic, she begins to experience muscle spasms, hyperthermia, and changes in mental status. Which of the following agents was she most likely prescribed after discontinuing paroxetine?

    (A) Buspirone
    (B) Diazepam
    (C) Imipramine
    (D) Phenobarbital
    (E) Tranylcypromine

24. An 18-month-old child is brought to the physician by her distraught parents because of a sore throat, difficulty breathing, and a barking cough for the past day. On physical examination, the toddler is found to have some respiratory stridor and a runny nose but is not in acute distress. The rest of the examination is unremarkable. Which of the following is the most appropriate treatment for this patient?

    (A) Amantadine
    (B) Bronchoalveolar lavage
    (C) Emergency department admittance
    (D) Penicillin
    (E) Supportive therapy

25. A 36-year-old woman comes to the physician because of dysphagia. Physical examination shows clawlike hands secondary to "tightened" skin; small, flat red skin marks around the upper extremities; and three small (< 2.5-cm diameter) subcutaneous nodules in her right forearm. Her hands are very sensitive to cold weather, and she wears winter gloves in air-conditioned stores to prevent her hands from cramping up and getting pale. In her chart, you notice that she tested positive for an antinuclear antibody, specifically anticentromere antibody, 2 years ago. Which of the following is the most likely diagnosis?

    (A) Achalasia
    (B) CREST syndrome
    (C) Polyarteritis nodosa

(D) Rheumatoid arthritis

(E) Systemic lupus erythematosus

26. A clinical laboratory technician is processing serum samples for HIV diagnostics. In order to confirm a positive enzyme-linked immunosorbent assay result, the technician performs a Western blot, assaying for the presence of antibodies to three different HIV proteins in the patient's serum. HIV infection is confirmed by the presence of antibodies to two of three HIV proteins. Which of the following is the most correct interpretation of the Western blot shown?

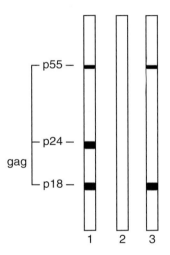

Reproduced, with permission, from USMLERx.com.

(A) The patient does not have HIV

(B) The patient's sample was most likely contaminated with positive control antibodies

(C) The positive control did not work; the blot must be redone

(D) The Western blot confirms a diagnosis of HIV

(E) The Western blot reveals that there are no antibodies to the HIV proteins in the patient's serum

27. A 24-year-old man presents to his primary care physician for a routine physical examination before beginning a new job. While performing a routine testicular examination, the physician notes a nodule on the left testicle. The patient is subsequently diagnosed with a seminoma and is treated by an oncologist. A short while after beginning treatment, the patient returns to his primary care physician with complaints of a 1-week history of cough and shortness of breath. His physician orders an x-ray film of the chest that shows bilateral interstitial infiltrates. Which of the following chemotherapeutic agents is this patient most likely using for treatment of his seminoma?

(A) Bleomycin

(B) Cisplatin

(C) Paclitaxel

(D) Vinblastine

(E) Vincristine

28. After a very difficult delivery 2 months ago, a new mother presents with complaints of amenorrhea, hair loss, weight gain, cold intolerance, constipation, puffy eyes, and flaky skin. Her blood pressure is 118/60 mm Hg, and her laboratory studies show an Na^+ level of 133 mEq/L, a K^+ level of 5.1 mEq/L, and a thyroid-stimulating hormone (TSH) level of 2.0 μU/mL. Physical examination is otherwise unremarkable. Which of the following is the most probable mechanism behind these symptoms?

(A) Antimicrosomal antibodies

(B) Ectopic thyroid-stimulating hormone secretion

(C) Hemorrhage and shock

(D) Subacute thyroiditis

(E) Thyroid-stimulating antibodies

29. Which of the following cell surface receptors is correctly paired with the immune cell that expresses it?

(A) B lymphocytes–CD3

(B) Cytotoxic T lymphocytes–CD19

(C) Dendritic cells–B-cell receptor

(D) Helper T lymphocytes–CD8

(E) Macrophages–CD4

(F) Natural killer cells–CD16

(G) RBCs–major histocompatibility complex class I

30. A 3-year-old boy is brought to the pediatrician because of worsening proptosis and decreased visual acuity and pain in his right eye. Past medical history is notable for the diagnosis of glaucoma shortly after birth, and the eye has been refractory to standard medical therapies. Physical examination shows café au lait spots, freckling in the axillary and inguinal regions, and iris hamartomas. Given the most likely diagnosis, which of the following additional signs might be expected on physical examination?

(A) Bilateral acoustic neuromas
(B) Bilateral renal cell carcinomas
(C) Cystic medial necrosis of the aorta
(D) Leptomeningeal angioma
(E) Sphenoid dysplasia

31. A 10-year-old boy is brought into the emergency department after falling from his bicycle. He presents with a large, painfully swollen knee; aspiration shows gross hemarthrosis. On further questioning, the patient's parents say that he bruises easily and that he had an episode of prolonged bleeding after losing a tooth 1 month ago. His maternal uncle had similar bleeding difficulties. After further testing, the patient is diagnosed with an X-linked recessive disorder. Which of the following laboratory schemes, relative to normal, corresponds to the patient's disorder?

Choice	Platelet Count	Bleeding Time	Prothrombin Time	Partial Thromboplastin Time
A	Normal	Normal	Normal	↑
B	Normal	↑	Normal	Normal
C	Normal	↑	Normal	↑
D	↓	↑	Normal	Normal
E	↓	↑	↑	↑

(A) A
(B) B
(C) C
(D) D
(E) E

32. A 35-year-old man comes to the physician because of a fever, headache, malaise, and a cough and sore throat. The causative virus is established and the patient is given zanamivir. Which of the following is the mechanism of action of zanamivir?

(A) Blocks viral penetration and uncoating
(B) Inhibits the activity of an enzyme that allows budding virions to be released from the host cell membrane
(C) Inhibits the activity of a viral surface protein that binds to the cell surface receptor and initiates infection
(D) Inhibits viral DNA polymerase, preventing viral replication
(E) It is a nucleoside analog that causes inhibition of guanine nucleotide synthesis, preventing viral protein synthesis

33. A 32-year-old woman presents to the emergency department with a temperature of 38.7° C (101.7° F), petechiae covering her abdomen, and mental status changes. On questioning, her husband states that "she had been fine 3 weeks ago but got sick real fast." Physical examination shows severe weakness, petechiae and ecchymoses on the abdomen and back, and pale conjunctiva. A laboratory study shows severe anemia and thrombocytopenia with leukocytosis. The peripheral blood smear demonstrates the presence of abundant myeloblasts. Which of the following chromosomal translocations is most likely involved in this disorder?

(A) t(8;14) c-myc activation
(B) t(9;22), bcr-abl
(C) t(11;22), EWS gene
(D) t(14;18), BCL1/PRAD1
(E) t(15;17), PML-RAR-α

34. A 17-year-old girl who is 6 weeks pregnant presents to the emergency department with abdominal pain and vaginal bleeding. Ultrasound shows no fetal heartbeat and incomplete fetal development, and the pregnancy is terminated by aspiration to remove the fetal tissue. On questioning, the patient reports that she has been taking high doses of her mother's ulcer medication for her own heartburn. Which of the following medications did this patient most likely take?

(A) Cimetidine
(B) Magnesium hydroxide
(C) Misoprostol
(D) Omeprazole
(E) Sucralfate

35. A 43-year-old man with a history of hypercalcemia and bilateral hemianopsia presents to the emergency department with muscle weakness, lethargy, and watery diarrhea. He reports brief episodes of complete paralysis in his lower extremities. The pH of the patient's nasogastric suction fluid is increased. An abdominal mass is noted on CT scan. The patient's family history is positive for numerous endocrine organ abnormalities. Which of the following is the most likely cause of this patient's symptoms?

(A) Gastrinoma
(B) Insulinoma
(C) Medullary thyroid carcinoma
(D) Pancreatic adenocarcinoma
(E) VIPoma

36. A 67-year-old former professional football player comes to the physician complaining of intense pain in his groin. Laboratory tests show an elevated leukocyte count; liver function tests are slightly elevated. He has an irreducible inguinal mass. Which of the following vessels is just lateral to this mass?

(A) Common femoral artery
(B) External iliac artery
(C) Inferior epigastric artery
(D) Superior epigastric artery
(E) Superior vesical artery

37. A 60-year-old Scandinavian woman presents to her doctor with a 2-month history of progressive fatigue. She also says that she has been feeling tingling and numbness in her lower extremities bilaterally and that she has felt "wobbly" lately. She does not have any significant past medical history. Her pulse is 101/min, and she has decreased lower extremity vibratory sensation and reflexes. Her laboratory studies show a hemoglobin level of 9 g/dL and a mean corpuscular volume of 110 mm³. Her peripheral blood smear is shown in the image. The pathogenesis of this patient's nutrient deficiency results from which of the following factors?

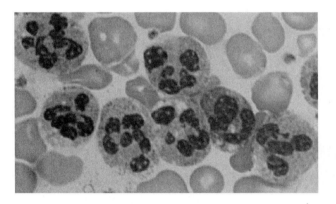

Reproduced, with permission, from Lichtman MA, Beutler E, Kipps TJ, Seligsohn U, Kaushansky K, Prchal JF. *Williams Hematology*, 7th ed. New York, McGraw-Hill, 2006: Color Plate VI-8.

(A) Abnormal neural crest cell migration
(B) Antibodies against parietal cells
(C) Bacterial overgrowth of colon
(D) Diet deficient in leafy vegetables
(E) Embolus to the superior mesenteric artery

38. A 37-year-old white man with end-stage liver disease secondary to hepatitis C presents to the emergency department confused and lethargic. He has ascites, spider angiomata, and asterixis. Bowel sounds are normal. Laboratory studies show the following results:

Aspartate aminotransferase: 46 U/L
Alanine aminotransferase: 55 U/L
Alkaline phosphatase: 100 U/L
Bilirubin, total serum: 1.4 mg/dL
Prothrombin time: 38 sec
Albumin: 2.0 g/dL

Which of the following is the most appropriate acute treatment of this patient's condition?

(A) Lactulose
(B) Liver transplantation
(C) Lorazepam
(D) Neomycin
(E) Restricted protein diet

39. A 45-year-old woman presents to her physician for a follow-up examination after being diagnosed with HIV. She says that she has been experiencing occasional pelvic pain and a vaginal discharge. She also complains of a fever and chills and adds that she feels as though she has the flu. On pelvic examination, the patient is found to have cervical motion tenderness and discharge that are highly suggestive of gonorrhea. On further questioning, the patient says that she has also had genital herpes in the past. She is informed of the potential risk of transmitting these diseases to other partners. Which of the following is a reportable disease in all states?

(A) Genital herpes
(B) Gonorrhea
(C) HIV
(D) Influenza
(E) Scarlet fever

40. A 7-year-old girl comes to the dermatologist for the removal of a malignant melanoma. Her face, legs, and arms are covered with freckles. She also suffers from severe persistent sunburns. Which of the following is the most likely cause of these findings?

(A) A defect in base excision repair
(B) A defect in mismatch repair
(C) A defect in proofreading enzymes
(D) Exposure to benzo(a)pyrene
(E) Exposure to ionizing radiation

41. A researcher at a pharmaceutical company develops an assay that can detect and quantify very low levels of human chorionic gonadotropin (hCG) in the blood by binding with high affinity to the β subunit. Which of the following hormones may interfere with the ability of this assay to achieve an accurate measure of hCG levels in the blood?

(A) ACTH
(B) Gonadotropin-releasing hormone
(C) Growth hormone
(D) Melanocyte-stimulating hormone
(E) Thyroid-stimulating hormone

42. A 3-month-old boy who was born at full term presents to the pediatrician for evaluation of his congenital heart condition. His 39-year-old mother is healthy. She states that the pregnancy was notable for a decreased level of α-fetoprotein. The boy has flat facies, prominent epicanthal folds, and a simian crease on each hand. This child most likely has a heart condition that involves tissue derived from which of the following structures?

(A) Bulbus cordis
(B) Neural crest cells
(C) Primitive atrium
(D) Primitive ventricle
(E) Truncus arteriosus

43. A 27-year-old man walks into the emergency department in an agitated state. He complains of severe abdominal pain and eventually becomes combative, requiring five-point restraint. His vital signs show elevated blood pressure and tachycardia. When a straight catheter is inserted, reddish urine enters the Foley bag. The urine is negative for RBCs, and a toxicity screen is negative. His doctor suspects a porphyria; laboratory tests for urine porphobilinogen are positive. Which of the following enzyme deficiencies is responsible for this patient's disorder?

(A) Aminolevulinate dehydratase
(B) Aminolevulinate synthase
(C) Ferrochelatase
(D) Heme oxygenase
(E) Porphobilinogen deaminase
(F) Uroporphyrinogen III cosynthase
(G) Uroporphyrinogen decarboxylase

44. A patient with adult T-lymphocyte leukemia receives a bone marrow transplant from an unrelated donor. Despite an immunosuppressive posttransplant treatment regimen, over the course of several weeks the patient develops a severe cutaneous rash and intractable diarrhea. Blood tests were normal except for alanine aminotransferase (1032 U/L), aspartate aminotransferase (829 U/L), lactate dehydrogenase (634 U/L), and alkaline phosphatase (446 U/L). Which of the following is the most likely etiology of the patient's current symptoms?

(A) Acute graft rejection
(B) Graft-versus-host disease mediated by alloreactive donor T lymphocytes
(C) Graft-versus-host disease mediated by alloreactive recipient T lymphocytes
(D) Hyperacute graft rejection
(E) Recurrence of leukemia

45. A 59-year-old man with a history of obesity, myocardial infarction, retinal detachment, and foot ulcers presents to the emergency department with numbness and tingling in his lower extremities. He has been receiving dialysis for the past 2 years. His hemoglobin A_{1c} level is increased. Which of the following describes the glomerular pathology most likely seen on light microscopy of this patient's kidneys?

(A) Diffuse capillary and basement membrane thickening
(B) Enlarged hypercellular glomeruli with neutrophils
(C) Nodular glomerulosclerosis with thickened basement membrane
(D) Segmental sclerosis with hyalinosis
(E) Wire-loop appearance with subendothelial basement membrane deposits

46. A full-term newborn girl is noted to be hypotensive at birth. Despite intravenous fluid support, the baby remains hypotensive. During the medical workup, the following data are obtained:

Na^+: 127 mEq/L
K^+: 5.5 mEq/L
Cl^-: 92 mEq/L
HCO_3^-: 18 mEq/L
17-Hydroxyprogesterone: 74 nmol/L (normal 7–45 nmol/L)

Which of the following is most likely to be found on further examination and workup?

(A) Biopsy of the gonads reveals the presence of testicular tissue
(B) Chromosome analysis shows a 47,XXX karyotype
(C) Endocrinology tests reveal a 5-α-reductase deficiency
(D) Physical examination reveals an enlarged clitoris and partially fused labioscrotal folds
(E) Radiographic examination shows evidence of ovarian dysgenesis

47. A 27-year-old pregnant woman with no significant past medical history comes to the clinic for a routine prenatal visit. She is 30 weeks pregnant and on questioning has no complaints other than mild fatigue. Laboratory evaluation of a blood sample shows a total thyroxine (T_4) level of 15.0 μg/dL and a thyroid-binding globulin (TBG) level of 40 μg/dL. Which of the following most likely represents the remainder of this patient's thyroid function tests?

Choice	Thyroid-Stimulating Hormone	Free Thyroxine
A	↑	↑
B	↑	Normal
C	Normal	↑
D	Normal	Normal
E	↓	↑

(A) A
(B) B
(C) C
(D) D
(E) E

48. An infant is brought to the pediatrician 13 days after birth because of a purulent yellow discharge oozing out of his eyes. He has swelling of his eyelids and inflammation of the conjunctivae. It is noted that the newborn did not receive erythromycin eye drops, usually given to all newborns at birth. Which of the following organisms is most likely responsible for this infant's conjunctivitis?

(A) *Chlamydia psittaci*
(B) *Chlamydia trachomatis*
(C) *Neisseria gonorrhoeae*
(D) *Trypanosoma brucei gambiense*
(E) *Ureaplasma urealyticum*

49. Various thrombolytic therapies are used in patients with cerebrovascular accidents; a meta-analysis investigates the time to resolution of symptoms with three different therapies. The investigators have calculated the mean time to symptom resolution on drug 1, drug 2, and drug 3. They would like to perform a parametric statistical analysis of the data. Which test would be appropriate for this task?

(A) Analysis of variance
(B) Chi-square test
(C) Dependent t-test
(D) Independent t-test
(E) Wilcoxon's test

50. A 16-year-old boy with a history of epistaxis, frequent bruising, and heavy bleeding during dental procedures comes to his physician with new onset of gastrointestinal bleeding in the setting of aspirin use for a sprained ankle. Physical examination shows mild bleeding in his gingiva as well as a swollen, tender right ankle. Laboratory blood studies show normal platelet counts, normal prothrombin time, increased partial thromboplastin time, and prolonged bleeding time. Which of the following diseases is the most likely diagnosis?

(A) Bernard-Soulier syndrome
(B) Glanzmann's thrombasthenia
(C) Hemophilia A
(D) Hemophilia B
(E) Thrombotic thrombocytopenic purpura
(F) Von Willebrand's disease

1. **The correct answer is C.** Malpractice is civil litigation as a result of the **4 D's** on the part of the physician: **D**ereliction of **D**uty **D**irectly causing **D**amage to the patient. The physician in this case prescribed a treatment that was not a deviation from standard treatment. This was not negligence on the part of the physician.

Answer A is incorrect. This choice is not correct because the treatment did directly cause the death of this patient.

Answer B is incorrect. The patient was indeed harmed by the actions of this physician.

Answer D is incorrect. The patient had an established physician-patient relationship with the patient so he had an obligation to treat the patient; therefore, this choice is not correct.

Answer E is incorrect. A skilled lawyer may produce a civil suit, but legally this is not a case of malpractice.

2. **The correct answer is D.** The patient has renal artery stenosis leading to secondary hyperaldosteronism. The constriction in the right renal artery is causing hypoperfusion of the right kidney leading to an increase in renin production. The increased renin production is causing an increase in aldosterone levels, resulting in high blood pressure, hypernatremia, and hypokalemia. Thus, levels of both aldosterone and renin would be increased in this patient.

Answer A is incorrect. Decreased levels of aldosterone and renin would be an unlikely combination in a patient unless both renin-angiotensin system dysfunction and adrenal dysfunction are present.

Answer B is incorrect. A decreased aldosterone and an increased renin level is seen in patients with primary adrenal hypofunction, such as occurs in patients with Addison's disease. The renin-angiotensin system kicks into overdrive in these patients as a response to the low aldosterone levels.

Answer C is incorrect. An increased aldosterone level paired with a decreased renin

level would be seen in a patient with primary hyperaldosteronism, such as in a patient with an aldosterone-secreting adenoma or adrenal hyperplasia. These patients have a decreased level of renin due to the negative feedback effect of increased aldosterone levels on the renin-angiotensin system.

Answer E is incorrect. Changes in aldosterone and renin levels would be expected in this patient.

3. **The correct answer is D.** Osmotic demyelination can result from overaggressive treatment of hyponatremia. This patient's hyponatremia is almost certainly the result of the syndrome of inappropriate secretion of ADH (SIADH) secondary to herpes encephalitis. The patient's sodium increased 20 mEq/L in the span of 7 hours, which indicates overly aggressive use of hypertonic saline to reverse the hyponatremia. Correction of hyponatremia to the normal range should be no more rapid than 1 mEq/L per hour, or osmotic demyelination can result. This is because as the hyponatremia develops, cerebral edema is combated through the loss of osmoles by the cells within the central nervous system. When the Na^- is corrected too quickly, the rise in tonicity is faster than the rate at which the organic osmoles can be either resynthesized or transported back into the cell, which results in cell shrinking and death. The clinical manifestations occur several days after the event and include dysarthria, dysphagia, and flaccid quadriparesis that can become spastic, and if severe, can progress to "locked-in" syndrome, in which the patient retains full awareness but can move only the extraocular muscles.

Answer A is incorrect. Cerebral edema occurs with acute hyponatremia as water flows freely across the blood-brain barrier and cell membranes and into brain cells to compensate for the drop in serum Na^+. However, cerebral edema does not typically accompany overly aggressive treatment of hyponatremia with hypertonic saline, but rather the opposite, when cell shrinking and death occurs as a result of water leaving the cells.

Answer B is incorrect. Diffuse axonal injury occurs in the setting of central nervous system trauma or angular acceleration or both and results in disruption of the axon at the nodes of Ranvier. Diffuse axonal injury does not occur with electrolyte abnormalities.

Answer C is incorrect. Intracerebral hemorrhage can occur as a result of hypertension, arteriovenous malformations, anticoagulation, thrombolysis, or amyloid angiopathy; however, it does not occur as a result of hyponatremia or the associated treatment.

Answer E is incorrect. Uncal herniation can result only from focal processes within the cranial vault, such as intracranial hemorrhage, but does not occur with diffuse processes associated with electrolyte abnormalities.

4. **The correct answer is D.** The muscarinic acetylcholine receptor, as well as the α_1-adrenergic and histamine$_1$ receptors, activates phospholipase C to cleave phosphatidylinositol biphosphate. Inositol triphosphate increases calcium ions for use in calmodulin activity, and diacylglycerol activates protein kinase C. This is done through the Gq receptor.

Answer A is incorrect. The γ-aminobutyric acid receptor is a neurotransmitter-activated ion-channel–linked receptor.

Answer B is incorrect. The dopamine$_1$ receptor is a Gs receptor and functions to increase adenyl cyclase activity. The dopamine$_2$ receptor is a G$_i$ receptor and inhibits adenyl cyclase activity.

Answer C is incorrect. The insulin receptor is an enzyme-linked receptor.

Answer E is incorrect. The serotonin receptor, like the γ-aminobutyric receptor, is an ion-linked receptor.

5. **The correct answer is B.** The patient has multiple myeloma. The big clues to the diagnosis are pathologic fractures, lytic lesions on x-ray, Bence Jones protein in the urine, and an M spike on serum protein electrophoresis. One possible consequence of multiple myeloma is systemic amyloidosis, as the plasma cells secrete misfolded aggregates of amyloid secondary to immunoglobulin light chain overproduction. These are deposited in the kidney and, in early stages, in the mesangium and subendothelial space; they stain positive with Congo red, with apple green birefringence in polarized light. Later in the course of the disease, they obliterate the glomerulus. These patients present with heavy proteinuria that progresses to renal insufficiency and uremia.

Answer A is incorrect. This describes rapidly progressive glomerulonephritis, which is caused by a variety of conditions, including Goodpasture's syndrome.

Answer C is incorrect. This is the description of focal segmental glomerulosclerosis, which occurs in HIV infection, heroin addiction, and sickle cell disease or in response to other events that cause scarring in the kidney (such as IgA nephropathy).

Answer D is incorrect. Minimal change disease (lipoid nephrosis) is characterized by normal-appearing glomeruli under light microscopy but foot process effacement under the electron microscope. It is common in children and presents with nephrotic syndrome. It is highly responsive to treatment with steroids.

Answer E is incorrect. The description of ovoid hyaline masses is characteristic of the Kimmelstiel-Wilson nodules seen in advanced diabetic glomerulosclerosis.

6. **The correct answer is C.** α_1-Antitrypsin deficiency (chromosome 14) produces a panacinar emphysema that is characterized by destruction of everything distal to the terminal bronchiole, including the respiratory bronchioles. Normally, α_1-antitrypsin is released into the bloodstream and travels to the lung where it protects the lungs from the destructive actions of common illnesses and exposures (e.g., tobacco smoke or respiratory irritants in the environment). The lack of α_1-antitrypsin leads to progressive lung damage by proteases and

eventually causes emphysema. Symptoms include chronic cough and shortness of breath that initially occurs only upon exertion and then gradually occurs at rest as well. These presentations usually develop over 15–20 years, but can eventually lead to respiratory failure and premature death.

Answer A is incorrect. α_1-Antitrypsin deficiency does not affect the bronchi.

Answer B is incorrect. α_1-Antitrypsin deficiency does not affect the larynx.

Answer D is incorrect. α_1-Antitrypsin deficiency affects everything distal to the terminal bronchiole.

Answer E is incorrect. α_1-Antitrypsin deficiency does not affect the trachea.

7. **The correct answer is A.** Patients with cirrhosis are at risk for hepatic encephalopathy, which in chronic liver disease is frequently a reversible delirious state. Hepatic encephalopathy can be precipitated by several different factors, including hypokalemia, azotemia, alkalosis, and hypovolemia, all of which can be induced by diuretics. Hydrochlorothiazide is especially known for causing hypokalemia.

Answer B is incorrect. As with all medications used in hepatically impaired patients, metformin should be used with caution. However, the hydrochlorothiazide is the most likely cause of this patient's delirium.

Answer C is incorrect. As with all medications used in hepatically impaired patients, metoprolol should be used with caution. However, the hydrochlorothiazide is the most likely cause of this patient's delirium. β-Blockers are used in patients with chronic liver disease to treat portal hypertension.

Answer D is incorrect. As with all medications used in hepatically impaired patients, ranitidine should be used with caution. However, the hydrochlorothiazide is the most likely cause of this patient's delirium.

Answer E is incorrect. Testosterone should be used with caution in patients with impaired liver function, but the diuretic is the most likely cause of this patient's delirium.

8. **The correct answer is E.** This patient has clinical and physical findings associated with pneumonia. Foul-smelling, fatty stools plus frequent pneumonia suggest cystic fibrosis. *Pseudomonas aeruginosa* is frequently associated with pneumonia in patients with cystic fibrosis.

Answer A is incorrect. *Chlamydia pneumoniae* can cause upper and lower respiratory tract infections, especially bronchitis and pneumonia, but it is not particularly associated with cystic fibrosis.

Answer B is incorrect. *Haemophilus influenzae* primarily causes upper respiratory tract infections such as otitis media, sinusitis, and epiglottitis. It can also cause pneumonia, but usually in an adult with chronic obstructive lung disease.

Answer C is incorrect. Pneumonia caused by *Klebsiella* is most frequently found in people with predisposing conditions such as advanced age, chronic respiratory disease, and alcoholism. It is characterized by thick, bloody sputum, sometimes called currant jelly sputum.

Answer D is incorrect. *Mycoplasma pneumoniae* causes atypical pneumonia, sometimes called walking pneumonia. Patients show few symptoms of infection with this type of infection, and it is not thought to be particularly associated with cystic fibrosis.

Answer F is incorrect. Respiratory syncytial virus (RSV) causes atypical pneumonia and is not thought to be associated with cystic fibrosis.

Answer G is incorrect. *Streptococcus pneumoniae* causes typical pneumonia, but infection with this organism, although possible, is not usually associated with cystic fibrosis.

9. **The correct answer is B.** During hemorrhage, blood loss leads to an increase in the renin-angiotensin-aldosterone (RAA) system. Whereas low concentrations of angiotensin II (AT II)

have the effect of preferentially constricting the efferent arteriole, high concentrations such as those in hemorrhage vasoconstrict both afferent and efferent arterioles. Renal prostaglandins are produced in response to increased sympathetic activity and act to vasodilate both afferent and efferent arterioles. This effect, although opposite to that of AT II, is protective for renal blood flow such that overall the glomerular filtration rate is reduced while the kidneys sustain adequate blood flow to maintain function.

Answer A is incorrect. The effects of prostaglandins are vasodilation of both efferent and afferent arterioles.

Answer C is incorrect. Low concentrations of AT II would tend to preferentially vasoconstrict the efferent arteriole, leading to an increase in glomerular filtration rate (GFR). Hemorrhage induces increased renin-angiotensin-aldosterone system activity, and vasoconstriction of both afferent and efferent arterioles leads to a reduction in GFR.

Answer D is incorrect. Angiotensin II vasoconstricts both A and B, while prostaglandins vasodilate both A and B.

Answer E is incorrect. Angiotensin II vasoconstricts (not vasodilates) both A and B, and prostaglandins vasodilate both A and B, with an overall effect of reducing glomerular filtration rate.

10. **The correct answer is D.** The patient described above is probably under the influence of a central nervous system (CNS) stimulant such as methamphetamine. Labetalol is a nonselective α and β antagonist that would block many of the dangerous peripheral side effects of CNS stimulants, such as hypertension and cardiac stimulation. Other appropriate medications that could be administered under these conditions would be antipsychotic agents (to control the agitation and psychotic symptoms) and diazepam (to control possible seizures).

Answer A is incorrect. Atropine is a muscarinic antagonist that would be an appropriate therapy for an overdose by an acetyl-

cholinesterase inhibitor. A patient presenting with an acetylcholinesterase inhibitor overdose would have miotic pupils and bradycardia.

Answer B is incorrect. Flumazenil is a benzodiazepine receptor antagonist. It is used in cases of benzodiazepine overdose.

Answer C is incorrect. Fluoxetine is a selective serotonin reuptake inhibitor antidepressant. It would not be indicated in the case of central nervous system stimulant overdose.

Answer E is incorrect. Physostigmine is an acetylcholinesterase inhibitor that might be used for an antimuscarinic drug overdose, such as with atropine, scopolamine, or Jimson weed. An antimuscarinic overdose can look similar to a central nervous system stimulant overdose, with at least one important exception. The hyperthermia seen with an antimuscarinic overdose is accompanied by hot and dry skin (because of blockade of the sympathetic cholinergics to the sweat glands). Stimulant overdose is often characterized by profuse sweating. Tachycardia, hypertension, hyperthermia, mental changes, and mydriasis are common to both.

Answer F is incorrect. Sumatriptan is a 5-HT_1 agonist used to treat migraines. Sumatriptan toxicity can present with chest discomfort and tingling.

11. **The correct answer is D.** This patient most likely has pellagra, caused by a niacin deficiency. Isoniazid impairs the conversion of tryptophan to niacin, and therefore its use can cause symptoms of niacin deficiency. Pellagra is characterized by the **3 "D's":** **D**ermatitis, **D**iarrhea, and **D**ementia (and beefy glossitis, as described in the vignette).

Answer A is incorrect. A deficiency of ascorbic acid (vitamin C) would cause scurvy, which would present with swollen gums, bruising, anemia, and poor wound healing.

Answer B is incorrect. A deficiency of biotin would cause pruritic skin (dermatitis) and enteritis, but the above presentation, which includes beefy glossitis and dementia, is more characteristic of niacin deficiency.

Answer C is incorrect. A deficiency of folic acid would cause a macrocytic, megaloblastic anemia and would include symptoms such as fatigue. It would not result in this patient's presentation.

Answer E is incorrect. A deficiency of riboflavin (vitamin B_2) would cause angular stomatitis, cheilosis, and corneal vascularization.

Answer F is incorrect. A deficiency of thiamine (vitamin B_1) would cause beriberi and Wernicke-Korsakoff syndrome. Signs of beriberi include polyneuritis, cardiac pathology, and edema. Wernicke-Korsakoff syndrome is associated with dementia and a confabulating patient.

Answer G is incorrect. A deficiency of vitamin D would cause rickets in children and osteomalacia (soft bones) in adults, along with symptoms such as hypocalcemic tetany.

12. **The correct answer is A.** Anti-CD3 antibodies that bind to CD3 and trigger destruction of T lymphocytes (via phagocytes or complement-mediated lysis) would be most useful in this scenario, as CD8+ T lymphocytes are the main effectors mediating acute allograft rejection. Note that monoclonal antibodies may be triggering, depleting, or blocking, and therefore it is absolutely necessary to characterize which of these effector functions they elicit, as those three scenarios would have three very different therapeutic applications.

Answer B is incorrect. Cytotoxic T lymphocytes express CD8, while helper T lymphocytes express CD4. While targeting CD4 T lymphocytes may be partially effective, it would be more useful to deplete all T lymphocytes with an anti-CD3 monoclonal antibody.

Answer C is incorrect. CD14 is a common macrophage cell surface marker.

Answer D is incorrect. CD16 is a common natural killer–cell surface marker.

Answer E is incorrect. CD19 is a common B-lymphocyte surface marker.

13. **The correct answer is B.** Prostatic carcinoma is the most common cancer in males. Metastasis can occur via hematogenous spread, often to the vertebral column, following the path of venous drainage of the prostate. An increased alkaline phosphatase level in the serum can be a sign of increased bone turnover caused by the metastatic tumor growth. Only this answer choice explains both the high alkaline phosphatase and prostate-specific antigen levels.

Answer A is incorrect. Hepatitis may increase alkaline phosphatase levels, as inflammation of the liver may obstruct parts of the biliary tree. However, hepatitis would not explain the increased prostate-specific antigen level.

Answer C is incorrect. A paraneoplastic syndrome occurs when a tumor aberrantly produces a hormone; antidiuretic hormone production by small-cell lung carcinoma is one example. In this case, the alkaline phosphatase is not coming from the tumor itself, and there is no syndrome described.

Answer D is incorrect. Although severe anaplasia may be present in the prostate biopsy, tumor grade and differentiation are not associated with elevated alkaline phosphatase levels unless bony metastasis has occurred.

Answer E is incorrect. Enlargement of the prostate leading to urethral obstruction can occur with benign prostatic hyperplasia as well as with prostatic adenocarcinoma, but the obstruction itself would not explain the laboratory results.

14. **The correct answer is A.** This patient is presenting with a ruptured ectopic pregnancy, which occurs when a blastocyst implants in an inappropriate location, most commonly the ampulla of the uterine tube. This typically presents as described in the question stem and constitutes a medical emergency. The most common risk factors are pelvic inflammatory disease, or PID (usually gonorrheal), prior appendicitis or endometriosis, and previous abdominal surgery.

Answer B is incorrect. This describes appropriate implantation of a blastocyst in a normal pregnancy and is therefore not directly associated with pathology.

Answer C is incorrect. This describes the likely etiology of acute appendicitis. This will present with right lower quadrant (RLQ) abdominal pain but typically begins with diffuse periumbilical pain that later migrates to the RLQ. This condition is not associated with prior PID, a missed period, or elevated human chorionic gonadotropin (hCG), and will typically produce a fever.

Answer D is incorrect. This describes endometriosis. Although this can be associated with irregular bleeding and abdominal/pelvic pain, it does not typically result in missed periods, shocklike signs, or elevated human chorionic gonadotropin (hCG).

Answer E is incorrect. When two sperm fertilize a single ovum, a partial hydatidiform mole is formed. Like a ruptured ectopic pregnancy, this will produce vaginal bleeding and an elevated human chorionic gonadotropin (hCG) but will not cause acute shocklike signs and is not associated with prior PID. It will also cause a rapid increase in uterine size.

15. **The correct answer is C.** Fructokinase converts fructose to fructose-1-phosphate. This is the first step in fructose metabolism, and it is deficient in patients with essential fructosuria.

Answer A is incorrect. Aldolase B converts fructose-1-phosphate to dihydroxyacetone-phosphate and glyceraldehydes, the second step in fructose metabolism. This enzyme is deficient in patients with fructose intolerance.

Answer B is incorrect. Aldolase B converts fructose-1-phosphate to glyceraldehydes and dihydroxyacetone-phosphate, the second step in fructose metabolism. This enzyme is deficient in patients with hereditary fructose intolerance.

Answer D is incorrect. Glyceraldehyde-3-phosphate dehydrogenase converts glyceraldehyde-3-phosphate to 1,3-bisphosphoglycerate, one of the steps that fructose metabolites undergo in glycolysis.

Answer E is incorrect. Triose kinase converts glyceraldehyde to glyceraldehyde-3-phosphate.

16. **The correct answer is E.** By inhibiting the voltage-dependent calcium channels in cardiac muscle and slowing the rate of recovery, diltiazem will prolong phase 0 and phase 2 of the cardiac action potential. As a result, the PR interval will be prolonged, especially in the atrioventricular nodal cells, which is why this medication is indicated to prevent nodal arrhythmias.

Answer A is incorrect. Diltiazem decreases cardiac chronotropy because it slows the recovery of the slow calcium channels. Nifedipine does not have this effect.

Answer B is incorrect. Because it inhibits calcium ion influx, diltiazem reduces cardiac inotropy.

Answer C is incorrect. By the same mechanism of PR prolongation, diltiazem will decrease the conduction velocity of the action potential in the myocardial cells.

Answer D is incorrect. By inhibiting calcium influx in vascular smooth muscle cells, calcium channel blockers will decrease vascular tone, which is the source of their efficacy as antihypertensive medications. Nifedipine is the calcium channel blocker that is more effective on vessel receptors, whereas diltiazem and verapamil have more cardiac function.

17. **The correct answer is E.** Erection is controlled by the parasympathetic nerves at S2–4. The parasympathetic nerves exit the spinal cord in the cranial and sacral regions. The neurotransmitter secreted by parasympathetic nerves is acetylcholine, which acts at end organs, the neuromuscular junction, and the adrenal gland to produce its effect. In the penis, the parasympathetic nerves act to relax the smooth muscle, compressing the tunical veins and generating erection. Parasympathetic nerves cause erection, whereas sympathetic nerves cause ejaculation. Remember: **Point**

and Shoot. A second mnemonic: S2-3-4 keeps the penis off the floor.

Answer A is incorrect. Parasympathetic nerves that exit in the cranial region do not contribute to erection.

Answer B is incorrect. Sympathetic nerves control ejaculation, not erection.

Answer C is incorrect. Sympathetic nerves control ejaculation, not erection. Sympathetic nerves travel in the sympathetic chain along the spinal cord and exit the spinal column in the thoracic and lumbar regions. Norepinephrine is the neurotransmitter of the sympathetic nervous system and typically acts at end organs in opposition to parasympathetic effects. In the penis, the sympathetic nervous system causes seminal fluid to enter the urethra followed by contraction of the cavernosus muscles, leading to ejaculation.

Answer D is incorrect. Sympathetic nerves control ejaculation, not erection.

18. **The correct answer is A.** Lambert-Eaton syndrome is associated with oat (small) cell carcinoma, while a similar disorder, myasthenia gravis, is associated with thymoma.

Answer B is incorrect. Systemic lupus erythematosus is associated with multiple symptoms, and is usually seen in women between 14 and 45 years of age.

Answer C is incorrect. Myasthenia gravis is similar to Lambert-Eaton syndrome, but is not associated with oat cell carcinoma.

Answer D is incorrect. Rheumatoid arthritis is seen mostly in females, and presents with symmetric morning stiffness and systemic symptoms (fever and fatigue).

Answer E is incorrect. Secondary tuberculosis is uncommon except in immunocompromised patients. Because the biopsy came back as oat cell carcinoma, tuberculosis is highly unlikely.

19. **The correct answer is E.** Degraded tetracycline is associated with Fanconi's syndrome, a disorder of proximal tubule function resulting in decreased absorption of particular molecules in the proximal tubules.

Answer A is incorrect. Diffuse cortical necrosis is not associated with either Fanconi's syndrome or tetracycline.

Answer B is incorrect. Glomerulonephritis is not associated with either Fanconi's syndrome or tetracycline.

Answer C is incorrect. Kidney stones are not associated with either Fanconi's syndrome or tetracycline.

Answer D is incorrect. Renal papillary necrosis is not associated with either Fanconi's syndrome or tetracycline.

20. **The correct answer is E.** Patients with somatization disorder present with many physical complaints. To be diagnosed, they must have had at least eight symptoms, including at least two gastrointestinal symptoms, four pain symptoms, one sexual symptom, and one pseudoneurotic symptom. The patient finds the symptoms to be disabling out of proportion to the examination. These patients tend to be female with onset before the age of 30, and many patients also meet the criteria for a personality disorder.

Answer A is incorrect. Patients with body dysmorphic disorder have a severely distorted body image. All they see are imagined or minor physical flaws. They tend to obsess over their appearance, frequently look in mirrors, compare the flawed features with other people, and perform grooming rituals in order to hide the flaw. Onset tends to be in the late teens.

Answer B is incorrect. Patients with conversion disorder typically present with the sudden onset of loss of a single sensory or motor function, usually after a stressful life event. These patients tend to be adolescents or young adults, live in a rural area, lack education, and be of low socioeconomic status. The loss of function is not under voluntary control, and pain is not the predominant aspect of their complaint.

Answer C is incorrect. Patients with hypochondriasis misinterpret normal body symptoms and worry excessively about physical illness despite negative tests and positive reassurance. The diagnosis is made after their worries persist for more than 6 months. These patients tend to be middle-aged, and the incidence is roughly equal between men and women.

Answer D is incorrect. Patients with pain disorder complain of intense pain that is not explained by organic disease and lack symptoms other than pain. They tend to be in their 30s and 40s.

21. **The correct answer is C.** Langerhans cells are stellate cells with an oval or irregular pale nucleus, pale cytoplasm, and characteristic cytoplasmic granules. These Birbeck granules are seen on electron microscopy as striated rodlike structures attached to a vesicle; they resemble tennis rackets. Langerhans cells are found in all layers of the epidermis, but mainly in the stratum spinosum. They are derived from bone marrow and function in the immune process by binding and processing antigens from the skin. After antigen uptake, they migrate to regional lymph nodes, where they mature into paracortical interdigitating dendritic cells and present antigens to T lymphocytes.

Answer A is incorrect. Clear cells are nonsecretory cells that line the secretory portion of sweat glands. They are involved in transepithelial salt and fluid transport.

Answer B is incorrect. Dark cells are pyramidal cells that line most of the luminal surface of the sweat gland. Their role is to secrete glycoproteins.

Answer D is incorrect. Melanocytes produce melanin, which is the chief factor responsible for the pigmentation of skin and hair.

Answer E is incorrect. Merkel's cells are sensory mechanoreceptors responsible for touch sensation. They respond to pressure and are usually present in the thick skin of palms and soles.

22. **The correct answer is E.** Sphingomyelinase converts sphingomyelin to cerebroside. Deficiency of sphingomyelinase in Niemann-Pick disease causes accumulation of sphingomyelin and cholesterol in parenchymal and reticuloendothelial cells.

Answer A is incorrect. α-Galactosidase A converts ceramide trihexoside to lactosyl cerebroside. This enzyme is deficient in Fabry's disease.

Answer B is incorrect. β-Galactosidase converts galactocerebroside to cerebroside. This enzyme is deficient in Krabbe's disease.

Answer C is incorrect. Hexosaminidase A converts ganglioside M_2 to ganglioside M_3. This enzyme is deficient in Tay-Sachs disease.

Answer D is incorrect. β-Galactosidase converts galactocerebroside to cerebroside. This enzyme is deficient in Krabbe's disease.

23. **The correct answer is E.** This patient is experiencing serotonin syndrome, a constellation of symptoms that includes hyperpyrexia, muscle rigidity, cardiovascular collapse, and mental status changes. This syndrome is a well-known complication of combining selective serotonin reuptake inhibitors and monoamine oxidase (MAO) inhibitors in the same drug regimen. Tranylcypromine, the only MAO inhibitor included among the choices, is the only agent of those listed that could have caused this syndrome when combined with paroxetine.

Answer A is incorrect. Buspirone is an anxiolytic used in the treatment of generalized anxiety disorders. It would not cause serotonin syndrome when combined with a selective serotonin reuptake inhibitor.

Answer B is incorrect. Diazepam, a benzodiazepine, is used to treat anxiety and status epilepticus, but does not lead to serotonin syndrome when combined with a selective serotonin reuptake inhibitor.

Answer C is incorrect. Imipramine, a tricyclic antidepressant (TCA) used to treat bed-wetting, depression, and chronic pain, is not indicated for anxiety. Additionally, the combination of TCAs and selective serotonin reuptake inhibitors has not been associated with serotonin syndrome, although both medications affect serotonin concentrations.

Answer D is incorrect. Phenobarbital is a barbiturate used to treat anxiety and seizures. It does not cause serotonin syndrome when combined with selective serotonin reuptake inhibitors.

24. **The correct answer is E.** The most likely diagnosis is croup, which is most commonly caused by parainfluenza virus. Croup is an infection of the upper airway causing narrowing that leads to inspiratory wheezing and a barking cough. Most cases of croup require only supportive therapy as treatment. Severe cases may require supplemental oxygen, corticosteroids, and epinephrine. While parainfluenza is the most common agent responsible for croup, it can also be caused by influenza, respiratory syncytial virus, and measles.

Answer A is incorrect. Amantadine is an antiviral that has a narrow spectrum and is used to treat influenza type A. While influenza can cause croup, it is not the most common cause of this disease.

Answer B is incorrect. Bronchoalveolar lavage is used to sample the lower respiratory tract in severe pneumonia, in the diagnosis of a lung tumor, and in the assessment of fibrosing alveolitis, among other indications.

Answer C is incorrect. Admission to the emergency department may be called for if the child is in acute respiratory distress.

Answer D is incorrect. Penicillin can be used to treat streptococcal pharyngitis, which presents with red, swollen tonsils and pharynx and a high fever.

25. **The correct answer is B.** This patient has CREST syndrome. It is a variant of scleroderma (progressive systemic sclerosis), which is a disease characterized by extensive fibrosis throughout the body, most notably of the skin. **CREST** stands for **C**alcinosis (skin nodules

formed from the deposition of calcium salts), **R**aynaud's phenomenon (intermittent ischemia, pallor, pain, or paresthesias of the fingers, nose, ears, or toes brought on by cold or stress and alleviated by heat), **E**sophageal dysfunction, **S**clerodactyly, and **T**elangiectasias (small focal red skin marks from abnormally dilated blood vessels). Ninety-six percent of patients with anticentromere antibody have CREST syndrome.

Answer A is incorrect. Achalasia is characterized by aperistalsis of the esophagus, incomplete relaxation of the lower esophageal sphincter (LES) with swallowing, and increased tone of the LES even in its resting state. While achalasia also presents with difficulty swallowing, this diagnosis does not subsume the other symptoms this patient presented with.

Answer C is incorrect. Polyarteritis nodosa, a necrotizing immune complex vasculitis that usually affects small or medium-sized muscular arteries, commonly presents with fever, malaise, myalgias, and hypertension. Findings may include pericarditis, myocarditis, palpable purpura, and cotton-wool spots (white or grey opacities in the retina).

Answer D is incorrect. Rheumatoid arthritis is an autoimmune disorder of synovial joints and often presents with morning joint stiffness, subcutaneous joint nodules (particularly in the proximal interphalangeal joints), and symmetric joint involvement. Eighty percent of patients test positive for rheumatoid factor, and the disease may include systemic symptoms such as fever, pleuritis, and pericarditis.

Answer E is incorrect. Systemic lupus erythematosus is diagnosed by the presence of four of the 11 symptoms summarized by the mnemonic **"BRAIN SOAP, MD"**: **B**lood dyscrasias (such as hemolytic anemia or thrombocytopenia), **R**enal disorder, **A**rthritis, **I**mmunologic disorder (such as anti-DNA antibody and anti-Smith antibody), **N**eurologic disorder, **S**erositis (such as pleuritis or pericarditis), **O**ral ulcers, **A**ntinuclear antibody (elevated titers in the absence of drugs associated with drug-induced lupus syndrome), **P**hotosensitivity, **M**alar rash, and **D**iscoid rash.

26. **The correct answer is D.** A positive enzyme-linked immunosorbent assay (ELISA) result must be confirmed by Western blot. The Western blot is a highly specific test with a very low false-positive rate, such that a positive reaction for two of the three commonly tested HIV antigens indicates disease. The Western blot technique is generally performed as follows: (1) Run three HIV antigens on a protein gel. (2) Transfer proteins to the nitrocellulose membrane. (3) Add the patient's serum. If the patient is infected, then antibodies to HIV antigens will be present and will bind to the HIV antigens on the membrane. (4) Add secondary enzyme-linked anti-Ig antibody. (5) Add substrate for enzyme and observe for product. As shown in the figure, it is wise to add a positive control lane where a known concentration of anti-HIV antigen antibodies are added; additionally, a negative control lane where antibodies that are known not to bind the HIV antigen is included. If the positive control demonstrates three bands, one can be assured that the assay was successful; if the negative control demonstrates no bands, cross-contamination is unlikely. The Western blot shown in this question demonstrates that the patient's serum contains antibodies that bind two of three HIV antigens. Thus, the patient would receive a diagnosis of HIV infection.

Answer A is incorrect. The Western blot is positive.

Answer B is incorrect. There is no reason to believe contamination has occurred. In fact, if the positive control antibodies were mistakenly loaded in the patient's sample lane, one would expect that there would be three bands present in that lane.

Answer C is incorrect. Both the positive and negative control worked well, as three bands are clearly present in the positive control lane, and no bands are evident in the negative control lane.

Answer E is incorrect. The bands seen on the Western blot indicate that there are HIV-reactive antibodies in the patient's serum.

27. **The correct answer is A.** Bleomycin acts by forming superoxide or hydroxide radicals that attack the DNA bonds, causing strand breakage. Its primary use is in the treatment of testicular tumors. Unfortunately, it commonly causes pulmonary toxicity that can progress to fibrosis. Other adverse effects include skin changes and alopecia.

Answer B is incorrect. A Cisplatin is a platinum compound that causes DNA strand cross-linkage, preventing new DNA synthesis. It is used in combination with bleomycin and vinblastine to treat testicular cancer but does not cause pulmonary toxicity. Its adverse effects include persistent vomiting and nephrotoxicity.

Answer C is incorrect. Paclitaxel is a microtubule inhibitor that promotes dysfunctional polymerization, resulting in cell death. It is used to treat ovarian and breast cancer, not testicular cancer. Major adverse effects of paclitaxel include hypersensitivity and neutropenia.

Answer D is incorrect. Vinblastine is a microtubule inhibitor that blocks polymerization in order to cause cell death. It is used in conjunction with bleomycin and cisplatin to treat testicular cancers but does not cause pulmonary symptoms. Its adverse effects include cellulitis, alopecia, and bone marrow suppression.

Answer E is incorrect. Vincristine is a microtubule inhibitor with the same mechanism of action as vinblastine. It is used to treat acute lymphoblastic leukemia, Wilms' tumor, and lymphomas, not testicular carcinoma. Its adverse effects include cellulitis and peripheral neuropathies.

28. **The correct answer is C.** R Low thyroid (indicated by the constellation of signs and symptoms described in the vignette, or myxedema) and thyroid-stimulating hormone (TSH) levels indicate a secondary pituitary hypothyroidism.

Sheehan's syndrome results from hemorrhage and shock of the pituitary gland after hypotension from postpartum hemorrhage. Gonadotropin levels decline first, followed by TSH and ACTH. This results in amenorrhea and myxedema, as well as in hypotension and electrolyte imbalances due to adrenocortical insufficiency.

Answer A is incorrect. Antimicrosomal antibodies are found in Hashimoto's hypothyroidism. This results in high compensatory thyroid-stimulating hormone levels. Hashimoto's may or may not be associated with goiter but does not affect electrolyte levels.

Answer B is incorrect. Ectopic thyroid-stimulating hormone (TSH) secretion may arise exogenously or endogenously from malignancies such as struma ovarii, an ovarian monodermal germ cell tumor that secretes TSH. This condition would be associated with high TSH levels.

Answer D is incorrect. De Quervain's thyroiditis is a self-limiting subacute hypothyroidism that occurs following a flulike viral illness. Patients present with a tender thyroid gland, jaw pain, and elevated thyroid-stimulating hormone levels.

Answer E is incorrect. Thyroid-stimulating or thyroid-stimulating hormone–receptor antibodies are associated with Graves' disease, which may present during pregnancy or the postpartum period. This would result in hyperthyroidism, presenting as menorrhagia, weight loss, heat intolerance, sweats, diarrhea, and exophthalmos.

29. **The correct answer is F.** CD16 (also called Fc-γ RIII) is an important cell surface receptor found on natural killer (NK) cells. As an Fc receptor, CD16 can bind to antibodies coating virally infected cells. CD16 recognizes the Fc portion of certain IgG subclasses, and once bound, intracellular signaling results in the release of perforin and granzymes, thereby killing the virally infected cells. This mechanism of NK Fc receptor-mediated destruction is called antibody-dependent cell-mediated cytotoxicity.

Answer A is incorrect. CD3 is a key component of the T-lymphocyte receptor complex and is thus expressed by T lymphocytes.

Answer B is incorrect. Helper T lymphocytes express CD4; cytotoxic T lymphocytes express CD8.

Answer C is incorrect. Dendritic cells do not express the B-cell receptor. B cells do.

Answer D is incorrect. Helper T lymphocytes express CD4; cytotoxic T lymphocytes express CD8.

Answer E is incorrect. Helper T lymphocytes (not macrophages) express CD4.

Answer G is incorrect. RBCs do not express any major histocompatibility complex.

30. **The correct answer is E.** This patient demonstrates several findings classic for neurofibromatosis type 1 (also known as von Recklinghausen's disease), which include café au lait spots, two or more neurofibromas, optic glioma, iris hamartomas (Lisch's nodules), a positive family history (autosomal dominant inheritance), or a distinctive bony lesion such as sphenoid dysplasia or scoliosis. Patients demonstrate 95% of the criteria by age 8 and all of the criteria by age 20. These patients also demonstrate increased tumor susceptibility. The gene is located on the long arm of chromosome 17.

Answer A is incorrect. Bilateral acoustic neuromas are characteristic of neurofibromatosis type 2. The *NF2* gene is located on chromosome 22. It is much less common than type 1 and typically manifests with multiple central nervous system tumors.

Answer B is incorrect. Bilateral renal cell carcinoma occurs in von Hippel–Lindau disease, an autosomal dominant disease that is characterized by hemangioblastomas of the retina, cerebellum, and medulla. About half of patients develop bilateral renal cell carcinomas. The disease is associated with the deletion of the *VHL* gene located on chromosome 3, which is a tumor suppressor gene.

FULL-LENGTH EXAM

Test Block 3

Answer C is incorrect. Cystic medial necrosis of the aorta leading to aortic insufficiency and dissecting aortic aneurysm is associated with Marfan's syndrome, a connective tissue disorder caused by the autosomal dominant inheritance of a defective fibrillin gene.

Answer D is incorrect. Leptomeningeal angioma is associated with Sturge-Weber syndrome (SWS), which is a rare congenital vascular disorder of unknown etiology affecting capillary-sized blood vessels. Its characteristic features include angiomas and a facial port-wine stain. Only a small portion of patients with port-wine stains at birth have SWS.

31. **The correct answer is A.** Hemophilia (types A and B) is an X-linked recessive disorder, with affected male individuals inheriting a defective copy of the X chromosome from heterozygous (asymptomatic) mothers. It is caused by a deficiency in factor VIII (hemophilia A) or factor IX (hemophilia B) of the clotting cascade. Platelet number and bleeding time are normal because there is no deficiency of platelet function. Prothrombin time measures activity of factors VII, X, V, prothrombin, and fibrinogen, thus it is also normal in hemophilia. Partial thromboplastin time (PTT) measures activity of factors VIII, IX, XI, and XII in addition to factors X, V, prothrombin, and fibrinogen. PTT is therefore elevated in the case of factor VIII or IX deficiency.

Answer B is incorrect. This profile describes qualitative platelet defects such as Bernard-Soulier disease and Glanzmann's thrombasthenia. Since there is no clotting factor deficiency, prothrombin time and partial thromboplastin time are normal.

Answer C is incorrect. This profile describes von Willebrand's disease. Von Willebrand's factor promotes platelet adhesion to damaged endothelium, therefore its deficiency prolongs bleeding time. It also serves as a carrier for factor VIII, so partial thromboplastin time is also prolonged in this disorder.

Answer D is incorrect. This profile describes thrombocytopenia. Since there is no clotting factor deficiency, prothrombin time and partial thromboplastin time are normal. Since platelets are low, bleeding time is prolonged.

Answer E is incorrect. This profile describes disseminated intravascular coagulation. In this disorder, widespread intravascular coagulation consumes platelets and clotting factors, resulting in lab findings indicative of a deficiency in all elements of the clotting machinery.

32. **The correct answer is B.** Zanamivir is used in the treatment of both influenza A and influenza B. The mechanism of action is inhibition of the neuraminidase enzyme, which is critical to the influenza life cycle. First, hemagglutinin binds to neuraminic acid on host cells, allowing infection of the cell. After entering the cell, the virus replicates, and progeny viral assembly takes place in the cytoplasm. The virions bud from the cell membrane while bound to neuraminic acid. Neuraminidase cleaves the neuraminic acid, releasing the virions from the host. Zanamivir prevents the release of progeny virions by blocking neuraminidase.

Answer A is incorrect. Amantadine blocks viral penetration and uncoating. It is used to treat influenza A and rubella, as well as idiopathic Parkinson's disease.

Answer C is incorrect. Hemagglutinin binds to neuraminic acid, initiating infection.

Answer D is incorrect. Acyclovir inhibits viral DNA polymerase. It is used to treat herpes simplex virus, varicella-zoster virus, and Epstein-Barr virus.

Answer E is incorrect. Ribavirin is a guanine analog that blocks viral protein synthesis. It is used to treat respiratory syncytial virus.

33. **The correct answer is E.** The disease that is described in this patient is acute myelogenous leukemia (AML), which is characterized by acute onset of myelosuppression and the presence of increased myeloblasts in the peripheral smear and bone marrow. One subtype of AML is acute promyelocytic leukemia with abnormal presence of t(15;17), which encodes for a

fusion protein of the retinoic acid receptor with the promyelocytic leukemia gene. This fusion protein renders these cancer cells sensitive to treatment with all-trans retinoic acid, causing differentiation of myeloblasts into mature granulocytes. Combination treatment with retinoic acid and chemotherapy leads to overall response rates of 70–80% in this disease.

Answer A is incorrect. In general, chromosomal translocations involving chromosome 14 commonly occur in B-lymphocyte lymphomas, as the locus for immunoglobulin production is on chromosome 14. This translocation is associated with Burkitt's lymphoma and induces overproduction of the c-myc oncogene.

Answer B is incorrect. Translocation t(9;22), encoding bcr-abl, also known as the Philadelphia chromosome, is found in over 90% of chronic myelogenous leukemia (CML) and also in some acute leukemias, where it is associated with a poor prognosis. The bcr-abl fusion protein is a constitutively active tyrosine kinase that drives the cells to express a cancerous phenotype. Treatment of CML with imatinib mesylate, a specific bcr-abl kinase inhibitor, may control disease growth for several years without cytotoxic chemotherapy.

Answer C is incorrect. Translocation t(11;12), found in Ewing's sarcoma, results in production of the EWS transcription factor, which induces the overexpression of various oncogenes such as c-myc. Ewing's sarcoma is a bone tumor that presents as a rapidly enlarging mass in the diaphysis of long bones. It most commonly occurs in children.

Answer D is incorrect. In general, chromosomal translocations involving chromosome 14 will involve lymphomas, as the locus for immunoglobulin production is on chromosome 14. Translocation t(14;18) is associated with mantle cell lymphoma, a type of non-Hodgkin's lymphoma with a particularly poor prognosis. This fusion protein encodes cyclin D1, a protein involved in G1- to S-phase progression of the cell cycle.

34. **The correct answer is C.** Misoprostol is a prostaglandin E1 analog that can be used to prevent nonsteroidal anti-inflammatory drug–induced peptic ulcers. It is also used as a medical abortifacient in many countries, particularly Latin American countries, and is therefore strictly contraindicated in pregnant women.

Answer A is incorrect. Cimetidine is an H_2 antagonist and is associated with inhibition of the cytochrome P-450 system.

Answer B is incorrect. Magnesium hydroxide is an antacid and is associated with diarrhea.

Answer D is incorrect. Omeprazole is a proton pump inhibitor and is associated with atrophic gastritis due to hypergastrinemia and carcinoid tumors.

Answer E is incorrect. Sucralfate binds to ulcers, allowing a physical protective barrier, and has no known significant adverse effects.

35. **The correct answer is E.** This patient has clinical evidence of multiple endocrine neoplasia (MEN) type 1, which can cause tumors in the "3 P's": the **P**ituitary gland, the **P**arathyroid gland, and the **P**ancreas. The MEN 1 syndrome follows an autosomal dominant pattern of inheritance, thus this patient's family history of multiple endocrine organ abnormalities further supports this diagnosis. In this patient, parathyroid involvement is suggested by hypercalcemia; and a pituitary adenoma is most likely causing his bilateral hemianopsia. This patient has signs and symptoms consistent with elevated levels of vasoactive intestinal peptide (VIP). VIP acts on the gut mucosa to promote Na^+ secretion, causing a secretory diarrhea. VIP also stimulates K^+ secretion in the colon, causing hypokalemia, which can lead to the muscle weakness, tetany, and even periodic paralysis seen in this patient. Finally, VIP inhibits gastric acid secretion, leading to hypochlorhydria, which can be tested by an elevated pH on nasogastric suction fluid. The majority of VIPomas arise within the pancreas and are one type of pancreatic tumor seen in MEN 1.

Answer A is incorrect. Gastrinomas are non–β islet cell tumors that commonly arise from the pancreas and secrete gastrin, leading to hypersecretion of hydrochloric acid. Although gastrinomas do cause diarrhea and are associated with multiple endocrine neoplasia I, the pH of the nasogastric suction fluid would be decreased, not increased, in a patient with a gastrinoma.

Answer B is incorrect. Insulinomas are islet cell tumors that secrete insulin. These tumors are associated with Whipple's triad: hypoglycemia, symptoms of hypoglycemia that include mental status changes, and relief of symptoms upon glucose administration.

Answer C is incorrect. Medullary thyroid carcinoma is associated with increased levels of calcitonin, which rarely causes hypocalcemia and muscle weakness in these patients. Medullary thyroid carcinoma is associated with multiple endocrine neoplasia (MEN) 2A and 2B but not with MEN 1.

Answer D is incorrect. Although an abdominal mass noted on CT scan could be a pancreatic adenocarcinoma, the patient's symptoms point to the diagnosis of VIPoma.

36. **The correct answer is C.** This man has a strangulated direct inguinal hernia. Direct inguinal hernias are hernias within the floor of Hesselbach's triangle, where the hernia sac does not traverse the internal ring but herniates directly through the abdominal wall. They are more common in older people, as they are acquired defects from mechanical breakdown over the years. The lab values, consistent with mesenteric ischemia, and the irreducibility, point to a strangulated hernia. Hesselbach's triangle is bounded by the inferior epigastric vessels laterally, the lateral border of the rectus abdominis muscle medially, and the inguinal (or Poupart's) ligament inferiorly.

Answer A is incorrect. The common femoral artery is a continuation of the external iliac artery distal to the inguinal ligament.

Answer B is incorrect. The external iliac artery is the source of the inferior epigastric artery. It continues inferolaterally beyond that branch point.

Answer D is incorrect. The superior epigastric arteries branch off the internal thoracic arteries near the inferior edge of the sternum. They mainly supply the rectus abdominis muscles before anastomosing with the inferior epigastric arteries.

Answer E is incorrect. The superior vesical arteries are medial to the inferior epigastric artery and branch off the umbilical artery. They supply the upper part of the bladder and the ureter.

37. **The correct answer is B.** In order to answer this question correctly, it is important to acknowledge that the vitamin deficiency is B_{12}, that the etiology is pernicious anemia, and that the pathogenesis involves antibodies against parietal cells. Pernicious anemia is a vitamin B_{12} deficiency associated with chronic atrophic gastritis. Autoantibodies are directed against gastric parietal cells, leading to an intrinsic factor deficiency. Without intrinsic factor, vitamin B_{12} is not absorbed in the ileum of the gut. Pernicious anemia is more common among women of Northern European descent; patients may present with fatigue, dyspnea, and tachycardia. They may also present with neurologic symptoms due to abnormal myelin production, which differentiates it from folate deficiency; such symptoms include mental status changes, paresthesias, and difficulty with gait. A peripheral blood smear will show macrocytic red cells with hypersegmented polymorphonuclear leukocytes, consistent with megaloblastic anemia (as seen in the image). Treatment includes vitamin B_{12} injections.

Answer A is incorrect. Abnormal neural crest cell migration leads to Hirschsprung's disease, which is a congenital aganglionic motility disorder affecting the large bowel. Patients present with obstructive symptoms such as megacolon and not with vitamin B_{12} deficiency.

Answer C is incorrect. The colon is not the site of vitamin B_{12} absorption, and bacterial overgrowth there, such as with *Clostridium dif-*

ficile, will produce symptoms such as diarrhea, flatulence, and weight loss.

Answer D is incorrect. Green leafy vegetables contain folate, not vitamin B_{12}. Folate is an essential cofactor in nucleic acid synthesis and commonly leads to megaloblastic anemia as seen in the image. However, folate deficiency does not explain the neurologic symptoms experienced by this patient.

Answer E is incorrect. An embolus to the superior mesenteric artery can lead to an acute bowel infarction, a life-threatening problem. Patients typically present with abdominal pain, bloody stools, fever, and peritoneal signs, not with signs of vitamin B_{12} deficiency.

38. **The correct answer is A.** This patient has developed cirrhosis of the liver from chronic hepatitis C infection. Physical findings of jaundice, spider angiomata, and ascites are consistent with portal hypertension, which often results from increased portal venous pressure due to cirrhosis. Increased prothrombin time and low albumin with a moderate increase in liver enzymes are typical findings in patients with end-stage cirrhosis. This patient also manifests signs of hepatic encephalopathy, including asterixis (flapping tremor), confusion, and lethargy. Hepatic encephalopathy is an alteration in mental function secondary to ammonia buildup in bodily fluids. Ammonia is toxic to the central nervous system if it is not detoxified into urea by hepatic synthesis. In the absence of bowel obstruction, the most effective way to rapidly lower the ammonia level in a patient with hepatic encephalopathy is treatment with lactulose, which serves both as a means of acidifying the colon, thereby decreasing ammonia production, and as a laxative, thus shunting ammonia out of the gastrointestinal tract.

Answer B is incorrect. Although this patient may benefit from liver transplantation, it is not an acute treatment strategy.

Answer C is incorrect. Lorazepam, as well as other benzodiazepines that are metabolically cleared by the liver, should not be used and can actually worsen the encephalopathy.

Answer D is incorrect. While neomycin can be used as an adjunct to decrease ammonia production by gut flora, it is not first-line therapy. Neomycin works by destroying the gut flora that normally produce ammonia.

Answer E is incorrect. While a restricted protein diet should be standard in all patients with end-stage liver disease, it will not acutely decrease ammonia concentrations.

39. **The correct answer is B.** Gonorrhea is a reportable illness in all states. Gonorrhea is caused by sexually transmitted gram-negative cocci. Other examples of reportable illnesses in all states include hepatitis A and B, *Salmonella* and *Shigella* infections, syphilis, AIDS, tuberculosis, and chickenpox.

Answer A is incorrect. Although genital herpes is sexually transmitted, it is not reportable in most states. Genital herpes is caused by the herpes simplex virus.

Answer C is incorrect. HIV is not a reportable illness in all states; however, AIDS is a reportable illness. Of note is the fact that physicians are not required to maintain confidentiality when an HIV-positive patient intentionally and maliciously puts another person at risk through unprotected sex.

Answer D is incorrect. Influenza is caused by an orthomyxovirus, which is an RNA virus. It is the cause of the flu; however, it is not reportable in all states.

Answer E is incorrect. Scarlet fever is caused by *Streptococcus pyogenes* (group A β-hemolytic *Streptococcus*); however, it is not reportable in most states.

40. **The correct answer is A.** This patient has xeroderma pigmentosum, a disease characterized by extreme sensitivity to sunlight, skin damage, and a predisposition to malignancies such as melanoma. The disease results from a defective excision repair mechanism for ultraviolet light–damaged DNA.

Answer B is incorrect. The mismatch repair mechanism replaces segments of DNA that include mismatched bases. Hereditary nonpolyposis colorectal cancer is caused by defects in mismatch repair.

Answer C is incorrect. A defect in proofreading enzymes would not cause xeroderma pigmentosum. It would affect DNA replication in all body tissues, not just those exposed to UV light.

Answer D is incorrect. Benzo(a)pyrene is a carcinogen found in cigarette smoke. This carcinogen binds to DNA and forms bulky adducts with guanine residues. Bulky lesions are repaired by nucleotide excision.

Answer E is incorrect. Ionizing radiation, such as x-rays, removes electrons from atoms and molecules such as DNA. This causes chromosome breakage, translocations, and point mutations. Bloom's syndrome and ataxia-telangiectasia are rare autosomal recessive genetic disorders that are hypersensitive to ionizing radiation. Patients with xeroderma pigmentosum are hypersensitive to UV light.

41. **The correct answer is E.** hCG, thyroid-stimulating hormone (TSH), luteinizing hormone, and follicle-stimulating hormone are all composed of an identical α subunit paired with a β subunit that is unique to each of these hormones. Hence, any of these may interfere with the accurate detection and measurement of hCG by this hypothetical assay. TSH is the only hCG structural homologue listed among the answer choices.

Answer A is incorrect. ACTH does not share structural homology with hCG and should not interfere with the assay.

Answer B is incorrect. Gonadotropin-releasing hormone does not share structural homology with hCG and should not interfere with the assay.

Answer C is incorrect. Growth hormone does not share structural homology with hCG and should not interfere with the assay.

Answer D is incorrect. Melanocyte-stimulating hormone does not share structural homology with hCG and should not interfere with the assay.

42. **The correct answer is C.** Based on the physical findings and the low α-fetoprotein during pregnancy, this child most likely has Down's syndrome caused by trisomy 21. Down's syndrome is associated with many defects of embryology; the most common cardiac abnormality is an atrial septal defect of the septum primum, present in 45% of patients. The atrial septum develops as an outgrowth of the wall of the primitive atrium. The primitive atrium also develops into the trabeculated part of both atria. The second most common heart defect in children with Down's syndrome is ventricular septal defect, appearing in 35% of patients.

Answer A is incorrect. The bulbus cordis gives rise to the smooth part of both ventricles. These are not commonly malformed in children with Down's syndrome.

Answer B is incorrect. The neural crest cells give rise to many structures, including the aorticopulmonary septum, which divides the truncus arteriosus into the aorta and pulmonary trunk. Several malformations related to this structure exist, including a persistent truncus arteriosus, transposition of the great vessels, and tetralogy of Fallot. However, the most likely cardiac defect in a patient with Down's syndrome is an atrial septal defect.

Answer D is incorrect. The primitive ventricle gives rise to the trabeculated part of both ventricles and the interventricular septum. Malformations of these structures are possible but are not the most likely cardiac defect in children with Down's syndrome.

Answer E is incorrect. The truncus arteriosus gives rise to the aorta and pulmonary trunk. Malformations of these structures are not common in children with Down's syndrome.

43. **The correct answer is E.** Acute intermittent porphyria (AIP) and porphyria cutanea tarda (PCT) are the two most common porphyrias seen clinically. AIP is a defect in the enzyme porphobilinogen (PBG) deaminase, also called uroporphyrinogen I (URO I) synthase. AIP is the third enzyme in the heme synthetic pathway and results in aberrant accumulation of

aminolevulinate (ALA) and PBG. In contrast, PCT is a defect in the enzyme uroporphyrinogen decarboxylase, the fifth step in the heme pathway, which causes an accumulation of uroporphyrinogen but not ALA or PBG. In this case, the patient presents with symptoms most consistent with AIP, which is manifested by acute intermittent attacks between periods of disease remission. Symptoms during acute attacks are marked by neurovisceral symptoms—most commonly abdominal pain, muscle weakness, and psychiatric manifestations such as anxiety, paranoia, and depression—and by high PBG levels in urine, which in severe cases can present as red port wine–colored urine. No increased photosensitivity is seen with this disease. In contrast, PCT presents with photosensitivity and chronic, blistering lesions of sun-exposed skin in the absence of neuropsychiatric signs.

Answer A is incorrect. Aminolevulinate (ALA) dehydratase deficiency is associated with ALA dehydratase porphyria, which resembles acute intermittent porphyria.

Answer B is incorrect. Aminolevulinate synthase deficiency is associated with X-linked sideroblastic anemia.

Answer C is incorrect. Ferrochelatase deficiency results in anemia and porphyria.

Answer D is incorrect. Heme oxygenase catalyzes the oxidation of heme to biliverdin.

Answer F is incorrect. Uroporphyrinogen III cosynthase deficiency is associated with congenital erythropoietic porphyria, which resembles porphyria cutanea tarda.

Answer G is incorrect. Uroporphyrinogen decarboxylase deficiency is responsible for porphyria cutanea tarda.

44. **The correct answer is B.** Graft-versus-host disease (GVHD) is an unwanted side effect of bone marrow transplantation whereby donor T lymphocytes recognize the recipient as foreign and mount an immune response. The organs most often affected are the gut, skin, and liver. Human leukocyte antigen matching of the donor and recipient can help reduce the sever-

ity of GVHD, but the disease may still occur due to a minor histocompatibility mismatch.

Answer A is incorrect. Acute graft rejection is a potential side effect of solid organ transplant and is mediated by the recipient's cytotoxic T lymphocytes. The recipient of a bone marrow transplant undergoes myeloablative therapy before transplant, and therefore it is not expected that the patient would have significant numbers of T lymphocytes.

Answer C is incorrect. Graft-versus-host disease is mediated by donor T lymphocytes; recipient T lymphocytes are ablated before transplant.

Answer D is incorrect. Hyperacute graft rejection is a potential side effect of solid organ transplant and is mediated by preformed recipient antibodies.

Answer E is incorrect. The clinical scenario described is more suggestive of graft-versus-host disease than recurrence of leukemia.

45. **The correct answer is C.** This patient has symptoms and a diagnosis consistent with type 2 diabetes mellitus. Type 2 diabetes mellitus can cause a number of health problems, including small vessel disease, retinopathy, nephropathy, large vessel atherosclerosis, coronary artery disease, peripheral vascular occlusive disease, cerebrovascular disease, neuropathies, and cataracts. Hyperglycemia in these patients, as reflected by the increased hemoglobin A_{1c} level, can be attributed to a number of causes, including peripheral insulin resistance, impaired insulin processing, dysfunctional glucose detection by β cells, or impaired intracellular signaling. On light microscopy, kidneys affected by diabetes demonstrate nodular glomerulosclerosis, also known as Kimmelstiel-Wilson disease, and a thickened glomerular basement membrane.

Answer A is incorrect. Diffuse capillary and basement membrane thickening is associated with membranous glomerulonephritis.

Answer B is incorrect. Enlarged hypercellular glomeruli with neutrophils can be found in acute poststreptococcal glomerulonephritis.

Answer D is incorrect. Segmental sclerosis with hyalinosis is seen in focal segmental glomerulosclerosis.

Answer E is incorrect. Glomeruli demonstrating a wire-loop appearance with subendothelial basement membrane deposits are seen in lupus nephropathy.

46. **The correct answer is D.** The baby suffers from 21-α-hydroxylase deficiency, the most common cause of congenital adrenal hyperplasia and the underlying cause of the girl's virilism. Without functioning 21-α-hydroxylase, the precursor molecule 17-hydroxyprogesterone accumulates. 21-α-Hydroxylase deficiency also causes salt wasting with hypotension, hyponatremia, and hyperkalemia. Congenital adrenal hyperplasia is a common cause of female pseudohermaphroditism, a condition in which patients may have ambiguous genitalia but have a 46,XX karyotype.

Answer A is incorrect. In true hermaphroditism, both ovarian and testicular tissue can be found within the gonads. However, in 21-α-hydroxylase deficiency, the ovaries develop normally—it is the adrenal glands that cause the male-looking genitalia.

Answer B is incorrect. A 47,XXX karyotype would not cause congenital adrenal hyperplasia, salt wasting, or pseudohermaphroditism. Most women with an extra X chromosome are asymptomatic; an extra Barr body can be seen microscopically.

Answer C is incorrect. A deficiency in 5-α-reductase is a cause of male pseudohermaphroditism and is also known as testicular feminization syndrome. A lack of 5-α-reductase means that testosterone cannot be converted to dihydrotestosterone, the necessary hormone in the masculinization of genitalia.

Answer E is incorrect. Ovarian dysgenesis, the "streak ovary," is found in Turner's syndrome (45,XO). It does not cause salt wasting or virilism. Patients with Turner's present with poorly developed secondary sexual characteristics and amenorrhea.

47. **The correct answer is D.** A decrease in thyroid-stimulating hormone level is consistent with an increase in free T_4, but the vignette is not consistent with a history of primary hyperthyroidism. Additionally, an increase in total T_4 is not necessarily indicative of thyrotoxicosis, as total T_4 can also be affected by changes in TBG levels.

Answer A is incorrect. While an increase in thyroid-stimulating hormone levels would result in an increase in free T_4 and TBG, this does not normally occur during pregnancy and would result in the signs and symptoms of thyrotoxicosis.

Answer B is incorrect. While normal free T_4 is consistent with elevated total T_4 and TBG levels, an elevated thyroid-stimulating hormone level is not consistent with these laboratory findings or with the clinical history presented in the vignette.

Answer C is incorrect. During pregnancy, there is a physiologically normal increase in TBG levels in the blood, resulting in an increase in total T_4; free T_4 and thyroid-stimulating hormone remain normal. Patients remain asymptomatic despite this laboratory abnormality and require no treatment.

Answer E is incorrect. An increase in free T_4 would be consistent with thyrotoxicosis, but the vignette does not present any of the signs and symptoms that are consistent with this diagnosis.

48. **The correct answer is B.** Swollen eyelids, conjunctival inflammation, and yellow purulent discharge are symptoms of conjunctivitis. The newborn was colonized by *Chlamydia trachomatis* during his passage through the birth canal. It tends to develop a few days to several weeks after birth. Since *C. trachomatis* is the most common sexually transmitted disease in the United States, all newborns receive erythromycin eye drops prophylactically.

Answer A is incorrect. *Chlamydia psittaci* causes psittacosis. This disease causes symptoms similar to atypical pneumonia. The bacteria are spread through poultry and birds.

Answer C is incorrect. *Neisseria gonorrhoeae* causes gonorrhea. In infants, it causes gonococcal ophthalmic conjunctivitis but does not cause inclusion conjunctivitis.

Answer D is incorrect. *Trypanosoma brucei gambiense* is transmitted by a bite of a tsetse fly and causes African sleeping sickness.

Answer E is incorrect. *Ureaplasma urealyticum* can produce nongonococcal urethritis. This organism has the ability to convert urea into ammonia and carbon dioxide.

49. **The correct answer is A.** Analysis of variance, sometimes referred to as ANOVA, compares the mean values of three different populations. The test may be performed using one or two variables. In this case, the only variable would be the drug used. An additional variable could be the gender of the patient receiving the drug.

Answer B is incorrect. A chi-square test is not a parametric statistical test but a categorical test, which can only be used if both the dependent and independent variables are categorical and not numerical in nature. An example of categorical data would be race, where no numerical data exists, as opposed to age, for which numerical values are recorded. The chi-square test is used to check for differences between two or more percentages or proportions of categorical outcomes. For example, the chi-square could be used to compare myocardial infarction rates between the sexes. Both variables are nonnumerical: either the person has an myocardial infarction or not, and they are either female or male.

Answer C is incorrect. A dependent t-test is used to analyze the mean of one group at two different times, which is not the design of this study.

Answer D is incorrect. An independent t-test is used to analyze the mean in two groups at one time, which is not the design of this study.

Answer E is incorrect. Wilcoxon's test is not a parametric test. Parametric tests assume a normal (Gaussian or bell-shaped) distribution of data around the mean. In contrast, nonparametric tests such as Wilcoxon's are used when a distribution is abnormal, as occurs with unknown confounders, systematic error, small sample size, or true coincident error.

50. **The correct answer is F.** von Willebrand factor (vWF) is a large multimeric protein that possesses two major functions in hemostasis: (1) it acts as a bridging molecule for platelet adhesion, and (2) it is a carrier protein for factor VIII. Von Willebrand's disease (vWD) is the most common inherited bleeding disorder and is divided into three major subtypes, depending on the degree to which these two biological functions are affected. The most common subtype is type I vWD (accounting for 70% of cases) and presents with a quantitative decrease in vWF multimers as well as decreased factor VIII (due to increased clearance of this factor). Functionally, this results in defects in platelet function (causing prolonged bleeding time) as well as coagulation (causing prolonged partial thromboplastin time).

Answer A is incorrect. Bernard-Soulier syndrome reflects a defect in platelet adhesion due to a defect in the GPIb receptor (the primary von Willebrand factor receptor). Without this receptor, platelet adhesion to the site of bleeding fails, platelet activation and aggregation does not occur, and prolonged bleeding time results.

Answer B is incorrect. Glanzmann's thrombasthenia reflects a defect in platelet aggregation due to a defect in the GPIIb/IIIa receptor (which binds both von Willebrand factor and fibrinogen). In this case, platelet adhesion occurs; however, platelet aggregation and formation of the platelet-ligand-platelet matrix is defective, resulting in prolonged bleeding time.

Answer C is incorrect. Hemophilia A is an X-linked deficiency of factor VIII. This is the second most commonly inherited bleeding disorder and results in prolonged partial thromboplastin time with normal platelet function (bleeding time).

Answer D is incorrect. Hemophilia B is an X-linked deficiency of factor IX. This is the third most commonly inherited bleeding disorder and is identical to hemophilia A in its clinical presentation. In vivo, factor IXa and factor VIIIa are associated on the platelet membrane.

Answer E is incorrect. Thrombotic thrombocytopenic purpura (TTP), in contrast to the other answer choices, results in enhanced thrombosis. TTP is caused by either the congenital absence or the antibody-induced inhibition of the von Willebrand factor (vWF)-cleaving protease. As a result, very large high-molecular-weight vWF multimers are present in the circulation. This causes enhanced platelet adhesion but does not activate the coagulation cascade (hence prothrombin and partial thromboplastin time are normal). Microangiopathic hemolysis with schistocytes and thrombocytopenia is often present in this disorder.

Test Block 4

1. A 2-year-old boy who started treatment for absence seizures 2 weeks ago presents to the physician with blistering around his nose and mouth. On examination it is noted that there is extensive shedding of the skin. Which of the following agents most likely caused this result?

(A) Carbamazepine
(B) Ethosuximide
(C) Phenytoin
(D) Topiramate
(E) Valproic acid

2. A 15-year-old girl presents to the physician with underdeveloped breasts and hirsutism. Her medical history includes menarche at age 12 and normal menses since then; her blood pressure is 90/55 mm Hg. The enzyme deficient in this patient is needed for the production of which of the following hormones?

(A) Aldosterone
(B) Estradiol
(C) Estrone
(D) Progesterone
(E) Testosterone

3. A 4-year-old child whose family arrived in the United States from China last month is brought to the pediatrician for a checkup. On physical examination, the patient is found to be short, potbellied, and pale with a puffy face, a protruding umbilicus, and a protuberant tongue. The child shows clear signs of significant mental retardation. Which of the following laboratory tests should be ordered for this patient and what are the likely results?

(A) Pituitary function tests: increased growth hormone and ACTH levels
(B) Pituitary function tests: increased growth hormone level, decreased ACTH level
(C) Thyroid function tests: decreased thyroid-stimulating hormone, increased triiodothyronine and thyroxine levels
(D) Thyroid function tests: increased thyroid-stimulating hormone, decreased triiodothyronine and thyroxine levels

(E) Thyroid function tests: increased thyroid-stimulating hormone, increased triiodothyronine and thyroxine levels

4. A 59-year-old woman was recently admitted to the hospital because of oral ulcers and diffuse crusted, denuded, erythematous plaques on her torso and upper arms (see image). She has tested positive for anti–epithelial cell antibodies. Which of the following is the most likely diagnosis?

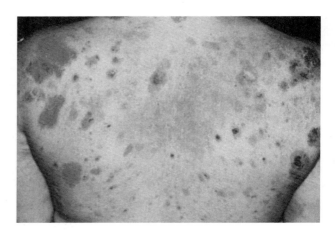

Reproduced, with permission, from Kasper DL, Braunwald E, Fauci AS, Hauser SL, Longo DL, Jameson JL, and Isselbacher KJ, eds. *Harrison's Principles of Internal Medicine*, 16th ed. New York, McGraw-Hill, 2004: Fig. 49-1A.

(A) Bullous pemphigoid
(B) Eczema
(C) Erythema multiforme
(D) Impetigo
(E) Pemphigus vulgaris

5. A 28-year-old woman has a 1-year history of recurrent abdominal pain relieved by defecation. She reports that her diarrhea has gotten worse in the last 2 weeks, since she started a new job. Her examination is unremarkable except for mild abdominal tenderness. Her laboratory studies show the following results:

Hemoglobin: 13.0 g/dL
Hematocrit: 39%

WBC count: 6,000/mm^3

Platelet count: 200,000/mm^3

Erythrocyte sedimentation rate: 8 mm/hr

Which of the following pharmacologic therapies would be most appropriate in the treatment of this patient's symptoms?

(A) Bactrim

(B) Bismuth

(C) Loperamide

(D) Metronidazole

(E) Octreotide

(F) Omeprazole

6. A 46-year-old man comes to the clinic with a cough that is occasionally productive of blood, diffuse muscle and joint pain in the upper extremities, and blood in his urine for the past several days. On further questioning, the patient reveals that he has had chronic sinusitis for the past several years. The patient has a low-grade fever and nasal ulcerations. Laboratory studies show a markedly elevated erythrocyte sedimentation rate, and staining for antibodies to cytoplasmic antigens of neutrophils is positive. Biopsy of a nasal ulceration reveals vasculitis and necrotizing granulomas. Which of the following is the most likely diagnosis?

(A) Alport's syndrome

(B) Giant cell (temporal) arteritis

(C) Goodpasture's syndrome

(D) Takayasu's arteritis

(E) Wegener's granulomatosis

7. A peripheral T lymphocyte engages peptide-bound class II major histocompatibility complex molecules on the surface of an antigen-presenting cell. No other contact is made between cell surface molecules present on the T lymphocyte and the antigen-presenting cell. Which of the following can be concluded about this peripheral T lymphocyte?

(A) The T lymphocyte will be activated and fully able to perform effector functions

(B) The T lymphocyte will be activated but unable to perform effector functions

(C) The T lymphocyte will cause the antigen-presenting cell to undergo apoptosis

(D) The T lymphocyte will clonally expand

(E) The T lymphocyte will undergo anergy

8. The *ras* oncogene is the most common abnormality in human cancer and is involved in approximately 30% of tumors. To which of the following families of molecules does *ras* belong?

(A) Cyclin-dependent kinases

(B) Epidermal growth factor receptor

(C) Guanosine triphosphate–binding proteins

(D) Non-receptor–associated tyrosine kinase

(E) Transcriptional activators

9. A 22-year-old white man with metastatic testicular carcinoma is undergoing treatment with high doses of cisplatin. Which class of drugs is most likely to suppress his chemotherapy-related nausea?

(A) Benzodiazepines

(B) Cholinergic antagonists

(C) Dopamine receptor antagonists

(D) Histamine receptor antagonists

(E) 5-HT$_3$ antagonists

10. A 3-year-old girl is brought to her pediatrician because of a progressive loss of motor function and a decline in her cognitive abilities. On physical examination, it is noted that the patient has decreased deep tendon reflexes, truncal ataxia, and a decreased attention span in comparison to the child's last visit 6 months ago. The physician knows that her pathology is due to an abnormal accumulation of cerebroside sulfate in her brain, peripheral nerves, kidney, and liver. A deficiency of which of the following enzymes leads to this condition?

(A) Arylsulfatase A

(B) β-Galactosidase

(C) α-Galactosidase A

(D) Hexosaminidase A

(E) Sphingomyelinase

11. A 35-year-old woman comes to the physician with right-handed paralysis, ataxia, and incontinence for the past 36 hours. The patient states that she has had generalized right-sided weakness for years along with episodes of sensory numbness and/or motor paralysis. The episodes normally last a few days, and the last episode occurred 18 months ago. Her left hand became so weak that she could not write with it. MRI of the brain is significant for periventricular white matter plaques. Which of the following signs and symptoms commonly occurs in patients with this disease?

(A) Forceful, spastic involuntary movements of the limbs and/or facial muscles; onset is gradual, but spasms are permanent
(B) Permanent bilateral resting tremor of the upper extremities
(C) Permanent progressive paralysis of respiratory muscles
(D) Spasm of digital arteries, causing blanching, numbness, and pain to the fingers whenever the patient is exposed to cold temperatures
(E) Vision loss in one eye, usually lasting a few days

12. A researcher studying a pedigree of familial type 1 diabetes mellitus discovers a mutation in the K^+ channel expressed in the cell membrane of pancreatic acinar β cells. This mutation impairs closing of the K^+ channel. The efficacy of which of the following agents would be most profoundly affected by this mutation?

(A) Acarbose
(B) Glargine
(C) Glipizide
(D) Metformin
(E) Troglitazone

13. A 47-year-old woman presents to her family practitioner because of depression. About this time last year, her husband died of pancreatic cancer 6 months after being diagnosed. She has returned to work but says that she still cries and feels sad most of the time. She also says that she continues to experience insomnia most nights of the week. She feels guilty that she is alive while he is dead. Her physical examination is unremarkable except that she weighs about 1.3 kg (2.9 lb) less than she did last year. Which of the following symptoms is an indication of an abnormal grief reaction in this patient?

(A) Continuing insomnia
(B) Feelings of sadness
(C) Guilty feelings
(D) Returning to work
(E) Weight loss

14. A 27-year-old woman is brought to the emergency department with an intense headache, unilateral weakness, and blurred vision that began after she was ejected from her vehicle in a motor vehicle accident. Paramedics report that she was ambulatory and cooperative at the scene of the crash but was unable to tell them what had happened. The patient had an episode of projectile vomiting while in the ambulance, and her mental status has deteriorated since then. On examination, the patient's blood pressure is 150/88 mm Hg with a pulse of 56/min; she has right-sided mydriasis. The patient's motor examination is 5/5 on the right side and 3/5 on the left side in both upper and lower extremities, with brisk reflexes on the left side. A CT scan of the head shows a hyperdense extra-axial fluid collection on the right side and a nondepressed temporal bone fracture on the same side. Injury to which of the following is the most likely cause of the patient's presentation?

(A) Inferior cerebral veins
(B) Middle meningeal artery
(C) Posterior ethmoidal artery
(D) Sigmoid sinus
(E) Superior sagittal sinus

15. An infant with severe jaundice that is not corrected by phototherapy is in danger of developing kernicterus. This can occur in infants with Crigler-Najjar syndrome, a genetic disorder in which there is a near-complete deficiency of glucuronyl transferase. Which of the following laboratory findings would you expect to see in blood tests in an infant with Crigler-Najjar syndrome?

(A) Decreased hematocrit
(B) Decreased indirect bilirubin
(C) Increased direct bilirubin
(D) Increased indirect bilirubin
(E) Increased reticulocyte count

16. A 72-year-old man who receives treatment for congestive heart failure presents to the emergency department with vomiting, abdominal pain, and changes in his color vision. He is confused and does not remember the names of his medications. His ECG is shown in the image. Which of the following could have caused this patient's symptoms?

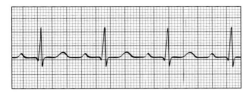

Reproduced, with permission, from USMLERx.com.

(A) Recent decrease in his digoxin dosage
(B) Recent decrease in his verapamil dosage
(C) Recent increase in his enalapril dosage
(D) Recent increase in his furosemide dosage
(E) Recent increase in his spironolactone dosage

17. A 78-year-old man has a 3-day history of diarrhea, left lower quadrant abdominal pain, and fever. His leukocyte count is slightly elevated,

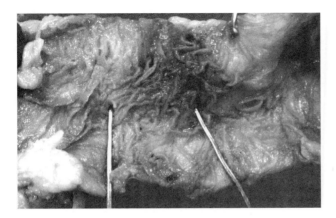

Image courtesy of PEIR Digital Library (http://peir.net)

his hematocrit level reveals slight anemia, and his platelets are normal. A biopsy is obtained and shown in the image. Which of the following is the most likely diagnosis?

(A) Angiodysplasia
(B) Crohn's disease
(C) Diverticulitis
(D) Ischemic bowel disease
(E) Ulcerative colitis

18. A 36-year-old man who is HIV-positive presents to the physician with fever, cough, headaches, and myalgias. Questioning reveals that the man has just returned from a visit with his brother, who lives in Mississippi. No action is taken at the time, and the patient is sent home. A few weeks later, the patient returns to the hospital with a lung disease resembling tuberculosis. Microscopic examination of the patient's sputum reveals a fungus with a captain's-wheel appearance. This patient is most likely infected with which of the following types of fungus?

(A) *Blastomyces*
(B) *Cryptococcus neoformans*
(C) *Histoplasma*
(D) *Mucor*
(E) *Tinea versicolor*

19. A 29-year-old woman comes to her primary care physician for a routine examination. Her past medical history is significant for narcolepsy, which is being treated by a neurologist. Which of the following medications is most likely to reduce excessive daytime sleepiness in this patient?

(A) Atomoxetine
(B) Desmopressin
(C) Imipramine
(D) Lorazepam
(E) Modafinil

20. A 44-year-old woman with end-stage renal disease on hemodialysis presents to the physician with abdominal pain. Laboratory tests are positive for HBsAg, IgM anti-HBc, and HBeAg antibodies, and negative for anti-HBs and anti-HBe antibodies. Which of the following is the appropriate treatment for this patient's disease?

    (A) Lamivudine and interferon-α
    (B) Lamivudine and interferon-β
    (C) Ribavirin and interferon-α
    (D) Ribavirin and lamivudine
    (E) Ribavirin and pegylated interferon

21. A previously healthy 20-year-old college student presents to the student health office complaining of a 1-week history of fatigue and dark-colored urine. On physical examination, his blood pressure is 155/90 mm Hg and his serum creatinine level is 4.4 mg/dL. Urinalysis shows 3+ blood and red cell casts without protein, glucose, or ketones. A kidney biopsy shows crescentic changes of the glomerulus. Which of the following is the most likely diagnosis?

    (A) Diabetic nephropathy
    (B) Membranoproliferative glomerulonephritis
    (C) Minimal change disease
    (D) Rapidly progressive glomerulonephritis
    (E) Systemic lupus erythematosus

22. A healthy 26-year-old woman delivers a single chorion and placenta but two amniotic sacs following a normal, full-term delivery. Which of the following is the most likely cause of these findings?

    (A) Chorioamnionitis
    (B) Complete hydatidiform mole
    (C) Dizygotic twins
    (D) Monozygotic twins
    (E) Sheehan's syndrome

23. A 54-year-old alcoholic is brought to the emergency department by fire rescue after being found lying face down in the street. He is incoherent and is unable to walk in a straight line. His pulse is 110/min, his blood pressure is 135/80 mm Hg, and his respiration rate is 20/min. Physical examination reveals a di-

aphoretic man with generalized weakness passing in and out of consciousness. A glucose fingerstick test shows a glucose level of 45 g/dL. This patient's hypoglycemia most likely resulted from an elevated ratio of which of the following?

    (A) NADH:NAD⁺
    (B) NAD⁺:NADH
    (C) NADPH:NADP
    (D) NADP:NADPH
    (E) Pyruvate:lactate

24. Eukaryotic genes can contain thousands of nucleotides that define the sequence. Not all the nucleotides are actually used to code for corresponding RNA molecules. Genes are divided into introns and exons based on whether or not a region of DNA within a gene is transcribed into messenger RNA. A mutation in a eukaryotic cell is shown below. The mutation is located at the 5′ end of an intron. This change is most likely to affect which of the following processes?

Normal	5′ TTCGUTCCGACT 3′
Mutant	5′ TTCAUTCCGACT 3′

    (A) Capping
    (B) Hybridization
    (C) Polyadenylation
    (D) Splicing
    (E) Transcription

25. A 20-year-old college student complains to student health services of severe fatigue and lethargy. She reports a recent mononucleosis infection that has resolved. Physical examination shows scleral icteral jaundice, cervical lymphadenopathy, and splenomegaly. The tips of her fingers are purple. Laboratory testing shows a decreased hemoglobin level and appropriate reticulocytosis. A heterophile test is positive. A Coombs' test is negative for IgG or IgM but is positive for complement. Which of the following is the most likely diagnosis?

(A) Aplastic anemia
(B) Disseminated intravascular coagulation
(C) IgG-mediated (warm) hemolytic anemia
(D) IgM-mediated (cold) hemolytic anemia
(E) Paroxysmal nocturnal hemoglobinuria

26. A clinical laboratory receives a sample of amniotic fluid from a 37-year-old female patient. The patient's doctor has requested a workup for potential genetic diseases. The laboratory isolates some of the DNA from the sample and proceeds to run tests to determine if any genetic diseases are present. In order to produce the most DNA possible for further testing, which of the following procedures should be performed?

(A) Enzyme-linked immunosorbent assay
(B) Ligase chain reaction
(C) Northern blot
(D) Polymerase chain reaction
(E) Southern blot

27. A 71-year-old Russian man comes to the physician complaining of a 4-month history of fatigue, low-grade fevers, night sweats, and cough. He became extremely worried yester-

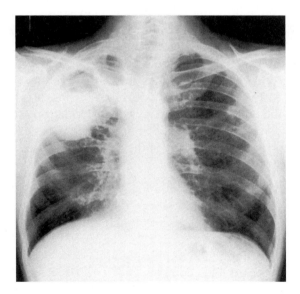

Reproduced, with permission, from Doherty GM, Way LW. *Current Surgical Diagnosis and Treatment*, 12th ed. New York, McGraw-Hill, 2006: Fig. 18-19.

day when he noticed blood in his sputum. On physical examination, he is extremely thin, with enlarged, nontender left-sided cervical lymph nodes. His x-ray film of the chest is shown. Which of the following organisms is the most likely cause of this patient's illness?

(A) *Legionella pneumophila*
(B) *Mycobacterium tuberculosis*
(C) *Mycoplasma pneumoniae*
(D) Respiratory syncytial virus
(E) *Streptococcus pneumoniae*

28. A 47-year-old woman presents to the physician with weight gain, fatigue, and lethargy. She says her appetite has decreased recently, and she has been constipated. Laboratory findings show a thyroid-stimulating hormone (TSH) level of 54 µU/mL, a total triiodothyronine (T_3) level of 57 ng/dL, and a thyroxine (T_4) level of 0.3 µg/dL. A thyroid biopsy shows an enlarged, symmetric, and firm thyroid. A histologic study shows a significant lymphocyte and plasma cell infiltrate with occasional germinal center formation. Follicles contain little colloid, while the follicular epithelial lining is replaced with Hürthle cells. Genetic testing indicates that the patient is HLA-DR5 and HLA-B5-positive. Which of the following autoantibodies would most likely be found in this patient?

(A) Anti–basement membrane antibodies
(B) Anti–epithelial cell antibodies
(C) Antimicrosomal antibodies
(D) Antimitochondrial antibodies
(E) Antineutrophil antibodies

29. A 66-year-old man presents to his primary care physician for a regular check-up, although it is 2 months earlier than the regularly scheduled appointment. His past medical history is significant for hypertension, type 2 diabetes mellitus, peripheral vascular disease, and coronary artery disease status post–myocardial infarction. His current medications are propranolol, captopril, aspirin, lovastatin, metformin, fluoxetine, and sublingual nitroglycerin. On further questioning, he admits to wanting a prescription for sildenafil. Which of his medications is unsafe to take with sildenafil?

(A) Aspirin
(B) Captopril
(C) Fluoxetine
(D) Lovastatin
(E) Metformin
(F) Nitroglycerin
(G) Propranolol

30. A 64-year-old woman is brought to her primary care physician by her daughter because she is concerned that she has been progressively losing her vision. The patient emigrated from Southeast Asia 1 week ago. The daughter says that her mother's poor vision worsens at night, causing her to frequently run into the bedroom wall. Her nutrition was poor in Asia. On physical examination, her conjunctivae are found to be notably dry with a small build-up of keratin debris. The physician diagnoses the patient with vitamin A deficiency. Which of the following syndromes is the result of another fat-soluble vitamin deficiency?

(A) Iron-deficiency anemia
(B) Megaloblastic anemia
(C) Osteomalacia
(D) Pellagra
(E) Wernicke's syndrome

31. A 62-year-old woman has sudden onset of stabbing epigastric pain and hematemesis of bright red blood. She has a history of heartburn and has been taking over-the-counter antacids for most of her adult life. She has no history of liver disease. In the emergency department, she is stabilized with intravenous fluids and sent for esophagogastroduodenoscopy. A bleeding ulcer is visualized on the posterior duodenum approximately 2 cm from the pylorus. Which of the following vessels is the most likely source of the bleeding?

(A) Gastroduodenal artery
(B) Left gastric artery
(C) Left gastroepiploic artery
(D) Right gastric artery
(E) Right gastroepiploic artery

32. A 70-year-old woman is hospitalized for a change in mental status. During the course of her hospitalization, she develops a urinary tract infection and her urinary catheter is removed. Urine cultures show a gram-negative bacillus that is determined to be *Enterobacter cloacae*. This infection should be treated with which of the following agents?

(A) Ciprofloxacin
(B) Gentamicin
(C) Imipenem
(D) Penicillin G
(E) Piperacillin-tazobactam

33. A 30-year-old darkly pigmented African-American man comes to the physician with loss of pigment on both hands resulting in white macules that create the appearance of white gloves. The patient is otherwise asymptomatic and states that he has had this condition for the past several years. A skin biopsy is taken from the macules and viewed on electron microscopy. Which of the following best describes the function of the structure affected or absent in this patient?

(A) To connect epithelial cells to underlying extracellular matrix
(B) To function as light touch sensory receptors
(C) To function as pressure and coarse touch sensory receptors
(D) To serve as antigen-presenting cells during certain immune responses
(E) To synthesize melanin and secrete it to keratinocytes

34. A 3-month-old infant presents with failure to thrive, poor feeding, and lethargy. A physical examination reveals an enlarged liver and jaundice. Laboratory analysis reveals an elevated blood galactitol level. Which of the following could correctly describe the levels of intermediates of galactose metabolism in this patient?

(A) Decreased galactose
(B) Decreased galactose-1-phosphate
(C) Decreased uridine diphosphoglucose
(D) Elevated glucose-1-phosphate
(E) Increased glycogen

35. A 54-year-old man presents to the emergency department with chest pain of 10 minutes' duration that began while he was mowing the lawn. The pain radiates to his left shoulder but does not compromise his ability to move his left shoulder or hand. He takes no medications. An ECG taken in the emergency department is shown in the image. The patient is given an aspirin. Additionally, which of the following medications should be given to the patient to alleviate his symptoms?

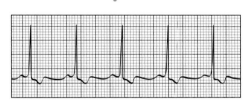

Reproduced, with permission, from USMLERx.com.

(A) Acetaminophen
(B) Digoxin
(C) Enalapril
(D) Hydrochlorothiazide
(E) Nifedipine
(F) Quinidine
(G) Sublingual nitroglycerin

36. A 32-year-old man presents with progressive dementia and sudden, jerky, purposeless movements. On evaluation, the patient is noted to be depressed. The patient states that his father, who died at age 50, had a similar condition as a young man. Huntington's disease is sus-

pected. Which of the following is the location of the lesion?

(A) Amygdala
(B) Caudate nucleus
(C) Lateral corticospinal tracts
(D) Locus ceruleus
(E) Nucleus basalis of Meynert
(F) Mammillary bodies

37. A new genetic test for cystic fibrosis was developed and tested on 100 neonates known to have the disease. It returns a positive result in 98 of the neonates and a negative result in the other 2 neonates. Which of the following can be concluded from this data about the new test?

(A) It has an incidence of 98%
(B) It has a negative predictive value of 98%
(C) It has a positive predictive value of 98%
(D) It has a prevalence of 98%
(E) It has a sensitivity of 98%
(F) It has a specificity of 98%

38. A 51-year-old man with HIV infection presents to the clinic with a 4-month history of increasing cognitive decline characterized by increasing apathy and mental slowing. He has a past medical history significant for several infections with *Pneumocystis jiroveci* (formerly *P. carinii*) pneumonia and had a recent CD4 count of 112/μL. Physical examination is notable for impaired saccadic eye movements, diffuse hyperreflexia, frontal release signs, and dysdiadochokinesia. A lumbar puncture is normal with the exception of a total protein concentration of 72 mg/dL and an elevated level of IgG. An MRI shows global cerebral atrophy with multiple ill-defined areas of white matter enhancement on T2-weighted images. Which of the following is the most likely cause of this patient's cognitive decline?

(A) Central nervous system lymphoma
(B) Cytomegalovirus encephalitis
(C) Disseminated *Mycobacterium avium* complex
(D) HIV-associated dementia
(E) Toxoplasmosis

39. To perform its unique function, the sperm cell has adapted many common cellular organelles into highly specialized structures, such as its powerful flagellum and its acrosome. The acrosome is derived from which of the following common organelles?

    (A) Centriole
    (B) Golgi apparatus
    (C) Mitochondrion
    (D) Nucleus
    (E) Plasma membrane

40. A 56-year-old man who is undergoing chemotherapy for colorectal carcinoma develops profound nausea and vomiting 4 hours after receiving treatments. The drug most likely to relieve the patient's symptoms functions by which of the following mechanisms?

    (A) Acetylcholine antagonist
    (B) Dopamine agonist
    (C) Norepinephrine reuptake inhibitor
    (D) Serotonin agonist
    (E) Serotonin antagonist

41. A 67-year-old man presents to his primary care physician with a 1-year history of increasing weakness and weight loss. Physical examination shows hepatosplenomegaly and generalized lymphadenopathy. A laboratory study shows leukocytosis. A peripheral blood smear shows increased lymphocytes that are destroyed during slide preparation. Which of the following normal cell types does the neoplastic cell in this condition most closely resemble?

    (A) B lymphocyte
    (B) Metamyelocyte
    (C) Plasma cell
    (D) Promyelocyte
    (E) T lymphocyte

42. A second-year medical student is under a lot of stress due to her impending biochemistry examination. She knows that her psychological stress causes an increase in her endogenous glucocorticoid levels. Glucocorticoids induce the enzyme phosphoenolpyruvate carboxykinase, among others. In which of the following pathways does this enzyme function?

    (A) Citric acid cycle
    (B) Gluconeogenesis
    (C) Glycogenolysis
    (D) Lipogenesis
    (E) Pentose phosphate pathway

43. After 3 days of flulike symptoms, a patient is feeling unsteady on her feet and dizzy when she attempts to stand up. During her illness she has eaten very little, has had frequent emesis, and is not interested in drinking fluids. A metabolic alkalosis is suspected. What is the most likely etiology of this acid-base disturbance?

    (A) Consumption of antacids
    (B) Decreased hydrogen excretion in the distal tubule
    (C) Increased bicarbonate reabsorption by the proximal tubule
    (D) Production of ADH
    (E) Volume depletion and increased H+ excretion in the distal tubule

44. If either the ulnar or radial arteries are occluded, which arteries ensure adequate collateral arterial flow in the hand?

    (A) Anterior and posterior interosseous
    (B) Arcuate
    (C) Common and proper palmar digitals
    (D) Deep and superficial dorsalis pedis
    (E) Deep and superficial palmar arch

45. An obese 35-year-old woman presents to her physician with a 6-month history of amenorrhea. Her blood pressure is 128/88 mm Hg, and her laboratory studies show a luteinizing hormone (LH) level of 300 mIU/mL, a follicle-stimulating hormone level of 5 mIU/mL, and a thyroid-stimulating hormone (TSH) level of 0.7 µU/mL. She also complains of increased hair growth. Physical examination reveals a normally developed woman, and a pelvic examination shows enlarged ovaries bilaterally. Her pregnancy test is negative Which of the following additional findings is most commonly associated with her condition?

    (A) Abdominal striae
    (B) Exophthalmos

(C) Galactorrhea
(D) Hyperglycemia
(E) Weak pulses in the lower extremities

46. A 4-year-old girl is brought to the emergency department by ambulance late at night. Her caretaker reports that the child refuses to bear weight on her left leg and reports that she fell down the stairs this morning. The child is unable to give a story of the accident. X-ray film of the leg shows a spiral fracture of her left femur along with evidence of old fractures in the ribs. Which of the following is the most likely diagnosis?

(A) Child abuse
(B) Normal play injury
(C) Osteogenesis imperfecta
(D) Osteosarcoma
(E) Vitamin D deficiency

47. A 1-month-old boy presents to the pediatrician with bilious vomiting, an intolerance of feeding, and bloody diarrhea. His disorder resulted from incomplete rotation of the midgut during fetal development. An x-ray film of this patient's abdomen is shown. Which of the following is the most likely diagnosis?

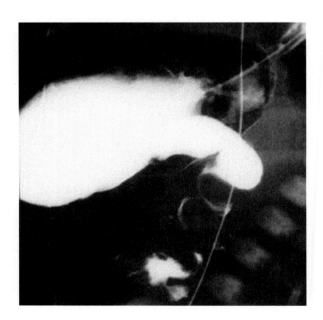

Image courtesy of PEIR Digital Library (http://peir.net).

(A) Hirschsprung's disease
(B) Meckel's diverticulum
(C) Omphalocele
(D) Vitelline fistula
(E) Volvulus

48. Antiviral agents used in the treatment of herpesvirus infections are effective only during the acute phase of infection and are ineffective during the latent phase. Which of the following medications is a guanosine analog used in the treatment of active herpesvirus infection?

(A) Acyclovir
(B) Didanosine
(C) Lamivudine
(D) Stavudine
(E) Zalcitabine
(F) Zidovudine

49. A 35-year-old woman presents with a fever of 38.2° C (100.8° F), night sweats, fatigue, and a weight loss of 4.5 kg (10 lb) over the past 6 months. A CT scan demonstrates mediastinal lymphadenopathy in multiple contiguous nodes. A biopsy of the nodes shows Reed-Sternberg cells with reactive lymphocytes, and a diagnosis of Hodgkin's disease is made. Which of the following histologic profiles would be indicative of the best prognosis for a patient with Hodgkin's disease?

(A) Few lymphocytes, many Reed-Sternberg cells
(B) Heterogeneous mixture of lymphocytes, eosinophils, plasma cells, and Reed-Sternberg cells
(C) Many lymphocytes, few Reed-Sternberg cells
(D) Many lymphocytes, few Reed-Sternberg cells, fibrous bands, nodular appearance
(E) Many lymphocytes, many macrophages, no Reed-Sternberg cells

50. A 25-year-old white woman of Ashkenazi Jewish descent presents to the physician with a 3-week history of lower abdominal cramps and intermittent bloody stools two times per day. She has not been febrile and reports no sick contacts, unusual food exposures, or travel history. She has an aunt with similar symptoms. Gross pathologic findings from a patient with similar symptoms are shown in the image. Her laboratory studies show the following results:

Hemoglobin: 13.0 g/dL

Hematocrit: 39%

WBC count: 6,000/mm^3

Platelet count: 200,000/mm^3

Erythrocyte sedimentation rate: 35 mm/hr

Which of the following is the most appropriate treatment for this patient's condition?

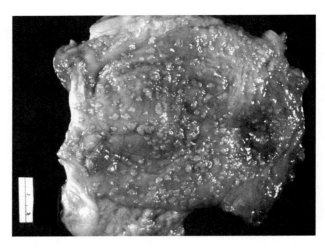

Image courtesy of PEIR Digital Library (http://peir.net).

(A) Ciprofloxacin
(B) Emergent surgery
(C) Infliximab
(D) Loperamide
(E) Oral steroids
(F) Sulfasalazine

1. **The correct answer is B.** Ethosuximide is the only agent that is both used for absence seizures and associated with Stevens-Johnson syndrome. Ethosuximide is an antiepileptic indicated for absence seizures. A rare but severe adverse effect is drug-induced Stevens-Johnson syndrome. This is characterized by blistering of the nasal, oral, and genital mucosa as well as the conjunctivae. Erythema, palpable purpura, and epidermal necrolysis may also ensue.

Answer A is incorrect. Carbamazepine can cause diplopia, induction of the cytochrome P-450 system, blood dyscrasias, and liver toxicity.

Answer C is incorrect. Phenytoin toxicity causes nystagmus, diplopia, ataxia, gingival hyperplasia, and hirsutism.

Answer D is incorrect. Topiramate can cause mental dulling, kidney stones, and weight loss.

Answer E is incorrect. Valproic acid is also indicated for absence seizures, but adverse effects include gastrointestinal distress and a rare but fatal hepatotoxicity.

2. **The correct answer is A.** 21-α-Hydroxylase deficiency constitutes the most common form of congenital adrenal hyperplasia. It is marked by deficits in glucocorticoid and mineralocorticoid synthesis coupled with increased sex steroid production due to the increased flow of precursors, such as pregnenolone and progesterone, through androgen-yielding pathways. The resultant low serum cortisol and mineralocorticoid levels (aldosterone) and high sex steroid levels manifest clinically as hypotension, hyponatremia, hyperkalemia, volume depletion, masculinization, and female pseudohermaphroditism.

Answer B is incorrect. Estradiol is the most potent of the estrogens. It functions to stimulate ovarian follicle development, endometrial proliferation and myometrial excitability, development of female reproductive tract and secondary sexual characteristics, breast development, luteinizing hormone surge, feedback inhibition of follicle-stimulating hormone, and hepatic synthesis of transport proteins. 17-α-Hydroxylase is necessary for the synthesis of estradiol, but 21-α-hydroxylase is not.

Answer C is incorrect. Estrone is one of the estrogens and is less potent than estradiol. Like the other estrogens, estrone stimulates ovarian follicle development, endometrial proliferation and myometrial excitability, development of female reproductive tract and secondary sexual characteristics, breast development, luteinizing hormone surge, feedback inhibition of follicle-stimulating hormone, and hepatic synthesis of transport proteins. 17-α-Hydroxylase is necessary for the synthesis of estrone, but 21-α-hydroxylase is not.

Answer D is incorrect. Progesterone is produced by the corpus luteum, placenta, adrenal cortex, and testes. Elevation of progesterone is indicative of ovulation. The functions of progesterone include stimulation of endometrial glandular secretions, ovulation, spiral artery development, maintenance of pregnancy, decreased myometrial excitability, production of thick cervical mucus that inhibits sperm entry into the uterus, increased body temperature, inhibition of gonadotropins (luteinizing hormone, follicle-stimulating hormone); and uterine smooth muscle relaxation. 17-α-Hydroxylase is necessary for the synthesis of progesterone, but 21-α-hydroxylase is not.

Answer E is incorrect. Testosterone is an androgen, the most potent of which is dihydrotestosterone. The androgens stimulate development of the male reproductive tract, male secondary sexual characteristics, and the pubertal growth spurt. They are responsible for increased anabolic effects, such as increased muscle mass and red blood cell production; they mediate normal spermatogenesis; and they increase libido. 17-α-Hydroxylase is necessary for the synthesis of testosterone, but 21-α-hydroxylase is not.

3. **The correct answer is D.** This patient is likely suffering from endemic cretinism due to a deficiency in dietary iodine, a disorder that is still common in parts of the world, including China. Lack of dietary iodine leads to deficient thyroid hormone production and thus hypothyroidism. Thyroid hormone is critical during development and thus children who grow up in iodine-deficient areas may manifest skeletal and central nervous system abnormalities, including short stature and mental retardation. Unfortunately for this child, once the syndrome is clinically apparent, it cannot be reversed. Thyroid function tests would show decreased levels of triiodothyronine and thyroxine, and increased levels of thyroid-stimulating hormone secondary to the lack of negative feedback on the pituitary, thus confirming the diagnosis of primary hypothyroidism.

Answer A is incorrect. Cretinism is caused by deficient production of thyroid hormone. While decreased negative feedback on the anterior pituitary leads to elevated thyroid-stimulating hormone levels, the levels of growth hormone and ACTH secretion by the pituitary would not be affected.

Answer B is incorrect. Cretinism is caused by deficient production of thyroid hormone. While decreased negative feedback on the anterior pituitary leads to elevated thyroid-stimulating hormone levels, the levels of growth hormone and ACTH secretion by the pituitary would not be affected.

Answer C is incorrect. Elevated T_3 and T_4 levels, with decreased thyroid-stimulating hormone (TSH) levels, would be seen in primary hyperthyroidism. This could be caused by autonomous TSH secretion, as in a toxic adenoma or by autoimmune antibody stimulation of the thyroid gland, as in Graves' disease.

Answer E is incorrect. An elevated thyroid-stimulating hormone (TSH) level, along with elevated thyroid hormone levels, suggests production of TSH that is unresponsive to negative feedback from the increased levels of thyroid hormone. These lab values could be seen in a patient with a TSH-secreting pituitary ade-

noma, but would not be expected in a patient with cretinism, who would have elevated TSH levels, but decreased levels of triiodothyronine and thyroxine.

4. **The correct answer is E.** This patient has pemphigus vulgaris, a potentially fatal autoimmune disorder characterized by easily ruptured superficial vesicles that often crust and erode. It is thought to be due to IgG antibody against epidermal cell membrane.

Answer A is incorrect. In bullous pemphigoid, patients have skin vesicles that are filled with a clear fluid; however, unlike pemphigus vulgaris, patients have IgG antibody against epidermal basement membrane. The bullae generally heal without scarring and do not rupture as easily as do the vesicles of pemphigus vulgaris.

Answer B is incorrect. Eczema is characterized by itchy, red papulovesicular skin that, through excessive scratching, can become denuded and prone to bacterial superinfection.

Answer C is incorrect. Erythema multiforme is characterized by a combination of macules, papules, vesicles, bullae, and "target lesions" (spreading halos of erythema and central clearing) that often symmetrically affect the extremities.

Answer D is incorrect. Impetigo is a common skin infection caused by staphylococci or streptococci. It often presents as shallow skin erosions that have honey-crust-appearing edges.

5. **The correct answer is C.** This young woman has irritable bowel syndrome (IBS). IBS, a diagnosis of exclusion, is an idiopathic functional disorder characterized by abdominal pain and changes in bowel habits that increase with stress (e.g., starting a new job) and are relieved with bowel movements. A normal complete blood count, erythrocyte sedimentation rate, and physical exam are consistent with this benign disease. Most people with this condition need reassurance from their physicians. However, pharmacologic treatment with antidiarrheals such as loperamide (an opioid)

may be used in patients with diarrhea-predominant IBS.

Answer A is incorrect. Bactrim (trimethoprim-sulfamethoxazole) is an antibiotic used to treat conditions of infectious origin. Bactrim is not used for the treatment of irritable bowel syndrome.

Answer B is incorrect. Bismuth is an agent used in peptic ulcers. This drug binds to the ulcer base, providing physical protection from acid. It has no clinical use in irritable bowel syndrome.

Answer D is incorrect. Metronidazole is an antibiotic that is effective against anaerobes, protozoans, and gram-negative bacteria. It has no role in irritable bowel syndrome treatment.

Answer E is incorrect. Octreotide, a somatostatin analog, may be useful in carcinoid syndrome and acromegaly. It has no known benefit in irritable bowel syndrome treatment.

Answer F is incorrect. Omeprazole is a proton pump inhibitor that is useful in therapy for gastroesophageal reflux disease, gastritis, and peptic ulcer disease. It has no use in treatment of irritable bowel syndrome.

6. **The correct answer is E.** This patient has Wegener's granulomatosis, a disease characterized by necrotizing, granulomatous vasculitis affecting several organs, most notably the upper respiratory tract, lung, and kidney. The hematuria is suggestive of glomerulitis. The presence of granulomas and the dramatic response to immunosuppressive therapy suggest that this disease process may be immunologic in origin. Elevated serum cytoplasmic antineutrophil cytoplasmic antibody is found in 90% of patients and is highly specific for the disease. Other clinical findings include skin rashes, muscle pains, and fever.

Answer A is incorrect. Patients with Alport's syndrome may have hematuria, but the hallmarks are ocular disorders and nerve deafness from defective synthesis of collagen type IV.

Answer B is incorrect. Giant cell (temporal) arteritis is a type of vasculitis that affects the ar-

teries of the head (especially, of course, the temporal arteries). The highlights of this disease can be remembered by the mnemonic **JOE,** because patients get **J**aw pain and **O**cular disturbances from ischemia to the arteries supplying them. Patients also often have markedly elevated **E**rythrocyte sedimentation rates. The disease is often associated with the presence of polymyalgia rheumatica.

Answer C is incorrect. Goodpasture's syndrome is a type II hypersensitivity reaction against collagen type IV, found in the lungs and the kidneys. The disease commonly presents with concurrent hemoptysis and hematuria. Exposure to hydrocarbon solvents (such as those found in the dry-cleaning industry) and cigarette smoking have been associated with an increased risk of developing Goodpasture's syndrome.

Answer D is incorrect. Takayasu's arteritis is a vasculitis characterized by fibrotic thickening of the aortic arch (it also affects the pulmonary arteries, the branches of the aortic arch, and the rest of the aorta in up to one-third of patients). Clinically, patients often have lower blood pressure and weaker pulses in the upper extremities than in the lower extremities; some patients also have ocular disturbances as well.

7. **The correct answer is E.** This is a phenomenon known as peripheral tolerance. It is an important factor because deletion of self-reactive T lymphocytes within the thymus ("central tolerance") is not completely efficient at removing all self-reactive T lymphocytes. Thus, one mechanism of peripheral tolerance is that of anergy: when a T lymphocyte receives the first signal (peptide-major histocompatibility complex) but no second signal (costimulation, such as CD28-B7 ligation), that T lymphocyte undergoes a reprogramming known as anergy, wherein it is subsequently made refractory to any future stimulation. Note that an anergic T lymphocyte cannot be activated later even if costimulation is present.

Answer A is incorrect. This is not true.

Answer B is incorrect. A T lymphocyte that becomes anergic does not undergo activation.

Answer C is incorrect. This is not true.

Answer D is incorrect. The T lymphocyte will not clonally expand.

8. **The correct answer is C.** The *ras* family of proteins, like the G proteins, bind guanosine triphosphate and guanosine diphosphate.

Answer A is incorrect. Cyclin-dependent kinases direct progression of cells through the cell cycle. They are activated by cyclins.

Answer B is incorrect. The oncogenes *erb* and *HER2* are examples of oncogenes that encode growth factor receptors.

Answer D is incorrect. *abl* is an example of a proto-oncogene with tyrosine kinase activity. In chronic myeloid leukemia, *abl* on chromosome 9 is translocated to chromosome 22, fusing it with *bcr* and creating a hybrid tyrosine kinase with potent activity.

Answer E is incorrect. The *myc* protein is an example of a transcriptional activator that binds DNA, activating many growth-related genes.

9. **The correct answer is E.** The most effective drugs for the treatment of chemotherapy-induced nausea are the serotonin 5-HT$_3$ antagonists. This class includes ondansetron, dolasetron, and granisetron. These drugs can cause fatigue, headache, constipation, urinary retention, and dizziness; however, setrons are generally not very toxic.

Answer A is incorrect. Benzodiazepines include lorazepam and diazepam. They may be effective in treatment of the anticipatory nausea associated with chemotherapy, but they are not as effective as the 5-HT$_3$ antagonists.

Answer B is incorrect. Cholinergic antagonists include scopolamine. These drugs are not used for the treatment of chemotherapy-induced nausea. They are used for motion sickness.

Answer C is incorrect. Dopamine receptor antagonists include chlorpromazine and haloperi-

dol. They are used to treat schizophrenia and psychosis.

Answer D is incorrect. Histamine receptor antagonists include diphenhydramine and promethazine. They are used for acid reflux and allergies.

10. **The correct answer is A.** Arylsulfatase A converts sulfatide to galactocerebroside. This enzyme is deficient in patients with metachromatic leukodystrophy, an autosomal recessive lysosomal storage disease in which patients cannot degrade sulfatides, leading to accumulation of cerebroside sulfate in both neuronal and nonneuronal tissues. There is abnormal myelination with widespread loss of myelination in the central nervous system and peripheral nerves, leading to the clinical signs. Metachromatic granules can be seen on histologic examination.

Answer B is incorrect. β-Galactosidase converts galactocerebroside to cerebroside. This enzyme is deficient in Krabbe's disease.

Answer C is incorrect. α-Galactosidase A converts ceramide trihexoside to lactosyl cerebroside. This enzyme is deficient in Fabry's disease.

Answer D is incorrect. Hexosaminidase A converts ganglioside M$_2$ to ganglioside M$_3$. This enzyme is deficient in Tay-Sachs disease.

Answer E is incorrect. Sphingomyelinase converts sphingomyelin to cerebroside. This enzyme is deficient in Niemann-Pick disease.

11. **The correct answer is E.** This patient most likely has multiple sclerosis, a central nervous system (CNS) demyelinating disorder characterized by neurologic lesions that produce signs and symptoms that are separated by both time (i.e., episodes greater than 1 month apart) and anatomic location within the white matter of the CNS. By definition, multiple sclerosis episodes produce symptoms that last longer than 24 hours. The exact etiology is unknown, but there is evidence supporting a role of autoimmune antibodies that attach to CNS myelin-secreting oligodendrocytes. Episodes of

optic neuritis (temporary unilateral vision loss) occur in 15–20% of multiple sclerosis patients. Over 90% of patients have multiple periventricular plaques found on MRI of the brain.

Answer A is incorrect. Chorea, the condition described in this answer, is not particularly associated with multiple sclerosis.

Answer B is incorrect. Permanent bilateral resting tremors of the upper extremities are not particularly associated with multiple sclerosis. Intention tremors and ataxia (denoting cerebellar disease) are commonly associated with multiple sclerosis.

Answer C is incorrect. Permanent progressive paralysis of the respiratory muscles is not particularly associated with multiple sclerosis.

Answer D is incorrect. Raynaud's phenomenon, the condition described in this answer, is not particularly associated with multiple sclerosis.

12. **The correct answer is C.** Glipizide is a sulfonylurea that acts by stimulating the closing of K^+ channels expressed in the cell membrane of pancreatic acinar β cells. It causes cellular depolarization and then Ca^{2+} influx, which in turn triggers insulin release. Hence, a mutation that impairs closing of the β cell K^+ channels would profoundly reduce the efficacy of the sulfonylureas.

Answer A is incorrect. Acarbose is an α-glucosidase inhibitor that acts at the intestinal brush border to decrease the absorption of starches and other polysaccharides. This agent would be effective in maintaining glycemic control in someone with type 1 diabetes when used in combination with exogenous insulin and other nonsulfonylurea hypoglycemics.

Answer B is incorrect. Glargine is a long-acting synthetic insulin that provides a continuous baseline level of insulin in the blood. This agent would be appropriate for use in this patient in combination with a short- or intermediate-acting insulin to cover the glycemic loads associated with meals and snacks.

Answer D is incorrect. Metformin is an oral hypoglycemic agent that is thought to inhibit gluconeogenesis and glycolysis, resulting in decreased blood glucose concentrations. This agent would be effective in helping to maintain glycemic control in someone with type 1 diabetes when used in combination with exogenous insulin and other nonsulfonylurea hypoglycemics.

Answer E is incorrect. Troglitazone is a thiazolidinone that acts to sensitize peripheral tissues to insulin and increase target cell response; it does not act on pancreatic acinar cells. This agent would be effective in helping to maintain glycemic control in someone with type 1 diabetes when used in combination with exogenous insulin and other nonsulfonylurea hypoglycemic medications.

13. **The correct answer is A.** Continuing insomnia is an indication of an abnormal grief reaction. Pathologic grief presents with a picture similar to that of a major depressive episode and is characterized by vegetative symptoms. The symptoms are excessively intense and/or prolonged.

Answer B is incorrect. Feelings of sadness are normal and can persist for a long time. They can even recur as anniversary reactions. Suicidal thoughts or attempts are indicative of pathologic grief.

Answer C is incorrect. Guilty feelings are also normal. They are abnormal if the feelings are intense and include feelings of worthlessness.

Answer D is incorrect. Returning to work is a healthy outcome in a grieving person. Failure to resume normal activities is abnormal.

Answer E is incorrect. Weight loss of 1.3 kg (2.9 lb) or less is not worrisome. A weight loss of 3.6 kg (8.0 lb) or more would be worrisome for pathologic grief.

14. **The correct answer is B.** Such an injury is consistent with a significant mechanism of injury such as ejection from a vehicle at a high

rate of speed. The patient was able to talk with the police at the scene of the accident but was unable to recall how the accident occurred, which likely demonstrates an initial loss of consciousness followed by normal mentation and subsequent deterioration of consciousness. This lucid interval is classically seen with an epidural hematoma. The patient's neurologic findings are consistent with the extra-axial blood collection on the right side caused by injury to the middle meningeal artery after it was injured during the fracture of the right temporal bone. An urgent neurosurgical consult is indicated for immediate evacuation of the clot to prevent the herniation syndrome from worsening.

Answer A is incorrect. Injury to the inferior cerebral veins would result in subarachnoid bleeding. Bleeding from such an injury does not result from a fracture of the temporal bone and is unlikely to cause the rapid deterioration evident in this case because it has a slower rate of bleeding. However, subarachnoid bleeding is frequently seen in the setting of trauma and could be an associated finding with the epidural hematoma.

Answer C is incorrect. The posterior ethmoidal artery supplies the anterior superior nose and nasal septum with blood; its tearing would not result in an epidural hematoma secondary to a temporal bone fracture.

Answer D is incorrect. Injury to the sigmoid sinus would result in a subarachnoid hemorrhage. Thus such a finding is inconsistent with an injury to the temporal bone, the lucid interval in this patient's history, and the CT findings.

Answer E is incorrect. Injury to the superior sagittal sinus would also result in a subarachnoid hemorrhage, but this is a far less likely cause of this patient's deterioration than an epidural hematoma.

15. **The correct answer is D.** In Crigler-Najjar syndrome, the absence of glucuronyl transferase results in an inability to conjugate bilirubin, leading to an unconjugated hyperbilirubinemia (high indirect bilirubin). The jaundice

will become more severe as bilirubin accumulates, and at high levels will result in brain damage. Two entities have been identified: type 1 (autosomal recessive) and type 2 (autosomal dominant). A partial glucuronyl transferase deficiency is found in Gilbert's syndrome.

Answer A is incorrect. While the patient may have abnormalities in hematocrit, they would not be due to a glucuronyl transferase deficiency.

Answer B is incorrect. If an enzyme for conjugation is lacking, unconjugated (indirect) bilirubin will increase, not decrease.

Answer C is incorrect. Because the enzyme missing is used for conjugating bilirubin, direct bilirubin will decrease, not increase.

Answer E is incorrect. A hemolytic anemia would cause an increased reticulocyte count and also increase bilirubin level, which would result in jaundice. While this would further complicate the infant's condition, hemolytic anemia is not the cause of Crigler-Najjar syndrome, nor is it associated with that syndrome.

16. **The correct answer is D.** This patient presents with symptoms of digoxin toxicity. Additionally, his ECG shows first-degree atrioventricular block, a sign of digoxin toxicity. Digoxin toxicity is fairly common given the narrow therapeutic-toxic range of this medication, which is commonly prescribed medication for congestive heart failure. An increase in furosemide would result in increased K^+ secretion in the nephron, which could cause hypokalemia, a state that potentiates the effects of digoxin.

Answer A is incorrect. A decrease in digoxin dosage would not cause an overdose of digoxin.

Answer B is incorrect. Verapamil, a calcium channel blocker, does not affect digoxin levels and thus could not cause digoxin toxicity.

Answer C is incorrect. Enalapril, an angiotensin-converting enzyme inhibitor, has no direct or indirect effect on digoxin levels.

Answer E is incorrect. Spironolactone is a K$^+$-sparing diuretic; thus, an increase in spironolactone dose would cause hyperkalemia because less K$^+$ would be secreted. Hyperkalemia would then reduce the effect of digoxin. The typical ECG in hyperkalemia includes peaked T waves, PR-interval prolongation, and widening of the QRS.

17. **The correct answer is C.** Diverticulitis is inflammation of diverticula, often in the sigmoid colon. It is related to retention of material within a diverticulum and fecalith formation. Diverticulitis typically manifests as left lower quadrant pain with fever, anorexia, and diarrhea and presents most commonly in older people. Diverticulitis should be distinguished from diverticulosis, which simply refers to the presence of diverticula. Diverticula occur when pressure causes herniation of the colonic wall through its own muscularis propria. A low-fiber diet is a known risk factor for diverticulosis. Occasionally, a diverticulum may cause rupture of a nutrient artery where it penetrates the muscularis propria; this results in bright red, painless bleeding from the rectum. However, only 20% of patients with diverticula experience hemorrhage. Thus, hemorrhage from diverticula is not always associated with diverticulitis, and diverticulitis may occur in the absence of bleeding.

Answer A is incorrect. Angiodysplasia is a dilation of small vessels in the intestinal mucosa and submucosa, most commonly involving the ascending colon. It manifests only as gastrointestinal bleeding, either as hematemesis or as guaiac-positive stool, and does not involve abdominal pain. Histologically, these lesions are seen as distorted, dilated, thin-walled vessels.

Answer B is incorrect. Crohn's disease is a chronic inflammatory condition that manifests as abdominal pain with or without diarrhea, fever, and perianal fistulas. Unlike ulcerative colitis, it can involve the entire gastrointestinal tract and affects all layers of the intestinal wall. Also unlike ulcerative colitis, it can affect noncontiguous regions of the intestine, resulting in skip lesions. Histologically it often has a cob-blestone appearance due to submucosal edema with mucosal elevation.

Answer D is incorrect. Ischemic bowel disease usually presents as pain disproportionately elevated in comparison to physical examination findings. Nausea, vomiting, and anorexia are common. It can result in intestinal transmural, mural, or mucosal infarction and, ultimately, necrosis.

Answer E is incorrect. Ulcerative colitis is an inflammatory bowel disease that often presents with rectal bleeding and diarrhea. Histologically it is characterized by an inflamed and edematous colon with a pseudopolypoid appearance. Unlike Crohn's disease, it involves only the colon and affects only the mucosal and submucosal layers. The most characteristic lesions are crypt abscesses and ulceration.

18. **The correct answer is C.** Histoplasmosis does not typically lead to any symptomatic presentation. When symptoms are present, they usually manifest as a flulike illness with fever, cough, headaches, and myalgias. Histoplasmosis can result in a lung disease resembling tuberculosis and widespread disseminated infection affecting the liver, spleen, adrenal glands, mucosal surfaces, and meninges. Histoplasmosis occurs most commonly in the Mississippi and Ohio River valleys.

Answer A is incorrect. Blastomycosis can present with flulike symptoms, fevers, chills, productive cough, myalgia, arthralgia, and pleuritic chest pain. Some patients will fail to recover from an acute infection and progress to develop chronic pulmonary infection or widespread disseminated infection. Fluconazole or ketoconazole are used for the treatment of local blastomycosis, and amphotericin B is used for the treatment of systemic infections.

Answer B is incorrect. *Cryptococcus neoformans* infection does not often present with any symptoms in an immunocompetent host. However, in an immunocompromised individual, it can present with meningoencephalitis. *Cryptococcus* is a heavily encapsulated yeast that is not dimorphic. The fungus is found in soil and pigeon droppings.

Answer D is incorrect. Mucor species is a mold with irregular nonseptate hyphae branching at wide angles (> 90 degrees). Symptoms of *Mucor* infection include an allergic reaction and infarction of distal tissue due to fungal proliferation in the walls of blood vessels. The disease is mostly seen in patients with ketoacidotic diabetes and leukemia. High doses of amphotericin B are used to treat mucormycosis.

Answer E is incorrect. *Malassezia furfur* infection causes tinea versicolor. Symptoms of this infection include hypopigmented skin lesions that occur in hot and humid weather. Topical miconazole or selenium sulfides (Selsun) are used to treat *M. furfur*.

19. **The correct answer is E.** Narcolepsy is a genetically based disorder that involves the derangement of rapid eye movement sleep and sleep-wake control and results in the sudden onset of sleep with or without cataplexy (sudden collapse while awake). Stimulants (e.g., amphetamines and methylphenidate) have been used with success but involve side effects. More recently, the advent of modafinil (Provigil) has increased the options for treatment of excessive daytime sleepiness in these patients. Although its mechanism has not been fully elucidated, it seems to possess a safer side-effect profile than stimulants.

Answer A is incorrect. Atomoxetine (Strattera) is a selective norepinephrine reuptake inhibitor that has shown greater efficacy than placebo in treating attention-deficit/hyperactivity disorder in adults. It has not been used or evaluated in the treatment of narcolepsy.

Answer B is incorrect. Desmopressin is a synthetic vasopressin analog that is used to decrease urine output by retaining water and concentrating urine in the distal tubules. With respect to sleep disorders, it is used in the treatment of enuresis but not narcolepsy.

Answer C is incorrect. Tricyclic antidepressants (TCAs) such as imipramine have been used as treatments for cataplexy and sleep paralysis in narcoleptic patients. However, TCAs are not first-line therapy for excessive daytime sleepiness.

Answer D is incorrect. Lorazepam is an intermediate-acting benzodiazepine used in the treatment of panic attacks and anxiety. It would increase daytime sleepiness in a narcoleptic patient.

20. **The correct answer is A.** This patient has acute hepatitis B infection. Abdominal pain, positive hepatitis B surface antigen, and presence of IgM anti-HBc antibody are consistent with the diagnosis. The correct combination therapy for hepatitis B is lamivudine and interferon-α. Lamivudine is a reverse transcriptase inhibitor that blocks the action of an enzyme that is necessary in hepatitis replication. It is also used as an HIV medication. Interferon-α is thought to block viral replication and thereby inhibit hepatitis replication.

Answer B is incorrect. Interferon-β is not used in the treatment of hepatitis.

Answer C is incorrect. Ribavirin, in combination with pegylated interferon, is used in the treatment of hepatitis C. Lamivudine, in combination with interferon-α, is used in the treatment of hepatitis B.

Answer D is incorrect. Ribavirin, in combination with pegylated interferon, is used in the treatment of hepatitis C. Lamivudine, in combination with interferon-α, is used in the treatment of hepatitis B.

Answer E is incorrect. Ribavirin, in combination with pegylated interferon, is used in the treatment of hepatitis C.

21. **The correct answer is D.** Rapidly progressive (crescentic) glomerulonephritis (RPGN) is a renal disease with a rapid course (weeks to months) to renal failure. It is characterized by extensive capillary damage leading to accumulation of cells and fibrinous changes in Bowman's space, together with the characteristic "crescent" seen on biopsy. Renal insufficiency is present at diagnosis in almost all cases. The

urinalysis typically reveals a nephritic picture of hematuria, red cell casts, and a variable degree of proteinuria. RPGN is a heterogeneous autoimmune disease caused by anti–glomerular basement membrane (as in Goodpasture's syndrome) immune complex deposition or by the progression of the ANCA-positive vasculitides (e.g., Wegener's granulomatosis).

Answer A is incorrect. Diabetes nephropathy is the most common cause of kidney failure in the United States. The histologic morphology is characterized by an increase in mesangial matrix and marked nodular accumulations known as Kimmelstiel-Wilson nodules with diffuse glomerulosclerosis. Urinalysis would show glucose if this were the etiology.

Answer B is incorrect. Membranoproliferative glomerulonephritis is an uncommon autoimmune disorder that affects young individuals (8–30 years old). The diagnosis is based on the histologic finding of mesangial proliferation and thickening of the capillary walls with mesangial interposition, which creates a tram-track appearance on light microscopy.

Answer C is incorrect. Minimal change disease is the most common cause of nephrotic syndrome in children. It usually presents as massive proteinuria and hyperlipidemia secondary to disruption of the epithelial foot process, which decreases the ability of the kidney to retain serum proteins, such as albumin. The primary histopathologic finding is diffuse epithelial foot process fusion on electron microscopy.

Answer E is incorrect. Systemic lupus erythematosus (SLE) is a chronic autoimmune disease that affects multiple organ systems, including the kidney. SLE affects young adults (women more than men) and usually presents with a combined nephritic and nephrotic picture. Histologically, SLE kidneys have a peculiar wire-loop appearance with subendothelial basement membrane deposits.

22. **The correct answer is D.** This woman has had a normal delivery of monozygotic (identical) twins. Monozygotes may also develop sep-

arately, producing two amniotic sacs, two placentas, and two chorions, but this would not be distinguishable from dizygotic twins. In the case of a single chorion and placenta, the pregnancy must have developed from a single zygote.

Answer A is incorrect. Chorioamnionitis is typically caused by an infection ascending from the cervix or vagina following a premature membrane rupture. It requires early delivery and has a high risk of mortality for the fetus and would not, therefore, be considered a normal delivery.

Answer B is incorrect. A complete hydatidiform mole would not produce a normal delivery. Gross pathology shows a single enlarged placenta with edematous villi resembling grapes. Clinically, it produces a significant increase in human chorionic gonadotropin, vaginal bleeding, and fast uterine growth. It confers a 2–3% risk of choriocarcinoma. Complete moles have no embryo present and are exclusively of paternal derivation.

Answer C is incorrect. Dizygotic twins would produce two chorions and two placentas, as well as two amniotic sacs.

Answer E is incorrect. Sheehan's syndrome is postpartum anterior pituitary necrosis resulting from hypotension and infarction following blood loss in pregnancy. It causes the gradual loss of anterior pituitary function. It has no relation to multiple amniotic sacs.

23. **The correct answer is A.** This patient is suffering from hypoglycemia related to his alcohol use. Ethanol is metabolized to acetaldehyde, which is then metabolized to acetate (acetaldehyde dehydrogenase). During both steps of ethanol metabolism, reduced nicotinamide adenine dinucleotide (NADH) is generated from nicotinamide adenine dinucleotide (NAD$^+$). With an elevated NADH:NAD$^+$ ratio in the liver, pyruvate is diverted to lactate, while oxaloacetate is diverted to malate, thus inhibiting gluconeogenesis. The metabolism of ethanol is also responsible for the hepatic fatty changes seen in chronic alcoholics (increased fatty acid synthesis).

Answer B is incorrect. An elevated nicotinamide adenine dinucleotide:reduced nicotinamide adenine dinucleotide ratio (NAD^+: NADH) does not result from alcohol metabolism. In any event, lactate would generate pyruvate, and gluconeogenesis would not be inhibited.

Answer C is incorrect. Reduced nicotinamide adenine dinucleotide phosphate (NADPH) is produced by the pentose pathway. NADPH is used for fatty acid synthesis and to reduce glutathione. Glutathione helps prevent oxidative damage to cells by reducing hydrogen peroxide. An elevated NADPH:nicotinamide adenine dinucleotide ratio would not inhibit gluconeogenesis.

Answer D is incorrect. An elevated nicotinamide adenine dinucleotide phosphate:reduced nicotinamide adenine dinucleotide phosphate ratio (NADP:NADPH) results from a faulty pentose shunt. NADPH is used for fatty acid synthesis and to reduce glutathione. The above presentation and decreased gluconeogenesis are consistent with an elevated reduced nicotinamide adenine dinucleo-tide: nicotinamide adenine dinucleotide ratio.

Answer E is incorrect. An elevated lactate: pyruvate ratio would be seen in alcohol intoxication rather than an elevated pyruvate:lactate ratio. During alcohol metabolism, the elevated reduced nicotinamide adenine dinucleo-tide: nicotinamide adenine dinucleotide ratio leads to diversion of pyruvate to lactate.

24. **The correct answer is D.** Introns are noncoding regions of RNA that are spliced out of mature mRNA. Almost all introns begin and end with 5′ GU——— AG 3′. A mutation in one of those nucleotides affects splicing. This type of mutation is one of those found in thalassemia.

Answer A is incorrect. Capping of the mRNA occurs at the 5′ end as it is being transcribed. A mutation at the 5′ end of an intron would not affect capping.

Answer B is incorrect. Hybridization is a process in which single-stranded DNA basepairs with a complementary sequence. A mutation at the 5′ end of an intron would not affect hybridization.

Answer C is incorrect. A poly(A) tail is added to the 3′ end of RNA after transcription. Poly(A) polymerase uses ATP as a precursor for adding adenosine one at a time. A mutation at the 5′ end of an intron would not affect polyadenylation.

Answer E is incorrect. Transcription of the DNA into RNA would not be affected by this mutation.

25. **The correct answer is D.** This patient's presentation is suggestive of IgM-mediated (cold) hemolytic anemia secondary to recent Epstein-Barr virus (EBV) infection. Mononucleosis, which is caused by EBV, is associated with IgM antibodies directed at the i (lowercase) antigen found on RBCs. In contrast, *Mycoplasma pneumoniae* infection typically yields a hemolytic anemia in which IgM antibodies are directed at the I (uppercase) antigen. IgM binds in the periphery at lower temperatures, binding complement, but IgM then falls off the RBCs as it returns to the central circulation. Agglutination of RBCs in the periphery can lead to the gray/purple discoloration seen in this patient's fingers.

Answer A is incorrect. Aplastic anemia results in pancytopenia, malaise, and severe infection. This disorder is a hypoproliferative anemia and would not have appropriate reticulocytosis as is seen in this patient.

Answer B is incorrect. Acute disseminated intravascular coagulation (DIC) results in bleeding and shock. Chronic DIC results in thrombosis and clotting.

Answer C is incorrect. Coombs' test for IgG-mediated (warm) hemolytic anemia is positive for IgG. Warm hemolytic anemia is associated with autoimmune disease, lymphoproliferative disorders, and drug abuse.

Answer E is incorrect. Paroxysmal nocturnal hemoglobinuria is caused by a defect in the RBC's protection mechanism against complement-mediated lysis. Loss of the enzyme PIG-

A, which is required for glycosylphosphatidyli-nositol anchoring of decay-accelerating factor, results in episodic acute intravascular hemoly-sis and thrombosis.

26. **The correct answer is D.** Polymerase chain reaction is a laboratory procedure used to ex-ponentially amplify DNA. It results in the pro-duction of many copies of a desired fragment of DNA for subsequent use in other molecular tests.

    Answer A is incorrect. Enzyme-linked im-munosorbent assay is a test of antigen-antibody hybridization used to detect an antigenic match in a patient's blood sample.

    Answer B is incorrect. Ligase chain reaction is a technique performed on mutant alleles for the purpose of detecting single-point muta-tions.

    Answer C is incorrect. A Northern blot is used to detect RNA through RNA-DNA hy-bridization.

    Answer E is incorrect. A Southern blot is used to detect DNA by DNA-DNA hybridiza-tion. It is performed after amplified DNA has been obtained.

27. **The correct answer is B.** The symptoms of fever, fatigue, night sweats, lymphadenopathy, and hemoptysis are consistent with the diagno-sis of tuberculosis (TB). The causative agent of TB is *Mycobacterium tuberculosis*. Primary tu-berculosis infections are only rarely symptom-atic in patients with normal immune function due to rapid containment by resident alveolar macrophages and infiltrating monocytes and lymphocytes. Symptomatic primary infection is mostly seen in the elderly, children, and im-munocompromised individuals.

    Answer A is incorrect. *Legionella pneumo-phila* causes an atypical pneumonia and is as-sociated with environmental water sources. It does not cause the symptoms described in the question.

    Answer C is incorrect. *Mycoplasma pneumo-niae* causes atypical pneumonia with cough and shortness of breath, and is visible as bilat-eral infiltrates on an x-ray film. The symptoms described in this patient are not consistent with this disease.

    Answer D is incorrect. Respiratory syncytial virus is an etiologic agent of bronchiolitis in children, pneumonia in the elderly, and severe pneumonia culminating in respiratory failure in immunocompromised individuals.

    Answer E is incorrect. *Streptococcus pneumo-niae* causes acute pneumonic symptoms reach-ing a crescendo within days, not weeks or months. Infection would not involve several months of fatigue, night sweats, and weight loss.

28. **The correct answer is C.** The patient is suffer-ing from Hashimoto's thyroiditis, an autoim-mune disorder of the thyroid that is a common cause of hypothyroidism. Other classic signs and symptoms of this disorder include cold in-tolerance; hypoactivity; decreased appetite; weakness; decreased reflexes; dry, cool skin; and coarse, brittle hair. Laboratory values demonstrate an increased thyroid-stimulating hormone level (the most sensitive test for pri-mary hypothyroidism) and decreased total T_3 and T_4 levels. The thyroid gland is usually goitrous and firm, while histology reveals a significant lymphocyte and plasma cell infil-trate with germinal center formation, colloid-sparse follicles, and Hürthle cells. Like pa-tients with Graves' disease, patients with Hashimoto's thyroiditis frequently have a his-tory or family history of autoimmune disease. There is an increased incidence of Hashimoto's thyroiditis in HLA-DR5 and -B5 individuals. Antimicrosomal antibodies, also called anti–thy-roid peroxidase antibodies, are associated with Hashimoto's thyroiditis.

    Answer A is incorrect. Anti–basement mem-brane antibodies are associated with Goodpas-ture's syndrome.

    Answer B is incorrect. Anti–epithelial cell an-tibodies are associated with pemphigus vul-garis.

    Answer D is incorrect. Antimitochondrial an-tibodies are associated with primary biliary cir-rhosis.

Answer E is incorrect. Antineutrophil antibodies are associated with vasculitides such as Wegener's granulomatosis and polyarteritis nodosa.

29. **The correct answer is F.** Sexual desire does not wane with aging, and physicians should be prepared to deal with sexually related questions from older patients. This patient has several risk factors for erectile dysfunction, including a history of diabetes, peripheral vascular disease, use of antihypertensive medications, and use of antidepressants. As is common for many older patients, this man is on several prescription medications. The only one that can significantly interact with sildenafil is the sublingual nitroglycerin. The combination can lead to severe hypotension and cardiovascular collapse.

Answer A is incorrect. Aspirin and sildenafil have no known dangerous interactions.

Answer B is incorrect. Captopril and sildenafil have no known dangerous interactions. However, the captopril is probably contributing to his erectile dysfunction.

Answer C is incorrect. Fluoxetine and sildenafil have no known dangerous interactions. However, the fluoxetine is probably contributing to his erectile dysfunction.

Answer D is incorrect. Lovastatin and sildenafil have no known dangerous interactions.

Answer E is incorrect. Metformin and sildenafil have no known dangerous interactions.

Answer G is incorrect. Propranolol and sildenafil have no known dangerous interactions. However, the propranolol may be contributing to his erectile dysfunction.

30. **The correct answer is C.** Like vitamin A, vitamins D, K, and E are all fat-soluble, and their absorption is dependent on the gut (ileum) and pancreas. Vitamin D deficiency impairs intestinal absorption of calcium and phosphate and can lead to a number of diseases, such as rickets, osteoporosis, and osteomalacia. Osteomalacia can present with bone pain and muscle weakness with reduced bone density on ra-

diographic examination. Hypophosphatemia, low calcidiol, and elevated alkaline phosphatase levels are commonly seen. Treatment is aimed at the specific etiology of the deficiency and can also include vitamin D supplementation and correction of the low phosphate (and possibly low calcium) levels.

Answer A is incorrect. Vitamin C plays an important role in the absorption of iron by keeping it in a reduced state. Its deficiency can cause symptoms such as swollen gums, anemia, and bruising, but it too is a water-soluble vitamin.

Answer B is incorrect. Megaloblastic anemia is commonly caused by a deficiency of vitamin B_{12} or folate, both of which have a role in DNA synthesis. Both are water-soluble vitamins.

Answer D is incorrect. Pellagra results from a deficiency of vitamin B_3 and is characterized by bilateral dermatitis (redness, thickening, and scaling), diarrhea, and dementia. Vitamin B_3 (niacin) is water-soluble.

Answer E is incorrect. Wernicke's syndrome is commonly seen in alcoholics with poor nutrition and is caused by a deficiency in vitamin B_1 (thiamine), which is a water-soluble vitamin. Patients present with ophthalmoplegia, nystagmus, and confusion.

31. **The correct answer is A.** The gastroduodenal artery arises from the celiac trunk and passes posterior to the duodenum. When an ulcer in the posterior duodenum erodes through the intestinal wall, it commonly erodes into this vessel. This requires urgent surgical repair, as an arterial bleed can rapidly lead to exsanguination and hemodynamic instability. Ulcers that occur in the anterior duodenum have a greater tendency to perforate than bleed.

Answer B is incorrect. The left gastric artery is a branch of the celiac trunk and supplies the superior lesser curvature of the stomach. It has anastomoses with the right gastric artery.

Answer C is incorrect. The left gastroepiploic artery supplies the greater curvature of the stomach and arises from the splenic artery, which arises from the celiac trunk.

Answer D is incorrect. The right gastric artery branches from the gastroduodenal artery proximal to the pylorus and supplies the lesser curvature of the stomach.

Answer E is incorrect. The right gastroepiploic artery branches from the gastroduodenal artery after it emerges inferior to the duodenum. It supplies the greater curvature of the stomach and has anastomoses with the left gastroepiploic artery.

32. **The correct answer is C.** *Enterobacter* species can cause pneumonia, urinary tract infections, and surgical site infections. Many strains have developed antibiotic resistance through the production of a β-lactamase that confers resistance to even the penicillin/penicillinase inhibitor combinations. Due to the high level of resistance, imipenem is commonly used for treatment, as is trimethoprim-sulfamethoxazole. Imipenem is a broad-spectrum, β-lactamase-resistant antibiotic.

Answer A is incorrect. Ciprofloxacin is a fluoroquinolone antibiotic used to treat gram-negative rods and some gram-positive organisms. Fluoroquinolones such as levofloxacin are used to treat upper respiratory infections and urinary tract infections.

Answer B is incorrect. Gentamicin is a macrolide antibiotic used to treat gram-negative bacilli. Adverse effects include nephrotoxicity and ototoxicity. Gentamicin is effective in treating *Enterobacter*, but it is not as efficacious as imipenem, which is the first-line choice.

Answer D is incorrect. Penicillin G is not effective against *Enterobacter*. It is an intravenous β-lactam antibiotic useful in treating gram-positive bacteria as well as some gram-negative cocci and spirochetes. The most common adverse effect is a hypersensitivity reaction.

Answer E is incorrect. Piperacillin-tazobactam (Zosyn) is a combination of an extended-spectrum penicillin with a penicillinase in-

hibitor. It is used to treat *Pseudomonas* infections as well as gram-negative rods. Like penicillin, it can cause hypersensitivity reactions.

33. **The correct answer is E.** This patient has vitiligo, a disorder characterized by partial or total absence of melanocytes within the epidermis. Studies have suggested an autoimmune connection to the disease process, citing associations to antibodies against tyrosinase, antigens that co-migrate with tyrosinase, or other antigens on melanocytes. Melanocytes produce skin pigment by synthesizing melanin and secreting it to keratinocytes.

Answer A is incorrect. Hemidesmosomes serve to connect epithelial cells to the underlying extracellular matrix.

Answer B is incorrect. Meissner corpuscles are found in the dermis of the palms, soles, and digits; they function as light sensory touch receptors.

Answer C is incorrect. Pacinian corpuscles are found in deep layers of skin (at ligaments, joint capsules, serous membranes, and mesenteries) and function as pressure and coarse touch sensory receptors.

Answer D is incorrect. Langerhans cells are found in the epidermis and function as antigen-presenting cells during certain immune responses.

34. **The correct answer is B.** Elevated galactitol is the cause of clinical symptoms in patients with galactosemia. Galactose is utilized in glycolysis and gluconeogenesis by a two-step conversion to glucose-1-phosphate. The first step is catalyzed by the enzyme galactokinase, which phosphorylates galactose to galactose-1-phoisphate. Decreased galactose-1-phosphate is the correct answer because galactosemia, and the damaging elevated galactitol that follows, can occur in glucokinase deficiency. This deficiency is between the conversion of galactose to galactose 1-phosphate and would lead to relatively decreased galactose-1-phosphate. Galactose reduction by aldose reductase is then increased, forming galactitol.

Answer A is incorrect. Galactose would be elevated.

Answer C is incorrect. Classic galactosemia is caused by a deficiency of this uridyltransferase and would theoretically lead to a build up of galactose-1-phosphate, uridine diphosphoglucose, and galactose, and decreased glucose-1-phosphate and decreased glucose-1-phosphate. None of these choices is given.

Answer D is incorrect. Glucose-1-phosphate is the final product of galactose metabolism before glycolysis and would be decreased in all types of galactosemia.

Answer E is incorrect. Glucose-1-phosphate is an intermediate in glycogen pathways and the final product of galactose metabolism. However, galactosemia does not result in glycogen level fluctuations.

35. **The correct answer is G.** The patient presents emergently with symptoms of acute coronary syndrome, or ACS (either unstable angina or acute myocardial infarction): new-onset chest pain that radiates and was prompted by increased activity. The ST segment depression on the ECG indicates myocardial ischemia. Because the situation is emergent, treatment must have a rapid onset, and nitroglycerin is the drug of choice because it will both reduce the use of oxygen by the heart and increase the oxygen supply to the heart. Nitroglycerin will reduce preload by causing venodilation and will also increase the oxygenation of myocardial cells by dilating the coronary vessels. Sublingual nitroglycerin is the route of administration with the quickest onset.

Answer A is incorrect. Acetaminophen would not be indicated in this clinical situation; the patient has already been given an aspirin, which is indicated for its antiplatelet activity.

Answer B is incorrect. Digoxin is a cardiac glycoside that increases cardiac inotropy and is thus contraindicated in the setting of acute coronary syndrome because it will increase the oxygen demands of the heart.

Answer C is incorrect. Enalapril is an angiotensin-converting enzyme (ACE) inhibitor and thus has no role in the treatment of acute coronary syndrome. If an acute myocardial infarction had occurred in this patient, then an ACE inhibitor would be prescribed for maintenance therapy to reduce ventricular remodeling.

Answer D is incorrect. Hydrochlorothiazide is a diuretic that has no role in the emergent treatment of acute coronary syndrome.

Answer E is incorrect. Nifedipine is a calcium channel blocker that causes arterial vasodilation. It can be used emergently in cases of vasospasm but is not the first-line drug in cases of acute coronary syndrome.

Answer F is incorrect. Quinidine is a class IA antiarrhythmic and thus has no role in treating acute coronary syndrome.

36. **The correct answer is B.** Huntington's disease is associated with atrophy of the caudate nucleus.

Answer A is incorrect. Klüver-Bucy syndrome, clinically manifested by hyperorality, hypersexuality, and disinhibited behavior, is associated with bilateral obliteration of the amygdala.

Answer C is incorrect. Amyotrophic lateral sclerosis, more commonly known as Lou Gehrig's disease, is associated with degeneration of the lateral corticospinal tracts.

Answer D is incorrect. Parkinson's disease is characterized histologically by neuronal depletion and depigmentation of cells in the locus ceruleus.

Answer E is incorrect. Alzheimer's disease is marked by a decreased number of neurons in the nucleus basalis of Meynert.

Answer F is incorrect. Wernicke's encephalopathy, which is most commonly seen in malnourished alcoholics, is associated with atrophy of the mammillary bodies.

37. **The correct answer is E.** Sensitivity is the probability that, given a disease, a test for that disease will correctly diagnose it. It is calculated by dividing the number of true positives (98) by the total number with the disease (100) = 98%.

Answer A is incorrect. Incidence is the number of new cases of a disease in a population per unit time.

Answer B is incorrect. Negative predictive value is the probability that, given a negative test result, the subject is actually free of the disease being tested. It is calculated by dividing the number of true negatives by the total number of subjects who tested negative. Since this experimental group included no healthy control subjects, one cannot determine the positive predictive value.

Answer C is incorrect. Positive predictive value is the probability that, given a positive test result, the patient actually has the disease. It is calculated by dividing the number of true positives by the total number of subjects who tested positive. Since this experimental group included no healthy control subjects, one cannot determine the positive predictive value.

Answer D is incorrect. Prevalence is the total number of disease cases in a population at a given time.

Answer F is incorrect. Given that the test was only performed on subjects known to have the disease, one cannot infer specificity from these data. Specificity is the probability that given a healthy subject, a given test returns a negative result. Thus, it is calculated by dividing the number of false-negatives by the total number of disease-free subjects on which the test was performed.

38. **The correct answer is D.** HIV-associated dementia (also known as acquired immunodeficiency syndrome dementia complex) presents with memory loss, gait disorder, and spasticity. It represents the most common direct central nervous system complication of HIV-1 disease and generally occurs later in the course of illness. Early symptoms may be subtle and may include depressive symptoms and apathetic withdrawal before development of later symptoms, which include global dementia and motor deficits. As the dementia progresses, patients experience difficulty with smooth limb movement, dysdiadochokinesia, impaired sac-

cadic eye movements, hyperreflexia, and frontal release signs. Imaging studies are imperative to rule out mass lesions; 20–40% of patients will demonstrate nonenhancing, poorly demarcated areas of increased T2 signal intensity in the deep white matter. The symptoms must be distinguished from typical focal neurologic signs and symptoms that may be evident in patients with mass lesions. Elevated levels of protein and IgG on cerebrospinal fluid examination are present in approximately 45% and 80% of cases, respectively.

Answer A is incorrect. Central nervous system (CNS) lymphoma typically affects patients with AIDS whose CD4 counts are < 50/μL with one or more enhancing lesions on MRI (50% multiple; 50% single). It can present with many overlapping signs and symptoms, but is less insidious and typically causes more focal signs earlier in the course of the illness. CNS lymphoma can present with a positive polymerase chain reaction for Epstein-Barr virus within the cerebrospinal fluid.

Answer B is incorrect. Cytomegalovirus (CMV) encephalitis can mimic HIV-associated dementia, but is usually more rapidly progressive and is typically concurrent with more generalized CMV infections. MRI typically demonstrates enhancing periventricular white matter lesions in cortical and subependymal regions.

Answer C is incorrect. Disseminated *Mycobacterium avium* complex is a late-stage complication of acquired immunodeficiency syndrome and is associated with CD4 counts under 50/μL. It typically presents with constitutional signs and symptoms that include fever, night sweats, lymphadenopathy, hepatosplenomegaly, weight loss, and pancytopenia. The symptoms are more generalized and severe than those in HIV-associated dementia.

Answer E is incorrect. Space-occupying lesions secondary to toxoplasmosis infection begin to occur with CD4 counts below 100/μL and typically appear as enhancing central nervous system (CNS) lesions (which may be multiple) on MRI, with positive serologies.

FULL-LENGTH EXAM

Test Block 4

Treatment is typically with sulfadiazine and pyrimethamine, with imaging studies repeated after a few weeks. If no regression has occurred, the diagnosis should be reconsidered, and CNS lymphoma should become the most likely diagnosis.

39. **The correct answer is B.** The Golgi apparatus develops into the sperm's acrosome, a structure that covers the anterior two-thirds of the nucleus and contains enzymes such as hyaluronidase that permit the sperm to penetrate the zona pellucida of the egg at fertilization.

    Answer A is incorrect. The centrioles initiate the formation of the sperm's flagellum and then migrate to the neck of the developing sperm to form the connecting piece, which unites the nucleus with the flagellum. The centrioles, however, do not play a role in the development of the acrosome.

    Answer C is incorrect. Mitochondria are specialized in the sperm only in the sense that a high concentration of mitochondria is necessary to supply sufficient energy to the sperm. The mitochondria are located in the middle piece of the sperm's tail.

    Answer D is incorrect. The sperm's nucleus contains condensed chromatin and is connected via the connecting piece to the flagellum. However, the acrosome develops from the Golgi apparatus, not the nucleus.

    Answer E is incorrect. The plasma membrane must migrate posteriorly during spermiogenesis in order to cover the developing flagellum; however, it does not form the acrosome.

40. **The correct answer is E.** The first-line therapy for treating severe nausea and vomiting due to chemotherapy is ondansetron. It is the strongest available antiemetic, surpassing more common agents, such as metoclopramide, in its ability to decrease symptoms. The mechanism of action of ondansetron is blockade of serotonin 5-HT$_3$ receptors. Adverse effects of ondansetron are headache and constipation.

Answer A is incorrect. Anticholinergic drugs include atropine, benztropine, scopolamine, and ipratropium. These drugs decrease parasympathetic activity by blocking muscarinic receptors. Scopolamine is commonly used to treat motion sickness but would not be the first-line therapy for chemotherapy-induced nausea and vomiting.

Answer B is incorrect. Dopamine agonists include bromocriptine, L-dopa, pramipexole, and amantadine. These drugs are mainly used for the treatment of Parkinson's disease and are not indicated for nausea and vomiting.

Answer C is incorrect. Tricyclic antidepressants (TCAs) such as imipramine and amitriptyline act by inhibiting presynaptic reuptake of norepinephrine, thus augmenting their effect on postsynaptic receptors. TCAs are primarily used to treat depression. Their adverse effects include sedation, β-blocking effects, and anticholinergic properties.

Answer D is incorrect. Serotonin agonists include selective serotonin reuptake inhibitors such as paroxetine and sertraline, which are antidepressants.

41. **The correct answer is A.** The stem is a description of a typical case of chronic lymphocytic leukemia (CLL), the leukemia counterpart of small lymphocytic lymphoma (SLL). The hallmark of CLL is the presence of smudge cells, which are fragile lymphocytes that are destroyed during slide preparation. These cells most closely resemble B lymphocytes and can occasionally produce a small monoclonal M spike of immunoglobulin.

    Answer B is incorrect. Metamyelocytes are increased in leukemias of myeloid lineage, such as chronic myelogenous leukemia (CML) and subsets of acute myelogenous leukemia (AML). The blood smear, which shows increased lymphocytes and smudge cells, essentially rules out CML.

    Answer C is incorrect. Plasma cells are the neoplastic cell in multiple myeloma, which typically presents with bone pain, lytic lesions, hypercalcemia, and renal failure.

Answer D is incorrect. Promyelocytes are increased in acute promyelocytic leukemia (APL), a subset of AML distinguished by t(15;17) translocation. APL responds uniquely to differentiation therapy. The blood smear does not demonstrate increased promyelocytes.

Answer E is incorrect. Abnormal lymphoblasts of T-lymphocyte origin are increased in T-lymphocyte leukemias (such as acute lymphocytic leukemia) and T-lymphocyte lymphomas (note T-ALL is not the same as T-lymphocyte lymphomas).

42. **The correct answer is B.** Phosphoenolpyruvate carboxykinase (PEPCK) functions as a regulatory enzyme in gluconeogenesis. It acts in the cytosol to convert oxaloacetate to phosphoenolpyruvate.

Answer A is incorrect. The regulatory enzyme in the citric acid cycle is citrate synthase.

Answer C is incorrect. The regulatory enzyme in glycogenolysis is phosphorylase.

Answer D is incorrect. The regulatory enzyme in lipogenesis is acetyl-CoA carboxylase.

Answer E is incorrect. The regulatory enzyme in the oxidative branch of the pentose phosphate pathway is glucose-6-phosphate dehydrogenase.

43. **The correct answer is E.** This patient is suffering from dehydration, as demonstrated by her symptoms of unsteadiness suggestive of orthostatic hypotension. Her frequent emesis results in the loss of large quantities of protons from the body in the form of stomach acid. In addition, rapid loss of bicarbonate-free fluids such as stomach contents or urine can result in a net increase in plasma bicarbonate concentration; this effect is termed *contraction alkalosis*. Finally, volume depletion leads to stimulation of the renin-angiotensin-aldosterone system, causing (1) an angiotensin-mediated increase in hydrogen secretion via the sodium-hydrogen antiporter in the proximal tubule,

and (2) an aldosterone-triggered influx of sodium (and water) and an efflux of potassium and protons in the distal tubule. The loss of protons and buildup of bicarbonate in this patient causes metabolic alkalosis.

Answer A is incorrect. Consumption of antacids can contribute to metabolic alkalosis but is not the cause in this patient.

Answer B is incorrect. Dehydration causes an increase, not decrease, in hydrogen excretion in the distal tubule.

Answer C is incorrect. Total bicarbonate reabsorption in the setting of metabolic alkalosis and volume depletion is likely to be reduced. Acutely, volume depletion will result in a net decrease in the filtered load of bicarbonate, despite an increase in bicarbonate concentration. In addition, increased plasma levels of bicarbonate will impair the ability of the proximal tubule cells to secrete acid necessary for bicarbonate reabsorption. Although angiotensin II stimulation serves to partially counteract these effects, the proximal tubule is not the primary site of acid loss in this patient.

Answer D is incorrect. ADH does not have direct effects on acid-base status because the aquaporin channels it mobilizes to the cell membrane are permeable only to water.

44. **The correct answer is E.** The superficial arch is a continuation of the ulnar artery and forms anastomoses with branches of the radial artery, while the deep arch is a continuation of the radial artery that forms anastomoses with branches of the ulnar artery. Together, these palmar arches ensure good collateral flow to the hand even if the radial artery becomes occluded. The Allen test is a way to determine if there is adequate arterial supply to the hand if the radial artery is occluded. This test is performed prior to inserting a catheter into this artery for blood pressure monitoring purposes or during coronary procedures. The radial and ulnar arteries are occluded while the patient makes a fist. The hand is relaxed and will appear pale. The pressure on the ulnar artery is released and the hand is visualized for uniform

pink color return and normalization of the pulse oximetry reading within 8–10 seconds.

Answer A is incorrect. The interosseous arteries branch from the radial and ulnar arteries proximal to the wrist, forming anastomoses between the two arteries more proximal in the arm.

Answer B is incorrect. The arcuate artery is a branch of the dorsal artery of the foot and gives off perforating branches to the plantar artery. This artery helps ensure collateral flow in the foot so that if either the posterior or anterior tibial artery becomes occluded, the foot will have adequate circulation.

Answer C is incorrect. The palmar digital arteries branch from the palmar arches to supply the fingers.

Answer D is incorrect. The dorsalis pedis is found in the foot.

45. **The correct answer is D.** The condition described in this vignette is polycystic ovarian disease (Stein-Leventhal syndrome), which is a syndrome of multiple ovarian cysts, amenorrhea, infertility, obesity, and hirsutism caused by excess LH and androgens. In some women, this is associated with insulin resistance and hyperinsulinemia, which increases androgen production and, secondarily, LH production. The insulin resistance also leads to hyperglycemia.

Answer A is incorrect. Abdominal striae are signs of adrenocortical excess or Cushing's syndrome. This syndrome includes central obesity, muscle wasting, virilization, hypertension, round facies, buffalo hump, and striae due to high levels of glucocorticoids, mineralocorticoids, and androgens secondary to adrenal hyperplasia. Ovaries are not affected. The name Cushing's disease applies when these effects are due to elevated levels of ACTH.

Answer B is incorrect. Exophthalmos, or bulging eyes, is a sign of Graves' hyperthyroidism. Hyperthyroidism can present with amenorrhea, fine hair growth, restlessness, heat intolerance, diarrhea, and tachycardia.

However, high thyroid levels usually result in low TSH levels and do not affect the ovaries.

Answer C is incorrect. Amenorrhea and galactorrhea are signs of hyperprolactinemia. Prolactin is controlled by dopamine secretion from the hypothalamus and inhibits gonadotropin secretion. This would not explain the high level of LH, elevated androgen levels, or enlarged ovaries.

Answer E is incorrect. Weak pulses in the lower extremities is a sign of coarctation of the aorta, which is associated with Turner's syndrome. Turner's syndrome is the most common cause of primary amenorrhea, and patients present with short stature, webbed neck, and infantile genitalia. Ovaries are replaced with fibrous streaks.

46. **The correct answer is A.** The suspicion of child abuse arises when the injury and the story of the injury do not match. The physician should look for signs such as multiple bruises in varying states of healing, old fractures on x-ray, subdural hematoma, retinal detachment/hemorrhage, and cigarette burns. Spiral fractures generally do not occur with a simple fall down the stairs. Child abuse must be reported in all states in the United States.

Answer B is incorrect. Normal play is an insufficient explanation for a serious injury such as a spiral fracture of the femur.

Answer C is incorrect. Children with osteogenesis imperfecta can certainly present with spiral fractures due to seemingly benign accidents; however, the time delay from the accident to presentation in the emergency department, as well as the healed rib fractures, is more suspicious for child abuse.

Answer D is incorrect. Fracture can be a complication associated with osteosarcoma; however, osteosarcomas are generally seen in male adolescents. The common finding on x-ray is a lytic lesion with or without soft tissue calcification in the proximal tibia or distal femur.

Answer E is incorrect. Rickets can present with fractures of the long bones; however, they tend to be greenstick fractures. These children are also typically bowlegged or knock-kneed due to the softening of the bony structure associated with vitamin D deficiency.

47. **The correct answer is E.** Volvulus is a common result of malrotation of the midgut but may also be associated with other congenital anomalies, such as Meckel's diverticulum and Hirschsprung's disease. Malrotation occurs when the midgut undergoes only partial rotation during development; normally, between weeks 10 and 12 the midgut rotates a total of 270 degrees counterclockwise. When malrotation leads to intestinal twisting and vascular congestion or ischemia, volvulus can result. The presentation of volvulus varies depending on the age of the child and the severity of the twisting but is generally associated with vomiting, bloody diarrhea, abdominal distention, and tenderness to palpation. In the x-ray film, note the twisting and overdistention of the colon with its coffee-bean shape and lack of septa and haustra, all indicative of obstruction due to volvulus. This is a dangerous condition, since ischemia can lead to gangrene and midgut necrosis; necrosis of the entire midgut is incompatible with life. Definitive treatment is corrective surgery.

Answer A is incorrect. Hirschsprung's disease may cause a similar radiograph and symptoms of obstruction but would not cause symptoms of ischemia and is not the result of malrotation. Rather, it is the result of a failure of neural crest cells to migrate, leading to aganglionosis of the distal colon.

Answer B is incorrect. Meckel's diverticulum, like malrotation, is associated with volvulus but is not itself a result of malrotation. This blind pouch near the terminal ileum instead represents a remnant of the vitelline duct. It is often asymptomatic but may become inflamed and ulcerated.

Answer C is incorrect. An omphalocele is a shiny gray sac protruding from the base of the umbilical cord. It is the result of failure of a midgut loop to return to the abdominal cavity after the normal physiologic umbilical hernia-

tion that occurs around week 6. It is evident in the newborn, not at 1 month, and would not result in the symptoms described here.

Answer D is incorrect. Vitelline fistula results from the full persistence of the vitelline duct. It leads to fecal discharge from the umbilicus, which would surely be noted on physical examination. It is not the result of malrotation and does not produce the x-ray image shown.

48. **The correct answer is A.** Acyclovir is a guanosine analog used in the treatment of active herpesvirus infections. Acyclovir causes premature DNA chain termination and limits the length of a herpes outbreak, although it does not change the frequency with which they occur.

Answer B is incorrect. Didanosine (ddI) is an antiretroviral drug also classified as a nucleoside analog.

Answer C is incorrect. Lamivudine (3TC) is a nucleoside reverse transcriptase inhibitor that inhibits the reverse transcriptase of HIV and hepatitis B.

Answer D is incorrect. Stavudine (d4T) is a nucleoside analog of thymidine that inhibits reverse transcriptase when biotransformed to its active form.

Answer E is incorrect. Zalcitabine (ddC) is a nucleoside analog that inhibits viral reverse transcriptase when converted to its active form.

Answer F is incorrect. Zidovudine, didanosine, zalcitabine, stavudine, and lamivudine are all drugs used in the treatment of HIV and AIDS. Zidovudine is a pyrimidine (nucleoside) analog that is converted to its active form in the host cell.

49. **The correct answer is D.** The presence of many lymphocytes and few Reed-Sternberg cells with collagen bands that circumscribe the lymphoid tissue into discrete nodules is consistent with the nodular sclerosing subtype of Hodgkin's disease (HD). This is the subtype with the best prognosis, and it is also the most common. Nodular sclerosing Hodgkin's lymphoma is more common in women. This his-

tologic picture also resembles the lymphocyte predominance subtype, which is much less common but has an excellent prognosis and is also found in women.

Answer A is incorrect. Any type of Hodgkin's disease (HD) involving many Reed-Sternberg cells and no or few lymphocytes describes the rare lymphocyte depletion subtype. This has the worst prognosis of any type of HD and is generally present in elderly men with disseminated disease.

Answer B is incorrect. The heterogenous mixture of many mononuclear cells, many Reed-Sternberg cells, and many lymphocytes is consistent with mixed cellularity Hodgkin's disease. This subtype is more common in men and more likely to be diagnosed at a later stage. The overall prognosis is good.

Answer C is incorrect. Lymphocyte predominance is a rare subtype of Hodgkin's disease most often seen in men younger than 35 years. Histologically, it is characterized by numerous lymphocytes. Reed-Sternberg cells are difficult to find; more commonly large lymphohistiocytic cells called popcorn cells are seen.

Answer E is incorrect. Hodgkin's disease is characterized by the presence of Reed-Sternberg cells. Without Reed-Sternberg cells, the diagnosis of Hodgkin's disease cannot be made.

50. **The correct answer is F.** Based on the presenting symptoms of abdominal pain, bloody stools, Ashkenazi Jewish ancestry, and family history, this patient is suffering from inflammatory bowel disease (IBD), most likely ulcerative colitis. The image shows classical diffuse mucosal inflammation with pseudopolyps. Infectious etiologies of diarrhea are less likely given the patient's absence of fever, left shift, sick contacts, and foreign travel. Increased erythrocyte sedimentation rate is also consistent with diagnosis of IBD. Sulfasalazine is first-line therapy for ulcerative colitis. It is metabolized to 5-aminosalicylic acid in the digestive tract and decreases inflammation locally. Adverse effects include renal insufficiency and increased risk of bleeding.

Answer A is incorrect. Ciprofloxacin may be useful in the treatment of ulcerative colitis complicated by strictures and infections of the gastrointestinal tract; however, it is not first-line treatment for inflammatory bowel disease.

Answer B is incorrect. Surgery, specifically colectomy in the case of ulcerative colitis, should be reserved for patients who have failed medical therapy.

Answer C is incorrect. Infliximab, a monoclonal antibody against tumor necrosis factor-α, is used for the treatment of severe ulcerative colitis following failure of more conservative therapies.

Answer D is incorrect. Loperamide, an antidiarrheal, should be used only in mild ulcerative colitis. While it may be useful for treatment of mild symptoms, it is not first-line therapy. Caution for development of fulminant colitis and/or toxic megacolon should preclude the use of antidiarrheals in patients with severe disease.

Answer E is incorrect. Oral steroids are used for treatment of moderate-severity ulcerative colitis that is refractory to first-line therapy. This patient is suffering from mild disease and may benefit from the addition of oral steroids if sulfasalazine therapy fails.

Test Block 5

1. A young couple presents to a fertility clinic because they have been unable to conceive despite trying for the past 18 months. On examination, the 27-year-old husband is found to have small testes and mild gynecomastia. He is 188 cm (6′2″) tall and weighs 64.4 kg (142 lb) (body mass index = 18.2 mg/kg^2). Further cytogenetic testing reveals the presence of an additional X chromosome in his cells. Which of the following laboratory results is consistent with this man's condition?

(A) Decreased follicle-stimulating hormone
(B) Decreased thyroid-stimulating hormone
(C) Increased ammonia
(D) Increased luteinizing hormone
(E) Increased testosterone

2. A 65-year-old man with cancer gives his best friend durable power of attorney. As his condition worsens, he goes into respiratory failure and is intubated. He is now on a ventilator in a coma. The friend believes the patient would have wished for life support to be withdrawn. The patient's son, however, believes the father would have wanted extreme measures taken to maintain his life. What is the legal course of action?

(A) Advise the friend to listen to the son's wishes
(B) Appoint a new power of attorney
(C) Keep the patient on life support
(D) Poll all the family members present
(E) Withdraw life support

3. Three days after eating in a fast-food hamburger restaurant, a 12-year-old boy develops abdominal pain, a fever of 39.6° C (103.3° F), and bloody diarrhea. He is admitted to the hospital. His stool smear shows many leukocytes; a Gram's stain shows many gram-negative rods. The organism forms pink colonies on Mac-Conkey agar. The responsible organism is thought to be associated with development of which of the following conditions?

(A) Fever, migratory polyarthritis, and carditis
(B) Fever, new murmur, small erythematous lesions on the palms, and splinter hemorrhages on the nail beds
(C) Petechial rash and bilateral hemorrhage into the adrenal gland
(D) Symmetric ascending muscle weakness beginning in the distal lower extremities
(E) Thrombocytopenia, anemia, and uremia

4. A 65-year-old man suffers an acute myocardial infarction. His right coronary artery is stented, and the patient is started on a cardioprotective regimen of drugs. Three weeks later, his laboratory studies show the following results:

Alanine aminotransferase (ALT): 62 U/L
Aspartate aminotransferase (AST): 42 U/L
Bilirubin, total: 1.4 mg/dL
Albumin: 3.6 g/dL

Which of the following agents was most likely included in this patient's drug regimen?

(A) Aspirin
(B) Clopidogrel
(C) Lisinopril
(D) Metoprolol
(E) Pravastatin

5. A 42-year-old African-American woman with a history of sarcoidosis presents to a neurologist with evidence of a Bell's palsy. The muscles involved in this condition are derived from which of the following embryologic structures?

(A) First branchial (pharyngeal) arch
(B) Fourth branchial (pharyngeal) pouch
(C) Second branchial (pharyngeal) arch
(D) Third branchial (pharyngeal) pouch
(E) Thyroglossal duct

6. A 60-year-old man is found to have advanced adenocarcinoma of the stomach. The tumor is centered at the pyloric zone just near the pyloric sphincter, on the lesser curvature. By mass effect, the neoplasm impinges on the omental (epiploic) foramen. Which of the following signs and symptoms is most likely to be

seen in this patient due to the mass effect of the tumor?

(A) Anemia
(B) Constipation
(C) Hoarseness
(D) Jaundice
(E) Seizures

7. A mutant strain of *Escherichia coli* expresses the protein products of the lactose operon in the presence of both glucose and lactose. However, no protein products are produced when the *E. coli* is grown only with glucose. Based on this observation, where is the mutation most likely located?

(A) Cyclic adenosine monophosphate–receptor protein
(B) Inducer-binding site
(C) Promoter
(D) Repressor
(E) RNA polymerase

8. A 14-month-old boy presents with recurrent viral and fungal infections, congenital heart defects, tetany, and anatomic malformations in the neck. The abnormal cells in his spleen would be found in which of the following areas?

(A) Periarterial lymphoid sheath
(B) Splenic artery
(C) Splenic capsule
(D) Splenic vein
(E) White pulp follicles

9. Prior to the advent of antibiotics, patients suffering from life-threatening bacterial infections often received injections of serum from horses that were immunized with the disease-causing bacteria. A severe adverse event with this treatment occurred 7–10 days later and included fevers, rash, arthritis, and glomerulonephritis. Today, the same adverse event is seen with certain drugs or with delivery of large amounts of foreign protein. Why does it take 7–10 days for symptoms to occur?

(A) It usually takes the immune system 7–10 days to mount a mature antibody response against foreign proteins

(B) Symptoms begin to occur much earlier, but they often go unnoticed for 1 week
(C) Symptoms occur when the life-threatening bacterial infection worsens; this happens about 1 week after an unsuccessful course of treatment
(D) The foreign protein or drug must be metabolized before the immune system recognizes it, which takes about 1 week
(E) This is a T-cell–mediated adverse effect, and it takes about 1 week to activate the T cells

10. A woman whose mother had cancer in both breasts develops breast cancer at age 26 years. Her identical twin sister would like to know how likely it is that she, too, will develop the disease, and she decides to undergo testing for mutations in the *BRCA* gene. This gene allows tumorigenesis by which of the following mechanisms?

(A) Dominant-negative effect
(B) Gain of function
(C) Imprinting
(D) Loss of function
(E) Viral insertion

11. A 6-year-old boy with recurrent otitis media is being treated with prophylactic antibiotics by his pediatrician. His father notices he has been bruising easily on his legs and bleeding heavily when he brushes his teeth. He had a nosebleed 2 days ago that took 30 minutes to stop bleeding. Examination reveals splinter hemorrhages in the fingertips. A micronutrient deficiency is suspected. Which of the following describes the correct function of the micronutrient the boy is missing?

(A) It is required to carboxylate glutamic acid residues in inactive clotting molecules
(B) It is required to counter exchange with sodium in a common membrane pump
(C) It is required to hydroxylate proline residues in procollagen synthesis
(D) It is required to maintain prothrombic antibiotic-sensitive intestinal flora
(E) It is required to reduce antithrombic antibiotic breakdown intermediates

12. A 3-year-old boy is brought to his pediatrician with difficulty breathing and wheezing. His mother states that he recently had a cold. The boy has a heart rate of 95/min, a blood pressure of 130/85 mm Hg, a respiratory rate of 20/min, and an oxygen saturation of 94%. The boy appears to be having difficulty breathing, and on lung examination, wheezing can be heard bilaterally throughout. The boy's mother adds that he had similar episodes of wheezing after his previous colds. Which of the following is contributing to this child's symptoms?

    (A) Cyclooxygenase
    (B) Leukotriene B_4
    (C) Leukotriene C_4
    (D) Prostaglandin I_2
    (E) Thromboxane A_2

13. A 26-year-old Mexican immigrant presents to the clinic with a 3-month history of right upper quadrant abdominal pain. The patient denies any history of fever, vomiting, or diarrhea in the last 6 months. An ultrasound of the right upper quadrant reveals a well-circumscribed circular lesion that is 3 cm in diameter. Laboratory findings are as follows:

    WBC count: 9000/mm^3
    Segmented neutrophils: 56%
    Band forms: 4%
    Eosinophils: 10%
    Basophils: 0.6%
    Lymphocytes: 26%
    Monocytes: 3%

    Which of the following is the most likely morphology of the offending agent?

    (A) Aerobic gram-negative bacteria
    (B) Nonmotile gram-negative bacteria
    (C) Pear-shaped protozoan
    (D) Tapeworm
    (E) Trophozoite

14. A 25-year-old woman presents with hypersecretion from the organ shown in the image. Increased levels of which of the following neurotransmitters might cause this patient's condition?

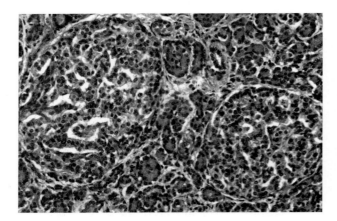

Image courtesy of PEIR Digital Library (http://peir.net).

    (A) Acetylcholine
    (B) GABA
    (C) Glycine
    (D) Norepinephrine
    (E) Serotonin

15. A 57-year-old man is brought to the emergency department in respiratory failure and dies shortly after his arrival. Paramedics report that the patient's examination was initially notable for meningeal signs and left-sided hemiplegia and hyperreflexia; he then vomited and became obtunded. The patient had reported suffering from a severe headache for the past 5 hours but had no history of neurologic disease and had not experienced any traumatic events recently. According to the wife's report, the patient's only medical problem was chronic renal insufficiency because "like his father, he has large kidneys." Given the patient's presentation and past medical history, which of the following is the most likely cause of death?

    (A) Disruption of the middle meningeal artery
    (B) Disruption of the sigmoid sinus
    (C) Hypertensive cerebrovascular disease
    (D) Rupture of a saccular aneurysm
    (E) Thromboembolization of the middle cerebral artery

16. A 3-year-old boy presents to his pediatrician with irritability, an ataxic gait, and regression of speech to single words. During the interview, the patient is constantly putting objects

in his mouth. Laboratory values are significant for a hemoglobin level of 8.3 g/dL. Which of the following etiologies should be suspected in this patient?

(A) Acetaminophen toxicity
(B) Aspirin toxicity
(C) Button battery ingestion
(D) Lead poisoning
(E) Organophosphate absorption
(F) Tricyclic antidepressant overdose

17. A mother brings her 1-month-old infant to the pediatrician. She says the baby is crying more than usual and is vomiting and does not want to eat. Meningitis is suspected, and a lumbar puncture is done, which shows the following results:

Opening pressure = 240 mm H₂O (normal = 100–200 mm H₂O)
WBC count: 1200/mm³
Protein: 200 mg/dL
Glucose: 30 mg/dL
Gram's staining reveals gram-positive rods

Which of the following organisms is most likely responsible for this infant's meningitis?

(A) *Escherichia coli*
(B) Herpes simplex virus
(C) *Listeria monocytogenes*
(D) *Neisseria meningitides*
(E) *Streptococcus agalactiae*

18. A 10-year-old boy with chronic granulomatous disease (CGD) suffers from chronic recurrent gut inflammation, which modestly improves with cyclosporine therapy. The patient's father wants to know how a child with an immunodeficiency disease like CGD could also have an autoimmune disease. Deficiencies in which of the following immunologic processes or molecules provides a logical link between chronic granulomatous disease and autoimmune gut inflammation?

(A) Antibodies
(B) IgA
(C) IgM
(D) Lysosomes
(E) Neutrophils

19. A 22-year-old woman presents to the emergency department with low blood pressure, hyponatremia, lethargy, anorexia, loss of pubic and axillary hair, and inability to nurse her newborn twins. Her past medical history is significant for a recent spontaneous vaginal delivery of twins complicated by postpartum bleeding. A CT scan of the head is performed and shows no tumors or masses. Which of the following sets of laboratory values is most likely to be seen in this patient?

CHOICE	CORTISOL	PROLACTIN	THYROID-STIMULATING HORMONE
A	↑	↑	↑
B	No change	No change	No change
C	No change	↑	No change
D	No change	↓	No change
E	↓	↓	↓

(A) A
(B) B
(C) C
(D) D
(E) E

20. Genetic analysis of multiple members in a family shows that they all have the same mutant gene. However, not all members display the characteristic phenotype; some members are more obviously affected than others. This is an example of which of the following?

(A) Anticipation
(B) Dominant-negative mutation
(C) Incomplete penetrance
(D) Mosaicism
(E) Pleiotropy

21. A 16-year-old boy with sickle cell disease has complained of a weak right leg for the past 10 days. He is unable to put much weight on it. On physical examination, the area over the right tibia is found to be swollen and erythematous. The organism responsible for this patient's infection most likely has which of the following features that makes it particularly pathogenic?

(A) Capsule
(B) Flagella
(C) Lack of cell wall
(D) Mycolic acids
(E) Pili

22. A 44-year-old woman comes to her physician complaining of a 2-month history of increasing fatigue but denies any other symptoms. On further questioning, the patient admits to a long history of alcoholism and says that she has a "horrible diet." Physical examination is unremarkable. Laboratory studies are significant for a hemoglobin level of 8 g/dL and a mean corpuscular volume of 110 mm³. A folic acid deficiency is suspected. Which of the following is the function of folic acid?

(A) Catalyze γ-carboxylation of glutamic acid residues
(B) Coenzyme for one-carbon transfer
(C) Cofactor for norepinephrine synthesis
(D) Constituent of visual pigments
(E) Increase intestinal calcium and phosphate absorption

23. A 32-year-old woman with a history of schizophrenia presents to the physician with amenorrhea and a milky discharge from both nipples. A pregnancy test is negative. Laboratory results show an increased level of prolactin, decreased gonadotropin levels, and normal thyroid function tests. Which of the following medications is the most likely cause of this patient's symptoms and laboratory findings?

(A) Amantadine
(B) Bromocriptine
(C) Cabergoline
(D) Chlorpromazine
(E) Lithium

24. A 20-year-old woman is referred to an endocrinologist for lack of menarche. On physical examination, breast tissue is found to be present, no cervix is palpable, the vagina ends in a blind pouch, and small atrophic testes are palpated in the inguinal canal. Laboratory studies reveal elevated levels of testosterone, estrogen, and luteinizing hormone. The karyotype is 46,XY. Which of the following is responsible for this patient's condition?

(A) CGG triplet repeat expansion
(B) Deficiency of 5-α-reductase
(C) Deletion of the X-linked dystrophin gene
(D) Excessive early gestational androgenic exposure
(E) Unresponsive testosterone receptors

25. A 40-year-old man has a cholecystectomy while undergoing surgery to remove a small intestine adenocarcinoma. While the gallbladder typically functions in the storage of bile, in which of the following locations is bile produced?

(A) Brush border of colon
(B) Brush border of terminal ileum
(C) Liver—hepatocytes
(D) Liver—Kupffer cells
(E) Liver—space of Disse

26. A 26-year-old woman is diagnosed with a congenital uterine malformation after several miscarriages. The gross specimen shown in the image is from a patient with the same uterine

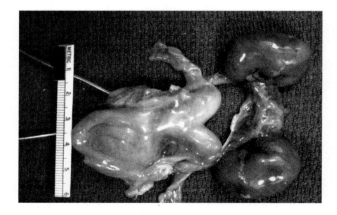

Image courtesy of PEIR Digital Library (http://peir.net).

malformation who died of unrelated causes. Which of the following is the most likely etiology of this malformation?

(A) Complete lack of fusion of the paramesonephric (müllerian) ducts
(B) Excessive resorption of mesonephric (wolffian) ducts
(C) Failure of the vaginal plates to canalize
(D) Incomplete fusion of mesonephric (wolffian) ducts
(E) Incomplete fusion of paramesonephric (müllerian) ducts

27. A previously healthy 5-year-old boy is brought to the pediatrician with a 3-day history of sore throat, conjunctivitis, rhinitis, and cough. His mother explains that more than 10 children in his class at school have similar symptoms, particularly conjunctivitis. No cultures are ordered, and the mother is assured that her son's illness will go away on its own. One week later, the mother reports that her son is healthy and back at school. Which of the following is the most likely causative agent in this child's illness?

(A) Adenovirus
(B) Coxsackie A virus
(C) Cytomegalovirus
(D) Herpes simplex virus type 1
(E) Rotavirus

28. A 40-year-old woman presents with progressive fatigue and bilateral joint inflammation characterized by pain, swelling, warmth, and morning stiffness. The patient says that the symptoms began in her hands over 1 year ago but have now begun to affect her knees. Which of the following agents would be useful in her treatment?

(A) Ceftriaxone
(B) Cyclophosphamide
(C) Methotrexate
(D) Probenecid
(E) Tamoxifen

29. An 83-year-old man is brought to the family physician by his daughter because the patient has become "increasingly forgetful." The patient himself has no complaints. The daughter states that her father's memory problems have been getting steadily worse for the past few months. His past medical history is remarkable only for mild hypertension. A neurologic examination is normal. A CT scan of the head shows mild cerebral atrophy. Which of the following is a treatable and reversible cause of this patient's memory problems?

(A) Alzheimer's dementia
(B) Hypothyroidism
(C) Multi-infarct dementia
(D) Normal aging
(E) Pick's disease

30. A 7-year-old girl presents with a 5-month history of persistent weakness despite taking vitamins and supplements. Her mother denies that she has a significant medical history of any kind. Physical examination is completely benign, with normal blood pressure and no peripheral edema. Laboratory studies show hyponatremia, hypokalemia, metabolic alkalosis, and an increased plasma renin level. Renal biopsy reveals juxtaglomerular cell hyperplasia. Bartter's syndrome, a defective cotransporter in the thick ascending loop of Henle, is suspected. Which of the following diuretics acts on the cotransporter defective in Bartter's syndrome?

(A) Acetazolamide
(B) Furosemide
(C) Hydrochlorothiazide
(D) Spironolactone
(E) Triamterene

31. A 6-year-old boy presents to the physician with poor exercise tolerance. Physical examination shows a wide pulse pressure and a murmur. He is diagnosed with a congenital disorder of a structure that shunts fetal blood from the pulmonary artery to the aorta. Which of the following therapies for the mother would have reduced the risk of having a child with this disorder?

(A) Amantadine
(B) Ganciclovir
(C) Pertussis vaccine
(D) Rubella vaccine
(E) Spectinomycin

32. A 53-year-old woman notices that her menstrual periods are becoming irregular, and sometimes she goes for 2 to 3 months without a period. She also complains of vaginal dryness and hot flashes. Blood tests reveal an estrogen level of 22 pg/mL, follicle-stimulating hormone level of 200 U/L, and luteinizing hormone level of 60 mIU/mL (without surge). Which of the following is responsible for this patient's symptoms?

(A) Decreased estrogen levels
(B) Decreased feedback on the anterior pituitary
(C) Decreased hormone inhibition
(D) Increased progesterone levels
(E) Increased testosterone levels

33. A 47-year-old man with a history of hyperparathyroidism presents to the physician with a thyroid mass. Laboratory studies show elevated serum calcitonin levels. The patient reports that multiple family members have had similar health problems. Which of the following is the most likely pathology of this patient's thyroid mass?

(A) Atrophic follicles with lymphocyte infiltrate and germinal centers
(B) Nests of enzyme-secreting tumor cells in an amyloid-filled stroma
(C) Papillary pattern with ground-glass nuclei and psammoma bodies
(D) Sheets of undifferentiated, pleomorphic cells

(E) Uniform follicles with sparse colloid and a large cell lining

34. A 27-year-old woman comes to the emergency department because of a slightly asymmetric smile and a swollen right knee and left shoulder for the past 2 days. While obtaining the patient's history, it is learned that 3 months ago she developed a painless, ring-shaped red mark on her left forearm that expanded outward and then went away. Two months ago, the patient had joint swelling of her left elbow, which lasted for 3 weeks and then resolved on its own. What is the most likely pathogen to have caused this constellation of findings?

(A) *Borrelia burgdorferi*
(B) *Neisseria gonorrhoeae*
(C) Parvovirus B19
(D) *Rickettsia rickettsii*
(E) *Streptococcus pyogenes*

35. A large study is conducted in a Middle Eastern country to observe the renal functionality of subjects with the nephritic disease shown in the following image. Which of the following is a common finding in this disease?

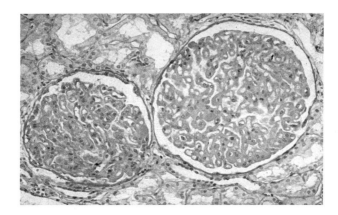

Image courtesy of PEIR Digital Library (http://peir.net).

(A) Foot process effacement
(B) Linear immunofluorescence
(C) Mesangial deposits of IgA
(D) Split basement membrane
(E) Subendothelial humps

36. A 27-year-old woman is involuntarily committed to a psychiatric ward. Her physicians note persistently elevated blood pressure with a mean arterial pressure of 120 mm Hg over a week. The patient has been asymptomatic. Her physicians would like to begin a standard treatment regimen but the patient refuses. She understands the risks, benefits, and outcomes that would result either with or without treatment. What has priority in the care of this patient?

    (A) Beneficence
    (B) Duty to other patients
    (C) Nonmaleficence
    (D) Patient autonomy
    (E) Physician autonomy

37. A 19-year-old woman with no significant past medical history presents to her primary care physician for a sports physical. Her examination is notable for a brachial artery pressure of 160/110 mm Hg and a weak femoral pulse. Prompted by the weak pulse, her physician measures her blood pressure in the lower extremity and finds it to be 80/40 mm Hg. An x-ray film of the chest shows rib notching. This woman is presenting with a congenital condition that places her at high risk for bacterial endocarditis and which of the following other conditions?

    (A) Acute lymphocytic leukemia
    (B) Boot-shaped heart
    (C) Cerebral hemorrhage
    (D) Cor pulmonale
    (E) Eisenmenger's syndrome

38. A 25-year-old man is brought to the emergency department by his next-door neighbor after being found unconscious. The neighbor reports having last seen the man working in his yard about 4 hours earlier. No medical history is available. On physical examination, the patient has a blood pressure of 60/40 mm Hg, a pulse of 150/min, and respirations of 10/min. Despite the efforts of the emergency department staff, the man cannot be resuscitated. On autopsy, he is noted to have extremely flexible joints and skin. Many bruises are noted on his thorax that were not present on admission. The

cause of death is determined to be rupture of the abdominal aorta. This patient suffered from defective synthesis of which of the following structural proteins?

    (A) Collagen
    (B) Elastin
    (C) Keratin
    (D) Myosin
    (E) Ubiquitin

39. A 6-hour-old baby boy who was born full-term and without complications now presents with cyanosis and dyspnea. Physical examination reveals absent breath sounds on the left with bowel sounds present in the left hemithorax. Heart sounds are distant on the left but heard well on the right. An x-ray film of the chest confirms the presence of bowel loops in the chest. These findings can all be explained by failed development of a single part of a specific structure. Which of the following is the most likely origin of the part of this structure that has failed to develop properly?

    (A) Bulbus cordis
    (B) Mesencephalon
    (C) Midgut loop
    (D) Pleuroperitoneal folds
    (E) Respiratory diverticulum

40. A 15-month-old boy is brought to the pediatrician by his parents because they have noticed that he has difficulty walking. On physical examination, the child exhibits a broad-based waddling gait. Laboratory studies show a serum Ca^{2+} level of 6.0 mg/dL, a serum phosphate level of 2.0 mg/dL, and a serum alkaline phosphatase activity of 85 U/L. Which of the following processes is most likely deficient in this child?

    (A) Degradation of serum alkaline phosphatase
    (B) Demineralization of osteoid matrix
    (C) Hydroxylation of proline and lysine in collagen synthesis
    (D) Intestinal absorption of Ca^{2+} and phosphate
    (E) Renal absorption of Ca^{2+} and phosphate

41. A 24-year-old tall, thin man complains of sudden unilateral pleuritic chest pain and shortness of breath after playing a game of basketball. Being suspicious of a spontaneous pneumothorax, an x-ray film is made, which confirms the suspicion. A chest tube is placed. Which of the following is a likely physical finding before chest tube placement?

(A) Bilateral chest expansion
(B) Bronchial breath sounds
(C) Hyperresonance on percussion
(D) Increased tactile fremitus
(E) Tracheal deviation toward the affected lung

42. A 20-year-old mother is unsure of the paternity of her new son. To determine the father of her child, a genetic test based on DNA restriction fragment length polymorphism was performed. Blood was drawn from the four men suspected to be the father (F1, F2, F3, F4) as well as from the mother (M) and the infant (C). DNA extracted from the samples was amplified using polymerase chain reaction and then treated with the restriction enzyme EcoRI. The resulting fragments were separated with gel electrophoresis and a Southern blot analysis was performed. According to the Southern blot shown, who is most likely the father of the child?

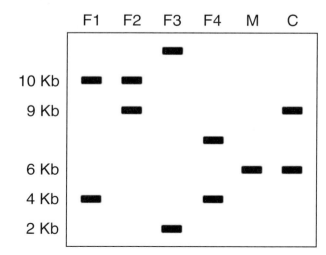

Reproduced, with permission, from USMLERx.com.

(A) F1
(B) F2
(C) F3
(D) F4

43. Taxonomists categorize the RNA viruses according to the shape of their nucleocapsid and the characteristics of their RNA. Which of the following pairs of RNA viruses have RNA that is described as double-stranded segmented?

(A) Bunyavirus and Orthomyxovirus
(B) Paramyxovirus and Morbillivirus
(C) Picornavirus and Calicivirus
(D) Rotavirus and Coltivirus
(E) Togavirus and Flavivirus

44. A 28-year-old woman comes to the physician's office complaining of anxiety and a recent 4.5-kg (9.9-lb) weight loss. Her physical examination is significant for an inability to fully cover her eyes with her eyelids and swelling on the anterior surface of both legs. The skin of her anterior legs appears dry and waxy and has several diffuse, slightly pigmented papules. Laboratory studies show low levels of serum thyroid-stimulating hormone and high levels of serum total thyroxine (T_4) and serum free T_4. Also, results of an antinuclear antibody test are negative, while those of a thyroid-stimulating immunoglobulin test are positive. Which of the following drug therapies should be used to treat this patient?

(A) Levothyroxine
(B) Mercaptopurine
(C) Procainamide
(D) Propofol
(E) Propylthiouracil

45. The symptoms of thiamine deficiency were first described over 4000 years ago. In adults, these symptoms commonly include polyneuropathy of the distal extremities, resulting in paresthesias and motor dysfunction. In addition to neuropathy, how else can isolated thiamine deficiency present in adults?

(A) Chronic infection

(B) Convulsions, hyperirritability, and jaundice

(C) Excessive diarrhea, dermatitis, and dementia

(D) Kidney failure

(E) Peripheral edema and congestive heart failure

46. Tubulointerstitial nephritis can be caused by infections and sarcoidosis but is more commonly associated with drug toxicity. The typical picture is that of acute renal failure after drug administration. Common findings are pyuria, hematuria, and WBC casts. The administration of which of the following drugs could lead to tubulointerstitial nephritis?

(A) Aspirin

(B) Cimetidine

(C) Imipenem

(D) Isoniazid

(E) Methicillin

47. A patient with long-standing renal failure secondary to focal segmental glomerulosclerosis undergoes parathyroid biopsy that shows marked hyperplasia. On physical examination, tapping over the cheek elicits facial muscle spasm. Which of the following sets of laboratory values will most likely be seen in this patient?

Choice	Parathyroid Hormone	Serum Ca²⁺	Serum Phosphate	Alkaline Phosphatase
A	↑	↑	↑	↑
B	↑	↑	↓	↑
C	↑	↓	↑	↑
D	↑	↓	↑	↓
E	↑	↓	↓	↑

(A) A

(B) B

(C) C

(D) D

(E) E

48. A 40-year-old nonsmoking woman comes to the physician complaining of a persistent cough and loss of weight and appetite over the past 3 months. On radiography, a well-demarcated subpleural mass is found on the right lung. Which of the following types of carcinoma does this patient most likely have?

(A) Adenocarcinoma of the lung

(B) Carcinoid of the lung

(C) Metastases to lung from a distant primary tumor

(D) Small-cell carcinoma of the lung

(E) Squamous cell carcinoma of the lung

49. A physician is studying the data from a trial of a new 3-hydroxy-3-methylglutaryl coenzyme A (HMG CoA) reductase inhibitor (statin). He notes muscle aches in 10% of patients. The medication can significantly lower LDL in patients at risk for coronary artery disease. The physician determines that he would need to treat five patients to prevent one from having a coronary event. He then calculates that there is approximately a 41% chance that at least one out of five patients will have muscle aches. Regarding this last figure, what type of calculation is this?

(A) Attack rate

(B) Clinical probability

(C) Prevalence

(D) Sensitivity

(E) Specificity

50. A 58-year-old man with a history of Berger's disease who recently underwent renal transplantation following several years of glucocorticoid treatment and hemodialysis presents to the emergency department unable to walk properly. His mentation is normal, and he denies any chest pain or shortness of breath. During the interview, he says that he has recently been taking a pill for "a bug I had." On physical examination, the patient is unable to plantar flex his right foot, and there is a large soft muscular mass high on his right calf. Which of the following medications has this patient most likely been taking?

(A) Amoxicillin
(B) Ceftriaxone
(C) Ciprofloxacin
(D) Erythromycin
(E) Metronidazole
(F) Penicillin G
(G) Vancomycin

1. **The correct answer is D.** The man has Klinefelter's syndrome, a common cause of male infertility. His karyotype is 47,XXY, thus accounting for the additional X chromosome found on cytogenetic analysis. In Klinefelter's syndrome, the testicles are nonfunctional, and therefore testosterone levels are decreased, resulting in a secondary increase in gonadotropin levels (follicle-stimulating hormone and luteinizing hormone) due to lack of negative feedback.

Answer A is incorrect. Because of testicular dysfunction, follicle-stimulating hormone secondarily becomes increased, not decreased, in Klinefelter's syndrome.

Answer B is incorrect. Thyroid-stimulating hormone, a measure of thyroid function, has no clinical application in diagnosing Klinefelter's syndrome.

Answer C is incorrect. Increased ammonia can be seen in hepatic encephalopathy. Hepatic disease can also cause hypogonadism and gynecomastia due to decreased clearance of estrogens. Ammonia levels are normal in Klinefelter's syndrome.

Answer E is incorrect. Klinefelter's syndrome causes testicular atrophy. This results in decreased, not increased, testosterone.

2. **The correct answer is E.** The appointed durable power of attorney is truly durable. The patient, in good state of mind, believed that the friend would make decisions with which he agreed. It is always appropriate to facilitate a discussion between people involved in the decision, but it is unethical to sway the friend by making the choice for him or telling him to listen to the patient's son.

Answer A is incorrect. The friend should be advised to decide what he believed the patient would have wanted.

Answer B is incorrect. A patient's chosen power of attorney can only be changed by the patient. If a patient is noncommunicative, the power of attorney cannot be changed.

Answer C is incorrect. The durable power of attorney is the ultimate decision maker and their decision to withdraw life support will be upheld.

Answer D is incorrect. The durable power of attorney was appointed as such to make decisions in accordance with the patient's wishes and should act accordingly. Input from family members is important and may be appropriate but is not legally necessary or in accordance with the patient's wishes.

3. **The correct answer is E.** *Escherichia coli* O157:H7 is an enterohemorrhagic bacterium that can cause bloody diarrhea, abdominal pain, and fevers. Hemolytic-uremic syndrome is associated with infection with this organism. It is characterized by a low platelet count (thrombocytopenia), anemia, and renal failure, often manifested by uremia.

Answer A is incorrect. Rheumatic fever is characterized by fever, migratory polyarthritis, and carditis. It may follow group A streptococcal pharyngitis.

Answer B is incorrect. Fever, a new murmur, Janeway lesions, and nail-bed hemorrhages are all signs of bacterial endocarditis. Acute endocarditis is caused by *Staphylococcus aureus*; subacute infection can be caused by viridans streptococci.

Answer C is incorrect. Waterhouse-Friderichsen syndrome is characterized by high fever, shock, purpura, and adrenal insufficiency classically associated with meningococcemia, although virtually any bacterial cause of septic shock can trigger the same findings.

Answer D is incorrect. Guillain-Barré syndrome is characterized by rapidly progressing ascending paralysis. It is thought to follow a variety of infectious diseases, such as cytomegalovirus, Epstein-Barr virus, HIV, and gastroenteritis caused by *Campylobacter jejuni*.

4. The correct answer is E. The HMG-CoA reductase inhibitors can cause an elevation of the transaminases, AST and ALT. Levels of these enzymes should be monitored following commencement of any statin. If the levels of AST and ALT increase, the drug should be discontinued.

Answer A is incorrect. Aspirin is associated with renal toxicity and gastrointestinal bleeds.

Answer B is incorrect. Clopidogrel is used to reduce the incidence of stent restenosis. It is associated with an increased risk of bleeding.

Answer C is incorrect. Lisinopril is an angiotensin-converting enzyme inhibitor and is associated with angioedema, cough, and hyperkalemia.

Answer D is incorrect. Metoprolol is a β-blocker that is important in the treatment of myocardial infarction but is not associated with elevation of hepatic enzymes. Its adverse effects include impotence, depression, bradycardia, and sedation.

5. The correct answer is C. A Bell's palsy is a lesion of cranial nerve VII (facial nerve) and affects the muscles of facial expression. These muscles are derived from the second branchial (pharyngeal) arch. Patients with sarcoidosis, tumors, diabetes, AIDS, and Lyme disease are at increased risk for Bell's palsy, although most cases are idiopathic. Important signs of Bell's palsy are ptosis and facial droop. The second arch also gives rise to the posterior belly of the digastric, the stylohyoid, and the stapedius muscles.

Answer A is incorrect. The first branchial arch gives rise to the muscles of mastication, the mylohyoid, the anterior belly of the digastric, the tensor veli palatini, and the tensor tympani. These muscles are innervated by cranial nerve V and are not affected by Bell's palsy.

Answer B is incorrect. The fourth branchial pouch gives rise to the superior parathyroid glands. It is implicated in DiGeorge's syndrome but is not related to Bell's palsy.

Answer D is incorrect. The third branchial pouch gives rise to the inferior parathyroid glands and the thymus. It is implicated in DiGeorge's syndrome but has no relation to Bell's palsy.

Answer E is incorrect. The thyroglossal duct connects the thyroid diverticulum to the foregut in the embryo but is obliterated during development. Its only remnant in the adult is the foramen cecum.

6. The correct answer is D. This question tests the concept of mass effect of tumors, as well as anatomy. These two topics are inseparable and are necessary to understanding the etiology of some symptoms seen in the context of neoplasms. The adenocarcinoma impinges on the omental foramen, which is formed partly by the hepatoduodenal ligament. This ligament contains the common bile duct along with the hepatic artery proper and the hepatic portal vein. Obstruction of the common bile duct would lead to cholestasis and subsequently conjugated hyperbilirubinemia.

Answer A is incorrect. Anemia may be a sign of gastrointestinal bleeding (seen with stomach or colonic cancers) or that bone marrow is dysfunctional and/or being replaced with malignant cells. Although anemia may be seen in this patient due to bleeding into the stomach, anemia is not a direct result of mass effect of the tumor.

Answer B is incorrect. Constipation may be a symptom of obstruction of the left colon.

Answer C is incorrect. Persistent hoarseness could be a manifestation of impingement of the recurrent laryngeal nerve. This symptom may be seen with thyroid or lung cancer.

Answer E is incorrect. Seizures may be a symptom of a tumor mass in the brain.

7. The correct answer is A. The lactose operon is an example of an inducible operon. Levels of glucose and lactose regulate gene transcription. In cells that do not have a supply of lactose, the operon is turned off by a repressor protein that binds to the operator and blocks

RNA polymerase. In the presence of lactose, the operon is on because lactose acts as an inducer. Lactose binds the repressor molecule and changes its shape so that it can no longer bind to the operator. When the cells are growing in the absence of glucose, transcription occurs. As glucose levels decrease, cyclic adenosine monophosphate (cAMP) levels rise and bind to the cAMP receptor protein (CRP). The CRP-cAMP complex binds to the operon and promotes the binding of RNA polymerase to the promoter. When the cells are exposed to glucose, transcription does not occur. Glucose decreases levels of cAMP so that there are less CRP-cAMP complexes. In this case, glucose fails to suppress transcription of the lactose operon. Therefore, the mutation is most likely located in the CRP.

Answer B is incorrect. Allolactose is the inducer of the lactose operon. Allolactose binds tightly to the repressor so that the repressor can no longer bind to the operator and block the RNA polymerase. If the inducer-binding site were mutated, the lactose operon would not be expressed in the presence of lactose.

Answer C is incorrect. A mutation in the promoter of the lactose operon is not consistent with the above observation. If the promoter were mutated, the ability of RNA polymerase to bind to it would be altered regardless of the presence of glucose or lactose.

Answer D is incorrect. In the absence of lactose, the lactose operon repressor binds to the operator and halts transcription. In this case, it is unlikely that the mutation is located in the repressor.

Answer E is incorrect. If RNA polymerase were mutated in these bacterial cells, all gene expression would be affected.

8. **The correct answer is A.** The patient described has many of the classic hallmarks of DiGeorge's syndrome, or thymic aplasia. Due to a 22q11 deletion that causes maldevelopment of the third and fourth pharyngeal pouches, this disease is marked by T-lymphocyte deficiency secondary to thymic aplasia.

Failure of parathyroid development creates a setting of hypocalcemia that leads to tetany. The periarterial lymphoid sheath (PALS) is a sheet of lymphoid tissue that surrounds the central arteries in the spleen. The PALS and the splenic red pulp contain T lymphocytes and would have different appearances in the setting of T-lymphocyte deficiency. This location of T lymphocytes allows pathogens in the blood to come in close contact with lymphoid cells for antigen recognition.

Answer B is incorrect. The splenic artery is the only artery supplying oxygen-rich blood to the spleen. This blood is important for carrying antigens to the lymphoid cells within the spleen. The splenic artery is not affected by DiGeorge's syndrome.

Answer C is incorrect. The splenic capsule is a layer of connective tissue that covers and holds the splenic tissue together. It is covered by a thin layer of mesothelium that is a covering of the visceral peritoneum over the spleen. It is not affected by DiGeorge's syndrome.

Answer D is incorrect. The splenic vein is the only vein that drains the spleen and it empties into the hepatic portal vessels. The splenic vein is not affected by DiGeorge's syndrome.

Answer E is incorrect. The splenic white pulp contains follicles of B lymphocytes. B lymphocytes are deficient in Bruton's agammaglobulinemia and selective immunoglobulin deficiencies, not in DiGeorge's syndrome.

9. **The correct answer is A.** This adverse effect, known as serum sickness, is mediated by immune complex formation and deposition (in the skin, they cause a rash; in the kidney, they cause glomerulonephritis). The patient mounts a humoral immune response against the foreign protein or drug, thus forming antibodies that bind with high avidity to the foreign protein. The induction of an affinity-matured antibody response usually takes 7–10 days and requires T-cell help.

Answer B is incorrect. This is not usually true. It takes about 1 week to mount a mature antibody response.

Answer C is incorrect. Symptoms are likely to occur after the body has had a chance to mount a humoral-mediated response. While symptoms may worsen if an infection worsens, this does not explain why there would be fevers, rash, arthritis, and glomerulonephritis 7–10 days after administration of a certain drug.

Answer D is incorrect. Since it takes time for the antibody-mediated response to be mounted, symptoms do not typically occur until this time.

Answer E is incorrect. While T-cell help is needed to make the pathogenic antibodies and thus immune complexes, this is a type III hypersensitivity reaction, which is mediated by antibodies, not T cells.

10. **The correct answer is D.** *BRCA1* and *BRCA2* are tumor suppressor genes. In order for tumors to develop from this type of gene, both alleles must be lost (complete loss of function).

Answer A is incorrect. Dominant-negative effects occur when the loss of one allele leads to disease because the body cannot produce enough of the necessary protein product from just one functioning allele. An example of this is osteogenesis imperfecta, caused by mutations in the *COL1A1* gene.

Answer B is incorrect. Oncogenes leading to tumorigenesis are gain-of-function mutations. Proto-oncogenes are mutated to cause an increased expression of the gene product or improper regulation, leading to uninhibited cellular proliferation. An example of this is the *c-myc* gene.

Answer C is incorrect. Genetic imprinting occurs when a different phenotype is present, depending on whether the mutation comes from the maternal or the paternal side. An example of this is the correlation of Angelman syndrome (maternal chromosome 15 mutation) and Prader-Willi syndrome (paternal chromosome 15 mutation).

Answer E is incorrect. Oncogenic viruses cause tumor formation through their insertion into the human genome within a cell. The viral DNA then allows unregulated cell growth and tumor production. An example of this occurs in Epstein-Barr virus.

11. **The correct answer is A.** Vitamin K–dependent gamma-glutamyl carboxylase converts glutamic acid residues to gamma-carboxyglutamic acid (GLA) residues. GLA residues are formed in clotting factors II, VII, IX, and X, as well as protein C and S. They function to bind the calcium which is required to activate the factors. Vitamin K deficiency is rare because it is synthesized by gut flora. This patient's deficiency is probably secondary to oral antibiotic use that destroyed those organisms. Deficiency is also seen in neonates who have sterile guts and a relatively new liver. Easy bruisability, melena, hematuria, and splinter hemorrhages can all be seen with vitamin K deficiency. Warfarin is a vitamin K analog used as an anticoagulant and is reversed with vitamin K.

Answer B is incorrect. This is the function of potassium, abbreviated as K, which has nothing to do with vitamin K.

Answer C is incorrect. The hydroxylation of proline and lysine residues requires the coenzyme ascorbic acid, or vitamin C. Deficiency results in a defective connective tissue syndrome called scurvy. Vitamin C has not been shown to cure the common cold or prevent coronary heart disease.

Answer D is incorrect. The antibiotics have resulted in a decrease in gut flora and subsequent synthesis of vitamin K. The intestinal flora themselves have no effect on blood clotting.

Answer E is incorrect. The antibiotics have resulted in a decrease in gut flora and subsequent synthesis of vitamin K. Metabolism of antibiotics does not generate significant antithrombic intermediates.

12. **The correct answer is C.** This child has the symptoms of asthma. Leukotriene (LT)C_4, LTD_4, and LTE_4 are bronchoconstrictors and are believed to contribute to symptoms of asthma. 5-Lipoxygenase is the enzyme that converts arachidonic acid to 5-hydroperoxy-

eicosatetraenoic acid, which is then used to produce leukotrienes.

Answer A is incorrect. Cyclooxygenase (COX) is the enzyme that catalyzes the formation of prostaglandins, thromboxanes, and prostacyclins. Nonsteroidal anti-inflammatory drugs, COX-2 inhibitors, and aspirin exert their effects by inhibiting the cyclooxygenase pathway.

Answer B is incorrect. Leukotriene B_4 is a neutrophil chemotactic agent. It is produced via the 5-lipoxygenase pathway; however, it does not cause bronchospasm.

Answer D is incorrect. Prostaglandin I_2 (PGI_2) inhibits platelet aggregation and vasoconstriction. PGI_2 is a product of the cyclooxygenase pathway.

Answer E is incorrect. Thromboxane A_2 stimulates platelet aggregation and vasoconstriction. It is a product of the cyclooxygenase pathway.

13. **The correct answer is D.** This patient has *Echinococcus granulosus*, presenting with a classic hydatid cyst lesion of the liver. Hydatid cysts contain larvae of the tapeworm *E. granulosus*, whose eggs are carried from the intestinal tract to the liver via the portal circulation. *Echinococcus* is a dog tapeworm that incidentally infects humans and causes walled-off granulomatous lesions that result in anaphylactoid reactions when they erupt. Treatment is surgical excision.

Answer A is incorrect. Aerobic gram-negative bacteria such as *Pseudomonas* species do not cause mass lesions.

Answer B is incorrect. Nonmotile gram-negative bacteria such as *Shigella* species do not cause mass lesions.

Answer C is incorrect. Although pear-shaped protozoans such as *Entamoeba histolytica* can cause hepatic abscesses, a patient with *E. histolytica* infection would present more acutely with a 1- to 2-week history of fever and abdominal pain. Less than one-third of patients infected with a liver abscess have concurrent diarrhea.

Answer E is incorrect. Trophozoites such as *Trichomonas* species present with dysuria and genital discharge.

14. **The correct answer is A.** The organ shown in the image is the pancreas. The pancreas is divided into lobules that contain acini, or clusters of exocrine cells. Within the lobules are islets of Langerhans, which contain the endocrine tissue of the pancreas. Pancreatic secretions are stimulated by the parasympathetic nervous system (PNS). The major neurotransmitter of the PNS is acetylcholine. Thus, increased levels of acetylcholine would lead to increased activity of the PNS and increased pancreatic secretions.

Answer B is incorrect. GABA is a major inhibitory neurotransmitter commonly found in the brain. It does not cause hypersecretion of the pancreas.

Answer C is incorrect. Glycine is an inhibitory neurotransmitter released by spinal interneurons. It does not cause hypersecretion of the pancreas.

Answer D is incorrect. Norepinephrine is the primary neurotransmitter for postganglionic sympathetic neurons. It does not cause hypersecretion of the pancreas.

Answer E is incorrect. Serotonin is a neurotransmitter in nuclei in the brainstem. It does not cause hypersecretion of the pancreas.

15. **The correct answer is D.** This patient has suffered a rupture of a saccular aneurysm. Although the etiology of these aneurysms is mostly unknown, an increased occurrence is found in patients with certain heritable conditions, such as polycystic kidney disease, connective tissue disorders, and coarctation of the aorta. Rupture of these aneurysms is associated with clinically significant subarachnoid hemorrhage that most often occurs in the fifth decade and involves the onset of severe headache followed by rapid deterioration in

mentation. Because the patient has renal insufficiency, "large kidneys," and a positive family history, polycystic kidney disease, which is associated with intracranial aneurysms, is the most probable etiology. The patient's severe headache and the nausea/vomiting with signs of nuchal rigidity and deteriorating level of consciousness are consistent with this diagnosis.

Answer A is incorrect. Disruption of the middle meningeal artery would result in an epidural hematoma, which is almost always the result of a traumatic event. It is frequently associated with skull fractures.

Answer B is incorrect. Disruption of the sigmoid sinus would result in a subarachnoid hemorrhage and would almost certainly be the result of a traumatic event, as is the case with epidural hematoma. The extremely rapid progression of symptoms is also uncharacteristic of venous bleeding that would result from injury to bridging veins.

Answer C is incorrect. Hypertensive cerebrovascular disease can result in massive hemorrhages, lacunar infarcts, and slit hemorrhages as well as hypertensive encephalopathy. However, in the absence of a history of hypertension, atherosclerotic disease, or diabetes, this is a less likely cause, especially given the patient's history of polycystic kidney disease.

Answer E is incorrect. Thromboembolization of the middle cerebral artery would result in a stroke syndrome with associated hemiplegia (affecting the arm and face more often than the leg), hemianesthesia, and possibly drowsiness or stupor. However, it would not result in a rapidly progressive decrease in mentation and death.

16. **The correct answer is D.** A diagnosis of lead poisoning should be considered in young patients living in an environment with high lead levels (such as old houses with lead paint) and with a history of pica (eating non-nutritive substances). These patients present with the findings described in this case, including irritability, anorexia, ataxia, and regression of speech.

These findings are due to acute encephalopathy secondary to lead poisoning as well as a microcytic anemia from inhibition of the heme synthetic pathway by lead. Treatment should include ethylenediamine tetraacetic acid or, for more severe cases, dimercaprol.

Answer A is incorrect. Acetaminophen toxicity can be a "time bomb" because patients may initially be asymptomatic. In the first 24 hours, nausea, vomiting, and malaise are common. At 24–48 hours, the patient's symptoms subside with possible right upper quadrant pain. At day 3–4, there is onset of jaundice and hepatic failure. N-acetylcysteine (Mucomyst) should be given within 8 hours of ingestion but is useful as late as 36 hours after ingestion.

Answer B is incorrect. Aspirin (salicylic acid) toxicity is associated with tinnitus, abdominal pain, vomiting, and tachypnea at low doses. At higher doses, respiratory alkalosis, metabolic acidosis, hypotension, coma, and death can occur. Urine can be alkalinized with sodium bicarbonate infusion to promote excretion of salicylate. Salicylate toxicity can be confused with diabetic ketoacidosis.

Answer C is incorrect. Button battery ingestion is a concern only if the battery becomes lodged in the esophagus, because leakage of alkali can lead to perforation. If the battery is past the esophagus, the child can be sent home and the parents can be instructed to screen for the battery in the patient's stool.

Answer E is incorrect. Organophosphate toxicity found in insecticides and carbamates can be absorbed through the skin. Symptoms include excess cholinergic activity (due to block of anticholinesterase by the organophosphate) leading to miosis, salivation, lacrimation, diarrhea, urination, and sweating. Treatment includes atropine and pralidoxime.

Answer F is incorrect. Tricyclic antidepressant overdose can result in anticholinergic symptoms such as hallucinations, dry mouth, flushing, urinary retention, and mydriasis ("mad as a hatter, dry as a bone, red as a beet"). However, the most severe complication of tricyclic antidepressant overdose is tachyarrhythmias, which can result in death.

17. **The correct answer is C.** The cerebrospinal fluid findings described in the question point toward a bacterial cause of the infant's meningitis. In infants between the ages of 0 and 3 months, the most common organisms causing meningitis are *Listeria monocytogenes*, *Escherichia coli*, and group B streptococcus. *Listeria monocytogenes* is the only gram-positive rod in the group.

Answer A is incorrect. *Escherichia coli* can cause bacterial meningitis in infants, but a Gram's stain of cerebrospinal fluid would show gram-negative rods.

Answer B is incorrect. Herpes simplex virus has also been shown to cause meningitis in infants. In viral meningitis, the cerebrospinal fluid findings would show far fewer leukocytes (11–500/mm^3), protein levels between 50 and 200 mg/dL, and normal glucose levels; a Gram's stain would not show any organisms.

Answer D is incorrect. *Neisseria meningitides* also causes bacterial meningitis but is commonly seen in older children.

Answer E is incorrect. *Streptococcus agalactiae* can cause bacterial meningitis in infants, but a Gram's stain of cerebrospinal fluid would show gram-positive cocci.

18. **The correct answer is E.** CGD is a disorder in which neutrophils are unable to completely eradicate certain phagocytosed bacteria and fungi. As a result, the chronic immune response to these lingering pathogens leads to the development of self-tissue damage. This answer provides a logical link between a correct description of chronic granulomatous disease (a disorder of neutrophil production of nicotinamide adenine dinucleotide phosphatase oxidase, which results in neutrophils that are unable to completely eradicate certain phagocytosed bacteria and fungi) and the development of autoimmune disease. This answer points to theories questioning why 50% of patients with chronic granulomatous disease

suffer a chronic gut inflammation that is similar to Crohn's disease.

Answer A is incorrect. Common variable immunodeficiency, the most common symptomatic primary antibody deficiency syndrome, is a disorder characterized by differing degrees of deficiency of antibody production, leading to recurrent sinopulmonary and gastrointestinal infections.

Answer B is incorrect. This choice is not the correct immunologic deficiency of CGD. The disorder characterized by a deficiency of IgA antibodies is called IgA deficiency, the most common primary immunodeficiency disease in the Western hemisphere.

Answer C is incorrect. Wiskott-Aldrich syndrome is an X-linked disorder that results in the body being unable to mount an IgM response to capsular polysaccharides or bacteria. It is associated with low levels of IgM, high levels of IgA, and normal levels of IgE.

Answer D is incorrect. Chédiak-Higashi syndrome is an autosomal recessive disease affecting a lysosomal trafficking regulator gene; it leads to defective microtubular function and lysosomal emptying of phagocytic cells. This disease is characterized by a partial oculocutaneous albinism, abnormally large granules found in many different cell types, and recurrent pyogenic staphylococcal and/or streptococcal infections.

19. **The correct answer is E.** The patient is most likely suffering from Sheehan's syndrome, a state of postpartum panhypopituitarism that can develop after severe uterine hemorrhage during or after childbirth. A lack of bloody supply to the enlarged pituitary leads to ischemic necrosis and destruction of hormone-producing tissue of the pituitary gland. Thus, patients with Sheehan's syndrome frequently have decreased levels of all hormones made in the anterior lobe of the pituitary gland, including a decreased prolactin level, which makes them incapable of breast-feeding after delivery.

Answer A is incorrect. Elevated cortisol, prolactin, and thyroid stimulating hormone would result in significantly different symptoms from those described in the patient above. Such a patient might have a hypothalamic hypersecretory lesion which would not be accompanied by the symptoms of lethargy, low blood pressure, and hyponatremia.

Answer B is incorrect. No change in cortisol; changes in prolactin and thyroid-stimulating hormone levels would not be expected in this patient.

Answer C is incorrect. An isolated increase in prolactin levels suggests a prolactinoma, which was not seen on CT scan, or treatment with a drug that decreases dopamine levels, such as chlorpromazine. An isolated increase in prolactin would not be expected to cause hypotension and hyponatremia.

Answer D is incorrect. An isolated decrease in prolactin levels would also not be expected to cause hypotension and hyponatremia.

20. **The correct answer is C.** Incomplete penetrance indicates that not all individuals with a mutant genotype exhibit the mutant phenotype. Treacher Collins syndrome is an example of a disease with incomplete penetrance.

Answer A is incorrect. Anticipation is the term used when a disease worsens or the age of onset of the disease is earlier in successive generations. Huntington's disease and fragile X syndrome (both of which involve trinucleotide repeats) show anticipation.

Answer B is incorrect. Dominant-negative mutation is a mutation in which the mutant product interferes with the function of the normal gene product, leading to pathology.

Answer D is incorrect. Mosaicism occurs when cells in the body have a different genetic makeup. Patients with Turner's syndrome can have a mosaic genotype, with some cells having 45,XO and some having 46,XX.

Answer E is incorrect. *Pleiotropy* is a term used when one gene has more than one effect on a person's phenotype.

21. **The correct answer is A.** Since sickle cell disease leads to autosplenectomy, a condition in which fibrosis results from repeated infarcts of the spleen due to adherence of sickled red blood cells. The spleen is unable to perform its normal functions, such as sequestering capsulated organisms. Since the spleen is the major defender against these organisms, patients without splenic function are susceptible to infection by encapsulated organisms such as *Staphylococcus aureus* and *Salmonella typhi*. The symptoms suggest that the boy has osteomyelitis of the tibia, and the most important determinant of virulence in sickle cell patients with osteomyelitis is the presence of a capsule. *S. aureus* is the most common cause of osteomyelitis in all groups, but *Salmonella* osteomyelitis has a particular association with sickle cell disease, and it is this association that is often tested on the USMLE Step 1 examination.

Answer B is incorrect. The flagellum of *Salmonella* is indeed a virulence factor that acts as an antigen that can be varied (antigenic variation or switching). However, it is not the presence of the flagellum that makes *Salmonella* more pathogenic in sickle cell patients.

Answer C is incorrect. *Mycoplasma* species are bacteria that lack a cell wall and that most often cause pneumonia (*M. pneumoniae*) or nongonococcal urethritis (also *Ureaplasma urealyticum*).

Answer D is incorrect. Mycolic acids are found in the outer cell membrane of mycobacteria. Mycobacteria can cause osteomyelitis, but autosplenectomy does not particularly put sickle cell patients at a higher risk.

Answer E is incorrect. Pili are structures on some bacteria that aid in adhesion to host cells.

22. **The correct answer is B.** Folic acid is a coenzyme for one-carbon transfer. It is involved in methylation reactions. A deficiency causes a macrocytic, megaloblastic anemia without neurologic symptoms. Folate is found in green

leafy vegetables and is not stored very long in the body. Therefore, nutrient deficiency can commonly lead to folate deficiency.

Answer A is incorrect. Vitamin K catalyzes γ-carboxylation of glutamic acid residues on various proteins involved in blood clotting. A deficiency would cause hemorrhage (particularly in neonates) with an elevated prothrombin time and activated partial thromboplastin time but a normal bleeding time.

Answer C is incorrect. Ascorbic acid (vitamin C) is a cofactor for the conversion of dopamine to norepinephrine. A deficiency causes scurvy, which is characterized by swollen gums, bruising, anemia, and poor wound healing.

Answer D is incorrect. Vitamin A (retinol) is a constituent of visual pigments. A deficiency causes night blindness and dry skin.

Answer E is incorrect. Vitamin D increases intestinal calcium and phosphate absorption. A deficiency causes rickets in children and osteomalacia in adults, along with hypocalcemic tetany.

23. **The correct answer is D.** Chlorpromazine is an antipsychotic used in the treatment of schizophrenia and psychosis. Chlorpromazine blocks dopamine D_2 receptors and thus blocks the effects of excess dopamine associated with schizophrenia. Because dopamine inhibits the secretion of prolactin, a dopamine antagonist such as chlorpromazine can cause hyperprolactinemia by decreasing the inhibitory effects of dopamine.

Answer A is incorrect. Amantadine is used for influenza A prophylaxis, and because it causes release of dopamine from intact nerve terminals, it is also used in the treatment of Parkinson's disease.

Answer B is incorrect. Bromocriptine is a dopamine agonist that decreases, rather than increases, prolactin levels and is actually used for the treatment of hyperprolactinemia.

Answer C is incorrect. Cabergoline, like bromocriptine, is a dopamine agonist that decreases prolactin levels.

Answer E is incorrect. Lithium is a first-line treatment for bipolar disorder. Its adverse effects include tremor, hypothyroidism, and nephrogenic diabetes insipidus. It is not used in the treatment of schizophrenia, nor does it cause elevated prolactin levels.

24. **The correct answer is E.** This patient has testicular feminization syndrome (androgen insensitivity), which is due to unresponsiveness on the part of the testosterone receptor protein to androgenic stimulation.

Answer A is incorrect. Fragile X syndrome, which is associated with congenital mental retardation, large ears, and macro-orchidism, is due to a CGG triplet repeat disorder.

Answer B is incorrect. A deficiency of 5-α-reductase presents with ambiguous genitalia until puberty, when there is masculinization of the genitalia. Testosterone and estrogen levels are normal.

Answer C is incorrect. Duchenne's muscular dystrophy, a disorder of skeletal muscle, is due to the deletion of the dystrophin gene.

Answer D is incorrect. Excessive exposure to androgenic steroids during early gestation leads to female pseudohermaphroditism (XX), a condition in which ovaries are present but the external genitalia are virilized.

25. **The correct answer is C.** Bile is produced in liver hepatocytes. Primary bile acids are synthesized by hepatocytes. They are then conjugated with taurine or glycine to form bile salts. In the gallbladder, bile is concentrated as solutes and water is reabsorbed.

Answer A is incorrect. Bacteria in the colon deconjugate and dehydroxylate bile acids.

Answer B is incorrect. The brush border of the terminal ileum is the site of uptake for conjugated and unconjugated bile acids. Bacteria in the terminal ileum also function to deconjugate and dehydroxylate bile acids.

Answer D is incorrect. Kupffer cells line the liver and remove waste from the blood.

Answer E is incorrect. The space of Disse in the liver is responsible for lymphatic drainage.

26. **The correct answer is E.** The image shows a bicornuate uterus in which the uterus has two horns entering a common vagina. The embryologic cause of this is incomplete fusion of the paramesonephric (müllerian) ducts. Normally, in the absence of müllerian-inhibiting substance, the paramesonephric (müllerian) ducts develop into the uterine tubes and fuse caudally to form a single uterus, cervix, and superior third of the vagina. A bicornuate uterus is associated with infertility and urinary tract abnormalities.

Answer A is incorrect. Complete lack of fusion of the paramesonephric (müllerian) ducts leads to a double uterus with a double vagina. However, in this patient and in the autopsy specimen, there is a common vagina due to partial fusion of the paramesonephric (müllerian) ducts.

Answer B is incorrect. In the male, the mesonephric (wolffian) duct develops into the seminal vesicles, epididymis, ejaculatory duct, and ductus deferens. In the female, the mesonephric (wolffian) duct is not stimulated to develop and it forms only vestigial structures (the appendix vesiculosa and the duct of Gartner), but the mesonephric (wolffian) duct is not resorbed.

Answer C is incorrect. If the vaginal plates fail to canalize, atresia of the vagina results. This leads to blockage of the vaginal lumen. The vaginal plates play no role in the development of the uterus, normal or bicornuate.

Answer D is incorrect. The mesonephric (wolffian) ducts play no role in the development of female reproductive organs and thus are unrelated to a bicornuate uterus. Normally, in the presence of müllerian-inhibiting substance and testosterone in the male, these ducts develop into the **S**eminal vesicles: **E**pididymis, **E**jaculatory duct, and **D**uctus deferens (remember the mnemonic **SEED**).

27. **The correct answer is A.** Adenovirus is a major cause of epidemic keratoconjunctivitis (pink eye). It is the fourth most common cause of childhood respiratory tract infections, after respiratory syncytial virus, parainfluenza, and rhinovirus. It is a naked, icosahedral, double-stranded linear DNA that results in a self-limited illness that requires no treatment.

Answer B is incorrect. Coxsackie A virus causes cold symptoms and rashes. It is also the causative agent of herpangina and hand, foot, and mouth disease.

Answer C is incorrect. Cytomegalovirus can reactivate and cause a variety of illnesses in the immunocompromised but is usually asymptomatic in healthy individuals.

Answer D is incorrect. Herpes simplex virus type 1 causes gingivostomatitis, herpetic keratitis of the eye, and encephalitis.

Answer E is incorrect. Rotavirus is the most common cause of diarrhea in infants < 3 years old.

28. **The correct answer is C.** This patient is presenting with signs suggestive of rheumatoid arthritis. Methotrexate, a folic acid analog antimetabolite that inhibits dihydrofolate reductase, is often used as treatment due to reduction of adenosine-mediated inflammatory changes. Other nononcologic uses of methotrexate include abortion, rheumatoid arthritis, psoriasis, and treatment of choriocarcinoma.

Answer A is incorrect. Ceftriaxone is a third-generation cephalosporin antibiotic that inhibits bacterial transpeptidase and cell wall synthesis. It is most commonly used to treat serious gram-negative infections, including meningitis and gonorrhea. Although gonorrhea can present with unilateral arthritis of the knee, this patient's clinical presentation is more consistent with rheumatoid arthritis. Ceftriaxone would therefore not be an effective treatment for this patient. Notably, tetracyclines **can** be used to inhibit the activity of metalloproteinases involved in joint destruction by the rheumatoid synovium, and are therefore effective agents in patients with early rheumatoid arthritis.

Answer B is incorrect. Cyclophosphamide is an alkylating agent that is useful in the treatment of non-Hodgkin's lymphoma and breast and ovarian carcinomas. It is also used as an immunosuppressant in systemic lupus erythematosus, multiple sclerosis, and autoimmune hemolytic anemia. It is not generally used as a treatment for rheumatoid arthritis.

Answer D is incorrect. Probenecid is an organic acid that is used most commonly for the treatment of chronic tophaceous gout or increasingly frequent gouty attacks. The drug acts at the anionic transport sites in the renal tubule to inhibit the reabsorption of uric acid, promoting its secretion. Gout normally presents with intermittent acute inflammatory arthritis, most often at only one site. In more chronic disease, more joints become involved and the intervals between attacks become shorter. Advanced gout results in chronic arthropathy, characterized by persistent asymmetric and asynchronous joint inflammation accompanied by uric acid deposits known as tophi, and can occasionally resemble rheumatoid arthritis. Nevertheless, the progressive and steady nature of this patient's disease strongly suggests a diagnosis of rheumatoid arthritis rather than gout. Probenecid would therefore be an ineffective pharmacologic therapy.

Answer E is incorrect. Tamoxifen is an estrogen receptor mixed agonist-antagonist that is most useful against estrogen-sensitive breast cancers.

29. **The correct answer is B.** Untreated hypothyroidism in the elderly, although uncommon, is a treatable cause of dementia. The workup for a patient with dementia includes a complete blood count, liver function tests, thyroid function tests, renal function tests, electrolytes, glucose, vitamin B_{12}, folate, rapid plasma reagin, HIV testing, and urinalysis along with an ECG, a CT/MRI, and/or an EEG if clinically indicated. Most of the time the diagnosis can be made by history alone, but it is important to rule out treatable causes of dementia. It is also important to talk with family members and friends because patients may not relate an accurate history.

Answer A is incorrect. Alzheimer's disease is not reversible. Its course can be temporarily slowed by cholinergic therapies such as donepezil, galantamine, and rivastigmine, but dementia and finally death are inevitable.

Answer C is incorrect. Multi-infarct dementia is irreversible. By the time a patient has had enough ministrokes to present clinically, the brain tissue is permanently damaged. Progression of the dementia can be slowed or even halted by antiatherogenic therapies such 3-hydroxy-3-methylglutaryl coenzyme A reductase inhibitors and antiplatelet agents, but a full recovery is not possible.

Answer D is incorrect. Normal aging is not a cause of dementia. The mild memory changes associated with aging are irreversible but do not qualify for a diagnosis of dementia.

Answer E is incorrect. Pick's disease is a non-reversible dementia that primarily affects the frontal cortex. It tends to occur in a younger age group than Alzheimer's disease, with most patients presenting before age 70. Generally, the first symptoms are personality changes, but in the end this disease is indistinguishable from Alzheimer's disease. Therapies for Alzheimer's disease are also used for the treatment of Pick's disease.

30. **The correct answer is B.** Furosemide is known as a loop diuretic that acts on the Na^+-K^+-$2Cl^-$ cotransporter on the thick ascending loop of Henle. It acts on the same cotransporter that is defective in Bartter's syndrome.

Answer A is incorrect. Acetazolamide acts at the proximal convoluted tubule, inhibiting carbonic anhydrase. It causes a reduction in total body HCO_3^-.

Answer C is incorrect. Hydrochlorothiazide is a thiazide diuretic that acts early in the distal tubule.

Answer D is incorrect. Spironolactone is a potassium-sparing diuretic that acts as a competitive aldosterone receptor antagonist in the cortical collecting tubule.

Answer E is incorrect. Triamterene is a potassium-sparing diuretic that blocks Na^+ channels in the cortical collecting tubule.

31. **The correct answer is D.** The child has a patent ductus arteriosus (PDA), identified in this question by its role in fetal circulation. This causes exercise intolerance, a wide pulse pressure, and a continuous "machinelike" murmur. Indomethacin may be used to close it in the neonate, but older children will require surgery or catheter placement. An important risk factor for a PDA is congenital rubella. Rubella is a mild, self-limited illness in adults but is one of the ToRCHeS organisms that can cross the placenta and cause congenital disease. There is no specific treatment for rubella, but a vaccine exists that can prevent maternal infection and thus significantly reduce the risk of a congenital PDA induced by rubella. Proper prenatal care includes screening for rubella antibodies and providing vaccination if the mother has not previously been exposed.

Answer A is incorrect. Amantadine is effective in the treatment and prevention of influenza A. It is commonly used in nursing home settings as prophylaxis during flu outbreaks. Influenza does not cross the placenta and is thus not a risk factor for a patent ductus arteriosus.

Answer B is incorrect. Ganciclovir is active against all herpesviruses, although its toxicity is much greater than that of acyclovir. Its use is therefore reserved for cytomegalovirus (CMV) infections in the immunocompromised, as CMV is not susceptible to acyclovir. CMV is one of the ToRCHeS organisms, but it typically causes mental retardation, microcephaly, and deafness; CMV does not commonly cause a patent ductus arteriosus.

Answer C is incorrect. While a vaccine does exist to prevent infection by *Bordetella pertussis*, this is not one of the organisms known to cause congenital disease and is not a risk factor for a patent ductus arteriosus. Infection causes whooping cough in the adult.

Answer E is incorrect. Spectinomycin effectively kills strains of *Neisseria gonorrhoeae* that are resistant to penicillin and tetracycline. Gonorrhea is an important cause of pelvic inflammatory disease, infertility, and ectopic pregnancies but does not cross the placenta and is not associated with a patent ductus arteriosus.

32. **The correct answer is A.** Menopause is the cessation of estrogen production due to a decreased number of available ovarian follicles. The average age of menopause onset is 51 years, with a normal range between 45–55 years. Remember, menopause causes **HAVOC**: **H**ot flashes, **A**trophy of the **V**agina, **O**steoporosis, and **C**oronary artery disease (CAD). Estrogen is necessary for the maintenance and development of the vagina and bone deposition, so a decrease leads to vaginal atrophy and osteoporosis. There is no direct link between estrogen and heart disease, but the incidence of CAD following menopause is two to three times higher than in premenopausal women, suggesting some protective effect of endogenous estrogen. Hot flashes are thought to be related to changes in the ability of the hypothalamus to recognize body temperature. As estrogen replacement therapy alleviates these symptoms, there may be a role for estrogen in body temperature regulation. Therefore, a decreased estrogen level will cause decreased maintenance of body organs and structures.

Answer B is incorrect. Menopause symptoms are not the result of decreased feedback at the level of the pituitary.

Answer C is incorrect. Menopause symptoms are not the result of inhibition by estrogen.

Answer D is incorrect. Decreased estrogen levels do not cause increased progesterone levels.

Answer E is incorrect. Decreased estrogen levels do not cause increased testosterone levels.

33. **The correct answer is B.** This patient has multiple endocrine neoplasia (MEN) type 2A, a condition characterized by tumors of the parathyroid gland, medullary carcinoma of the

thyroid, and tumors of the adrenal medulla. All MEN syndromes follow an autosomal dominant mode of inheritance with incomplete penetrance. Medullary carcinoma of the thyroid is a calcitonin-secreting tumor of parafollicular thyroid cells. Microscopically, the tumor consists of nests of tumor cells in an amyloid-filled stroma.

Answer A is incorrect. Atrophic follicles with prominent germinal center formation and lymphocyte infiltrate are characteristic of Hashimoto's thyroiditis.

Answer C is incorrect. A papillary branching pattern of epithelial cells with ground-glass nuclei and psammoma bodies (laminated concentric calcified spherules) is seen in papillary carcinoma of the thyroid, the most common form of thyroid cancer and the one with the best prognosis.

Answer D is incorrect. Sheets of undifferentiated pleomorphic cells are seen in anaplastic, or undifferentiated, thyroid cancer. This form of thyroid cancer is more common in older patients and has a very poor prognosis.

Answer E is incorrect. Follicular carcinoma of the thyroid can resemble normal thyroid tissue. It is composed of relatively uniform follicles lined with cells that are typically larger than those seen in a normal thyroid. Colloid is sparse.

34. **The correct answer is A.** This patient most likely has Lyme disease, a multisystemic infection/disorder caused by the spirochete *Borrelia burgdorferi* and commonly transmitted by a bite from the *Ixodes* tick. The expanding ring-shaped red mark is called erythema chronicum migrans and represents multiplication and spread from the primary bite site. This is the first stage of the disease and may be accompanied by flulike symptoms within 10 days of the bite. The swelling of the left elbow and then the left shoulder and right knee (i.e., migratory arthritis/joint/muscle pain) is caused by dissemination of the disease and may be accompanied by secondary annular skin lesions, cardiac disease (such as myocarditis or transient heart block), and/or neurologic disease (such as meningitis and cranial nerve palsies, which may explain her asymmetric smile, possibly caused by a seventh nerve, or Bell's, palsy). The second stage of the disease can occur weeks after the onset of the first stage. Ten percent of these patients progress to the third stage of the disease, weeks to months after the onset of the second stage. This stage is characterized by chronic arthritis and/or encephalitis that is believed to be an autoimmune response. The immune response in these patients is generally out of proportion to the number of organisms remaining in the patient.

Answer B is incorrect. *Neisseria gonorrhoeae* is a bacterium that can cause septic arthritis, which commonly occurs as an acute-onset fever accompanied by swelling of one to two joints.

Answer C is incorrect. Parvovirus B19 can cause a common childhood illness called fifth disease, also known as "slapped cheek disease" because infected children characteristically get a red maculopapular bilateral cheek rash (or erythema infectiosum—not to be confused with the erythema chronicum migrans of Lyme disease).

Answer D is incorrect. *Rickettsia rickettsii* is a bacterium commonly spread by a tick bite that can cause Rocky Mountain spotted fever. It is characterized by a rash that begins in the distal extremities and spreads proximally, as well as by fever, headache, and conjunctival redness.

Answer E is incorrect. *Streptococcus pyogenes*, also known as group A β-hemolytic streptococci, can lead to rheumatic fever, which can cause fever, myocarditis, arthritis, chorea, subcutaneous nodules, and/or rash. Symptoms usually occur 2–3 weeks after a pharyngitis infection from S. *pyogenes*.

35. **The correct answer is E.** Membranoproliferative glomerulonephritis (MPGN) is an uncommon autoimmune renal disorder that normally affects young individuals (ages 8–30 years). The diagnosis is based on histologic presentation, including mesangial proliferation, thick-

ening of the peripheral capillary walls by subendothelial "humplike" immune deposits (which can coalesce to give a ribbonlike appearance), and mesangial interposition into the capillary wall, giving rise to a tram-track appearance on light microscopy (type I). The mesangial cells interpose into the capillary wall in attempts to remove the deposits. MPGN is caused by a variety of factors. Primary MPGN is idiopathic and can be treated with aspirin and/or dipyridamole. Secondary MPGN can be caused by hepatitis C and B, cryoglobulinemia, lupus, rheumatoid arthritis, and malignancy. Due to significant complement activation, hypocomplementemia is a characteristic finding with all types of MPGN. Diagnosis is confirmed by kidney biopsy. The primary treatment goal for MPGN is to treat the underlying disease: antiviral treatments for hepatitis C and B and immunosuppression for lupus and other rheumatologic conditions.

Answer A is incorrect. Minimal change disease (lipoid nephrosis) is the most common cause of childhood nephrotic syndrome. It is characterized by lipid-laden renal cortices, and demonstrates normal-appearing glomeruli by light microscopy. However, on examination by electron microscopy, fusing of epithelial foot processes can be seen. This disease responds well to steroid therapy.

Answer B is incorrect. Goodpasture's syndrome (antiglomerular basement membrane disease) is caused by antibodies directed against antigens in glomerular basement and alveolar membranes. It demonstrates linear immunofluorescence by fluorescent antibody staining. It is manifest clinically by nephritic syndrome, pneumonitis with hemoptysis, and hematuria.

Answer C is incorrect. IgA nephropathy (Berger's disease) is a common cause of nephritic syndrome defined by deposition of IgA in the mesangium. It is most often characterized by a mild, postinfectious hematuria in children.

Answer D is incorrect. Alport's syndrome is hereditary nephritis associated with nerve deafness and ocular disorders such as lens disloca-

tion and cataracts. It is caused by a mutation in the gene for the α-5 chain of type IV collagen. And it demonstrates a split basement membrane on electron microscopy.

36. **The correct answer is D.** Patient autonomy in a legally competent patient is paramount. Understanding the risks and benefits of a treatment, as well as outcomes, with and without the treatment are defining characteristics of competence. A physician is obligated to respect patient autonomy over the principals of nonmaleficence and beneficence. Patients who are involuntarily admitted are done so for treatment of psychiatric conditions only. Even then, unless they pose a risk to themselves or others, competent patients can refuse psychiatric treatment.

Answer A is incorrect. Beneficence implies that an intervention is in a patient's best interest. All interventions have this characteristic in modern medicine but cannot be instituted without patient consent.

Answer B is incorrect. The duty to other patients involves patients who are a potential harm to other patients. Psychiatric patients have an increased potential to be physically dangerous to other patients as well as the normal potential to be a carrier of infectious disease. This patient's condition is not a threat to other patients.

Answer C is incorrect. Nonmaleficence implies that risks of a treatment are less than benefits. Such a treatment can be offered by physicians but cannot be instituted without patient consent.

Answer E is incorrect. Physician autonomy is not a defined concept.

37. **The correct answer is C.** A blood pressure in the upper extremity significantly greater than in the lower extremity, a weak to nonexistent femoral pulse, and rib notching on chest x-ray are all consistent with postductal coarctation of the aorta. This condition is associated with a high risk of bacterial endocarditis and cerebral hemorrhage. Postductal coarctation is caused by an abnormal constriction of the

aorta distal to the ductus arteriosus during fetal development.

Answer A is incorrect. Acute lymphocytic leukemia is associated with Down's syndrome, which is also associated with an increased risk of an atrial septal defect. However, this is not associated with coarctation of the aorta.

Answer B is incorrect. A boot-shaped heart refers to the cardiac silhouette produced in cases of isolated right ventricular hypertrophy, classically seen in tetralogy of Fallot. While aortic coarctation may theoretically lead to right ventricular hypertrophy, it will do so only after the left ventricle has hypertrophied and thus will not produce the boot-shaped silhouette.

Answer D is incorrect. Cor pulmonale is defined as heart failure secondary to lung disease. If lung disease produces pulmonary hypertension, it will lead to right-sided failure. Since aortic coarctation is not lung disease, it cannot be associated with cor pulmonale.

Answer E is incorrect. Eisenmenger's syndrome is the secondary development of cyanosis in conditions that produce a left-to-right shunt, such as ventricular septal defects. The increased blood flow in the pulmonary circulation leads to pulmonary hypertension, which raises the pressure on the right side of the heart, eventually reversing the shunt. Because blood is now shunted right to left, avoiding the pulmonary circulation, cyanosis develops. Aortic coarctation does not produce a left-to-right shunt and thus does not lead to Eisenmenger's syndrome.

38. **The correct answer is A.** Aortic aneurysms—both abdominal and thoracic—are sequelae of Ehlers-Danlos syndrome, a group of disorders characterized by joint hypermobility, skin hyperelasticity, easy bruising, and tissue weakness. The disorders can be traced to a genetic defect in collagen, which results in the observed joint laxity and poor tissue integrity.

Answer B is incorrect. Elastin is another structural protein found in the body. While collagen provides structural rigidity to the tissues, elastin allows them to distend and recoil. A defect in elastin synthesis might be observed as an increase in tissue rigidity as opposed to an increase in elasticity, as observed in this patient.

Answer C is incorrect. Keratin is a structural protein found in hair, nails, and skin. However, it is not a component of arterial walls and is not implicated in Ehlers-Danlos syndrome.

Answer D is incorrect. Myosin is a component of skeletal, cardiac, and smooth muscle. It interacts with actin to produce muscle contraction but is not implicated in Ehlers-Danlos syndrome.

Answer E is incorrect. Ubiquitin is a small protein responsible for regulating the cell cycle. It also has roles in apoptosis and DNA repair, but it is not a structural protein. A defect in ubiquitin would not produce the symptoms observed in this patient.

39. **The correct answer is D.** The clinical picture presented is one of a congenital diaphragmatic hernia with pulmonary hypoplasia. When bowel protrudes through the open diaphragm (usually on the left), the lungs cannot develop fully and the mediastinum is pushed to the right (explaining the heart sounds). This occurs most commonly as a result of the pleuroperitoneal folds either failing to fuse with the other components of the diaphragm or failing to develop altogether. The diaphragm derives from four fetal structures: the **S**eptum transversum, the **P**leuroperitoneal folds, the **B**ody wall, and the **D**orsal mesentery of the esophagus. This can be remembered by the mnemonic "Several Parts Build Diaphragm."

Answer A is incorrect. The bulbus cordis gives rise to the smooth part of both the right and left ventricles. While the heart is shifted due to the herniation, its development is normal.

Answer B is incorrect. The mesencephalon gives rise to the midbrain, which is not at all implicated in this scenario.

Answer C is incorrect. The midgut loop is the precursor to much of the gastrointestinal tract, from the jejunum to the proximal two-thirds of the transverse colon. While bowel is involved in this clinical scenario in that it herniates through the diaphragm, its development is perfectly normal and is not the underlying cause of the pathology.

Answer E is incorrect. The respiratory diverticulum is an outpouching of the foregut that is the first step in the development of the respiratory system, eventually enlarging to generate the lung bud. While the lungs are not properly developed in this scenario, it is the result of the diaphragmatic hernia and is not itself the underlying cause of the pathology. This can be deduced from the presence of bowel in the chest—this would not happen if the pathology were strictly in the development of the lungs.

40. **The correct answer is D.** The vignette describes a patient with rickets, the clinical syndrome that results from vitamin D deficiency. Hallmarks of this condition include a broad-based waddling gait, bending of long weight-bearing bones on radiographs, and hypocalcemia with low to normal serum phosphate and elevated alkaline serum phosphatase activity. Vitamin D functions in its active form, 1,25-dihydroxycholecalciferol, to increase intestinal absorption of Ca^{2+} and phosphate. A deficiency in this nutrient will result in a deficiency in intestinal Ca^{2+} and phosphate absorption.

Answer A is incorrect. A deficit in serum alkaline phosphatase degradation would result in increased alkaline serum phosphatase activity with hypercalcemia and hyperphosphatemia as a consequence. This is not consistent with the clinical manifestations of vitamin D deficiency described in this vignette.

Answer B is incorrect. A deficit in the demineralization of bone would result in brittle bones with an increased frequency of fractures, which is inconsistent with the syndrome described in the vignette.

Answer C is incorrect. A deficiency in the hydroxylation of proline and lysine in collagen synthesis is typically a result of ascorbic acid,

or vitamin C, deficiency. This usually results in the clinical syndrome known as scurvy, which is not consistent with this clinical scenario.

Answer E is incorrect. Although this patient does have vitamin D deficiency, vitamin D is not important in renal absorption of Ca^{2+} and phosphate. A deficiency in this process is typically the result of renal failure.

41. **The correct answer is C.** Since air is filling up the space previously occupied by the lung, there will be hyperresonance on percussion on the side of the lesion.

Answer A is incorrect. Primary pneumothorax presents with unilateral chest expansion, indicating that one side is not being filled with air during inspiration.

Answer B is incorrect. Lobar pneumonia may have bronchial breath sounds over the lesion, while pneumothorax will have decreased breath sounds over the lesion.

Answer D is incorrect. Lobar pneumonia would present with increased tactile fremitus, while pneumothorax will have absent tactile fremitus.

Answer E is incorrect. Bronchial obstruction would present with tracheal deviation toward the lesion side, while pneumothorax will have tracheal deviation away from the side with the lesion.

42. **The correct answer is B.** F2 is most likely the father of this child. The child could have received the 9-kb fragment from the mother (M) and the 6-kb fragment from F2.

Answer A is incorrect. F1 is unlikely to be the father of this child. The child could have received the 6-kb fragment from his mother (M), but he could not have received the 9-kb fragment from either the mother or F1.

Answer C is incorrect. F3 is unlikely to be the father of this child. The child could have received the 6-kb fragment from his mother (M), but he could not have received the 9-kb fragment from either the mother or F3.

Answer D is incorrect. F4 is unlikely to be the father of this child. The child could have received the 6-kb fragment from his mother (M), but he could not have received the 9-kb fragment from either the mother or F4.

43. **The correct answer is D.** Rotavirus and Coltivirus are two types of reoviruses. They have icosahedral nucleocapsids and are nonenveloped, double-stranded RNA viruses.

    Answer A is incorrect. Bunyavirus and Orthomyxovirus have helical nucleocapsids and are enveloped, single-stranded, segmented RNA viruses.

    Answer B is incorrect. Paramyxovirus and Morbillivirus are both from the Paramyxoviridae family. They have helical nucleocapsids and possess single-stranded, nonsegmented RNA.

    Answer C is incorrect. Picornavirus and Calicivirus are single-stranded, nonsegmented RNA viruses. They have icosahedral nucleocapsids and are nonenveloped.

    Answer E is incorrect. Togavirus and Flavivirus have icosahedral nucleocapsids and are enveloped with single-stranded, nonsegmented RNA.

44. **The correct answer is E.** This patient has Graves' disease, an autoimmune disorder resulting from the presence of elevated levels of thyroid-stimulating immunoglobulin (TSI), an IgG immunoglobulin that binds to and stimulates the TSH receptor of the thyroid gland, causing an increase in the production and release of thyroid hormone. The presence of TSI is relatively specific for Graves' disease. The three classic findings associated with Graves' disease are hyperthyroidism, ophthalmopathy (exophthalmos), and dermopathy/pretibial myxedema (i.e., non-pitting edema on the anterior surface of both legs, with overlying skin that is dry and waxy and may have several diffuse, slightly pigmented papules). Propylthiouracil is a peroxidase inhibitor used to treat hyperthyroidism. It blocks many of the steps of endogenous thyroid hormone synthesis and decreases peripheral conversion of T_4 to T_3.

Answer A is incorrect. Levothyroxine, a synthetic thyroxine analog, is not indicated for Graves' disease. Please note that this drug is indicated for certain cases of hypothyroidism.

Answer B is incorrect. Mercaptopurine, an adenine analog that functions as an immunosuppressant/antineoplastic drug, is not indicated for Graves' disease.

Answer C is incorrect. Procainamide, a class IA antiarrhythmic drug commonly used for ventricular arrhythmias, is not indicated for Graves' disease.

Answer D is incorrect. Propofol, a hypnotic agent used for anesthesia and sedation, is not indicated for Graves' disease.

45. **The correct answer is E.** Adult beriberi is classified as dry or wet. Dry beriberi includes the described polyneuritis while wet beriberi includes the polyneuritis plus cardiomegaly, cardiomyopathy, peripheral edema, and ultimately high-output cardiac failure. Infant beriberi manifests as tachycardia, vomiting, seizures, and death. Beriberi was first described in Chinese medical texts used where the diet of thiamine-deficient rice was the culprit.

Answer A is incorrect. Chronic infection is not a direct manifestation of vitamin B_1 deficiency.

Answer B is incorrect. Convulsions and hyperirritability are symptoms of vitamin B_6 deficiency. The additional symptom of jaundice suggests alcohol abuse and withdrawal, but the three are not seen in isolated thiamine deficiency.

Answer C is incorrect. While dry skin and disordered thought can also be seen in adult beriberi, diarrhea, dermatitis, and dementia are the triad associated with vitamin B_3 deficiency, called pellagra. It is worth noting that Wernicke-Korsakoff syndrome is associated with thiamine deficiency in malnourished alcoholics.

Answer D is incorrect. Kidney failure is not associated with vitamin B_1 deficiency.

FULL-LENGTH EXAM

Test Block 5

46. The correct answer is E. Tubulointerstitial nephritis can be caused by infections and sarcoidosis but is more commonly associated with drug toxicity. The typical picture is that of acute renal failure after drug administration. Common findings are pyuria, hematuria, and WBC casts. Drugs that can cause tubulointerstitial nephritis include sulfonamides, methicillin, furosemide, rifampin, and nonsteroidal anti-inflammatory agents (except for aspirin).

Answer A is incorrect. Aspirin acetylates and irreversibly inhibits cyclooxygenase (COX)-1 and COX-2 enzymes. It is an antipyretic, analgesic, anti-inflammatory, and antiplatelet drug. Aspirin is one nonsteroidal anti-inflammatory drug that does not lead to tubulointerstitial nephritis. Common toxicities of aspirin include gastric ulceration, bleeding, Reye's syndrome, tinnitus, and hyperventilation.

Answer B is incorrect. Cimetidine reversibly blocks histamine H_2 receptors and is used for the treatment of peptic ulcer, gastritis, and gastroesophageal reflux disease. Common toxicities of cimetidine include antiandrogenic effects and decreased renal excretion of creatinine. It is not associated with tubulointerstitial nephritis.

Answer C is incorrect. Imipenem is a broad-spectrum, β-lactamase–resistant carbapenem. It is associated with gastrointestinal distress, skin rash, and seizures, but not with tubulointerstitial nephritis.

Answer D is incorrect. Isoniazid decreases the synthesis of mycolic acids and is used for the treatment of tuberculosis. It is associated with neurotoxicity, hepatotoxicity, a systemic lupus erythematosus-like syndrome, and hemolysis if glucose-6-phosphate dehydrogenase deficient. Isoniazid is not associated with tubulointerstitial nephritis.

47. The correct answer is C. The patient is suffering from hyperparathyroidism secondary to renal disease, also known as renal osteodystrophy. Conversion of vitamin D to its active form is impaired in patients with renal disease. As a result, calcium absorption from the gut is de-creased, which then leads to an increase in levels of parathyroid hormone (PTH). Furthermore, the increase in phosphate levels due to the patient's renal disease leads to a decrease in calcium levels. The patient's labs, therefore, reflect an increased PTH, a decreased serum calcium level, and increased phosphate. The increase in PTH activates osteoclasts, leading to bone resorption and increased levels of alkaline phosphatase.

Answer A is incorrect. Patients with renal disease have decreased serum calcium levels secondary to impaired activation of vitamin D to $1,25(OH)_2D_3$. Lack of biologically active vitamin D results in decreased absorption of calcium from the gastrointestinal tract.

Answer B is incorrect. This set of lab values is characteristic of a patient with primary hyperparathyroidism. The primary difference between the lab results for a patient with primary versus secondary hyperparathyroidism is the relationship between parathyroid hormone (PTH) and serum calcium. Patients with primary hyperparathyroidism will have a resultant increase in serum calcium levels, while those with secondary hyperparathyroidism have a decreased serum calcium level, which then leads to the increase in PTH.

Answer D is incorrect. Increased levels of parathyroid hormone in patients with secondary hyperparathyroidism leads to osteoclast activation, increased bone resorption, and an increase in alkaline phosphatase.

Answer E is incorrect. Patients with renal disease have increased, not decreased, levels of phosphate.

48. The correct answer is A. The two most important points in this question are that the patient is a nonsmoker and that the lesion is located peripherally (subpleural mass). Lung cancers are typically divided into two types: small cell lung cancers and non–small cell lung cancer consisting of adenocarcinoma, squamous cell carcinomas, and other histologic types. These two types are treated with different chemotherapy regimens. The most common lung cancer subtype in nonsmokers and women in general (independent of smoking status) is adenocarcinoma. Adenocarcinomas are peripherally located and are more amenable to (possibly curative) surgical removal than other more centrally located primary lung tumors.

Answer B is incorrect. Carcinoid tumors are found in major bronchi and may cause carcinoid syndrome (flushing due to excessive histamine release).

Answer C is incorrect. Although metastases from other organs are by far the most common malignancy found in the lung, they would likely present as multiple foci rather than a single peripheral nodule.

Answer D is incorrect. Small-cell carcinoma of the lung is an undifferentiated tumor usually in a central location. It is clearly linked to smoking and tends to be widespread at diagnosis, with frequent brain metastases. Small-cell lung cancer is often not amenable to surgical removal and is treated primarily with chemotherapy and radiation.

Answer E is incorrect. Squamous cell carcinoma of the lung often presents as a centrally located hilar mass. This lung cancer subtype is more common in men, and it is clearly linked to smoking.

49. **The correct answer is B.** Clinical probability is the study of the likelihood of events. It is defined as the number of times an event occurs divided by the number of times it can occur. In this instance, there is a 90% probability that a patient will not have muscle aches. $1 - (0.9 \times 0.9 \times 0.9 \times 0.9 \times 0.9)$ equals approximately 41%.

Answer A is incorrect. Attack rate is applied in disease outbreaks in relation to exposure. An exposure is assigned an attack rate based on incidence rate in those exposed.

Answer C is incorrect. Prevalence of a disease is the number of people with a disease at a given time.

Answer D is incorrect. Sensitivity and specificity are measures of validity; although expressed in percentages, these terms are not related to clinical probability.

Answer E is incorrect. Sensitivity and specificity are measures of validity; although expressed in percentages, these terms are not related to clinical probability.

50. **The correct answer is C.** Although a rare occurrence, fluoroquinolones have been reported to cause tendinitis, particularly Achilles' tendinitis. Occasionally, the tendon will rupture, producing the clinical picture described in the stem. Those at increased risk for fluoroquinolone-induced tendinitis include those older than 50 years and those with a history of renal disease, hemodialysis, renal transplant, and glucocorticoid use.

Answer A is incorrect. Amoxicillin is not associated with tendinitis.

Answer B is incorrect. Ceftriaxone is not associated with tendinitis.

Answer D is incorrect. Erythromycin is not associated with tendinitis.

Answer E is incorrect. Metronidazole is not associated with tendinitis.

Answer F is incorrect. Penicillin G is not associated with tendinitis.

Answer G is incorrect. Vancomycin is not associated with tendinitis.

Test Block 6

1. A 45-year-old man presents to his physician with occasional burning mid-epigastric pain that is ameliorated when he eats food. The patient has been experiencing this symptom intermittently for the past 5 months. A drug that inhibits which of the following receptors would be helpful in treating this patient's symptoms?

   (A) α_1
   (B) β_1
   (C) β_2
   (D) Histamine$_1$
   (E) Histamine$_2$

2. A 24-year-old man presents to the emergency department with nausea, vomiting, a low-grade fever, and crampy abdominal pain that has gotten progressively worse over the past 12 hours. He is otherwise healthy except for a 6-month history of a bulge in his right groin that worsens with lifting but is not painful and is always reducible. The physician diagnoses a strangulated indirect hernia with resulting bowel obstruction and necrosis. Which of the following is the underlying cause of this type of hernia?

   (A) Congenital defect in diaphragmatic membrane
   (B) Enlarged external inguinal ring
   (C) Enlarged femoral ring
   (D) Patent processus vaginalis
   (E) Weak abdominal wall musculature

3. A 42-year-old man comes to the physician because of a 2-day history of a low-grade fever. He also says that he has been feeling weak and tired. He says that he went to the dentist last week and that he took the prophylactic medication prescribed by his doctor. His physical examination is unremarkable except for a grade III/VI blowing systolic murmur heard best at the apex. His laboratory findings are significant for a mild anemia. Which of the following organisms is most likely responsible for this man's condition?

   (A) *Clostridium difficile*
   (B) *Staphylococcus aureus*
   (C) *Staphylococcus epidermidis*
   (D) *Streptococcus mutans*
   (E) *Streptococcus pneumoniae*

4. A 70-year-old African-American man with a 50-pack-year history of smoking comes in complaining of shortness of breath. While sitting, the patient is leaning forward and breathing with his lips pursed. Auscultation of his lungs reveals decreased breath sounds. Emphysema, a lung condition that results in diffusion-limited gas exchange, is suspected. Which of the following statements describes diffusion-limited exchange?

   (A) It is illustrated by CO and O_2 under healthy, resting conditions
   (B) It is illustrated by N_2O and CO_2 concentrations in the blood at rest
   (C) It is only increased by an increase in blood flow
   (D) It is present when there is a decreased surface area for gas exchange
   (E) It is when oxygen equilibrates early along the length of the pulmonary capillary
   (F) It is when the gas partial pressure of alveolar air and pulmonary capillary blood equalizes

5. A 60-year-old man with recurrent bacterial sepsis is hospitalized in order to receive intravenous antibiotics. He is started on his fourth course of broad-spectrum antibiotics within the past month. Three days into the admission, his nurse notes that his venous access is oozing blood. Laboratory tests reveal a prolonged prothrombin time. Which of the following coagulation cofactors would be expected to be deficient first?

   (A) Factor II
   (B) Factor V
   (C) Factor VII
   (D) Factor X
   (E) Protein C
   (F) Protein S

6. A medical examiner is investigating the death of a 27-year-old man. He died of acute respiratory distress syndrome 1 day after presenting to the hospital with shortness of breath and a temperature of 38° C (100.4° F). His hospital course was notable for ventilation on 100% oxygen in the ICU and monitoring via a Swan-Ganz catheter. On the second hospital day, he developed extreme pulmonary edema and hypotension before he died. His family says that he had recently gone hiking and caving in an area known to be heavily populated with rodents. Which of the following is the most likely cause of death in this patient?

(A) Dengue virus
(B) Ebola virus
(C) Hantavirus
(D) Marburg virus
(E) Rhabdovirus

7. A 32-year-old woman presents to her primary care physician with a 3-week history of fever, weakness, and petechiae on her abdomen. A laboratory study shows the following results:

WBC count: 125,000/mm^3
Hemoglobin: 7.8%
Hematocrit: 23.4%
Platelet count: 17,000/mm^3

Peripheral blood smear demonstrates the following image. Which of the following is the correct diagnosis?

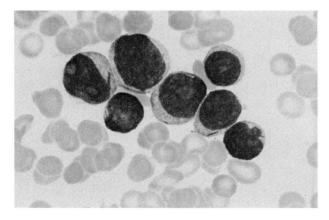

Image courtesy of PEIR Digital Library (http://peir.net).

(A) Acute lymphocytic leukemia
(B) Acute myelogenous leukemia
(C) Chronic lymphocytic leukemia
(D) Multiple myeloma
(E) *Streptococcus pyogenes* (group A) infection

8. Intravenous administration of drug X to an anesthetized animal produces an increase in its blood pressure. After administration of drug Y, readministration of drug X produces a decrease in the animal's blood pressure. Which of the following pairs of drugs could produce this sequence of events?

(A) Drug X—acetylcholine; drug Y—neostigmine
(B) Drug X—epinephrine; drug Y—phentolamine
(C) Drug X—isoproterenol; drug Y—atropine
(D) Drug X—norepinephrine; drug Y—propranolol
(E) Drug X—phenylephrine; drug Y—hexamethonium

9. An 82-year-old man comes to the physician because of a 3-week history of progressively worsening nonlocalizing, nonradicular low back pain that is not relieved by sitting or sleeping. He describes urinary hesitancy and a long history of benign prostatic hypertrophy that has recently worsened. Physical examination is notable for perianal hyperesthesia with slightly decreased rectal tone, a uniformly enlarged prostate, and diminished ankle jerk reflexes bilaterally. No pain is elicited with straight leg raises in the supine position. X-ray films of the thoracic and lumbosacral spine show moderate osteoarthritis. Laboratory studies are unremarkable. Which of the following is the most likely cause of the patient's symptoms?

(A) Conus medullaris tumor
(B) Lumbosacral disc herniation
(C) Spinal epidural abscess
(D) Spinal stenosis
(E) Vertebral osteomyelitis

10. A newborn girl presents to the neonatologist with an inability to swallow and coughing, choking, and vomiting when fed. Workup reveals a tracheoesophageal fistula. Which of the following symptoms would have been present during the mother's pregnancy with this child?

    (A) Abnormal vaginal bleeding
    (B) Hematosalpinx
    (C) Oligohydramnios
    (D) Polyhydramnios
    (E) Preeclampsia

11. A 53-year-old man is brought to the emergency department via ambulance after he began to feel heart palpitations. He has no significant past medical history. The ECG taken by paramedics is shown. Which of the following antiarrhythmic agents should this patient be given intravenously?

    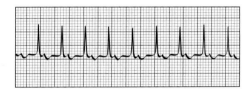

    Reproduced, with permission, from USMLERx.com.

    (A) Adenosine
    (B) Amiodarone
    (C) Bretylium
    (D) Lidocaine
    (E) Procainamide

12. A 67-year-old man presents to the emergency department with diaphoresis and crushing chest pain that radiates down his left arm. An ECG is performed and shows ST elevations and inverted T waves. His troponin level is high. He is taken to the cardiac catheterization unit, where he is diagnosed with an obstructive myocardial infarction due to a blockage in his left anterior descending artery (LAD). Which of the following best describes the area of myocardium supplied by the LAD?

    (A) Anterior wall and interventricular septum
    (B) Atrioventricular node and posterior septum
    (C) Left atrium and left ventricle
    (D) Right atrium and posterior wall
    (E) Right ventricle and apex

13. A 32-year-old man with a history of atrial fibrillation, gastroesophageal reflux disease, type 1 diabetes mellitus, and mitral valve stenosis was recently started on a new medication. He presents to the physician with easy bruising and palpable petechiae on his arms. He has been taking warfarin for 4 years without any complications. An ECG reading reveals a new arrhythmia. A coagulation panel shows the following results:

    Prothrombin time: 45 seconds
    Partial thromboplastin time: 38 seconds
    Platelet count: 300,000/mm^3
    Bleeding time: 7 minutes
    D-dimer: 0.4 µg/mL (normal < 0.5 µg/mL)

    Which of the following medications is most likely responsible for these symptoms?

    (A) Cimetidine
    (B) Insulin lispro
    (C) Metoprolol
    (D) NPH insulin
    (E) Omeprazole

14. A 40-year-old woman presents to the physician with a 5-year history of morning stiffness, intermittent low-grade fever, and fatigue. The morning stiffness is most pronounced in the distal joints of her arms and legs, and the pain improves throughout the day. The physician notes that there is swelling and redness of the proximal interphalangeal joints in both hands but not the distal interphalangeal joints. The patient reports that her maternal aunt and cousin both suffer from similar symptoms. Which of the following therapies, paired with a possible side effect of treatment, is most likely to directly benefit this patient?

(A) Abciximab–thrombocytopenia
(B) Aldesleukin–fever
(C) Etanercept–myelosuppression
(D) Etanercept–tuberculosis
(E) Infliximab–myelosuppression

(A) t(8;14)
(B) t(9;22)
(C) t(11;14)
(D) t(11;22)
(E) t(14;18)
(F) t(15;17)

15. A 25-year-old woman presents to her primary care physician because she has been having headaches. She states that these headaches have been occurring off and on for the past 3 months and adds that they have reached the point where she is worried that something might be wrong. She denies scotomata, numbness, tingling, or loss of consciousness. She also states that the headaches are relieved by sleep and nonsteroidal anti-inflammatory drugs. Her past medical history is unremarkable, and there is no family history of migraine headaches. On physical examination, no focal findings are elicited and the neurologic examination is normal. The patient is diagnosed with depression and given a prescription for antidepressants. Which of the following antidepressants most strongly inhibits norepinephrine uptake?

(A) Bupropion
(B) Escitalopram
(C) Fluoxetine
(D) Reserpine
(E) Sertraline
(F) Trazodone

16. A 13-year-old boy is brought to the physician because of swelling and pain of his right leg. He says he first noticed these symptoms about 3 months ago, but the pain has gotten much worse over the past few weeks. An x-ray film of the leg shows a large lytic lesion with an onion-skin appearance located midway along the femur. Malignancy is suspected, and a karyotype of the biopsied bone tumor cells is ordered. Which of the following chromosomal translocations would most likely be found in the karyotype of this patient?

17. A 19-year-old woman comes to the emergency department after losing a large amount of blood in a motor vehicle collision. The patient requires large amounts of intravenous fluids, blood replacement, and medications to maintain her blood pressure. On the third day of her hospitalization, she becomes severely acidotic with a tense, tender abdomen. Bowel ischemia is suspected. Which of the following is the most likely site of infarcted bowel?

(A) Cecum
(B) Hepatic flexure, large bowel
(C) Ileum
(D) Jejunum
(E) Splenic flexure, large bowel
(F) Stomach

18. A tall, lanky 13-year-old boy presents to the ophthalmologist with a sudden change in vision. Examination shows lens luxation. The patient has always been tall and thin for his age, and a family history reveals that his uncle died from a ruptured aortic aneurysm. On physical examination, the patient is found to have long and slender fingers, ligament laxity, an abnormal ratio of arm length to height, and a diastolic murmur over the aortic area. Which of the following is most likely deficient in this patient?

(A) Dihydrotestosterone receptor
(B) Dystrophin
(C) Fibrillin
(D) Glucose-6-phosphate dehydrogenase
(E) LDL receptor

19. A 35-year-old woman from Arizona comes to the physician with an x-ray film of her chest taken during a routine health insurance examination. The x-ray film shows bilateral hilar adenopathy. The patient is completely asymptomatic. Sarcoidosis is suspected. She was told that her serum levels of angiotensin-converting enzyme (ACE) were elevated. The sensitivity and specificity of using ACE levels to test for the disease in question are 80% and 50%, respectively. Assuming that sarcoidosis is highly prevalent among residents in the southeastern United States, how would the patient's place of residence affect the positive predictive value and negative predictive value of the test?

    (A) In areas of higher prevalence, both the positive predictive value and negative predictive value are higher
    (B) In areas of higher prevalence, both the positive predictive value and negative predictive value are lower
    (C) In areas of higher prevalence, the positive predictive value is higher and the negative predictive value is lower
    (D) In areas of higher prevalence, the positive predictive value is lower, and the negative predictive value remains the same
    (E) Regardless of the prevalence, the positive predictive value and negative predictive value are unchanged

20. Below is a short sequence of DNA showing the mutation that causes β-thalassemia. Which of the following DNA mutations causes β-thalassemia?

| Normal β globin allele | AAC CAG AGG |
| β⁰ globin allele (thalassemia) | AAC TAG AGG |

    (A) Frameshift mutation
    (B) Insertion mutation
    (C) Missense mutation
    (D) Nonsense mutation
    (E) Silent mutation

21. A pathologist examines a section of bronchial tissue obtained during a transbronchial biopsy performed on an individual who smokes. She notes that the bronchial lining consists of several layers of well-differentiated, organized squamous epithelia contained above the basement membrane. Which of the following terms best describes the pathologist's finding?

    (A) Anaplasia
    (B) Dysplasia
    (C) Hyperplasia
    (D) Metaplasia
    (E) Neoplasia

22. A 51-year-old man with a history of Cushing's syndrome undergoes surgery for resection of an adrenal adenoma. During the operation, the patient becomes hypotensive. Despite aggressive fluid resuscitation, the patient remains hypotensive and requires therapy with intravenous pressors to maintain his blood pressure. Which of the following medications should have been administered intraoperatively to avoid this complication?

    (A) Hydrocortisone
    (B) Octreotide
    (C) Phenoxybenzamine
    (D) Phenylephrine
    (E) Vasopressin

23. Following antibiotic treatment for a respiratory infection, a 35-year-old woman experiences vaginal itching along with a vaginal discharge that has a cheeselike consistency. Her doctor explains that the good bacteria of the vagina have been killed, in addition to the bacteria that were causing her respiratory infection. Lowering the population of the good bacteria made conditions favorable for other organisms already present in the vagina to overgrow and cause the symptoms she is currently experiencing. Species from which of the following genera normally make up a majority of the normal flora, or the good bacteria, in the vagina?

    (A) *Bacteroides*
    (B) *Candida*
    (C) *Lactobacillus*
    (D) *Staphylococcus*
    (E) *Trichomonas*

24. β-Thalassemia major results from a homozygous genotype that leads to complete absence of both of the β-globin chains. An intrauterine screening test has been used on 100,000 patients, 87 of whom tested positive for β-thalassemia major, with the remaining 99,913 testing negative. Of those 87 cases, 7 were shown to be false positives. Ultimately, 100 of those originally screened were found to have the disease. Which of the following is the correct sensitivity of the intrauterine screening test?

(A) 8%
(B) 80%
(C) 87%
(D) 92%
(E) 99.99%

25. A 30-year-old man presents to the emergency department complaining of shortness of breath, dizziness, nausea, and vomiting. He also says that his heart feels "like it is jumping out of my chest." Two days ago, while he was out for his daily run, he passed a burning house and stopped to help the residents evacuate. He made multiple trips into the house, inhaling a lot of smoke each time. He declined medical assistance because aside from a mild cough, he felt fine at the time. Yesterday, however, he felt fatigued and stayed in bed for most of the day. On examination, his pulse is 90/min, his blood pressure is 100/60 mm Hg, and his respiratory rate is 22/min. He is slumped in a chair in the examination room, taking deep gasps of air. The rest of the examination is unremarkable with the exception of bright red vessels in both of his eyes. What is the mechanism of action of the toxic agent that resulted in this patient's symptoms?

(A) Direct tissue injury
(B) Inhibition of cellular respiration
(C) Inhibition of cholinesterase
(D) Increased epinephrine release
(E) Interference with DNA synthesis

26. The human leukocyte antigen (HLA)-DR4 and HLA-DR3 molecules are known to confer greater-than-average susceptibility to type 1 di-

abetes. In fact, epidemiologic studies suggest that a carrier of both HLA-DR4 and HLA-DR3 is 50 times more susceptible to type 1 diabetes than a noncarrier. For the pedigree shown, what is the probability that the proband harbors both of these high-risk alleles (HLA-DR3 and HLA-DR4)? (Note that the two DR alleles possessed by the proband's grandparents are shown above their pedigree symbols.)

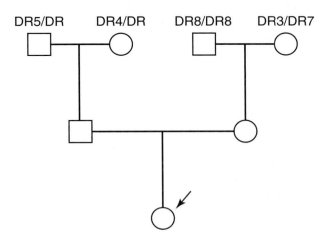

Reproduced, with permission, from USMLERx.com.

(A) 0
(B) 1/8
(C) 1/4
(D) 1/2
(E) 1

27. A 26-year-old woman and her husband have been trying to conceive a child for the past 14 months and have been unsuccessful. They visit the woman's obstetrician/gynecologist to learn more about their options for increasing their fertility. The physician decides to prescribe a medication for the woman that induces ovulation. Which of the following is a common adverse effect of this medication?

(A) Disturbances in color vision
(B) Nasal congestion
(C) Nausea and vomiting
(D) Vasomotor flushes
(E) Weight gain

28. An intoxicated man is found unresponsive in the woods and is brought to the emergency department. On examination, he is found to have bite marks on his lower left extremities. He is unable to explain how they appeared. Which of the following is the most likely recommended course of action?

   (A) Administer human immune globulin immediately, and follow up with injections of killed virus vaccine only if the patient develops symptoms
   (B) Administer human immune globulin immediately, and give a series of five injections of killed virus vaccine
   (C) Administer human immune globulin in a series of five doses
   (D) Administer killed virus vaccine immediately, and follow up with injections of human virus vaccine only if the patient develops symptoms
   (E) Administer killed virus vaccine immediately, and give a series of five injections of human immune globulin
   (F) Do nothing

29. An 82-year-old woman presents to the emergency department with a 3-week history of fever, weight loss, and malaise in the setting of hip and shoulder girdle pain that is most severe in the morning. She also reports a 1-week history of headaches and left-sided jaw pain that occurs at every meal. The patient's temperature is 38.2° C (100.8° F), her pulse is 104/min, and her blood pressure is 140/80 mm Hg. Laboratory studies show a hemoglobin level of 11.8 g/dL, a WBC count of 11,900/mm^3, and an erythrocyte sedimentation rate of 121 mm/hr. Physical examination is unremarkable except for moderate synovitis of the ankles and wrist. Which of the following procedures is most likely to be diagnostic in this patient?

   (A) Arthrocentesis
   (B) Mesenteric angiogram
   (C) Temporal artery biopsy
   (D) Testing for anti–double-stranded DNA and antinuclear antibody levels
   (E) Testing for rheumatoid factor and anti–cytidine cyclic phosphate levels

30. A patient with a known allergy to sulfa drugs presents to the emergency department with severe shortness of breath and rapid, shallow breathing. A pulmonary examination reveals bilateral crackles halfway up from the bases, and x-ray film of the chest shows pulmonary vascular redistribution and bilateral interstitial markings. The attending physician chooses to treat the patient with a high dose of a diuretic agent. Subsequently, the patient develops muscle weakness and difficulty hearing his wife's voice. Which of the following diuretics is this patient most likely taking?

   (A) Acetazolamide
   (B) Ethacrynic acid
   (C) Furosemide
   (D) Hydrochlorothiazide
   (E) Spironolactone

31. A 45-year-old man comes to the physician with a high temperature, neck stiffness, nausea, and vomiting. He is lethargic and shows definite signs of mental status changes. Physical examination shows a positive Kernig's sign and papilledema. The patient notes that he has just returned from a business trip in a town located on the Mississippi River. Which of the following is the most likely cause of his symptoms?

   (A) Eastern equine encephalitis virus
   (B) Japanese encephalitis virus
   (C) Poliovirus
   (D) St. Louis encephalitis virus
   (E) Western equine encephalitis virus

32. The hemoglobin tetramer is composed of two identical dimers, αb1 and αb2. The two polypeptide chains within each dimer are held tightly together primarily by hydrophobic interactions. In contrast, the two dimers, being held together by polar bonds, are able to move with respect to each other to assume either a taut or a relaxed form. Which of the following is correct regarding different forms of hemoglobin?

   (A) When in the relaxed form, hemoglobin is in its deoxy state and has high oxygen affinity
   (B) When in the relaxed form, the polypeptide chains move more easily and have low oxygen affinity

(C) When in the taut form, hemoglobin is in its deoxy state and has high oxygen affinity

(D) When in the taut form, hemoglobin is in its deoxy state and has low oxygen affinity

(E) When in the taut form, hemoglobin is in its oxygenated state and has high oxygen affinity

(F) When in the taut form, the polypeptide chains move more easily and have higher oxygen affinity

33. A 60-year-old man comes to the physician because of persistent headaches and increased clumsiness; he cites repeated collisions into door frames. He says that he has experienced decreased libido over the same period of time. This patient is most likely to also present with which of the following conditions?

(A) Bitemporal hemianopsia
(B) Dysphagia
(C) Hydrocephalus
(D) Right facial droop
(E) Right hand weakness

34. A 39-year-old man who is treated for schizophrenia begins to experience muscular rigidity, decreased perspiration, hyperthermia, and signs of autonomic instability. Which of the following drugs should be administered to the patient immediately?

(A) Dantrolene
(B) Diazepam
(C) Flumazenil
(D) Haloperidol
(E) Phenobarbital

35. The mother of a 3-year-old boy is referred to genetic counseling after her son is diagnosed with an enzyme deficiency. Recently, the mother noticed that her son has an abnormal facial appearance as well as pearly papular skin lesions over the scapulae and on the lateral upper arms and thighs, however, his corneas are clear bilaterally. She has also noticed that her son is hyperactive compared to other children of the same age. This patient carries a diagnosis of which of the following syndromes?

(A) Hunter's syndrome
(B) Hurler's syndrome

(C) Morquio's syndrome
(D) Sanfilippo's syndrome
(E) Sly syndrome

36. A 31-year-old man comes to the physician with a 5-day history of shortness of breath. The patient says that he also has had a nonproductive cough in the same time period. X-ray film of the chest reveals bilateral diffuse infiltrates, and laboratory results show a WBC count of $2500/mm^3$. An enzyme-linked immunosorbent assay is positive for HIV infection, and methenamine silver stain shows the causative organism. The patient is started on sulfamethoxazole-trimethoprim. Which of the following is the mechanism of action of the antibiotic used to treat this patient's infection?

(A) Blockade of ergosterol synthesis
(B) Blockade of the pathway that converts pteridine and PABA into nucleotides
(C) Cell wall synthesis
(D) Inhibition of the larger ribosomal subunit
(E) Inhibition of the small ribosomal subunit

37. A 24-year-old man is attempting to open a package with a knife, when he loses his grip and slices his finger with the knife. He goes to the emergency department, where the physician finds a laceration on the dorsal surface of the second digit of his left hand between the proximal interphalangeal (PIP) and distal interphalangeal (DIP) joints. The wound has stopped bleeding and looks clean, and the physician decides to put a couple of stitches in to help the healing process. Before he sutures up the patient, he wants to numb the area with lidocaine. Where should the physician inject the lidocaine?

(A) At the lateral aspect of the wrist
(B) At the medial aspect of the wrist
(C) On the dorsal surface of the digit near the DIP joint
(D) On the dorsal surface of the digit near the metacarpophalangeal joint
(E) On the lateral aspect of the forearm halfway between the wrist and the elbow

38. A 59-year-old man with type 2 diabetes presents to the emergency department with nausea, vomiting, and abdominal pain. On examination, his blood pressure is found to be 130/93 mm Hg, respirations are 32/min, and arterial oxygen saturation is 99%; he is disoriented to time and place. Laboratory results are as follows:

Na^+: 138 mEq/L
K^+: 4.2 mEq/L
Cl^-: 103 mEq/L
HCO_3^- : 8 mEq/L
Blood urea nitrogen: 25 mg/dL
Creatinine: 2.0 mg/dL
Glucose: 57 mg/dL

Which of the following medications has this patient most likely been taking?

(A) Acarbose
(B) Metformin
(C) Miglitol
(D) Tolbutamide
(E) Troglitazone

39. An outbreak of infection in a small village in Ghana has nearly wiped out an entire village. A group of scientists travels to Ghana to determine the cause of this disease. As a result of their work, they discover that a new toxin-producing bacterium caused the outbreak. The toxin appears to inhibit the cytoplasmic Na^+-K^+-ATPase pump. Which of the following compounds has a mechanism of action similar to that of the newly isolated toxin?

(A) Albuterol
(B) Botulinum toxin
(C) Cocaine
(D) Ouabain
(E) Procainamide

40. Mr. Smith is a 66-year-old man who was diagnosed with diabetes mellitus 15 years ago. Over the past 3 years his serum creatinine levels have increased from 1.3 to 2.2 mg/dL. In an effort to slow diabetes-induced damage to his kidneys, he was started on an angiotensin-converting enzyme inhibitor 2 years ago, without much change in his nephropathy. His most recent laboratory values:

Serum K^+: 5.5 mEq/L
Urine pH: 5.2
Serum Na^+: 140 mEq/L
HCO_3^-: 18 mEq/L
Cl^-: 110 mEq/L
Arterial blood pH: 7.33
pCO_2: 40 mm Hg

Which of the following conditions does this patient most likely have?

(A) Anion-gap metabolic acidosis
(B) Hyperreninemic hyperaldosteronism
(C) Type I renal tubular acidosis
(D) Type II renal tubular acidosis
(E) Type IV renal tubular acidosis

41. A pregnant woman comes to the physician for a checkup before the beginning of her third trimester. It is learned that she has been exposed to an infectious disease. Fortunately, the infections disease caused no morbidity to the fetus, and the resulting pregnancy is uncomplicated. The woman later gives birth to a healthy child. Of the following viruses, which was the woman most likely exposed to?

(A) Cytomegalovirus
(B) Epstein-Barr virus
(C) Herpes simplex virus
(D) HIV
(E) Rubella
(F) Syphilis
(G) Toxoplasmosis

42. Carcinoma in situ refers to neoplastic cells that have not yet invaded the basement membrane. Progression of the carcinoma to metastasis may be made possible by the aberrant expression of which of the following factors that allows the neoplastic cells to leave the primary site?

(A) Collagenase
(B) α-Fetoprotein
(C) γ-Glutamyl transpeptidase
(D) Keratin
(E) Mucin

43. A 41-year-old man comes to the physician complaining of crampy, bloating abdominal discomfort. He also reports changes in his bowel habits and recently noticed dark stool. His father, sister, and uncle all died of colorectal cancer. Which of the following is the most likely cause of these findings?

(A) A defect in base excision repair
(B) A defect in mismatch repair
(C) Exposure to benzo(a)pyrene
(D) Mutation of the *p53* gene
(E) The *bcr-abl* hybrid gene

44. A 75-year-old man comes to the physician because he recently began experiencing seizures. A CT scan shows an irregular ring-enhancing lesion with central necrosis. A biopsy taken from a mass in one of his cerebral hemispheres is shown in the image. Which of the following is the most likely diagnosis?

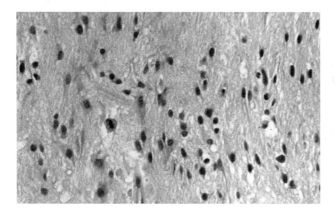

Image courtesy of PEIR Digital Library (http://peir.net).

(A) Glioblastoma multiforme
(B) Medulloblastoma
(C) Meningioma
(D) Neurilemmoma
(E) Oligodendroglioma

45. A 19-year-old college student developed sore throat, palatal petechiae, splenomegaly, fever, and generalized lymphadenopathy after she began dating her first serious boyfriend. The symptoms were self-limiting and lasted approximately 2–3 weeks. Upon presentation at the campus health clinic, a blood sample tests positive for heterophil antibodies and she is diagnosed with symptomatic primary Epstein-Barr virus (EBV) infection that clinically manifested as infectious mononucleosis. Which of the following innate immune cell types plays a direct and important role in controlling the early stages of her systemic response to EBV infection?

(A) Eosinophils
(B) Mast cells
(C) Megakaryocytes
(D) Microglia
(E) Natural killer cells
(F) Plasma cells
(G) Regulatory T lymphocytes

46. A 4-month-old girl who was born full-term presents to her pediatrician with an upper respiratory infection. Her mother notes that this is the fifth time her daughter has had an upper respiratory infection since birth. Her past medical history is significant for seizures shortly after birth. In addition to pulmonary findings, the physical examination is notable for oropharyngeal candidiasis that the patient's mother says has been occurring regularly. Laboratory studies are significant for hypocalcemia and lymphopenia. This child is presenting with a syndrome that is due to aberrant development of which of the following embryonic structures?

(A) First and second aortic arches
(B) First and second branchial arches
(C) Fourth and sixth pharyngeal arches
(D) Second and third branchial clefts
(E) Third and fourth branchial pouches

47. A major problem in hospitals is the risk of needle sticks and the accidental transmission of hepatitis C, hepatitis B, and HIV to health care personnel. Although different circumstances can make the likelihood of infection higher or lower, it is well known that the chance of infection transmission from a needle is not the same for each of these diseases. From greatest chance of infection to least, which of the following is the order of infection among these three diseases?

    (A) Hepatitis B, hepatitis C, HIV
    (B) Hepatitis B, HIV, hepatitis C
    (C) Hepatitis C, hepatitis B, HIV
    (D) Hepatitis C, HIV, hepatitis B
    (E) HIV, hepatitis B, hepatitis C

48. The inhaled anesthetics listed have the properties indicated in the chart. Which of the following statements best describes the properties of these drugs?

	MINIMUM ALVEOLAR CONCENTRATION	BLOOD SOLUBILITY
Drug A	7.3	0.5
Drug B	3.1	1.0
Drug C	2.0	0.1
Drug D	4.4	0.15

    (A) Drug A is more potent than drug D
    (B) Drug B is less soluble in blood than drug C
    (C) Drug C will have both the highest potency and the most rapid induction
    (D) Drug D will induce anesthesia more rapidly than drug C
    (E) Patients treated with drug B will recover more quickly from anesthesia than drug A

49. A 60-year-old man is referred to an oncologist by his primary care doctor after complaining of fatigue, shortness of breath, and a recent history of bruising. Physical examination is notable for marked splenomegaly as well as purpura on his arms and thighs. Laboratory studies show anemia, thrombocytopenia, and abnormal findings on peripheral blood smear, prompting a bone marrow biopsy. Biopsy is notable for the replacement of normal marrow elements by fibrosis with no evidence of malignancy. What would a peripheral blood smear in this patient likely show?

    (A) Acanthocytes
    (B) Macro-ovalocytes
    (C) Schistocytes
    (D) Spherocytes
    (E) Target cells
    (F) Teardrop cell

50. A mentally retarded 16-year-old visits her physician with her parents because she is pregnant. A urine and serum β-human chorionic gonadotropin test are positive. The parents would like the daughter to have an abortion. The patient would like to keep the pregnancy. What is the legal course of action?

    (A) Consult a judge for patient competency determination
    (B) Consult child protective services to have the baby taken at birth
    (C) No medical intervention to terminate the pregnancy
    (D) Perform an abortion to terminate the pregnancy
    (E) Repeat the urine and serum β-human chorionic gonadotropin

1. **The correct answer is E.** This patient's symptoms are consistent with those of a duodenal ulcer. A duodenal ulcer can be caused by hypersecretion of stomach acid, *Helicobacter pylori* infection, or use of nonsteroidal anti-inflammatory drugs. The initial treatment of a duodenal ulcer involves a trial of a histamine$_2$ blocker such as cimetidine. Activation of histamine$_2$ receptors leads to increased gastric acid production. Thus, by inhibiting the histamine$_2$ receptor, gastric acid secretion is decreased, allowing the ulcer to heal. Other treatments for ulcers involve inhibiting the H$^+$-K$^+$-ATPase pumps on parietal cells (using proton pump inhibitors such as omeprazole) or neutralizing stomach acid (using antacids). If a biopsy of the ulcer is positive for *H. pylori*, then the patient should be treated with a triple regimen of bismuth, metronidazole, and either amoxicillin or tetracycline.

Answer A is incorrect. Activation of α_1 receptors results in vasoconstriction and increased blood pressure. α_1 Receptors are typically found in blood vessel walls and are not involved in the production of gastric acid.

Answer B is incorrect. Activation of β_1 receptors leads to inotropy and chronotropy. β_1 Receptors are typically located in the heart, and stimulation of the receptors results in increased contractility (inotropy) and heart rate (chronotropy).

Answer C is incorrect. Activation of β_2 receptors located in blood vessel walls and respiratory epithelium leads to vasodilation and bronchodilation, respectively.

Answer D is incorrect. Activation of histamine$_1$ receptors results in pruritus, bronchoconstriction, and increased nasal and bronchial mucus production.

2. **The correct answer is D.** Indirect inguinal hernias are the most common type of hernia and are the result of a congenital defect of the processus vaginalis. If the processus vaginalis remains patent, this provides a potential space through the internal inguinal ring for abdominal contents to herniate. In autopsy specimens, up to 20% of men have some degree of patency of their processus vaginalis, so other factors contribute to the development of an indirect hernia. One factor is increased abdominal pressure (from lifting heavy objects, chronic cough, or constipation) that can force intestine into this space. Potential complications of any hernia include strangulation and infarction of bowel, as has occurred in this case.

Answer A is incorrect. A congenital defect in the development of the pleuroperitoneal membranes of the diaphragm would lead to a hiatal hernia, which is characterized by the esophageal-gastric junction pulling upward through the diaphragm into the thorax. A classic sign for this is the hourglass sign on abdominal radiographs.

Answer B is incorrect. An enlarged external inguinal ring can be seen in hernias but is not the cause of a hernia. The external ring is a superficial structure that is separated from the intestines by the thick abdominal wall. Abdominal contents must first penetrate the abdominal wall or enter the internal ring before reaching the external ring.

Answer C is incorrect. An enlarged femoral ring may predispose people to the development of a femoral hernia, which is characterized by abdominal contents entering the femoral sheath at the femoral canal.

Answer E is incorrect. A weakness in the abdominal wall musculature can lead to a direct inguinal hernia, where abdominal contents protrude directly through the abdominal wall, often seen in Hesselbach's triangle. Both direct and indirect hernias can exit through the external ring and enter the scrotum. The distinction between these two types of hernias lies in whether the abdominal contents enter the internal ring (indirect) or not (direct).

3. **The correct answer is D.** *Streptococcus mutans* is a viridans group streptococcus. Mem-

bers of this group of bacteria are known to cause subacute bacterial endocarditis. After the bacteria gain entry into the bloodstream, they seed the surface of a previously damaged heart valve. The bacteria slowly pile up and cause the slow development of low-grade fevers, fatigue, anemia, and a new heart murmur. This patient most likely had his mitral valve damaged by rheumatic fever, for which his doctor prescribed antibiotic prophylaxis before dental procedure.

Answer A is incorrect. *Clostridium difficile* causes severe nonbloody diarrhea associated with pseudomembranes. It is associated with previous antibiotic treatment. It does not cause bacteremia and, consequently, is virtually unknown as a cause of endocarditis.

Answer B is incorrect. *Staphylococcus aureus* causes acute bacterial endocarditis, which presents with an acute onset of high fever, other flulike symptoms, new-onset murmur, and petechiae.

Answer C is incorrect. *Staphylococcus epidermidis*, a common skin flora, most commonly causes endocarditis on prosthetic heart valves or right-sided valves in intravenous drug users.

Answer E is incorrect. *Streptococcus pneumoniae* is a rare cause of bacterial endocarditis in the post-antibiotic era.

4. **The correct answer is D.** Emphysema is an obstructive lung disease in which alveoli are destroyed. This decreases surface area for gas exchange, and illustrates diffusion-limited exchange.

Answer A is incorrect. Diffusion-limited exchange is illustrated by CO and O_2 during strenuous exercise.

Answer B is incorrect. N_2O and CO_2 under healthy, resting conditions are not illustrative of diffusion-limited exchange.

Answer C is incorrect. Diffusion-limited exchange is not related to blood flow, it is related to the borders of gas exchange (type I pneumocytes, basement membrane, and capillary endothelial cells).

Answer E is incorrect. Oxygen does not equilibrate by the time blood reaches the end of the capillary.

Answer F is incorrect. Gas partial pressure difference is maintained between alveolar air and pulmonary capillary blood.

5. **The correct answer is C.** Vitamin K is synthesized by the intestinal flora; therefore, long-term treatment with broad-spectrum antibiotics can induce a deficiency by clearing intestinal flora. Vitamin K is a necessary cofactor for hepatic production of clotting factors II, VII, IX, and X, and proteins C and S. Factor VII has the shortest half-life of all clotting factors (4–6 hours), which is why the prothrombin time (PT) is prolonged first in vitamin K deficiency.

Answer A is incorrect. Factor II (thrombin) does require vitamin K as a cofactor, but its half-life is 42–72 hours. Early factor II deficiency would result in prolongation of prothrombin time and partial thromboplastin time.

Answer B is incorrect. Vitamin K is not required for factor V synthesis and would not be deficient in this patient.

Answer D is incorrect. Factor X has a half-life of 27–48 hours; deficiency would not be seen early.

Answer E is incorrect. The half-life of protein C is comparable to factor VII at 9 hours and would become deficient soon after factor VII.

Answer F is incorrect. Protein S deficiency is unlikely early in the process due to its half-life of 60 hours.

6. **The correct answer is C.** Hantavirus pulmonary syndrome is a rare viral cause of acute respiratory distress syndrome (ARDS). Hantavirus has been found in rodents throughout the United States. It is thought to be transmitted from rodent droppings and saliva. ARDS presents as described in the question stem, with fever and respiratory distress, and is treated with ventilatory support.

Answer A is incorrect. Dengue virus is a mosquito-transmitted virus that causes a hemorrhagic fever. It is found in Asia and in South and Central America. Patients present with rash and bleeding from the mucous membranes.

Answer B is incorrect. Ebola virus and Marburg virus are members of the *Filovirus* genus, which cause hemorrhagic fever. Both are found only in central and southern Africa. They have an animal reservoir that has not been found. Treatment is supportive, and symptoms include massive hemorrhage from the mucous membranes accompanied by high fevers.

Answer D is incorrect. Ebola virus and Marburg virus are members of the Filovirus genus, which cause hemorrhagic fever. Both are found only in central and southern Africa. They have an animal reservoir that has not been found. Treatment is supportive, and symptoms include massive hemorrhage from the mucous membranes accompanied by high fevers.

Answer E is incorrect. Rhabdovirus is the causative agent of rabies. It is possible to become infected with rabies from a rodent; however, the incubation period is much longer (weeks to a year), and the later stages of the disease are classically acute encephalitis.

7. **The correct answer is B.** Acute myelogenous leukemia (AML) typically presents with rapid-onset symptoms of bone marrow suppression, including anemia (weakness), thrombocytopenia (petechiae), and poor immunity (susceptibility to infection) in the context of leukocytosis. The peripheral blood smear demonstrates myeloblasts with Auer rods, which are present in many cases of AML, particularly acute promyelocytic leukemia (type M3).

Answer A is incorrect. Acute lymphocytic leukemia (ALL) presents with clinical symptoms that are often indistinguishable from AML. Thus, the only way to tell these two apart with the information in the question is the image, which shows myeloblasts with Auer

rods. If it were ALL, the image would show lymphoblasts. Another clue to differentiating ALL from AML is the patient's age: Of course both AML and ALL can be seen in all age groups; however, AML is more common in adults 15–40 years old, whereas ALL is usually seen in patients younger than 15 years. ALL is also more common in individuals with Down's syndrome (mnemonic: We **ALL** fall **DOWN**).

Answer C is incorrect. Chronic myelogenous leukemia follows a more insidious course than AML, with symptoms of bone marrow suppression developing slowly. Additionally, it presents with fewer myeloblasts and increased neutrophils, myelocytes, and metamyelocytes.

Answer D is incorrect. Multiple myeloma can present with leukocytosis, but the peripheral blood smear would not show myeloblasts with Auer rods. Renal failure and lytic lesions in the bones are also common. Additionally, it follows a more chronic progressive course.

Answer E is incorrect. *Streptococcus pyogenes* (group A) infection can present with scarlet fever, which could produce symptoms similar to these. However, the presence of myeloblasts with Auer rods is diagnostic of acute myelogenous leukemia. In addition, the WBC count is not likely to be as high as in the leukemias.

8. **The correct answer is B.** Epinephrine is an agonist at α_1, α_2, β_1, and β_2 receptors; phentolamine is an antagonist at α_1 and α_2 receptors. Therefore, after the administration of phentolamine, epinephrine administration stimulates only β receptors, which results in decreased blood pressure. This is called epinephrine reversal because epinephrine originally increased blood pressure and then produced the opposite effect after phentolamine administration.

Answer A is incorrect. Acetylcholine stimulates the noninnervated muscarinic (M_3) receptors that are located on endothelial cells of the vasculature. Stimulation of these receptors releases endothelial-derived relaxing factor (nitric oxide), which produces a relaxation of the neighboring smooth muscle cells, leading to a decrease in blood pressure. Neostigmine, an acetylcholinesterase inhibitor, would simply prolong the action of acetylcholine at its receptors and would thus indirectly cause a decrease in blood pressure.

Answer C is incorrect. This choice should be eliminated because isoproterenol, a nonspecific β agonist, decreases blood pressure by stimulation of β_2 receptors in the vasculature. Epinephrine, norepinephrine, and phenylephrine all increase blood pressure, so the remaining answers must be eliminated by examining the effects of drug Y on drug X.

Answer D is incorrect. Norepinephrine is an agonist at α_1, α_2, and β_1 receptors; propranolol is a nonselective β antagonist. After administration of propranolol, norepinephrine can stimulate only α receptors, which will still cause vasoconstriction (primarily via α_1 stimulation in the vasculature) and therefore increase blood pressure.

Answer E is incorrect. Phenylephrine is an α_1 agonist, and hexamethonium is a nicotinic ganglionic blocker. Hexamethonium administration will eliminate the baroreceptor response after the second phenylephrine administration by blocking the peripheral ganglia. However, phenylephrine will still reach the α_1 receptors on the vasculature to produce an increase in blood pressure.

9. **The correct answer is A.** This patient is suffering from a cord compression syndrome due to a conus medullaris tumor. These tumors are relatively uncommon and can be very difficult to diagnose because they are difficult to differentiate from tumors of the cauda equina. Patients can manifest symptoms of one or both syndromes. Night and rest pain is an immediate red flag for metastatic disease, multiple myeloma, or spinal infections. The x-ray films and normal laboratory values help to make metastatic disease or myeloma less likely. The examination is consistent with conus medullaris syndrome because of the relatively rapid, bilateral onset of moderate back pain with a minimal radicular component and preserved ankle reflexes. These patients tend to have perianal numbness and urinary retention with an atonic rectal sphincter, as opposed to the saddle anesthesia more typically found in cauda equina syndrome. This patient's presentation warrants empiric steroids and emergent MRI.

Answer B is incorrect. The physical examination largely excludes the possibility of disc herniation as a cause of the patient's symptoms because of absent positive straight leg raises and pain that is neither aggravated by activity nor relieved by resting.

Answer C is incorrect. The triad for spinal epidural abscess includes back pain, fever, and progressive weakness. This patient does not have the second two symptoms, making abscess a less likely possibility.

Answer D is incorrect. Spinal stenosis is characterized by neurogenic claudication, or pain in the buttocks or back that is induced by walking or prolonged standing and relieved by rest; it may also include focal neurologic findings. However, it is a less likely diagnosis in this patient because his pain does not abate with sitting.

Answer E is incorrect. Vertebral osteomyelitis would most likely present in a patient that was suffering constitutional signs and symptoms, as opposed to the relatively focal findings presented in this case. Characteristically, a patient with osteomyelitis would have night sweats and fever. The patient would have symptoms that would point to the source of the hematogenous dissemination of the infectious agent to the spine (e.g., urinary tract infection).

10. **The correct answer is D.** A tracheoesophageal fistula will cause polyhydramnios during pregnancy, as the fetus is unable to swallow amniotic fluid. The defect occurs when the lateral walls of the foregut fail to fuse after separating from the trachea. Treatment is immediate surgical repair.

Answer A is incorrect. Abnormal vaginal bleeding is a nonspecific sign but is not associated with tracheoesophageal fistula.

Answer B is incorrect. Hematosalpinx refers to bleeding into the fallopian tubes most commonly caused by an ectopic pregnancy. It is not associated with tracheoesophageal fistula in the fetus.

Answer C is incorrect. Oligohydramnios occurs when fetal urine is not produced or cannot be excreted, as in bilateral renal agenesis. There is no evidence of urinary obstruction or renal defects in this case.

Answer E is incorrect. Preeclampsia is a syndrome of hypertension, albuminuria, and edema. Its etiology is not well understood, but it is not specifically associated with tracheoesophageal fistula.

11. **The correct answer is A.** Intravenous adenosine is the drug of choice in a case of acute supraventricular tachycardia (SVT), a condition that is evident on this patient's ECG. Because adenosine slows the conduction velocity and increases refractoriness at the AV node, it can convert an acute SVT into a normal rhythm.

Answer B is incorrect. Amiodarone, a class III antiarrhythmic, slows repolarization or phase 3 of the action potential. Because it does not cause atrioventricular nodal block, it is not indicated for patients in acute supraventricular tachycardia.

Answer C is incorrect. Bretylium, a class III antiarrhythmic, slows repolarization or phase 3 of the action potential and is not indicated for cases of acute supraventricular tachycardia because it does not achieve atrioventricular nodal block.

Answer D is incorrect. Lidocaine, a class IB drug, is indicated for ventricular arrhythmias because it has a greater effect on inactivated Na^+ channels. Because the action potential in atrial cells is short, lidocaine is not effective in treating atrial arrhythmias.

Answer E is incorrect. As a class IA antiarrhythmic, procainamide decreases Na^+ conduction and thus increases the duration of the action potential and the QT interval. However, it is not indicated in cases of supraventricular

tachycardia because it does not achieve atrioventricular nodal block.

12. **The correct answer is A.** The left anterior descending artery branches from the left main coronary artery as it approaches the atrioventricular junction. It descends toward the apex on the anterior wall of the heart between the right and left ventricles and supplies the anterior wall of both ventricles and most of the interventricular septum.

Answer B is incorrect. The right main coronary artery courses around to the posterior wall of the heart and supplies the atrioventricular node and posterior interventricular septum.

Answer C is incorrect. The circumflex artery branches from the left main coronary and courses superiorly posteriorly between the left atrium and ventricle to supply both of these areas.

Answer D is incorrect. The right main coronary artery branches from the aorta near the superior vena cava and hugs the right atrium as it courses toward the posterior side of the heart. It is the main supply to the right atrium and posterior wall of the heart.

Answer E is incorrect. The right marginal artery is a branch of the right main coronary on the inferior-anterior surface of the heart and supplies the right ventricle and apex.

13. **The correct answer is A.** Cimetidine is an H_2 blocker associated with P450 inhibition, antiandrogenic effects, decreased renal excretion of creatinine, and arrhythmias. As a result of P450 inhibition, cimetidine decreases hepatic metabolism of many drugs oxidized by the P450 system, including warfarin, increasing their systemic toxicities. This results in a prolonged prothrombin time.

Answer B is incorrect. Insulin lispro can cause hypoglycemia.

Answer C is incorrect. Metoprolol can be associated with decreased perception of hypoglycemia in diabetics. However, it does not affect warfarin levels.

Answer D is incorrect. NPH insulin can cause hypoglycemia or idiopathic allergic and anaphylactoid reactions.

Answer E is incorrect. Omeprazole is a proton pump inhibitor that is relatively free of adverse effects.

14. **The correct answer is D.** The patient is suffering from rheumatoid arthritis, an autoimmune disorder that targets the synovial lining of distal joints, leading to cartilage destruction, microscopic pannus formation, and eventual bony deformation. Both an antibody- and a T-lymphocyte–mediated immune response have been implicated in the pathogenesis of this disease. In particular, proinflammatory cytokines such as tumor necrosis factor (TNF)-α are believed to play an important role in the maintenance of the immune response within the joint. Etanercept is a recombinant TNF-α receptor:Fc fusion protein that binds TNF-α in vivo, thereby neutralizing its activity. Some patients respond quite well to this treatment, with both drops in subjective pain scores and objective improvements within the joints. Unfortunately, TNF-α plays a major role in the host defense response against certain pathogens, and the occurrence/reactivation of tuberculosis in some patients treated with anti-TNF therapy attests to this.

Answer A is incorrect. Abciximab is a monoclonal antibody that binds to the glycoprotein receptor IIb/IIIa on activated platelets, thus inhibiting interaction between platelets and fibrinogen. While thrombocytopenia is often a side effect of this treatment, abciximab is not an antirheumatic.

Answer B is incorrect. Aldesleukin is recombinant interleukin (IL)-2 and is used clinically as adjuvant therapy for renal cell carcinoma and metastatic melanoma. While fever is often a side effect of this treatment, it is unlikely that IL-2 therapy would benefit a patient suffering from rheumatoid arthritis; thus, this is not the correct answer choice.

Answer C is incorrect. Myelosuppression is not a common side effect of etanercept treatment.

Answer E is incorrect. Infliximab is a monoclonal antibody to tumor necrosis factor-α and has shown efficacy in the treatment of rheumatoid arthritis. Like etanercept, it acts to neutralize the effect of this proinflammatory cytokine. However, myelosuppression is not a common side effect of infliximab treatment.

15. **The correct answer is A.** Bupropion is an atypical antidepressant that inhibits neuronal uptake, mostly of norepinephrine and dopamine. It is also useful in smoking cessation. Bupropion differs from selective serotonin reuptake inhibitors in that it has few to no sexual side effects.

Answer B is incorrect. Escitalopram is a selective serotonin reuptake inhibitor.

Answer C is incorrect. Fluoxetine is a selective serotonin reuptake inhibitor.

Answer D is incorrect. Reserpine depletes catecholamines and serotonin. It can cause severe depression. It was originally developed for the treatment of hypertension.

Answer E is incorrect. Sertraline is a selective serotonin reuptake inhibitor.

Answer F is incorrect. Trazodone works by inhibiting serotonin reuptake and acting as a partial serotonin agonist. It is useful for the treatment of depression with insomnia. Male patients should be warned of the potential for priapism.

16. **The correct answer is D.** This is a case of Ewing's sarcoma, which can present with symptoms similar to an infection. However, the x-ray describes the classic location and appearance of the sarcoma. Ewing's sarcoma is a small blue cell tumor of childhood that arises in the medullary cavity in the diaphysis of long bones. It is most often found in boys younger than 15 years of age. The periosteal reaction results in reactive bone deposition in an onion-skin manner. The tumor cells carry the t(11;22) translocation, and this would be seen on karyotype.

Answer A is incorrect. t(8;14) is most commonly associated with Burkitt's lymphoma.

Answer B is incorrect. t(9;22), the Philadelphia chromosome, is most commonly associated with chronic myeloid leukemia.

Answer C is incorrect. t(11;14) is associated with mantle cell lymphoma.

Answer E is incorrect. t(14;18) is most commonly associated with *bcl-2* activation in follicular lymphomas.

Answer F is incorrect. t(15;17) is associated with the M3 type of acute myeloid leukemia. This type is treatable by all-trans retinoic acid.

17. **The correct answer is E.** The splenic flexure of the large bowel is vulnerable to ischemia from hypoperfusion because it lies at the junction of two vascular areas, the superior and inferior mesenteric arteries. This watershed phenomenon also occurs in the brain.

Answer A is incorrect. The cecum is supplied by the superior mesenteric artery; it is not a watershed area.

Answer B is incorrect. The hepatic flexure of the large bowel is supplied by the superior mesenteric artery; unlike the splenic flexure, it is not in a border zone between two vascular territories.

Answer C is incorrect. The ileum is supplied by the superior mesenteric artery; it is not in a watershed area.

Answer D is incorrect. The jejunum is supplies by the superior mesenteric artery; it is not a watershed area.

Answer F is incorrect. The stomach is richly supplied by the celiac trunk, it is not a watershed area.

18. **The correct answer is C.** This patient most likely has Marfan's syndrome. Marfan's syndrome is due to a defect in the fibrillin gene, manifested by a deficiency of fibrillin (a glycoprotein constituent of microfibrils).

Answer A is incorrect. Dihydrotestosterone receptor deficiency leads to testicular feminization syndrome (androgen insensitivity). Patients with this condition are normal-looking females with a rudimentary vagina.

Answer B is incorrect. Dystrophin deficiency is seen in Becker's and Duchenne's muscular dystrophy, both of which are progressive degenerative muscular conditions. They are manifested by increasing weakness and paralysis.

Answer D is incorrect. Glucose-6-phosphate dehydrogenase deficiency results in hemolytic anemia when a patient is exposed to oxidizing agents (e.g., fava beans, sulfonamides, or primaquine).

Answer E is incorrect. A deficient LDL receptor manifests as familial hypercholesterolemia, which leads to accelerated atherosclerosis.

19. **The correct answer is C.** Sarcoidosis is a systemic granulomatous disease of unknown origin that particularly involves the lungs. The pathologic hallmark is the presence of noncaseating granulomas. Bilateral hilar adenopathy can be the presenting sign in asymptomatic patients with sarcoidosis. Sarcoidosis is associated with increased levels of angiotensin-converting enzyme (ACE), but testing serum ACE levels does not provide a definitive diagnosis of sarcoidosis because of the relatively low specificity and sensitivity of the test. Nevertheless, for any given test, the positive predictive value (i.e., the probability that a positive test result is truly positive for the disease one is looking for) increases and the negative predictive value (i.e., the probability that a negative test result is a truly negative for the disease one is looking for) decreases as the prevalence of the disease increases. In the United States, sarcoidosis used to be strongly associated with residence in the southeastern United States; however, recent studies have suggested that the disease may be common in other areas as well.

Answer A is incorrect. For any given test, as the prevalence of the disease increases, the positive predictive value increases and the negative predictive value decreases.

Answer B is incorrect. For any given test, as the prevalence of the disease increases, the positive predictive value increases and the negative predictive value decreases.

Answer D is incorrect. For any given test, as the prevalence of the disease increases, the positive predictive value increases and the negative predictive value decreases.

Answer E is incorrect. For any given test, as the prevalence of the disease increases, the positive predictive value increases and the negative predictive value decreases.

20. **The correct answer is D.** A nonsense mutation occurs when a point mutation results in an early stop codon and a truncated protein. In this question, the substitution of thymine for cytosine formed a stop codon.

    Answer A is incorrect. A frameshift mutation is an insertion or deletion of nucleotides that results in a misreading of all codons downstream.

    Answer B is incorrect. An insertion mutation is an addition of one or more nucleotides to the DNA.

    Answer C is incorrect. A missense mutation is a point mutation that causes one amino acid to be replaced by a different amino acid.

    Answer E is incorrect. A silent mutation occurs when a point mutation does not change the amino acid sequence of the protein. The point mutation is often in the third position of the codon.

21. **The correct answer is D.** The pathologist has found an example of metaplasia, which is characterized by one adult cell type being replaced by another cell type. This change is reversible. Normal bronchi are lined with pseudostratified, columnar, ciliated epithelium. Squamous epithelia in the bronchi are not normal and are often a sign of environmental exposure and/or irritation (i.e., smoking).

    Answer A is incorrect. Anaplasia, an irreversible change, describes abnormal cells lacking differentiation. Anaplasia is not the answer, since the squamous cells appear organized and differentiated, although they are in an abnormal location.

    Answer B is incorrect. Dysplasia is abnormal growth with loss of cellular orientation, shape,

and size in comparison to normal tissue maturation. Dysplasia is not the answer, since the squamous cells appear organized and differentiated, although they are in an abnormal location.

Answer C is incorrect. Hyperplasia is an increase in number of the normal cell type.

Answer E is incorrect. Neoplasia describes a clonal proliferation of cells that is uncontrolled and excessive, and in this case the growth is confined above the basement membrane. There is no sign of metastasis, nor is there a sign of uncontrolled proliferation, as there are only a few layers of squamous cells. Like anaplasia, neoplasia is not reversible.

22. **The correct answer is A.** Patients with Cushing's syndrome secondary to a hyperfunctioning adrenal adenoma suffer from symptoms secondary to excessive levels of cortisol in the blood. This results in negative feedback of the cortisol onto the anterior pituitary, leading to adrenal suppression. Such patients require exogenous cortisol to maintain hemodynamic stability in response to stresses such as surgery. Prednisone administered intraoperatively would be the most appropriate agent to prevent hemodynamic instability due to hypocortisolemia.

    Answer B is incorrect. Octreotide is a somatostatin analog that can be used to inhibit secretion of growth hormone and prolactin from the anterior pituitary. It can also inhibit the secretion of gastrin, secretin, cholecystokinin, vasoactive intestinal polypeptide, insulin, glucagon, and pancreatic exocrine enzymes. Octreotide does not have any effect on adrenal cortisol secretion, nor does it have any intrinsic effect on the maintenance of hemodynamic stability.

    Answer C is incorrect. Phenoxybenzamine is an α-specific adrenergic antagonist that acts primarily to cause peripheral vasodilation. Like metoprolol, this agent acts to reduce blood pressure and hence would not be appropriate in the treatment of hypotension, regardless of the cause. Phenoxybenzamine is classically indicated for the treatment of hypertension secondary to pheochromocytoma.

Answer D is incorrect. Phenylephrine is an α-specific adrenergic agonist that primarily stimulates peripheral vasoconstriction, resulting in an increase in blood pressure. Like epinephrine, this agent is effective as a pressor in treating hypotension, but it is not the most appropriate selection because it does not address the primary problem of adrenal suppression.

Answer E is incorrect. Vasopressin acts both to increase water absorption in the renal collecting duct via increased expression of aquaporin channels, and to stimulate peripheral vasoconstriction, although this latter effect is observed only at supraphysiologic concentrations. Although this agent can be used to provide blood pressure support in the treatment of septic shock, it does not address the core problem of adrenal suppression and would not be the most effective agent in this case.

23. **The correct answer is C.** Lactobacilli make up a majority of the normal flora of the vagina. The composition of the normal flora varies from premenarchal, childbearing, and menopausal stages, but a key feature of the normal vaginal environment is a low pH (6.5–7), which inhibits growth of other, possibly pathogenic, organisms. This pH is likely maintained by the lactobacilli, and when numbers of these bacteria are reduced during the course of antibiotic treatment (with, for example, tetracycline), the vaginal pH may increase, making conditions favorable for the yeast *Candida albicans* to grow. Symptoms of a yeast infection are as described, and diagnosis is made by 10% potassium hydroxide preparation on which pseudohyphae are seen.

Answer A is incorrect. *Bacteroides* is an anaerobe and a major colonizer of the colon.

Answer B is incorrect. *Candida* is the yeast that is most likely to cause the symptoms described in the stem. Although many women are colonized with *Candida* (specifically *C. albicans*), most do not experience symptoms unless conditions in the vagina change to allow overgrowth of the organism.

Answer D is incorrect. Staphylococci are not a majority of the flora in the vagina but may be found around the external vaginal opening, as staphylococci are normal skin flora.

Answer E is incorrect. *Trichomonas* is a pathogenic protozoan and is never considered normal flora. It is responsible for causing symptoms of frothy, foul-smelling discharge, along with itching and burning on urination. Motile parasites are seen on wet mount.

24. **The correct answer is B.** The screening test results were positive in 80 of the 100 patients with β-thalassemia. Sensitivity = 80 / 100 = 80%.

Answer A is incorrect. Calculation error.

Answer C is incorrect. 87% is the answer one would arrive at if the seven false positives were not recognized.

Answer D is incorrect. Positive predictive value = 80/87 = 92%.

Answer E is incorrect. Sensitivity = 99,893/ 99,900 = 99.99%.

25. **The correct answer is B.** Cyanide modifies the iron within cytochrome oxidase (cytochrome aa_3) in the mitochondria, thereby abnormally interrupting the electron transport chain and halting cellular respiration. Tissues with the highest oxygen demands, such as the heart, brain, and liver, are most significantly affected because cyanide prevents oxygen from binding to cytochrome oxidase and serving as the final electron acceptor in the chain.

Answer A is incorrect. Substances such as ammonia or chlorine cause direct injury to exposed tissues. Symptoms include shortness of breath, severe throat pain, vomiting, and coughing up blood, but the ocular symptoms in this patient are not characteristic of this type of poisoning.

Answer C is incorrect. Sarin gas irreversibly inhibits acetylcholinesterase, resulting in an overload of acetylcholine at synapses. As a result, the body experiences a parasympathetic overload and flaccid paralysis. Symptoms of sarin poisoning depend on the degree of exposure and the form of the toxin; they resemble some of the symptoms this patient is experiencing. However, the circumstances of his injury point to a side effect of smoke inhalation as opposed to poisoning with a biological warfare agent.

Answer D is incorrect. While the patient's increased heart rate and tachypnea could be explained by an increase in sympathetic nervous system activity achieved by epinephrine release, this is not the mechanism of action of cyanide.

Answer E is incorrect. Alkylating or blister agents are so called because they penetrate the skin and mucous membranes and cause large blisters to form all over the exposed individual's body. The mechanism of action is interference with DNA synthesis. However, this patient lacks the characteristic dermal symptoms.

26. **The correct answer is B.** While HLA-DR3– and/or HLA-DR4–positive individuals are at increased risk for developing type 1 (insulin-dependent) diabetes, the causal nature of this association is still being researched. The DR locus is one of the class II major histocompatibility complex alleles, and therefore presents peptides to CD4+ T lymphocytes. It should also be noted that carriers of the DR2 allele are less susceptible to type 1 diabetes. The answer to this question can be resolved based on genetic principles: (1) The probability that the proband's mother is homozygous HLA-DR4 is 1/4. The probability that this allele is passed on to the proband is 1. Thus, the probability of both events is 1/4. (2) The probability that the proband's mother harbors one HLA-DR4 allele is 1/2. The probability that this allele is passed on to the proband is 1/2. Thus, the probability of both events is 1/4. (3) Therefore, the probability that the proband will inherit an HLA-DR4 allele from his mother is 1/4 + 1/4 = 1/2. (4) The probability that the proband's father harbors one DR3 allele is 1/2. The probability that this allele is passed on to the proband is 1/2. Thus, the probability of both events is 1/4. (5) Therefore, the probability that the proband will inherit a HLA-DR3 allele from his father is 1/4. The probability that HLA-DR3 is inherited from the father and that HLA-DR4 is inherited from the mother is = (1/4) × (1/2) = 1/8.

Answer A is incorrect. The probability is not zero.

Answer C is incorrect. The probability is not 1/4.

Answer D is incorrect. The probability is not 1/2.

Answer E is incorrect. The probability is not 1.

27. **The correct answer is D.** Clomiphene acts as an antiestrogen by binding receptor sites. It successfully treats women with anovulatory cycles but is not effective in women whose infertility is secondary to a pituitary abnormality. Other adverse effects of clomiphene include ovarian enlargement and visual disturbances.

Answer A is incorrect. Disturbances in color vision are an adverse effect of sildenafil, a muscle relaxant used to treat erectile dysfunction.

Answer B is incorrect. Nasal congestion, orthostasis, nausea, and headache may occur with cabergoline in the treatment of infertility due to hyperprolactinoma. Cabergoline is an ergoline derivative with potent inhibitory effects on prolactin secretion.

Answer C is incorrect. Nausea and vomiting are common adverse effects of estrogen therapy, not antiestrogen therapy. Estrogen therapy can be used for postmenopausal hormone therapy and hypogonadism.

Answer E is incorrect. Weight gain and fluid retention are adverse effects of gonadotropins, which can be used to increase ovarian follicular maturation.

28. **The correct answer is B.** This man may have been bitten by a rabid animal. The best prophylaxis for rabies infection is immediate administration of human rabies immune globulin to provide passive immunity, followed with a series of five injections of killed rabies virus vaccinations to develop active immunity. The idea is to provide immunity while the patient is still in the incubation period.

Answer A is incorrect. If the patient develops symptoms, the disease will have progressed to an incurable stage.

Answer C is incorrect. The administration of human rabies immune globulin is not the best course of action, because it does not provide long-term active immunity.

Answer D is incorrect. If the patient develops symptoms, the disease will have progressed to an incurable stage.

Answer E is incorrect. Providing the killed rabies virus vaccine first and following with a series of human rabies immune globulin does not give immediate passive immunity and is not the standard of care.

Answer F is correct. Although rabies is not curable after symptoms develop, it is possible to provide immunity to a patient who has been exposed before the virus replicates enough to cause disease. Therefore, doing nothing is not the appropriate response.

29. **The correct answer is C.** This patient has symptoms consistent with polymyalgia rheumatica (PMR) and giant cell arteritis (temporal arteritis). She requires immediate steroids for treatment and subsequent temporal artery biopsy to confirm the diagnosis. PMR occurs in 50% of patients with temporal arteritis and involves symmetrical aching of the proximal muscles and girdle stiffness. The elevated erythrocyte sedimentation rate indicates a generalized inflammatory process, and additional evidence is provided by the new-onset jaw claudication and constitutional symptoms that usually present in patients with temporal arteritis.

Answer A is incorrect. Analysis of joint fluid would be neither diagnostic nor possible in this patient because she is only currently suffering from synovitis of her wrists and ankles.

Answer B is incorrect. Mesenteric angiography is the primary imaging modality used to determine the presence of aneurysms and vessel narrowing in patients with polyarteritis nodosa (PAN). PAN is a necrotizing vasculitis that typically presents with constitutional signs as well as with myalgias, arthralgias, and fatigue. This patient's girdle stiffness and jaw claudication are not consistent with this diagnosis.

Answer D is incorrect. Testing for anti–double-stranded DNA and antinuclear antibody levels would be appropriate to diagnose lupus, which is uncommon in patients this age and does not involve jaw claudication.

Answer E is incorrect. Testing for rheumatoid factor and anti–cytidine cyclic phosphate levels would be appropriate to diagnose rheumatoid arthritis, which may produce symmetrical and proximal joint symptoms. However, rheumatoid arthritis does not cause jaw claudication and is not usually associated with an elevated erythrocyte sedimentation rate.

30. **The correct answer is B.** This patient has a typical presentation of acute pulmonary edema. Common causes include myocardial ischemia, acute aortic insufficiency, acute mitral regurgitation, renovascular hypertension, or acute decompensation of chronic congestive heart failure. Loop diuretics such as furosemide are the normal treatments of choice for this condition. Ethacrynic acid is a diuretic similar in action to furosemide but without sulfa adverse effects such as rash or acute interstitial nephritis, and is therefore used in persons with a sulfa allergy. Other adverse effects, including ototoxicity, metabolic alkalosis, hypokalemia, hyperglycemia, and hyperuricemia are shared with furosemide. The patient is suffering from ototoxicity and hypokalemia, leading to the hearing and muscle disturbances, respectively.

Answer A is incorrect. Acetazolamide causes hyperchloremic metabolic acidosis and neuropathy.

Answer C is incorrect. Furosemide has an adverse event profile very similar to that of ethacrynic acid, but also causes sulfa allergy, and thus would be contraindicated in this patient.

Answer D is incorrect. Hydrochlorothiazide causes hypokalemic alkalosis, hyponatremia, hyperglycemia, hyperlipidemia, hyperuricemia, and hypercalcemia as well as sulfa allergy.

Answer E is incorrect. Spironolactone causes hyperkalemia and antiandrogen effects.

31. **The correct answer is D.** St. Louis encephalitis virus is the most common cause of epidemic encephalitis in the United States. Treatment is supportive, since there are no antiviral medications for this virus. It can occur throughout the United States but is more prevalent in the Mississippi–Ohio River valley. The positive Kernig's sign suggests meningeal irritation. The sign is elicited by flexing the patient's leg at both the hip and knee; straightening the knee from this position elicits pain.

Answer A is incorrect. Eastern equine encephalitis virus is a member of the Togaviridae virus family. It is a mosquito-borne virus that causes encephalitis and is most prevalent in the eastern United States.

Answer B is incorrect. Japanese encephalitis virus is a flavivirus that causes encephalitis throughout Asia. It infects horses and pigs as well as humans.

Answer C is incorrect. Poliovirus is a member of the Picornaviridae family. It is an enterovirus that causes paralytic poliomyelitis.

Answer E is incorrect. Western equine encephalitis virus is a member of the Togaviridae virus family. It is a mosquito-borne virus that causes encephalitis and is most prevalent in the western United States and Canada.

32. **The correct answer is D.** The four polypeptide chains that make up hemoglobin are arranged in different relative positions, depending on whether the molecule is deoxyhemoglobin or oxyhemoglobin. The taut (T) form of hemoglobin is the deoxy form. The movement of the polypeptide chains is restricted and hemoglobin is in its low-oxygen-affinity state. When hemoglobin binds oxygen, certain bonds between the polypeptide chains are ruptured, leading to the relaxed (R) form. In the R form, the polypeptide chains have greater ability to move and also have a higher oxygen affinity. A good way to remember this fact is that you get very **T**ense when you can't breathe, but you **R**elax when you can.

Answer A is incorrect. In the relaxed (R) form, hemoglobin is in its oxygenated state and has high oxygen affinity.

Answer B is incorrect. When in the relaxed form, the polypeptide chains move more easily, allowing them to have higher, rather than lower, oxygen affinity.

Answer C is incorrect. In the taut (T) form, hemoglobin is in its deoxy state and has low, rather than high, oxygen affinity.

Answer E is incorrect. In its taut (T) form, hemoglobin is in its deoxy form with a low oxygen affinity.

Answer F is correct. Hemoglobin is in its deoxy state in the taut (T) form, rather than the relaxed form. In this state the movement of the polypeptide chains is restricted.

33. **The correct answer is A.** The vignette describes a presentation of prolactinoma, the most common tumor of the pituitary gland. Signs and symptoms are a consequence of excessive prolactin secretion and local mass effects, specifically compression of suprasellar structures in the brain. Among these structures is the optic chiasm, which is situated just superior to the pituitary gland. Early compression of the optic chiasm results in a superior bitemporal quadrantanopia due to impingement onto the lower surface of the chiasm, eventually leading to the classic finding of a bitemporal hemianopsia with further compression. This often causes patients to miss objects that present in their temporal fields, such as door frames.

Answer B is incorrect. Dysphagia can occur with compression or ischemia of the medulla or the motor cortex within the parietal lobe. A tumor of the pituitary generally would not result in this finding.

Answer C is incorrect. Hydrocephalus usually occurs due to obstruction of cerebrospinal fluid (CSF) outflow from the cerebral ventricular system or due to impaired CSF absorption by the arachnoid granulations. While obstruction of the CSF outflow is a plausible consequence of intracranial mass effect, compression of the optic chiasm, hypothalamus, and other structures immediately surrounding the pituitary gland would produce marked symptoms prompting presentation well before a pituitary adenoma could attain the size necessary to cause hydrocephalus.

Answer D is incorrect. Right facial drop can occur due to compression or ischemia of the motor cortex within the parietal lobe, as well as compression or damage to cranial nerve VII (Bell's palsy). However, a tumor of the pituitary generally would not result in this finding.

Answer E is incorrect. Right-handed weakness can occur as the result of tumor compression or infiltration into the motor cortex of the left parietal lobe. However, this finding is more likely in a transient ischemic attack or stroke of the same region. A tumor of the pituitary gland generally cannot cause this finding via local compression of surrounding structures.

34. **The correct answer is A.** This patient is likely suffering from neuroleptic malignant syndrome, a severe and potentially life-threatening extrapyramidal side effect of antipsychotic agents. Classic symptoms of this syndrome include hyperpyrexia, autonomic instability, and severe rigidity. Treatment requires rapid discontinuation of all neuroleptics, supportive care, and the administration of dantrolene, a skeletal muscle relaxant.

Answer B is incorrect. Diazepam is not indicated for the treatment of neuroleptic malignant syndrome.

Answer C is incorrect. Flumazenil, a competitive antagonist at the γ-aminobutyric acid receptor, is used to treat an overdose of benzodiazepines but is not indicated for the treatment of neuroleptic malignant syndrome.

Answer D is incorrect. Haloperidol, a neuroleptic agent, would worsen the symptoms of neuroleptic malignant syndrome and therefore should not be given.

Answer E is incorrect. Phenobarbital, a barbiturate, would not be helpful in a patient who is experiencing neuroleptic malignant syndrome.

35. **The correct answer is A.** Hunter's syndrome is an X-linked disorder that is caused by a deficiency of iduronate sulfatase. Although Hunter's syndrome and Hurler's syndrome are similar, Hunter's syndrome is notable for the absence of corneal clouding, which is present in Hurler's syndrome.

Answer B is incorrect. Hurler's syndrome is a severe disorder with a broad spectrum of clinical findings. It is generally diagnosed within the first year of life and is characterized by a variety of musculoskeletal abnormalities, corneal clouding, hepatosplenomegaly, and severe mental retardation.

Answer C is incorrect. Morquio's syndrome is typically diagnosed around the age of 1 year and is characterized primarily by short stature and joint laxity. Other musculoskeletal abnormalities are also associated with this autosomally transmitted disorder. Some patients demonstrate hepatosplenomegaly, mild corneal clouding, and valvular heart disease.

Answer D is incorrect. There are multiple enzyme deficiencies associated with Sanfilippo's syndrome, but this class of disorders is primarily distinguished by the central nervous system symptoms in these patients. Some of the physical abnormalities seen in the other mucopolysaccharidoses are also observed in Sanfilippo's patients, but the hallmarks of this disease are developmental delay and behavioral problems such as aggressive tendencies and hyperactivity that manifest in early childhood. Sleep disorders are also common in these patients, and the physical findings typically develop after the behavioral and sleep pattern abnormalities.

Answer E is incorrect. Patients with Sly syndrome have a defect in the beta-glucuronidase enzyme and are generally diagnosed as toddlers. The disorder is autosomal recessive, and the presentation can resemble that of Hurler's syndrome. Mental retardation is not a significant component of Sly syndrome, although various musculoskeletal abnormalities are common.

36. **The correct answer is B.** The patient described is infected with *Pneumocystis jiroveci* (formerly *carinii*) pneumonia, which is commonly associated with AIDS and immunosuppression. It is diagnosed with methenamine silver stain of lung biopsy tissue. *P. jiroveci* pneumonia is treated primarily with sulfamethoxazole-trimethoprim, but it can be treated with pentamidine or dapsone. Both sulfamethoxazole and trimethoprim inhibit the folate synthesis pathway. In the folate synthesis pathway, pteridine and PABA are converted to tetrahydrofolate, which is a component of nucleic acids and certain amino acids.

Answer A is incorrect. Many antifungal agents inhibit ergosterol synthesis, including fluconazole and terbinafine. Although *Pneumocystis jiroveci* (formerly *carinii*) is a fungus, antifungals that block ergosterol synthesis are not effective in the treatment of this infection.

Answer C is incorrect. Cell wall synthesis is blocked by many antibiotics, including penicillins, cephalosporins, and vancomycin. Pneumocystis jiroveci (formerly carinii) is a fungus and does not have a cell wall.

Answer D is incorrect. Inhibition of the larger ribosomal subunit (50S) is the mechanism of action of chloramphenicol, erythromycin, clindamycin, and linezolid. None of these is used to treat *Pneumocystis jiroveci* (formerly *carinii*) pneumonia.

Answer E is incorrect. Inhibition of the small ribosomal subunit (30S) is the mechanism of action for many antibiotics, including aminoglycosides and tetracyclines. None of these antibiotics is used for *Pneumocystis jiroveci* (*formerly* carinii) pneumonia.

37. **The correct answer is C.** This patient has injured his finger in an area that receives cutaneous innervation from the median nerve. Lidocaine is best injected near the DIP joint, which is still within the area supplied by the median nerve, to provide anesthesia.

Answer A is incorrect. The lateral aspect of the wrist is supplied by the radial nerve and will not provide anesthesia to the area of injury.

Answer B is incorrect. The medial aspect of the wrist is supplied by the ulnar nerve and will not provide anesthesia to the area of injury.

Answer D is incorrect. The dorsal surface of the digit near the metacarpophalangeal joint is supplied by the radial nerve and will not provide anesthesia to the area of injury.

Answer E is incorrect. The lateral aspect of the forearm is supplied by the lateral cutaneous nerve of the forearm and will not provide anesthesia to the area of injury.

38. **The correct answer is B.** This patient presents with a classic picture of anion-gap metabolic acidosis caused by lactic acidosis. The anion gap is calculated by $([Na^+] - [Cl^-] - [HCO_3^-])$ or in this case, $138 - 103 - 8$, or 27. Normal anion gap is between 10 and 12. Metformin is an oral hypoglycemic medication used by diabetic patients. As it reduces glucose levels, there is a risk for lactic acidosis that is increased in patients with renal or cardiovascular disease.

Answer A is incorrect. Acarbose is an α-glucosidase inhibitor leading to delayed hydrolysis of sugars and absorption of glucose. Toxicity is generally limited to gastrointestinal disturbances.

Answer C is incorrect. Miglitol is an α-glucosidase inhibitor leading to delayed hydrolysis of sugars and absorption of glucose. Toxicity is generally limited to gastrointestinal disturbances.

Answer D is incorrect. Tolbutamide is a sulfonylurea that stimulates endogenous insulin release and is associated with disulfiramlike effects. Second-generation sulfonylureas such as glyburide and glipizide are more commonly associated with hypoglycemia.

Answer E is incorrect. Troglitazone increases peripheral sensitivity to insulin, and adverse effects include hepatotoxicity and weight gain.

39. **The correct answer is D.** Ouabain is an Na^+-K^+-ATPase inhibitor similar to the newly isolated toxin. The Na^+-K^+-ATPase pump in cells is key to the creation of the electrochemical gradient that is needed in order for pumps on the cell surface to work correctly. Na^+-K^+-ATPase pumps are located throughout the body. For example, decreased activity of the Na^+-K^+-ATPase pump in vascular smooth muscle will lead to an increase in the cell sodium concentration due to less extrusion of sodium from the cell. The increase in cell sodium will diminish the gradient, favoring further sodium diffusion into the cell and thus reducing calcium efflux as well, which normally occurs by passive sodium-calcium exchange. The ensuing accumulation of calcium in the cell will then increase vascular resistance and raise systemic blood pressure. By contrast, inhibition of the Na^+-K^+-ATPase pump in the kidney will lead to decreased tubular sodium resorption.

Answer A is incorrect. Albuterol is a β_2 agonist. β_2 Receptors are located primarily in blood vessel walls and in the respiratory tract. Drugs that antagonize β_2 receptors are used in the treatment of asthma.

Answer B is incorrect. Botulinum toxin blocks the release of acetylcholine from presynaptic vesicles. Botulinum toxin is produced by *Clostridium botulinum*, a gram-positive anaerobic bacterium. Botulinum toxin is a neurotoxin that interferes with presynaptic release of acetylcholine from nerve endings and interrupts neuromuscular transmission. In addition, it exerts a blocking action on the parasympathetic nervous system and may inhibit other neurotransmitters or affect transmission of afferent neuronal impulses.

Answer C is incorrect. Cocaine is a catecholamine reuptake inhibitor. Since reuptake is the major mechanism by which neurotransmitters are removed from their active receptor sites, this inhibition results in potentiation of the response to sympathetic stimulation of innervated organs and to infused catecholamine.

Answer E is incorrect. Procainamide is a class Ia sodium channel blocker. It is used primarily as an antiarrhythmic drug. Procainamide decreases myocardial excitability and conduction velocity and may depress myocardial contractility by increasing the electrical stimulation threshold of the ventricle and His-Purkinje system as well as through direct cardiac effects.

40. **The correct answer is E.** Renal tubular acidosis (RTA) is a disorder of renal acidification characterized by non–anion-gap, hyperchloremic metabolic acidosis. There are several types of RTA. Type IV RTA is characterized by impaired ability to secrete sufficient acid into the urine due to hypoaldosteronism. The most common causes of this hyporeninemic hypoaldosteronism are diabetic nephropathy and chronic tubulointerstitial nephro-pathies. Hypoaldosteronism leads to decreased sodium reuptake in the distal convoluted tubule and collecting duct and therefore decreased excretion of potassium (and to some extent hydrogen ions) into the urine. The resulting hyperkalemia generates a shift in hydrogen ions to the extracellular fluid to maintain potassium balance, thus producing a metabolic acidosis. The alkalotic environment in the renal tubule cells, however, inhibits ammonia and hydrogen production and secretion, reducing the kidney's ability to excrete the generated acid. Specifically, low ammonia levels decrease the buffering capacity of the urine for hydrogen ions, and therefore the pH of the urine remains low although few hydrogen ions are secreted. Clinically, hypoaldosteronism therefore presents with elevated serum potassium levels, and urinary pH is < 5.5. Angiotensin-converting enzyme inhibitors, trimethoprim, and heparin can similarly reduce aldosterone production, producing an RTA IV picture.

Answer A is incorrect. This patient presents with a non–anion-gap metabolic acidosis. His anion gap (calculated as [serum Na^+] − [serum Cl^-] - [serum HCO_3^-]) is 12.

Answer B is incorrect. Hyperaldosteronism can promote alkalosis based roughly on the reversal of the arguments described in the correct answer.

Answer C is incorrect. In type I renal tubular acidosis, there is an inability to acidify urine due to inadequate transport of hydrogen ions (failure of the ATPase pump) or back diffusion of ions (increased tight junction permeability). Potassium levels are usually normal or reduced, and urine pH is > 5.5.

Answer D is incorrect. In type II renal tubular acidosis, impaired bicarbonate reabsorption in the proximal tubule is typically observed in childhood with other features of Fanconi's syndrome. Rickets and osteomalacia are commonly associated disorders.

41. **The correct answer is B.** Epstein-Barr virus, the virus that causes infectious mononucleosis, is a rare cause of congenital defects. The other answer choices make up the ToRCHeS diseases, a collection of serious infections of pregnancy that is associated with morbidity and mortality of the fetus and newborn. **ToRCHeS** stands for **T**oxoplasmosis, **R**ubella, **C**ytomegalovirus, **H**erpes/HIV, and **S**yphilis.

Answer A is incorrect. Congenital cytomegalovirus can result in hepatosplenomegaly, jaundice, and brain calcifications.

Answer C is incorrect. Herpes simplex virus can result in a variety of congenital defects, spontaneous abortion, and neonatal encephalitis.

Answer D is incorrect. Congenital HIV results in neonatal AIDS.

Answer E is incorrect. Congenital rubella infection can result in deafness, patent ductus arteriosus, pulmonary artery stenosis, cataracts, and microcephaly.

Answer F is incorrect. Congenital syphilis can result in cranial nerve VIII deafness, mulberry molars, saber shins, saddle nose, and Hutchinson's teeth.

Answer G is incorrect. Congenital toxoplasmosis infection can result in mental retardation and chorioretinitis.

42. **The correct answer is A.** Collagen is a major component of the basement membrane. Neoplastic cells bound to the basement membrane can potentially escape if they can break through it. Aberrant expression of collagenase and hydrolase can confer that ability. Metastasis occurs when these cells escape the confines of the basement membrane, find their way to the lymph or bloodstream, and subsequently adhere to tissues in another part of the body.

Answer B is incorrect. α-Fetoprotein is a normal serum protein produced by fetal yolk sac and liver. In the context of oncology, α-fetoprotein levels can be used to follow the progression of hepatocellular carcinoma.

Answer C is incorrect. γ-Glutamyl transpeptidase (GGT) participates in the transfer of amino acids across the cellular membrane and in the metabolism of glutathione. High concentrations are found in the liver, bile ducts, and kidney. A test for serum GGT is used to detect diseases of the liver, bile ducts, and kidney and to differentiate liver or bile duct (hepatobiliary) disorders from bone disease.

Answer D is incorrect. Keratin is a marker of epithelial differentiation and is not a factor in metastasis.

Answer E is incorrect. Mucin is a nitrogenous substance found in mucous secretions that serves as a lubricant that protects body surfaces. It is often produced by colonic-type adenocarcinomas.

43. **The correct answer is B.** This patient has hereditary nonpolyposis colorectal cancer, which can be caused by an inherited mutation in one of the five DNA mismatch repair genes. The mismatch repair mechanism replaces segments of DNA that include mismatched bases. Without this proofreading function, errors can accumulate in crucial areas, such as cancer suppressor genes and proto-oncogenes.

Answer A is incorrect. A defect in base excision repair results in xeroderma pigmentosum, a disease characterized by extreme sensitivity to sunlight, skin damage, and a predisposition to malignancies such as melanoma.

Answer C is incorrect. Benzo(a)pyrene is a carcinogen found in cigarette smoke. This carcinogen binds to DNA and forms bulky adducts with guanine residues. Bulky lesions are repaired by nucleotide excision.

Answer D is incorrect. The *p53* gene is a tumor suppressor gene that is mutated in more than 50% of all human cancers. Inheriting one mutant *p53* gene places a patient at high risk of developing many different types of cancer by sporadic mutation of the second normal allele. This is known as Li-Fraumeni syndrome.

Answer E is incorrect. The *bcr-abl* hybrid gene is the result of a translocation between chromosomes 9 and 22, t(9;22). Chronic myeloid leukemia is associated with t(9;22), or the Philadelphia chromosome.

44. **The correct answer is A.** Glioblastoma multiforme (GBM) is the most common primary intracranial neoplasm and is typically seen in older patients. Although this neoplasm arises from glial cells, it is impossible to differentiate the specific line. The characteristic features shown in the image include a central area of necrosis surrounded by a hypercellular zone called palisading necrosis. There is also a high degree of anaplasia and pleomorphism. The tumor as a whole shows vascular proliferation and areas of necrosis. Patients with GBM have a very poor prognosis regardless of management.

Answer B is incorrect. Medulloblastomas are tumors that preferentially affect children in the first decade of life and do not typically affect adults. The cells have a characteristic blue appearance and crowd together to form perivascular rosettes or pseudorosettes. They arise from the cerebellum, not the cerebral hemispheres, and commonly block the fourth ventricle, resulting in an obstructive hydrocephalus.

Answer C is incorrect. Meningiomas are the second most common primary intracranial tumors in adults and are typically benign and slow-growing. They commonly affect people in the fourth and fifth decades of life but can affect younger adults as well and are seen more frequently in women than men. They can arise from any portion of the meninges and classically exhibit calcified whorls called psammoma bodies on histologic examination.

Answer D is incorrect. Neurilemmomas are benign tumors arising from Schwann cells associated with cranial nerve VIII (appropriately, they are also called acoustic schwannomas). They are the third most common primary intracranial tumor in adults and, if bilateral, are associated with neurofibromatosis type 2. The two typical patterns seen histologically are either a compact palisading nuclei (Antoni A) or a loose arrangement of cells (Antoni B).

Answer E is incorrect. Oligodendrogliomas are generally benign, slow-growing tumors that arise from oligodendrocytes, which are found in the cerebral hemispheres. They are the fourth most common primary intracranial tumors and typically have the appearance of a fried egg with interspersed chicken wire.

45. **The correct answer is E.** Natural killer (NK) cells are a component of the innate immune system. These cells have a battery of germline-encoded activating and inhibitory receptors that can detect and distinguish virally infected cells from uninfected cells. For example, virally infected cells often express less major histocompatibility complex class I on their surface, and this absence is detected by the NK cell. Detection of a virally infected cell signals the NK cell to release cytotoxic granules onto the infected cell, and thus they play a direct and important role in controlling the early stages of systemic response to viral infection. It should be noted that individuals with defective NK-cell function are particularly susceptible to herpes virus infection. This suggests that NK cells play an important, nonredundant physiologic function in the control of this family of viral infections.

Answer A is incorrect. Eosinophils are important effector cells in host defense against parasites.

Answer B is incorrect. Mast cells control the early inflammatory response by release of potent vasoactive granules.

Answer C is incorrect. Megakaryocytes are resident bone marrow cells that give rise to platelets.

Answer D is incorrect. Microglias are tissue macrophages located within the central nervous system and do not play as direct a role in the control of systemic viral infections as natural killer cells do.

Answer F is incorrect. Plasma cells are antibody-producing B cells and an important component of the adaptive immune system.

Answer G is incorrect. Regulatory T lymphocytes are components of the adaptive immune response that have been shown to suppress effector T-lymphocyte functions in both an antigen-specific and antigen-nonspecific manner.

46. **The correct answer is E.** The child is presenting with DiGeorge's syndrome, which is due to abnormal development of the third and fourth branchial (pharyngeal) pouches. This leads to hypoplasia of the thymus and parathyroid glands. Without a properly functioning thymus, T-lymphocyte maturation fails, resulting in impaired cell-mediated immunity. Thus, patients with DiGeorge's syndrome often present with recurrent viral and fungal infections, as in this patient. Without adequate production of parathyroid hormone, these patients are often hypocalcemic, leading to tetany and seizures. DiGeorge's syndrome can be summarized by the mnemonic **CATCH-22**: Cardiac defects, Abnormal facies, Thymic hypoplasia, Cleft palate, and Hypocalcemia due to a microdeletion on chromosome **22**.

Answer A is incorrect. The first aortic arch gives rise to part of the maxillary artery, while the second aortic arch gives rise to the stapedial artery and the hyoid artery. They are not involved in DiGeorge's syndrome.

Answer B is incorrect. The first and second branchial arches play no role in DiGeorge's syndrome. For first-arch derivatives, think "M": Mandible, Malleus, sphenoMandibular ligament; muscles of Mastication (teMporalis, Masseter, Medial and lateral pterygoids). The first arch is associated with cranial nerve V. For second-arch derivatives, think "S": Stapes, Styloid process, Stylohyoid ligament; muscles of facial expression, Stapedius, Stylohyoid. Cranial nerve VII is associated with the second arch.

Answer C is incorrect. The fourth and sixth pharyngeal arches do not have a part in DiGeorge's syndrome. The fourth arch is responsible for muscles of the soft palate (but not the tensor veli palatini, a first arch derivative), the muscles of the pharynx (except the stylopharyngeus), the cricothyroid, and the aortic arch. Fourth-arch muscles are innervated by the superior laryngeal branch of cranial nerve X. The sixth arch produces the muscles of the larynx, except for the cricothyroid, as well as the pulmonary arteries. These muscles are innervated by the recurrent laryngeal branch of cranial nerve X.

Answer D is incorrect. The second through fourth branchial clefts form temporary sinuses but are obliterated before maturation. Thus, they have no derivatives in the adult.

47. **The correct answer is A.** The CDC reports that if stuck by an infected needle, there is up to a 30% chance of contracting hepatitis B, while there is only a 10% chance of contracting hepatitis C. OSHA reports that the chance of actually becoming infected with HIV if you are accidentally stuck with a needle used on an HIV patient is between 0.3% and 0.45%.

Answer B is incorrect. One has only a 0.3–0.45% chance of being infected with HIV if accidentally stuck, versus a 10% chance of infection if stuck with a hepatitis C–infected needle.

Answer C is incorrect. One has a 10% chance of being infected with hepatitis C if accidentally stuck, versus up to a 30% chance of infection if stuck with a needle contaminated with hepatitis B.

Answer D is incorrect. One has a 10% chance of being infected with hepatitis C if accidentally stuck, versus up to a 30% chance of infection if stuck with a hepatitis B–infected needle.

Answer E is incorrect. One has up to a 30% chance of being infected with hepatitis B if accidentally stuck, versus a 0.3–0.45% chance of being infected with HIV if accidentally stuck.

48. **The correct answer is C.** The potency of inhaled anesthetics is quantified as the minimum alveolar concentration (MAC). This is the concentration of inhaled gas that is needed to eliminate movement among 50% of patients who are challenged by surgical incision. For potent anesthetics, the MAC will be numerically small, meaning that it is inversely proportional to the anesthetic's potency. Drug C, which has the smallest MAC value, is thus the most potent. The blood solubility of an anesthetic is the physical property that determines both speed of induction and time to recovery. Drugs with low blood solubility, such as nitrous oxide, will rapidly induce anesthesia, and patients will recover quickly. In contrast, an anesthetic gas with high blood solubility, such as halothane, will have a longer time to induction and a slower time to recovery. Therefore, drug C, which has the lowest blood solubility, will have the most rapid induction.

Answer A is incorrect. The minimum alveolar concentration (MAC) for a drug is inversely related to its potency. Drug A has a larger MAC than drug D and will be less potent than drug D.

Answer B is incorrect. Drug B, with a solubility of 1.0 (100% soluble in blood), will dissolve completely in the bloodstream, whereas drug C, with its solubility value of 0.1, will be only 10% dissolved in blood. Drug B is more soluble than Drug C.

Answer D is incorrect. An anesthetic with greater blood solubility will have a more rapid induction time. Drug D, which is more soluble in blood than drug C, will therefore induce anesthesia less rapidly than drug C.

Answer E is incorrect. Recovery time from anesthesia is based on the blood solubility of a gas. Gases with high blood solubility result in slower recovery when compared with drugs that have lower blood solubility. Drug B has the highest blood solubility of all those that are listed and thus will have the slowest recovery time of all.

49. **The correct answer is F.** This patient presents with findings consistent with myelofibrosis (or agnogenic myeloid metaplasia), a clonal hematopoietic stem cell disorder resulting in chronic myeloproliferation and atypical megakaryocytic hyperplasia. These clonally expanded megakaryocytes secrete growth factors secondarily, which induces fibroblastic proliferation and bone marrow fibrosis. Fibrosis seen on bone marrow biopsy is diagnostic for myelofibrosis and leads to impaired hematopoiesis, severe anemia, and thrombocytopenia. The classical findings on peripheral blood smear are (1) a leukoerythroblastic smear (nucleated RBCs and left-shifted WBCs), (2) large, abnormal platelets, and (3) teardrop cells (also called dacryocytes).

Answer A is incorrect. Acanthocytes, spiny-shaped RBCs, are seen in A-β-lipoproteinemia.

Answer B is incorrect. Macro-ovalocytes are seen in megaloblastic anemia.

Answer C is incorrect. Schistocytes are seen in microangiopathic hemolytic anemias, including disseminated intravascular coagulation; thrombotic thrombocytopenic purpura; hemolysis, elevated liver enzymes, and low platelet count syndrome of pregnancy; and anemia secondary to artificial heart valves.

Answer D is incorrect. Spherocytes are consistent with autoimmune hemolytic anemia (Coombs' positive) or hereditary spherocytosis (Coombs' negative).

Answer E is incorrect. Target cells are seen in liver disease, thalassemia, and hemoglobin C.

FULL-LENGTH EXAM

Test Block 6

50. **The correct answer is C.** If the patient does not want an abortion, the physician does not perform one. It is appropriate to discuss all the options with the patient and the family, but ultimately it is the patient's decision.

Answer A is incorrect. Persons with mental retardation and diminished mental faculties usually retain competency to make medical decisions. Consulting a judge in this case is probably unnecessary.

Answer B is incorrect. There is no reason to suspect that the child will not be cared for appropriately, but a discussion of options for raising this child is reasonable.

Answer D is incorrect. In many states, a minor requires parental consent to have an abortion performed. However, decisions involving medical care of a pregnant minor, including the decision to have an abortion, are made by the patient.

Answer E is incorrect. A positive urine β-human chorionic gonadotropin (β-hCG) test implies significant elevation. This test is both sensitive and specific. An additional serum β-hCG elevation confirms any question of a pregnancy. It is not necessary to repeat these tests.

Test Block 7

1. A 23-year-old woman is 39 weeks pregnant with her first child when she begins to feel ill. She is mildly febrile, has pain on urination, and feels she must urinate approximately 10 times a day. With a long history of urinary tract infections, she quickly recognizes the symptoms. She begins taking medication left over from her last urinary tract infection and continues to use it through her delivery. At term, her baby has an Apgar score of 9 at 5 minutes, begins breast-feeding well, makes normal cooing noises, and has mild jaundice around the abdomen. Five days later, the mother brings the infant to the emergency department stating that the baby has become fussy, refuses feeding, and wails at a high pitch. He soon becomes extremely lethargic and stops producing urine. Which of the following medications did this patient's mother most likely take to treat her urinary tract infection?

(A) Amoxicillin
(B) Ampicillin
(C) Nitrofurantoin
(D) Ofloxacin
(E) Trimethoprim-sulfamethoxazole

2. A physician is performing blood work on another physician. Through the blood work, the physician discovers that the patient is HIV-positive. The physician is practicing medicine in a state that does not require routine reporting of HIV-positive results. What is the appropriate course of action regarding reporting of his HIV status?

(A) No reporting is necessary
(B) Report his status to his sexual partner
(C) Report his status to other patients
(D) Report his status to the appropriate medical association
(E) Report his status to the appropriate medical licensing board

3. A 9-year-old boy with no vaccine history presents with an erythematous maculopapular rash that erupted about 5 days after the onset of cough, conjunctivitis, coryza, high fever, and white spots on the buccal mucosa. In order for this patient to activate his T-lymphocytes to manage this infection (caused by a paramyxovirus), two signals are required. Which of the following types of cells are the most capable of providing both of these signals?

(A) Activated B lymphocytes, other T lymphocytes, and natural killer cells
(B) Activated CD8+ T lymphocytes, B lymphocytes, and dendritic cells
(C) Activated macrophages, epithelial cells, and B lymphocytes
(D) Activated macrophages, Langerhans cells, and B lymphocytes
(E) Activated macrophages, Langerhans cells, and natural killer cells

4. An Ashkenazi Jewish couple expecting their first child presents to the physician with concerns about their baby's health. The woman says that she had a sister who died at age 2 years. She says that her sister was healthy at birth but weakened over the first few months of her life and died of pneumonia. When questioned further, she says she remembers her sister having a "large head" as an infant. The man adds that he had an uncle who also died as a toddler. He had been told that the baby was blind and developed seizures toward the end of his life. Which of the following represents the likelihood that this couple's child will be affected by this condition?

(A) 3%
(B) 25%
(C) 50%
(D) 100%
(E) Same as the population prevalence

5. A 29-year-old woman who is 36 weeks pregnant presents to the emergency department experiencing contractions that are only 5 minutes apart. She is somewhat distraught because her first pregnancy 2 years ago ended in a mis-

carriage. Nevertheless, she delivers an apparently healthy baby boy. During the initial survey, the OB/GYN resident notes that the baby has good color and is crying loudly but seems unable to move either of his legs very well. X-rays reveal healing fractures bilaterally in the femoral shaft and new fractures in the right tibia. This infant would be expected to have mutations in the gene(s) for which of the following?

(A) Hydroxyapatite
(B) Type I collagen
(C) Type II collagen
(D) Type III collagen
(E) Type IV collagen
(F) Type X collagen

6. A 33-year-old man who is HIV-positive presents to the physician with a 3-week history of sore throat and dysphagia. On physical examination, his oral mucosa is erythematous and friable, with white patches that bleed when he picks at them. Laboratory tests reveal a CD4+ cell count of 100/μL (normal 440–1600/μL) and a CD8+ cell count of 300/μL (normal 180–850/μL). Which of the following pathogenic organisms is most likely responsible for this patient's condition?

(A) *Candida albicans*
(B) Cytomegalovirus
(C) Herpes simplex virus type 1
(D) JC virus
(E) *Pneumocystis jiroveci*

7. A 63-year-old man presents to his primary care physician complaining of weakness, weight loss, and left upper quadrant pain. Physical examination demonstrates diffuse lymphadenopathy and splenomegaly. A laboratory study shows lymphocytosis; peripheral blood smear shows increased neutrophils and metamyelocytes with the Philadelphia chromosome. A diagnosis of chronic myelogenous leukemia is made. Which of the following could be used in the treatment of this condition?

(A) Imatinib mesylate
(B) Infliximab

(C) Paclitaxel
(D) Propylthiouracil
(E) Tamoxifen

8. A 56-year-woman with a history of advanced cervical cancer that was treated with radiotherapy and chemotherapy is admitted to the hospital for worsening symptoms of abdominal pain and vomiting over a 3-day period. The patient's blood pressure is 108/75 mm Hg supine and 95/60 mm Hg standing. Laboratory studies are as follows:

pH: 7.64
BUN: 31 mg/dL
Creatinine: 1.2 mg/dL
Na+: 141 mEq/L
K+: 3.3 mEq/L
Cl-: 90 mEq/L
Total CO_2: 35 mEq/L
Urine pH: 5.1
Urine Na+: 10 mEq/L

Which of the following is the most likely cause of the acidic urine?

(A) The paraneoplastic effects of the cancer
(B) The patient has a history of chemotherapy
(C) The patient is hypokalemic
(D) The patient is in prerenal failure due to hypotension
(E) The patient's hypotension has led to a lactic acidosis

9. A 54-year-old woman with a history of breast cancer has had a surgical lumpectomy with radical axillary node dissection. A neck exploration was performed for an enlarged cervical node secondary to concern about metastatic disease. Several weeks into her subsequent radiation treatment, she presents with a swollen right arm and swollen fingers along with right facial edema that is most pronounced around the orbit. Which of the following is the most likely cause of these findings?

(A) Deep venous thrombosis of the cephalic vein
(B) Disruption of the right lymphatic duct
(C) Disruption of the thoracic duct
(D) Metastatic disease to the humerus
(E) Normal side effect of radiation

10. A 35-year-old woman patient in a psychiatric hospital is interviewed by a medical student. The patient has no complaints and feels "exuberantly jolly," although she is annoyed at being in the hospital. A history given by the patient's husband indicates that about 3 weeks ago, the woman began acting differently. She did not sleep more than 2 hours a night in the 2 weeks prior to admission. She also spent most of their life savings ($20,000) during this time. He says that this behavior is completely unlike her normal behavior. While in the hospital, the patient has required medication to sleep nightly. She has also exhibited loud speech and thoughts of grandiosity. Which of the following is the most likely diagnosis?

(A) Amphetamine intoxication
(B) Bipolar disorder
(C) Hyperthyroidism
(D) Schizoaffective disorder
(E) Schizophrenia

11. A 68-year-old white man with a history of diabetes mellitus, hypertension, increased cholesterol, sedentary lifestyle, and 40-year smoking history comes into the office complaining of severe substernal chest pressure that resolved when he sat down and relaxed. The patient states that he has "always" had episodes like this but they have not caused this much distress. Angina caused by silent myocardial is-

chemia is suspected. An ECG is performed and the patient is recommended to have an exercise stress test. Which of the following is a physiologic response to exercise?

(A) Decreased arterial pH with strenuous exercise
(B) Decreased O_2 consumption
(C) Increased hypoxic vasoconstriction
(D) No change in venous partial carbon dioxide pressure
(E) Pulmonary blood flow remains unchanged

12. A 12-year-old girl with severe anemia, neutropenia, and thrombocytopenia is brought to an inpatient pediatric unit by her mother. Bone marrow biopsy shows hypercellularity with fatty infiltration. The patient's mother says that she received a course of antibiotics 3 weeks ago. Which of the following medications is most likely to cause the findings seen in this patient?

(A) Chloramphenicol
(B) Ciprofloxacin
(C) Clindamycin
(D) Erythromycin
(E) Gentamicin
(F) Tetracycline

13. A couple has four children. Two of the children suffer from severe erythema and scaling on sun-exposed areas of their bodies. The other two children and both parents are unaffected. One of the affected children later develops melanoma, and the other develops squamous cell carcinoma. The two affected children most likely have a genetic defect in which of the following pathways?

(A) DNA excision repair
(B) Double-stranded DNA break sensing
(C) Glycolytic
(D) Heme synthesis
(E) Purine salvage pathway

14. An infant is born with a defect in his abdominal wall. Studies confirm that the discharge from this defect is urine. Which of the following is the postnatal derivative of the structure with the defect?

(A) Fossa ovalis
(B) Ligamentum teres hepatis
(C) Medial umbilical ligament
(D) Median umbilical ligament
(E) Nucleus pulposus

15. A physician is setting up to perform a therapeutic thoracentesis on a patient with stage IV ovarian cancer. She drapes the patient and inserts the needle in the midaxillary line on the right side, immediately superior to the tenth rib. Which of the following structures is she trying to avoid by inserting the needle here instead of higher in this intercostal space?

(A) Ninth intercostal nerve, artery, and vein
(B) Phrenic nerve
(C) Right pericardiophrenic artery and vein
(D) Right recurrent laryngeal nerve
(E) Tenth intercostal nerve, artery, and vein

16. A 55-year-old man is found to have a singular thyroid nodule during a routine visit to his primary care physician. Fine needle aspiration biopsy shows cells with large nuclei and a "ground glass" appearance of the cytoplasm. A section from the resected tumor is shown in the image; it demonstrates a laminated, concentric calcified deposit of infracted tumor cells, which is found in approximately 50% of thyroid cancers of this type. The patient is informed that this type of thyroid cancer has a

better prognosis than other forms of thyroid cancer and that resection of the mass is frequently curative. In which of the following tumors can the histologic finding shown in the image also be found?

(A) Adenocarcinoma of the lung
(B) Dysgerminoma
(C) Follicular carcinoma of the thyroid
(D) Medullary carcinoma of the thyroid
(E) Mesothelioma

17. A woman is concerned about her risks for developing cervical cancer. Which of the following factors poses the largest risk for developing cervical cancer?

(A) Alcoholism
(B) Early sexual activity
(C) Low-fiber diet
(D) Nulliparity
(E) Prolonged estrogen use

18. A 12-year-old boy with moderate mental retardation comes to the physician because of painful swollen joints. During the examination, the physician notices that the boy makes several uncontrolled spastic muscle movements. Past medical history includes a diagnosis of muscular hypotonia at 5 months of age. At 3 years of age, the patient was referred to a pediatric dentist for severe repetitive biting of his lip and tongue. Which of the following is the most likely cause of these findings?

(A) A deficiency of adenosine deaminase
(B) A deficiency of β-glucocerebroside
(C) A mutation of an enzyme in the de novo biosynthetic pathway
(D) Absence of hypoxanthine guanine phosphoribosyltransferase
(E) An excision repair enzyme deficiency

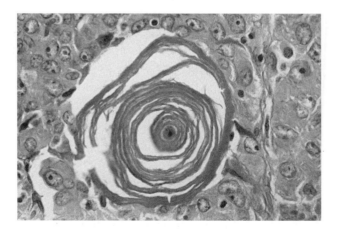

Image courtesy of Armed Forces Institute of Pathology.

19. A 40-year-old woman visits her physician with complaints of dry mouth, chronic cough, difficulty swallowing, and a "sandy" sensation in her eyes, especially in the morning. The patient's physical examination and review of systems are unremarkable except for low-grade fevers and recent onset of joint pain. Which of the following additional conditions is this patient most likely to develop?

(A) Dental caries
(B) Hyperglycemia
(C) Jaundice
(D) Septic joints
(E) Vision loss

20. A 45-year-old man who is of Scandinavian descent presents to the physician with hematuria, left-sided flank pain, and a palpable mass in his left flank. He undergoes a kidney biopsy and is diagnosed with renal cell carcinoma. Radiographic findings suggest metastatic disease to his lung. He is initiated on a chemotherapy regimen that includes an interleukin-2 (IL-2). Which of the following is the mechanism of action of interleukin-2 (IL-2)?

(A) Activation of lymphoid cells
(B) Blocking the ATP-binding site in the Bcr-Abl tyrosine kinase
(C) Causing a decreased blood supply to the tumor
(D) Directly interfering with tumor cell proliferation
(E) Inhibition of monoamine oxidase

21. When conducting a clinical trial on a new asthma drug, a nonblinded physician participating in the study has noticed benefits in patients who are taking the drug rather than the placebo. Knowing that the experimental drug is actually beneficial, he begins to unconsciously assign newly enrolled patients with more severe asthma to the experimental group rather than the placebo group. Which of the following types of bias is this?

(A) Late-look bias
(B) Length bias
(C) Recall bias

(D) Sampling bias
(E) Selection bias

22. A 60-year-old man who is being treated for multiple myeloma develops osteonecrosis of his maxilla. His presentation is significant for a molar tooth extraction site that has displayed poor healing 4 months after surgery. Localized swelling, exposed bone, erythema, and a purulent discharge are noted on intraoral examination. Which of the following drug classes is most likely associated with this lesion?

(A) Angiotensin converting enzyme inhibitors
(B) Bisphosphonates
(C) Cephalosporins
(D) Osmotic diuretics
(E) Vinca alkaloids

23. The sexually indifferent embryo contains several structures that will develop into male or female reproductive organs depending on hormonal influence. From which of the following embryonic structures is the clitoris derived?

(A) Genital tubercle
(B) Labioscrotal swellings
(C) Mesonephric (wolffian) duct
(D) Paramesonephric (müllerian) duct
(E) Urogenital folds

24. A town with 1000 citizens has a 10% prevalence of disease X. A screening test for disease X was just developed, with a sensitivity of 80% and a specificity of 70%. How many people without disease X will be falsely diagnosed positive by this screening test?

(A) 20
(B) 80
(C) 100
(D) 270
(E) 630

25. A 54-year-old woman has had longstanding rheumatoid arthritis. Her rheumatologist recently started her on methotrexate, a dihydrofolate reductase inhibitor. What effect does methotrexate have on dihydrofolate reductase?

(A) The maximum reaction rate is decreased
(B) The maximum reaction rate is increased

(C) The Michaelis-Menten constant is decreased

(D) The Michaelis-Menten constant is increased

(E) The Michaelis-Menten constant is unchanged

26. While watching television, an 82-year-old woman suffers an episode of lightheadedness that is associated with dysarthria and difficulty swallowing. She subsequently faints but awakens within a few seconds. This episode is most likely due to which of the following mechanisms?

(A) Dysrhythmia

(B) Hypoxia

(C) Orthostasis

(D) Vertebrobasilar insufficiency

(E) Vertigo

27. A 45-year-old man comes to the physician because of a fever of 39.6° C (103.2° F) that developed suddenly the previous night. On physical examination, the physician notes a new-onset murmur along with white spots on the retina. The appearance of his hands is shown in the image. Which of the following organisms is most likely responsible for this patient's symptoms?

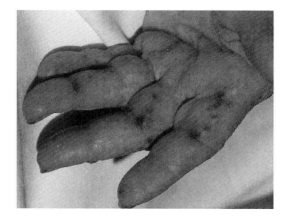

Reproduced, with permission, from Wolff K, Johnson RA,   D. *Fitzpatrick's Color Atlas & Synopsis of Clinical Dermatology,* 5th ed. New York, McGraw-Hill, 2005: Fig 22.38.

(A) *Neisseria meningitides*

(B) *Staphylococcus aureus*

(C) *Staphylococcus epidermidis*

(D) *Streptococcus pneumoniae*

(E) *Streptococcus viridans*

28. When a peripheral nerve fiber gets damaged or transected, the neuron attempts to repair the damage, initiating a series of metabolic and structural events collectively called the axon reaction. Wallerian degeneration is one example. Which of the following is the mechanism most likely involved in Wallerian degeneration?

(A) Degeneration of neuronal cell body

(B) Degeneration of neuronal target cells

(C) Degeneration of the axon distal to the lesion

(D) Degeneration of the axon proximal to the lesion

(E) Phagocytosis of local neuronal debris

29. A 47-year-old man with chronic asthma who has been treated with steroids for many years develops a productive cough, weight loss, and night sweats. Imaging studies reveal the presence of abscesses in the lungs and brain. Cultures show gram-positive filaments that are weakly acid-fast. Which of the following organisms is responsible for this patient's condition?

(A) *Actinomyces israelii*

(B) *Bacillus anthracis*

(C) *Mycobacterium tuberculosis*

(D) *Nocardia asteroids*

(E) *Streptococcus pneumoniae*

30. A 76-year-old woman presents to the emergency department with blurry vision and a headache that started 5 hours ago. She has a past medical history of chronic essential hypertension and asthma. She is afebrile with a pulse of 75/min and a blood pressure of 210/120 mm Hg. Which of the following medications should be prescribed immediately?

(A) Captopril

(B) Hydrochlorothiazide

(C) Labetalol

(D) Losartan

(E) Sodium nitroprusside

31. DNA is extracted from cells and cut by restriction enzymes. The resulting fragments of DNA are run on an electrophoresis gel. Bands of DNA are transferred from a gel to a nitrocellulose sheet, which is then treated with a labeled DNA probe. Which of the following laboratory techniques does this describe?

   (A) Enzyme-linked immunosorbent assay
   (B) Gel electrophoresis
   (C) Northern blot
   (D) Polymerase chain reaction
   (E) Sequencing
   (F) Southern blot
   (G) Western blot

32. A 15-year-old boy is brought to his pediatrician because he feels short of breath and has to stop and walk after brief runs. He underwent cardiac surgery when he was an infant for a congenital heart defect. An inspiratory chest x-ray shows the right hemidiaphragm is much higher than the left one. This boy's exertional dyspnea is probably caused by which of the following conditions?

   (A) Damaged left phrenic nerve
   (B) Damaged right phrenic nerve
   (C) Eisenmenger's syndrome
   (D) Left diaphragmatic hernia
   (E) Right diaphragmatic hernia

33. Nutrients such as fats and proteins are both produced by the body and consumed in the diet. In addition, several nutritional components are not able to be synthesized by the body and must be obtained in food. Which of the following substances can a healthy adult synthesize?

   (A) The fatty acids linolenic acid
   (B) The glucogenic amino acid histidine
   (C) The ketogenic amino acid leucine
   (D) The micronutrient folic acid
   (E) The micronutrient vitamin K

34. A 52-year-old man presents to the emergency department with a complaint of nocturia, dysuria, and crippling back pain. X-ray of the spine shows the following image. Laboratory values are notable for anemia, hypercalcemia,

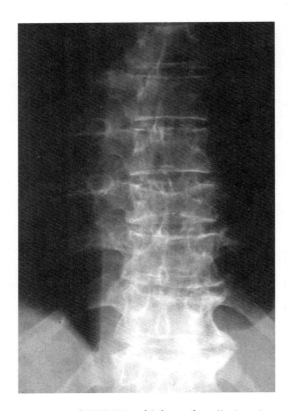

Image courtesy of PEIR Digital Library (http://peir.net).

and increased total protein. Which of the following is the typical cause of the increased total protein in this disease?

   (A) Inability to clear chylomicron particles from the blood
   (B) Increased production of albumin
   (C) Increased production of clotting factors and acute-phase reactants
   (D) Increased production of IgG molecules
   (E) Increased production of IgM molecules

35. A 42-year-old woman comes to the physician with red papular lesions along her arm, some of which have ulcerated. She reports that the lesions appeared 1 week ago, a day after working in her rose garden. Initially, there were only a couple of lesions on her right forearm. Since then, more lesions have appeared along her arm approaching her axilla. The physician makes a quick diagnosis and prescribes itraconazole. This patient is most likely infected with which of the following fungi?

(A) *Blastomyces* species
(B) *Coccidioides* species
(C) *Malassezia furfur*
(D) *Pneumocystis jiroveci*
(E) *Sporothrix schenckii*

36. A 3-year-old girl is brought to her pediatrician because she has a pyogenic infection. The patient is started on an antibiotic regimen. Over the next 24 hours, her condition deteriorates considerably and she is brought into the emergency department. Laboratory evaluation shows that the patient has a defect in the LFA-1 adhesion proteins on her neutrophils. This patient most likely has which of the following immune deficiencies?

(A) Chronic granulomatous disease
(B) Leukocyte adhesion deficiency syndrome
(C) Selective IgA deficiency
(D) Severe combined immunodeficiency
(E) Wiskott-Aldrich syndrome

37. A 20-year-old college student who is 4 weeks pregnant goes to her local Planned Parenthood to obtain information on her options for her pregnancy. She is interested in having an abortion, but is fearful of an operation and asks about medical abortion. She is told that mifepristone is a drug that can be used early in pregnancy to terminate gestation, with an efficacy around 85%. When administered with a particular drug, the efficacy rises to almost 100%. Which of the following is the coadministered drug?

(A) Clomiphene
(B) Diethylstilbestrol
(C) Ethinyl estradiol
(D) Progesterone
(E) Prostaglandin E_1

38. In a discussion with his therapist, a student at a local university reveals an affection for a fellow student that seems obsessive. He also notes he has an intent to purchase a gun but does not clearly state why. With whom **MUST** the physician be sure contact is made?

(A) Another physician who knows the fellow student
(B) Another physician who knows the patient
(C) Law enforcement authorities and the fellow student
(D) Law enforcement authorities only
(E) No one; do not break confidentiality
(F) The fellow student only

39. Anovulation in polycystic ovarian syndrome (PCOS) is due to a peripheral production of which of the following hormones, as represented on the graph?

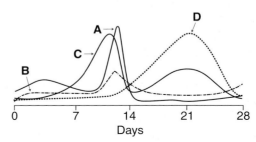

Reproduced, with permission, from USMLERx.com.

(A) A
(B) B
(C) C
(D) D

40. In order to ascertain the specific genetic defect in patients with cystic fibrosis, scientists obtained buccal smears from several patients and isolated DNA from these cells. The DNA was amplified by polymerase chain reaction and then sequenced. The region of the sequencing gel where the normal gene differs from the mutated gene is shown below. Which of the following types of DNA mutations caused this disease?

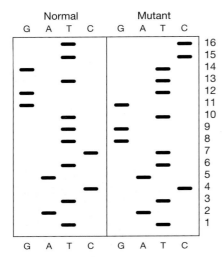

Reproduced, with permission, from USMLERx.com.

(A) Deletion mutation
(B) Frameshift mutation
(C) Insertion mutation
(D) Missense mutation
(E) Nonsense mutation
(F) Point mutation
(G) Silent mutation

41. A new experimental cancer drug for treating acute lymphocytic leukemia has just been discovered. The drug was designed to prevent microtubule spindle formation. The mechanism of action of this new drug is similar to which of the following?

(A) Cocaine
(B) Digoxin
(C) Mebendazole
(D) Neostigmine
(E) Procainamide

42. A 3-year-old girl is brought to the physician because of a lifelong history of multiple fractures, some from apparently minor trauma. In addition, her sclerae have a grayish hue. After a comprehensive work-up, the patient is diagnosed with osteogenesis imperfecta. Osteogenesis imperfecta is caused by a mutation in type I collagen synthesis. Which of the following types of genetic effect does this mutation exhibit?

(A) Anticipation
(B) Dominant negative
(C) Incomplete penetrance
(D) Mosaicism
(E) Pleiotropy

43. A 65-year-old man with a history of hypertension and hyperlipidemia comes to the physician because of constant, dull groin pain. The patient has noticed a slight decrease in his urine output but denies fever or hematuria. The right kidney is palpable in the right flank region. A CT scan of the pelvis is performed and confirms the diagnosis. Which of the following is the most likely cause of this patient's findings?

(A) Abdominal aortic aneurysm
(B) Right bladder calculus
(C) Right common iliac artery aneurysm
(D) Right ureteral calculus
(E) Urinary tract infection

44. A 5-year-old boy is expected to be discharged from the pediatric intensive care unit after sustaining an intraventricular hemorrhage following a motor vehicle accident. Maintenance fluids have been discontinued, and intravenous access has been kept open by flushing with heparin. The intern asks the third-year medical student to draw blood off the patient's intravenous line for coagulation studies. The third-year student, however, neglects to discard the first 5 cc of blood before collecting blood for the sample. He then sends this sample off to the hematology laboratory for a coagulation panel but neglects to tell the intern about the error. Which of the following laboratory results would be expected in this patient?

(A) Decreased activated partial thromboplastin time
(B) Decreased international normalized ratio
(C) Decreased prothrombin time
(D) Increased activated partial thromboplastin time
(E) Increased international normalized ratio
(F) Increased prothrombin time

45. A 43-year-old woman patient in a psychiatry ward is admitted from a medical floor after attempting suicide by medication overdose. She states that she recently broke up with her boyfriend, who disapproved of her cocaine and marijuana use. This is the fifth time they have broken up. She also states that she and her ex-boyfriend fought constantly; however, she adds that the only times she did not feel "empty" were when they were fighting. She also states that she has made "hundreds" of suicide attempts and has been hospitalized numerous times. Which of the following personality disorders best describes this patient?

(A) Avoidant
(B) Borderline
(C) Dependent
(D) Narcissistic
(E) Schizoid
(F) Schizotypal

46. An 82-year-old man is brought to the emergency department by ambulance with complaints of severe dyspnea and altered mental status. He is obtunded and tachypneic with moist mucous membranes, and his blood pressure is 70/40 mm Hg. Bilateral rales are auscultated, and a new soft decrescendo systolic murmur is heard at the apex of the heart, as is an S_4 gallop. Of the following, which medication would be most effective in this patient?

(A) Amrinone
(B) Dopamine
(C) Epinephrine
(D) Isoproterenol
(E) Phenylephrine

47. A construction worker accidentally drives a nail into his thigh with a nail gun. The nail is removed, but the area remains painful and edematous. A diagnosis of cellulitis is made. After a few days, the skin over the affected area becomes spongy and, on palpation, has a crackling consistency. A blood-tinged exudate is also observed. To which of the following organisms was this man most likely exposed?

(A) *Actinomyces israelii*
(B) *Bacillus anthracis*
(C) *Clostridium perfringens*
(D) *Clostridium tetani*
(E) *Sporothrix schenckii*

48. A 64-year-old woman presents to the physician with vaginal bleeding. After an extensive work-up, a small mass is found in the left adnexa. A biopsy of her left ovary is shown in the image. Which of the following is this patient's most likely diagnosis?

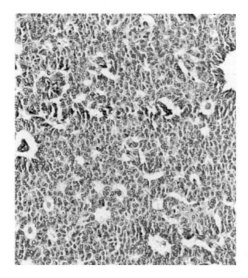

Reproduced, with permission, from Chandrasoma P, Taylor CR. *Concise Pathology*, 3rd ed. New York, McGraw-Hill, 1998: Fig. 52-15.

(A) Endometrioid tumor
(B) Granulosa cell tumor
(C) Krukenberg's tumor
(D) Serous cystadenocarcinoma
(E) Teratoma

49. A 54-year-old man was recently diagnosed with congestive heart failure and is started on a medication regimen to treat this condition. After 4 months, the patient returns to his cardiologist complaining that his "pecs" are getting bigger on both the right and left side, and he has an aching pain behind both nipples. Which of the following drugs is most likely responsible for this patient's symptoms?

    (A) Enalapril
    (B) Hydralazine
    (C) Metoprolol
    (D) Nitroglycerin
    (E) Spironolactone

50. A term infant is born after an uncomplicated pregnancy to a 35-year-old woman. On cutting the umbilical cord, the physician notes an abnormality that leads him to consult a pediatric cardiologist. Which of the following abnormalities did this physician most likely observe?

    (A) Single allantoic duct
    (B) Single umbilical artery
    (C) Single umbilical vein
    (D) Two umbilical arteries
    (E) Two umbilical veins

1. **The correct answer is E.** Trimethoprim-sulfamethoxazole is one of the most common treatments for simple urinary tract infections, most of which are caused by *Escherichia coli* in the general population. Sulfamethoxazole binds to, and will displace, unconjugated bilirubin from albumin. In a newborn, this can lead to kernicterus (bilirubin encephalopathy), a disorder of newborns caused by deposition of bilirubin in the brain. The basal ganglia are particularly affected. Common early symptoms include lethargy, poor feeding, and absent Moro reflex. If the infants survive, they can develop seizures, mental retardation, deafness, choreoathetoid movements, and decreased upward eye movements.

Answer A is incorrect. Amoxicillin is not associated with kernicterus.

Answer B is incorrect. Ampicillin is not associated with kernicterus.

Answer C is incorrect. Nitrofurantoin, commonly used to treat urinary tract infections, is not associated with kernicterus.

Answer D is incorrect. Ofloxacin is not associated with kernicterus.

2. **The correct answer is A.** All states have a requirement to report cases of AIDS, but not all states have a requirement to report HIV-positive results.

Answer B is incorrect. Reporting to a sexual partner is a requirement of all HIV patients, but a physician is only required to do so if he or she believes that the patient will not.

Answer C is incorrect. A physician who practices infection control is not at risk for infecting his other patients.

Answer D is incorrect. Medical associations do not require HIV-positive result reporting.

Answer E is incorrect. Medical licensing boards do not require HIV-positive result reporting.

3. **The correct answer is D.** T-lymphocyte activation requires two signals: (1) T-lymphocyte receptor recognition of major histocompatibility complex/peptide, and (2) CD28-B7 interaction. Professional antigen-presenting cells (APCs) are capable of delivering both of these signals. The three types of professional APCs are the dendritic cells, macrophages, and B lymphocytes. Langerhans cells are a type of dendritic cells present within the skin.

Answer A is incorrect. T lymphocytes and natural killer cells are not professional antigen-presenting cells.

Answer B is incorrect. T lymphocytes are not professional antigen-presenting cells.

Answer C is incorrect. Epithelial cells are not professional antigen-presenting cells.

Answer E is incorrect. Natural killer cells are not professional antigen-presenting cells.

4. **The correct answer is B.** Twenty-five percent of heterozygous parents' offspring will be affected with autosomal recessive diseases such as Tay-Sachs disease, which is the condition described in this couple's family histories.

Answer A is incorrect. Three percent is the approximate recurrence risk for the offspring of an individual with a multifactorial genetic disorder (e.g., cleft lip). This also applies to siblings of an affected child; each subsequent birth in a family with one affected child has a 3% risk of also being affected.

Answer C is incorrect. Fifty percent of heterozygous parents' offspring will be affected in autosomal dominant inheritance.

Answer D is incorrect. In the case of mitochondrial inheritance, 100% of an affected mother's children receive the disease, and none of an affected father's children receive it (children inherit their mother's mitochondrial DNA).

Answer E is incorrect. When a disease is due to somatic mutations, the chance of a child being affected will depend on the population prevalence of the somatic mutation that causes the disease to occur. There is no transmission from one generation to the next, and therefore it is not considered an inherited condition.

5. **The correct answer is B.** Osteogenesis imperfecta (OI) is an inherited defect in type I collagen. There is a spectrum of severity observed with OI, ranging from prepubertal fractures with mild deformity and normal stature to frequent childhood fractures and even severe in utero fractures that result in perinatal death.

Answer A is incorrect. Hydroxyapatite is a component of bone that is not implicated in osteogenesis imperfecta.

Answer C is incorrect. Type II collagen is found in cartilage, vitreous body, and nucleus pulposus. It is not related to osteogenesis imperfecta.

Answer D is incorrect. Type III collagen (reticulin) is found in skin, blood vessels, uterus, fetal tissue, and granulation tissue. It is not related to osteogenesis imperfecta.

Answer E is incorrect. Type IV collagen is found in basement membrane or basal lamina. It is not related to osteogenesis imperfecta.

Answer F is incorrect. Type X collagen is found at the epiphyseal plates. It is not related to osteogenesis imperfecta.

6. **The correct answer is A.** *Candida* esophagitis classically presents with sore throat and dysphagia with friable white plaques and erythematous mucosa present on physical examination. *Candida albicans* is an opportunistic fungal pathogen—also called thrush—that is most commonly found in the oropharynx of immunosuppressed patients. It can also be present as diaper rash in infants or as a diffuse mucocutaneous fungal infection in severely immunosuppressed individuals. Nystatin "swish and shallow" is often used for oral candidiasis; however, amphotericin B or fluconazole is used for serious systemic infection.

Answer B is incorrect. Cytomegalovirus esophagitis has a presentation similar to that of herpes simplex virus esophagitis, with punched-out mucosal lesions and inclusion bodies on microscopy.

Answer C is incorrect. Herpes simplex virus esophagitis presents with punched-out mucosal erosions characterized by cytoplasmic and intranuclear inclusion bodies on light microscopy.

Answer D is incorrect. Latent JC virus can be reactivated when a patient is immunosuppressed, developing into progressive multifocal leukoencephalopathy, a space-occupying irregular intracranial lesion best visualized on MRI.

Answer E is incorrect. *Pneumocystis jiroveci* (formerly *carinii*) infection classically causes a mixed alveolar and interstitial pneumonia in patients with CD4 counts below $400/\mu L$. It is associated with hypoxia, elevated LDH, and systemic symptoms such as fever and chills.

7. **The correct answer is A.** Imatinib mesylate is an oral inhibitor of the abnormal bcr-abl tyrosine kinase receptor produced in over 90% of chronic myeloid leukemia (CML) cases as a result of t(9;22) (the Philadelphia chromosome). Treatment of CML with imatinib mesylate results in blockade of the growth signals triggered by bcr-abl, resulting in quiescent disease and restoration of normal blood counts. Imatinib mesylate does not cure patients but renders their disease under control with a daily oral tablet. Imatinib mesylate as a first-line single agent for chronic-phase CML has been proven to prevent CML progression to accelerated or blast phase (acute leukemia transformation) in most patients for several years. Imatinib mesylate is the first successful targeted biological therapy for cancer and is the model drug for a new era of biologically targeted oncologic therapy.

Answer B is incorrect. Infliximab is a monoclonal antibody to tumor necrosis factor-α that is used in the treatment of refractory Crohn's disease.

Answer C is incorrect. Paclitaxel is an antimitotic agent that binds to tubulin and stabilized polymerized microtubules so that they cannot break down. It is used in ovarian and breast cancers.

Answer D is incorrect. Propylthiouracil is used in the treatment of hyperthyroidism and acts by blocking thyroid hormone synthesis and conversion of thyroxine to triiodothyronine.

Answer E is incorrect. Tamoxifen is a selective estrogen receptor modulator used in the treatment of breast cancer.

8. **The correct answer is C.** Acidic urine in the presence of metabolic alkalosis, known as paradoxical aciduria, is primarily a result of hypokalemia in the presence of volume contraction. The loss of hydrochloric acid due to vomiting leads to a transient increase in pH. The kidney responds by excretion of sodium and/or potassium bicarbonate. As the vomiting persists, the alkalemic and dehydrated patient tries to conserve sodium by activation of the renin-angiotensin-aldosterone system. Therefore, while bicarbonate excretion persists due to the alkalosis, it is primarily excreted with potassium rather than sodium due to the dehydration. Compensating by conserving sodium and excreting bicarbonate at the expense of potassium soon fails because in the presence of severe hypokalemia, the kidney begins to exchange hydrogen ions in the distal convoluted tubule in order to conserve potassium. Therefore, acidic urine in the setting of volume contraction and alkalosis is primarily due to the loss of potassium.

Answer A is incorrect. Cervical cancer is not associated with any common paraneoplastic effects.

Answer B is incorrect. A history of chemotherapy would have no effect on the present state of this patient's urine.

Answer D is incorrect. The patient is hypotensive, and her blood urea nitrogen/creatinine (BUN:Cr) ratio shows prerenal failure (defined as BUN/plasma creatinine > 20:1).

Renal failure leads to an inability to excrete hydrogen ions (as seen in renal tubular acidosis). Therefore, although she is suffering from prerenal disease due to a drop in her blood pressure, it does not account for the loss of hydrogen ions in her urine.

Answer E is incorrect. Lactic acidosis normally occurs in the setting of shock. There is reduced tissue oxygenation and, as the oxygen requirements of cells are not met, they begin to metabolize anaerobically, leading to a buildup of lactic acid and a subsequent metabolic acidosis. However, this patient is not in shock because her systolic blood pressures are > 90 mmHg and sufficiently perfusing her peripheral tissues. Therefore, she does not need to excrete hydrogen ions to counteract a metabolic acidosis.

9. **The correct answer is B.** Most of the lymph in the body is drained via the thoracic duct. It passes through the diaphragm with the aorta and azygous vein posteriorly at the level of T12. The right chest, back, arm, neck, and head, however, are drained via the right lymphatic duct, which empties into the angle between the internal jugular and subclavian veins. With symptoms of swelling in the right upper quadrant of the body, one must consider disruption of this structure, especially with a history of surgery in the axilla and neck.

Answer A is incorrect. Symptoms of deep venous thrombosis (DVT) include swelling, redness, and tenderness of the areas distal to the thrombosis. DVT can develop in the axillary or subclavian veins as a complication of venous catheters in these sites and may present as in this patient. A DVT in the cephalic vein, however, does not explain the facial edema.

Answer C is incorrect. The thoracic duct drains all the lymph in the body except that from the right upper quadrant, which includes the right arm and right side of the face.

Answer D is incorrect. Metastatic disease to bone is common in advanced breast cancer, and most metastatic disease occurs in the central skeleton (vertebrae, pelvis, ribs, upper legs, and arms). Bone metastases may cause pain and pathologic fractures but does not best explain the symptoms of swelling and edema in the face and arm.

Answer E is incorrect. Radiation has many adverse effects, including systemic effects, such as a decreased WBC count, as well as local effects, such as skin irritation. Local radiation to the right breast does not explain edema of the arm and face. These symptoms should prompt a more thorough workup.

10. **The correct answer is B.** The manic phase of bipolar disorder is characterized by an elevated, expansive, or irritable mood for more than 1 week; marked impairment in functioning socially, at work, or at home; and three or more of the following symptoms: inflated self-esteem/grandiosity, decreased need for sleep, increased rate of speech/talkativeness, flight of ideas/racing thoughts, distractibility, increased activity/psychomotor agitation, and an increase in pleasurable activities without regard for consequences.

Answer A is incorrect. Amphetamine intoxication can present with manic-type symptoms, but the duration of this patient's symptoms rules out drug intoxication. Routine drug screening would also confirm such findings.

Answer C is incorrect. Hyperthyroidism can present with agitation and decreased sleep, but patients with this disorder are unlikely to exhibit other symptoms of mania, including grandiosity and flight of ideas.

Answer D is incorrect. Schizoaffective disorder is schizophrenia with a prominent component of mood disorder, either depression or mania.

Answer E is incorrect. Schizophrenia typically does not have a clinical picture similar to that of bipolar disorder. Schizophrenia classically presents as a persisting chronic illness, often with residual psychotic symptoms, but it lacks the periodicity seen in bipolar disorder and usually has no evidence of manic symptoms.

11. **The correct answer is A.** With mild exercise, arterial pH does not change because the body is able to maintain aerobic metabolism. During strenuous exercise arterial pH is decreased secondary to anaerobic metabolism and generation of lactic acid.

Answer B is incorrect. During exercise, the increased O_2 need by the muscles is attained by increased O_2 consumption by the lungs through more rapid and deeper ventilation.

Answer C is incorrect. As a result of increased pulmonary blood flow, more pulmonary capillaries are perfused and more gas exchange occurs. The ventilation/perfusion ratio is more even throughout the lung during exercise.

Answer D is incorrect. Venous partial carbon dioxide pressure increases during exercise because the muscles give off excess CO_2 that is carried to the lungs by venous blood.

Answer E is incorrect. Pulmonary blood flow increases during exercise because cardiac output increases to ensure adequate O_2 delivery to muscles and CO_2 delivery to the lungs to be exhaled.

12. **The correct answer is A.** The answer is chloramphenicol, which is no longer widely used due to its toxicities, including gray baby syndrome and aplastic anemia. Aplastic anemia secondary to chloramphenicol is a rare, dose-independent adverse event that can occur after only a short course of therapy and can be fatal. The challenge with using this medication is that it is difficult to predict which patient will have this serious complication.

Answer B is incorrect. Ciprofloxacin (is associated with gastrointestinal upset, superinfections, skin rashes, headache, and dizziness. The most notable complications include tendonitis and tendon rupture in adults, and cartilage malformation in children and in utero.

Answer C is incorrect. Clindamycin is classically associated with intestinal colonization with *Clostridium difficile* (leading to pseudomembranous colitis).

Answer D is incorrect. Erythromycin is associated with gastrointestinal discomfort, cholestatic hepatitis, eosinophilia, and skin rashes. Azithromycin, a related macrolide, is better tolerated and has fewer adverse events.

Answer E is incorrect. Gentamicin is associated with nephrotoxicity and ototoxicity with prolonged use.

Answer F is incorrect. Tetracycline is associated with gastrointestinal distress, tooth discoloration, and inhibition of bone growth in children. Photosensitivity can also result, leading to sun-exposed tetracycline skin rash.

13. **The correct answer is A.** The condition described is xeroderma pigmentosum (XP), a genetic defect in the DNA excision repair pathway. In XP, there is a defective excision repair that results in the inability to repair thymidine dimers, which form in DNA exposed to ultraviolet light. XP is associated with dry skin, and individuals that have XP are much more likely to develop both melanoma and nonmelanoma skin cancers. Clinically, XP manifests as a sunburnlike reaction, and individuals with XP often die by age 30 years. XP is autosomal recessively inherited, which is demonstrated by the frequency of occurrence of XP in the vignette family.

Answer B is incorrect. A defect in double-stranded DNA break repair leads to ataxia-telangiectasia, which renders the individual's cells susceptible to x-ray damage. The primary features of ataxia-telangiectasia include progressive gait and truncal ataxia with onset between the ages of 1 and 4 years. The most common malignancies among these patients are leukemia and lymphoma.

Answer C is incorrect. The various glycolytic enzyme deficiencies are associated with hemolytic anemia and are not associated with an increased risk of cancer.

Answer D is incorrect. A defect in heme synthesis results in a type of porphyria and is not associated with an increased risk of cancer.

Answer E is incorrect. Purine salvage deficiencies such as adenosine deaminase deficiency (leading to severe combined immunodeficiency) and Lesch-Nyhan syndrome (excess uric acid production) do not lead to an increased risk of cancer.

14. **The correct answer is D.** This vignette describes an urachal cyst or sinus, which is a remnant of the allantois and continues to drain urine from the bladder. The allantoic duct eventually becomes the median umbilical ligament. Remember, "allaNtois" has an "N," as does "mediaN."

Answer A is incorrect. The fossa ovalis is the remnant of the foramen ovale, which allowed shunting of blood from the right to left atrium but did not communicate with the bladder.

Answer B is incorrect. The ligamentum teres hepatis is the remnant of the umbilical vein, which carried blood from the mother to the baby but did not communicate with the bladder.

Answer C is incorrect. The medial umbilical ligaments are the remnants of the fetal umbilical arteries, which carried blood from the baby to the mother but did not communicate with the bladder.

Answer E is incorrect. The nucleus pulposus is the remnant of the notochord, which induced differentiation during development but did not directly communicate with the bladder.

15. **The correct answer is A.** Ovarian cancer is difficult to detect, and unfortunately the presenting symptom may be large pleural effusions from metastatic disease. The intercostal vessels and nerve run in the intercostal groove on the inferior surface of each rib. When a thoracentesis is performed, the needle is always inserted immediately superior to a rib to avoid these structures.

Answer B is incorrect. The phrenic nerve is found deep in the thorax, running along the mediastinum and pericardium; it is too deep to be injured by thoracentesis.

Answer C is incorrect. The pericardiophrenic vessels travel with the phrenic nerve along the mediastinum and pericardium. These vessels are too deep to be injured by this procedure.

Answer D is incorrect. The recurrent laryngeal nerve is a branch of the vagus nerve and is found in the neck. This nerve can be injured during a thyroidectomy or other neck surgeries but is not in danger of being damaged during a chest procedure.

Answer E is incorrect. The needle here is inserted above the tenth rib, in the ninth intercostal space. The tenth intercostal vessels and nerve run below the tenth rib, in the tenth intercostal space.

16. **The correct answer is E.** The patient has papillary thyroid carcinoma, which accounts for approximately 80% of thyroid carcinomas and can usually be cured by resection of the primary tumor. The diagnosis can usually be made with a fine needle biopsy. The histologic finding depicted in the slide is a psammoma body, which is found in approximately 50% of papillary adenocarcinomas of the thyroid. Psammoma bodies are laminated, concentric calcified spherules that are also found in serous papillary cystadenocarcinoma of the ovary, meningiomas, and mesotheliomas.

Answer A is incorrect. Psammoma bodies are not found in adenocarcinomas of the lung. Well differentiated adenocarcinomas of the lung are characterized microscopically by mucin-producing glands lined by cuboidal or columnar cells, while poorly differentiated adenocarcinomas have a papillary or solid structure that usually does not produce mucin.

Answer B is incorrect. Dysgerminoma tumors of the ovary do not contain psammoma bodies; however, as previously mentioned, serous papillary cystadenocarcinoma of the ovary does. Dysgerminoma tumors of the ovary often have cells with clear cytoplasm in large sheets. The cells contain regular nuclei with a background of fibrous stroma.

Answer C is incorrect. Follicular carcinomas of the thyroid are less common but more malignant than papillary carcinomas of the thyroid. Unlike papillary carcinoma, in which

hematogenous metastasis is rare, follicular carcinomas commonly metastasize via the blood to lungs or bones. Histologically, follicular carcinomas tend to form acini or follicles lined with cells that are larger than those found in normal thyroid. Psammoma bodies are not found in follicular carcinoma.

Answer D is incorrect. Medullary carcinoma of the thyroid arises from the C cells of the thyroid, which produce calcitonin. It is a rare cancer of the thyroid and can be associated with multiple endocrine neoplasia (MEN) types IIA and IIB. Histologic examination of medullary carcinomas reveals sheets of tumor cells in an amyloid stroma. Psammoma bodies are not found in medullary carcinoma.

17. **The correct answer is B.** Risk factors for developing cervical cancer include early sexual activity, multiple sex partners, smoking, and low socioeconomic status. Furthermore, cervical cancer is almost always associated with human papillomavirus (HPV) infection. Cervical cancers are most often squamous cell and arise from disordered epithelial growth, classified as cervical intraepithelial neoplasia (CIN) 1, 2, or 3, depending on the extent of epithelial involvement from the basal layer. Papanicolaou smears have reduced the mortality of these cancers.

Answer A is incorrect. Alcoholism has little relation to cervical cancer but is strongly associated with chronic pancreatitis and pancreatic adenocarcinoma. Smoking is also a risk factor for these conditions.

Answer C is incorrect. A low-fiber diet has little relation to cervical cancer, but it is a risk factor for developing colorectal cancer. Other risk factors for developing colorectal cancer include villous adenomas, familial adenomatous polyposis, hereditary nonpolyposis colorectal cancer, inflammatory bowel disease, and a positive personal or family history.

Answer D is incorrect. Nulliparity is a risk factor for breast cancer. Other risk factors for breast cancer include gender, early first menarche (< 6 12 years), delayed first pregnancy

(> 30 years), late menopause (> 50 years), and a positive family history.

Answer E is incorrect. Prolonged estrogen use is a risk factor for endometrial carcinoma. Other risk factors for endometrial carcinoma include obesity, diabetes, and hypertension.

18. **The correct answer is D.** Lesch-Nyhan syndrome is an X-linked recessive disorder caused by a deficiency in the production of hypoxanthine guanine phosphoribosyltransferase that leads to the overproduction of purine and the accumulation of uric acid. This rare biochemical disorder is characterized clinically by hyperuricemia, excessive production of uric acid, and certain characteristic neurologic features, including self-mutilation, choreoathetosis, spasticity, and mental retardation.

Answer A is incorrect. A deficiency of adenosine deaminase would result in severe combined immunodeficiency disease (SCID), which prevents development of both the humoral and cell-mediated immune systems. Therefore individuals with SCID are faced with recurrent devastating bacterial, viral, and fungal infections.

Answer B is incorrect. A deficiency of β-glucocerebroside would result in Gaucher's disease. There are several types of Gaucher's disease based on the type of mutation, but most forms are marked by lipid-laden macrophages (termed *Gaucher cells*) that invade the bone marrow and cortex, leading to bone infarction, vertebral collapse, and anemia and thrombocytopenia.

Answer C is incorrect. This boy's findings can best be explained by Lesch-Nyhan syndrome, which is caused by a deficiency in the production of hypoxanthine guanine phosphoribosyltransferase, not a mutation of an enzyme in the de novo biosynthetic pathway, which would result in deficiencies in nucleotides needed for DNA synthesis. Symptoms may resemble conditions in which dietary deficiencies impede de novo nucleotide synthesis, such as megaloblastic anemia due to folic acid and/or vitamin B_{12} deficiency.

Answer E is incorrect. An excision repair enzyme deficiency would result in xeroderma pigmentosum, which is marked by dry and hyperpigmented skin that is extremely sensitive to exposure to ultraviolet radiation. Therefore, individuals with this disease are at increased risk for severe sunburns and skin cancer.

19. **The correct answer is A.** The patient's complaints of dry mouth, difficulty swallowing, "sandy" sensation in the eyes, and associated joint pain are consistent with the clinical presentation of Sjögren's syndrome. Sjögren's syndrome is characterized by dry eyes (keratoconjunctivitis sicca) and dry mouth (xerostomia) resulting from autoimmune destruction of lacrimal and salivary glands. It can occur as an isolated disorder or as an association with another autoimmune disease (secondary form). Among associated disorders, rheumatoid arthritis is the most common, explaining the recent onset of joint pain in this patient. Since patients with Sjögren's syndrome have decreased salivary secretions, the defense against pathogenic bacteria that cause dental caries is compromised.

Answer B is incorrect. Hyperglycemia is most commonly associated with insulin resistance and/or absence of insulin production associated with diabetes mellitus. It is not a common phenomenon in Sjögren's syndrome.

Answer C is incorrect. Jaundice is usually associated with pathologic processes involving liver or hemolytic anemias. These pathologies are relatively uncommon in Sjögren's syndrome.

Answer D is incorrect. Septic joints are usually a consequence of an infectious process and generally have no association with Sjögren's syndrome.

Answer E is incorrect. Although development of vision loss could be a potential consequence of Sjögren's syndrome due to the lack of lacrimal gland secretions, it is not the most likely condition that these patients will develop.

20. **The correct answer is A.** Interleukin-2 (IL-2) is a recombinant cytokine used for treatment of renal cell carcinoma and metastatic melanoma. IL-2 acts as a T-lymphocyte growth factor and assists the immune system by promoting the proliferation, differentiation, and recruitment of T lymphocytes, B lymphocytes, natural killer cells, and thymocytes.

    Answer B is incorrect. Interleukin-2 does not block the ATP-binding site in the Bcr-Abl tyrosine kinase; imatinib mesylate does.

    Answer C is incorrect. Interleukin-2 does not decrease the blood supply to the tumor.

    Answer D is incorrect. The chemotherapeutic affect of interleukin-2 does not involve interfering with tumor cell proliferation, but rather activating lymphoid cells.

    Answer E is incorrect. Interleukin-2 does not inhibit monoamine oxidase.

21. **The correct answer is E.** Selection bias occurs when patients in a study are not randomly assigned to a treatment group. This can occur because either the patients or the investigators select the group that an individual patient will enter.

    Answer A is incorrect. Late-look bias concerns information gathered at an inappropriate time of the study. It results in selection of patients of less severe disease because those with more severe disease died before detection.

    Answer B is incorrect. Length bias (and lead-time bias) occurs when a disease's characteristics are ignored. For instance, a disease with more aggressive symptoms may progress to death more quickly and be falsely underrepresented by a cross-sectional look for prevalence. In evaluating 1000 patients with thyroid biopsies on follow-up visits each month, it would appear that fewer patients with anaplastic carcinoma have survived each month. Looking in cross-section 1 year after biopsy without considering patients who have died, the prevalence of anaplastic carcinoma would be falsely decreased.

    Answer C is incorrect. Recall bias occurs when a patient's report of symptoms or past events is selective, either intentionally or not. It may be secondary to perceptions of the patient about their own treatment, disease, or symptom causes.

    Answer D is incorrect. Sampling bias occurs when a sample group is not representative of the population from which it is taken.

22. **The correct answer is B.** Bisphosphonates, such as pamidronate and zoledronic acid, are used in the treatment of metastatic bone diseases, such as osteoporosis and hypercalcemia in cancer patients. Bisphosphonates reduce osteoclast activity, leading to poor bone healing.

    Answer A is incorrect. Angiotensin converting enzyme (ACE) inhibitors, such as enalapril, inhibit angiotensin-converting enzyme and are utilized in the treatment of hypertension. ACE inhibitor toxicity can include cough, angioedema, proteinuria, taste changes, rash, and hyperkalemia. Osteonecrosis is not associated with use of ACE inhibitors.

    Answer C is incorrect. Cephalosporins are β-lactam antibiotics used to treat infections caused by gram-positive and gram-negative bacteria. Use of cephalosporins does not cause osteonecrosis.

    Answer D is incorrect. Osmotic diuretics such as mannitol are used to treat shock and drug overdose. Osmotic diuretics are not associated with causing osteonecrosis.

    Answer E is incorrect. The vinca alkaloids, such as vincristine and vinblastine, are microtubule inhibitors used in the treatment of testicular carcinoma and Hodgkin's and non-Hodgkin's lymphomas. Vinca alkaloids are not associated with osteonecrosis.

23. **The correct answer is A.** Up until the seventh week of development, the external genitalia, including the genital tubercle, labioscrotal swellings, and urogenital folds, is the same in both sexes and can develop into male or fe-

male structures, depending on hormonal influences. In the male, the genital tubercle develops into the glans penis; the labioscrotal swellings fuse to form the scrotum, and the urogenital folds become the penile urethra in the ventral shaft of the penis. In females, the absence of androgens ceases the growth of the genital tubercle and the presence of estrogens leads to the development of the clitoris; the labioscrotal swellings develop into the labia majora, and the urogenital folds become the labia minora.

Answer B is incorrect. The labioscrotal swellings normally develop into the labia majora in the female and the scrotum in the male.

Answer C is incorrect. The production of testosterone by the Sertoli cells of the testes causes the mesonephric (wolffian) ducts to develop into the seminal vesicles, epididymis, ejaculatory duct, and ductus deferens. The absence of testosterone in females leads to the regression of the mesonephric ducts.

Answer D is incorrect. The testes produce antimüllerian hormone, which leads to the regression of the paramesonephric (müllerian) ducts in a male. In a female, there is no antimüllerian hormone and the paramesonephric ducts develop into the fallopian tubes, the uterus, and the upper two-thirds of the vagina.

Answer E is incorrect. The urogenital folds fuse in the male to form the penile urethra and the ventral shaft of the penis; in the female, the unfused portions of the urogenital folds become the labia minora.

24. **The correct answer is D.** The question is asking for the number of false-positives. Specificity = true-negatives/(true-negatives + false-positives). False-positive signifies the number of people without disease X who will be falsely diagnosed by the screening test. In this case, 900 people do not have the disease, represented by true-negatives + false-positives. Using a specificity of 70%, the number of true-negatives is 630, while the number of false-positives

is 270. Thus, 270 people without disease X will be falsely diagnosed with this screening test (i.e., they will be false-positives).

Answer A is incorrect. The figure 20 is the number of people with the disease who will have an incorrect negative screening test result (i.e., false-negatives).

Answer B is incorrect. The figure 80 is the number of people who will have a correct positive screening test result (i.e., true-positives).

Answer C is incorrect. The figure 100 is the number of people in the town with disease X (i.e., the prevalence of disease X).

Answer E is incorrect. The figure 630 is the number of people who will have a correct negative screening test result (i.e., true-negatives).

25. **The correct answer is D.** Methotrexate is a competitive inhibitor of dihydrofolate reductase. The Michaelis-Menten constant (K_m) of an enzyme such as dihydrofolate reductase reflects the enzyme's affinity for a particular substrate (e.g., methotrexate). The K_m of an enzyme is the concentration of substrate required to achieve a reaction velocity equal to half of the maximum reaction rate (V_{max}). A competitive inhibitor binds reversibly to the same site that the substrate would normally occupy and thus competes with the substrate for that site. Therefore, in the presence of a competitive inhibitor, the concentration of methotrexate required to achieve half of V_{max} will be increased.

Answer A is incorrect. The maximum reaction rate of an enzyme is unchanged by a competitive inhibitor.

Answer B is incorrect. The V_{max} is the maximum rate or velocity in which substrate molecules are converted to product per unit time. At high substrate concentrations, the reaction rate levels off, reflecting the saturation of all available binding sites with substrate. The effect of a competitive inhibitor is reversed by increasing the concentration of substrate. At a sufficiently high substrate concentration, the reaction velocity reaches the V_{max} observed in the absence of inhibitor. Thus, the V_{max} of an enzyme is unchanged by a competitive inhibitor.

Answer C is incorrect. The Michaelis-Menten constant of an enzyme is increased by a competitive inhibitor.

Answer E is incorrect. The Michaelis-Menten constant of an enzyme is increased by a competitive inhibitor.

26. **The correct answer is D.** Syncope has an extremely broad differential and can be divided into cardiac, orthostatic/reflex, neurologic, and psychiatric categories, all of which result in reduced perfusion of the cerebrum, causing the syncopal episode. All of the answer choices can cause syncope except for vertigo, which is included in the differential diagnosis of syncope. Given her symptoms of dysarthria and difficulty swallowing, she probably suffered a transient ischemic attack as a result of decreased perfusion to the posterior circulation, which is known as vertebrobasilar insufficiency.

Answer A is incorrect. Cardiac dysrhythmias commonly cause syncope, but nothing in the history suggests a cardiac etiology.

Answer B is incorrect. Hypoxia can be a cause of syncope, but this episode occurred at rest and lacks any features that would be consistent with hypoxia as a cause (e.g., respiratory difficulties).

Answer C is incorrect. Hypovolemia can be a cause of syncope but tends to be associated with either hypotension or sudden changes in posture, neither of which have occurred in this patient.

Answer E is incorrect. Vertigo can be associated with syncope but is not a frequent cause of it. The lack of any description of the patient suffering from the abnormal sensation of motion makes this option unlikely.

27. **The correct answer is B.** *Staphylococcus aureus* causes acute bacterial endocarditis, which presents with an acute onset of high fever, other flulike symptoms, new-onset murmur,

petechiae, Roth's spots (white spots on the retina formed by microemboli), Janeway lesions (painless macules on the palms or soles), Osler's nodes (small, painful nodules on the pads of the fingers or toes), and nail-bed (subungual) hemorrhages. The bacteria can attack healthy valves and result in vegetations that are much larger than those of subacute bacterial endocarditis.

Answer A is incorrect. *Neisseria meningitidis* is not an etiologic agent of bacterial endocarditis.

Answer C is incorrect. *Staphylococcus epidermidis* most commonly causes endocarditis on prosthetic heart valves or right-sided valves in intravenous drug users.

Answer D is incorrect. *Streptococcus pneumoniae*, particularly in the postantibiotic era, is a much rarer cause of bacterial endocarditis. When it does occur, *S. pneumoniae* endocarditis is typically a sequela of pneumococcal pneumonia.

Answer E is incorrect. *Streptococcus viridans* causes subacute bacterial endocarditis. This disease presents with small vegetations on previously damaged valves. The onset of symptoms is more gradual, as compared to acute bacterial endocarditis.

28. **The correct answer is C.** When an axonal injury results from traumatic transection of the nerve, the fibers distal to the transection undergo wallerian degeneration. Wallerian degeneration is the process whereby peripheral nerve fibers (axons) distal to the site of damage undergo disintegration, necrosis, and degeneration. This type of degeneration often occurs following mechanical injury to the axon (i.e., transection).

Answer A is incorrect. Following a transection, the cell body is spared. Instead, the axon is affected by wallerian degeneration.

Answer B is incorrect. Target cells are cells that receive postsynaptic stimuli (i.e., neurotransmitters) from the damaged axons. The axons are affected by wallerian degeneration;

however, the target cells (i.e., neurons, endocrine cells, muscle cells) are spared.

Answer D is incorrect. In wallerian degeneration, the proximal fibers are spared.

Answer E is incorrect. Phagocytosis of local neuronal debris occurs following a transection, but it is not involved in wallerian degeneration. Neuroglial cells participate in the repair and removal of debris.

29. **The correct answer is D.** *Nocardia asteroides* is a filamentous gram-positive organism that is weakly acid-fast. Infection with this organism is typically seen in immunocompromised individuals, such as someone who has chronically taken steroids. It is commonly misdiagnosed as tuberculosis because of its acid-fast nature and its similar disease process.

Answer A is incorrect. *Actinomyces israelii* is also a filamentous organism but is not weakly acid-fast. It is part of the normal flora of the mouth and gastrointestinal tract. It is classically associated with "sulfur granules" seen on microscopy. It can cause abscesses and invasive infections, most commonly in the head/neck, oropharynx, and abdomen. It easily traverses tissue planes, so it is known for causing draining sinus tracts.

Answer B is incorrect. *Bacillus anthracis* can cause inhalation anthrax. It is not an acid-fast organism.

Answer C is incorrect. *Mycobacterium tuberculosis* causes tuberculosis, the symptoms of which are similar to the disease caused by *Nocardia asteroides*. Unlike *N. asteroides*, *M. tuberculosis* is an acid-fast bacillus.

Answer E is incorrect. *Streptococcus pneumoniae* causes pneumonia. It is a gram-positive coccus.

30. **The correct answer is E.** This patient has the signs and symptoms of hypertensive emergency; she has symptoms of end-organ involvement (blurry vision and headache) as well as a significantly elevated blood pressure. Sodium nitroprusside, a first-line medication for hypertensive emergencies, acts by direct vasodilation

of both arteries and veins. Although it can cause a reflex tachycardia due to its hypotensive properties, this patient's heart rate is not currently elevated, and she has no past medical history of cardiac disease.

Answer A is incorrect. Captopril is an angiotensin-converting enzyme inhibitor, which is an extremely effective medication in controlling chronic hypertension. However, it is not useful in acute hypertensive emergencies because its mechanism of action is too slow.

Answer B is incorrect. As a diuretic, hydrochlorothiazide is an effective medication for the treatment of chronic essential hypertension. However, due to its mechanism of action, it does not cause a rapid enough reduction in blood pressure and thus is not useful in an emergent situation.

Answer C is incorrect. Labetalol is also a first-line medication for hypertensive emergencies because it will decrease the blood pressure without the reflex tachycardia. However, the patient's past medical history of asthma means that labetalol is not as good a choice as nitroprusside.

Answer D is incorrect. As an angiotensin receptor blocker, losartan is a useful drug with which to control chronic hypertension; however, it has no role in acute management of hypertensive emergency because it takes too long to work.

31. **The correct answer is F.** This question describes a Southern blot. In a Southern blot procedure, DNA is separated with electrophoresis, denatured, transferred to a filter, and hybridized with a labeled DNA probe. Regions on the filter that base-pair with the labeled DNA probes can be identified when the filter is exposed to film that is sensitive to the radiolabeled probe.

Answer A is incorrect. Enzyme-linked immunosorbent assay (ELISA) is an immunologic technique used in laboratories to determine whether a particular antibody is present in a patient's blood. Labeled antibodies are used to detect whether serum contains antibodies against a specific antigen precoated on an ELISA plate. This is not the technique described above.

Answer B is incorrect. Gel electrophoresis uses an electric field to separate molecules based on their sizes. This is not the technique described above.

Answer C is incorrect. Northern blots are similar to Southern blots except that in Northern blotting, mRNA is separated by electrophoresis instead of DNA. This is not the technique described above.

Answer D is incorrect. Polymerase chain reaction is a laboratory technique used to produce many copies of a segment of DNA. In the procedure, DNA is mixed with two specific primers, deoxynucleotides and a heat-stable polymerase. The solution is heated to denature the DNA and is then cooled to allow synthesis. Twenty cycles of heating and cooling amplify the DNA over a million times. This is not the procedure described above.

Answer E is incorrect. Sequencing is a laboratory technique that utilizes dideoxynucleotides to randomly terminate growing strands of DNA. Gel electrophoresis is used to separate the varying lengths of DNA. The DNA sequence can then be read based on the position of the bands on the gel. This is not the technique described above.

Answer G is incorrect. In a Western blot procedure, protein is separated by electrophoresis and labeled antibodies are used as a probe. This technique can be used to detect the existence of an antibody to a particular protein.

32. **The correct answer is B.** An x-ray film of the chest indicates that the boy has a paralyzed right hemidiaphragm. It is possible for the phrenic nerve to become damaged during heart surgery, since it runs along the pericardium. It is not unusual for a patient to remain asymptomatic until starting to run long distances.

Answer A is incorrect. When a patient holds his or her breath during a chest x-ray, a contracted diaphragm will move downward, and a paralyzed diaphragm will paradoxically move upward because of the negative pressure generated on the left side of the thorax pulling the mediastinal structures towards the left.

Answer C is incorrect. Eisenmenger's syndrome is the cyanosis and symptoms that occur when a prior left-to-right shunt reverses and becomes a right-to-left shunt. Cyanosis does not occur in a left-to-right shunt because oxygenated arterial blood simply reenters the pulmonary circulation. After years of arterial blood overloading the right side of the heart, however, pulmonary pressures can increase above systemic pressures and the shunt reverses. When this occurs, deoxygenated blood enters systemic circulation and cyanosis results. Although the question states that this patient had a cardiac defect repaired in infancy, there is no evidence of cyanosis, which is the hallmark of Eisenmenger's syndrome.

Answer D is incorrect. An x-ray film of a left diaphragmatic hernia would also reveal abdominal viscera in the thoracic cavity, which is not reported in this scenario.

Answer E is incorrect. An x-ray film of a right diaphragmatic hernia would also reveal abdominal viscera in the thoracic cavity, which is not reported in this scenario.

33. **The correct answer is B.** The eight essential amino acids are leucine, lysine, isoleucine, phenylalanine, tryptophan, methionine, threonine, and valine. Arginine and histidine can be synthesized but can become essential during times of intense anabolic states such as infancy, growth spurts, and recovery from infection.

Answer A is incorrect. The essential fatty acids are linoleic and linolenic acid. They are ubiquitous in natural diets.

Answer C is incorrect. Both ketogenic amino acids are essential and begin with the letter "L" (leucine and lysine).

Answer D is incorrect. The body cannot synthesize the micronutrient folic acid, but symbiotic bacteria can synthesize folic acid from the precursor p-aminobenzoic acid. This is inhibited by sulfa antibiotics.

Answer E is incorrect. The body cannot synthesize vitamins (an exception is a limited synthesis of niacin from tryptophan metabolism); however, microflora in the gut synthesize vitamin K for human use.

34. **The correct answer is D.** This question describes the most common symptoms of multiple myeloma. The increased total protein could be further studied by ordering a serum protein electrophoresis, which would show increased gamma-globulin fraction. Multiple myeloma is a neoplastic proliferation of plasma cells, which produce immunoglobulins. The most common molecule that is produced by the plasma cells is IgG.

Answer A is incorrect. The inability to clear chylomicron molecules from the blood is the primary pathologic process in type I family dyslipidemias. However, these typically present at a young age with increased lipids, not increased total protein.

Answer B is incorrect. The production of albumin typically is normal in multiple myeloma.

Answer C is incorrect. There can be increased clotting factors and acute-phase reactants in a variety of conditions, but this is not the main cause of increased total protein in multiple myeloma.

Answer E is incorrect. IgM molecules are produced in Waldenström's macroglobulinemia, a condition related to multiple myeloma. Waldenström's typically presents with hyperviscosity syndrome, adenopathy, and hepatosplenomegaly. Hypercalcemia, lytic lesions, and renal insufficiency are much less common in this condition.

35. **The correct answer is E.** *Sporothrix schenckii* is the cause of sporotrichosis. When *S. schenckii* is introduced into the skin, usually by a thorn prick, it causes a local pustule or ulcer with nodules along draining lymphatics (ascending lymphangitis). *S. schenckii* is a dimorphic fungus that has cigar-shaped budding yeast visible in pus. Itraconazole or potassium iodide is used for the treatment of *S. schenckii* infection.

Answer A is incorrect. Blastomycosis can present with flulike symptoms, fevers, chills, productive cough, myalgia, arthralgia, and pleuritic chest pain. Some patients will fail to recover from an acute infection and progress to develop chronic pulmonary infection or widespread disseminated infection. Fluconazole or ketoconazole is used for the treatment of local blastomycosis infections, and amphotericin B is used for the treatment of systemic infections.

Answer B is incorrect. Coccidioidomycosis is the second most common fungal infection encountered in the United States. About 60% of these infections cause no symptoms, and in the remaining 40% of cases, the symptoms can range from mild to severe. Severe forms of the infection can present with blood-tinged sputum, loss of appetite, weight loss, a painful red rash on the legs, and change in mental status.

Answer C is incorrect. *Malassezia furfur* infection is the cause of tinea versicolor. Symptoms of this infection include hypopigmented skin lesions that occur in hot and humid conditions. *M. furfur* is treated with topical miconazole or selenium sulfide (Selsun).

Answer D is incorrect. *Pneumocystis jiroveci* (formerly *carinii*), like most fungal infections, does not present with any symptoms in the immunocompetent host. In children or patients afflicted with AIDS, cancer, or inherited immune deficiencies, *P. jiroveci* can present with pneumonia (PCP). Symptoms begin suddenly in this form of *Pneumocystis* pneumonia. The patient develops a fever and begins to cough and breathe abnormally fast. Often the patient's lips, fingernails, and skin turn blue or gray because the patient has difficulty drawing in air. On chest x-ray, the diffuse interstitial pneumonia gives a ground-glass appearance. PCP infection is treated with trimethoprim-sulfamethoxazole.

36. The correct answer is B. Leukocyte adhesion deficiency syndrome is caused by a defect in the LFA-1 adhesion protein on the surface of neutrophils. The disease usually presents with marked leukocytosis and localized bacterial infections that are difficult to detect until they have progressed to an extensive life-threatening level. Since neutrophils are unable to adhere to the endothelium and transmigrate into tissues, infections in patients with leukocyte adhesion deficiency syndrome act similarly to those observed in neutropenic patients.

Answer A is incorrect. Chronic granulomatous disease presents with an increased susceptibility to opportunistic bacterial infections. It results from defective neutrophil phagocytosis due to a lack of NADPH oxidase (or similar enzyme) activity. A negative nitroblue tetrazolium dye reduction test confirms the diagnosis of chronic granulomatous disease.

Answer C is incorrect. Selective immunoglobulin deficiency is a deficit in a specific class of immunoglobulins. IgA deficiency is the most common of these diseases. Since IgA is the most prominent immunoglobulin found in mucous membranes, patients suffering from a deficiency of it often present with sinus and lung infections.

Answer D is incorrect. Severe combined immunodeficiency is a defect in early stem cell differentiation that can have many causes. The typical presentation of this disease includes recurrent bacterial, viral, protozoal, and fungal infections.

Answer E is incorrect. Wiskott-Aldrich syndrome is an X-linked defect associated with elevated IgA levels, elevated IgE levels, normal IgG levels, and low IgM levels. It involves a defect in the ability to mount an IgM response to bacteria. Recurrent pyogenic infections, eczema, and thrombocytopenia are the typical triad of symptoms in this disease.

37. The correct answer is E. Mifepristone is a progestin antagonist with partial agonist activity. Progesterone is necessary to maintain a pregnancy, so mifepristone's interference with this hormone causes abortion of the fetus. Prostaglandin E_1 increases the efficacy of mifepristone by acting directly on the myometrium to induce contractions.

Answer A is incorrect. Clomiphene is an antiestrogen that is used to treat ovulatory dysfunction in women. It is a drug used for infertility, not pregnancy termination.

Answer B is incorrect. Diethylstilbestrol (DES) is a synthetic compound with estrogen-like activity that is used to treat primary hypogonadism. Clear cell cervical adenocarcinoma has been linked to DES use in patients' mothers during pregnancy.

Answer C is incorrect. Ethinyl estradiol is a synthetic estrogen analog that is used in combination oral contraceptives. The estrogen component of the combination pill suppresses ovulation using a constant low dose of estrogen for 21 days. High doses of ethinyl estradiol plus a progesterone such as norgestrel can be used for postcoital contraception, but not in combination with mifepristone.

Answer D is incorrect. Mifepristone is a progestin antagonist. The addition of exogenous progesterone would decrease its efficacy, not increase it.

38. The correct answer is C. Confidentiality must be maintained in most circumstances, but harm to other persons or patients themselves warrants breach of confidentiality. The information presented in this question is based on *Tarasoff vs. Regents of the University of California* (1976). This landmark case involved a situation as described in this question. A student's therapist notified the police verbally and in writing. The police questioned the student and found him to be harmless. Two months later, the victim (Tarasoff) was murdered. In a rehearing in the Supreme Court, they ruled that "confidentiality ends with public peril" and that third parties must be informed.

Answer A is incorrect. Notifying another physician is never necessary.

Answer B is incorrect. Notifying another physician is never necessary, regardless of their relationship with the potential perpetrator.

Answer D is incorrect. The physician must notify the potential victim.

Answer E is incorrect. This choice is perhaps the most seductive but is also the most frankly inappropriate. A physician has a legal obligation to protect the public from "peril" according to the Supreme Court of the United States, regardless of the breach of confidentiality required to do so.

Answer F is incorrect. The physician must also notify law enforcement officials.

39. **The correct answer is C.** Curve C represents estrogen. PCOS, or Stein-Leventhal syndrome, manifests with amenorrhea, infertility, obesity, and hirsutism due to increased peripheral estrogen production from elevated androgen levels. The consistently elevated estrogen levels suppress the luteinizing hormone (LH) surge that drives ovulation, corpus luteum formation, and endometrial proliferation. Menstruation occurs when estrogen and progesterone levels decrease due to the disintegration of the corpus luteum. Without the normal hormonal cycle, menstruation does not occur.

Answer A is incorrect. Curve A represents luteinizing hormone (LH). The LH surge, released by the anterior pituitary and normally driven by the gradual increase of estrogen secondary to follicular growth, triggers ovulation around day 14. Due to the consistently elevated levels of peripheral estrogen in PCOS, the LH surge is suppressed and ovulation does not occur, resulting in oligomenorrhea or amenorrhea. PCOS is not characterized by peripheral production of LH.

Answer B is incorrect. Curve B represents follicle-stimulating hormone (FSH). FSH and luteinizing hormone are released by the anterior pituitary and are normally suppressed by high estrogen and progesterone levels. PCOS is not characterized by peripheral production of FSH.

Answer D is incorrect. Curve D represents progesterone. Progesterone is released by the corpus luteum after normal ovulation. It helps prepare the endometrium for implantation and pregnancy. A decline in progesterone and estrogen levels results in menstruation. PCOS is not characterized by peripheral production of progesterone.

40. **The correct answer is A.** This is a deletion mutation. Bases 7–9 of the normal gene are missing from the mutant gene. Because three nucleotides are missing, there is no change in the reading frame.

Answer B is incorrect. A frameshift mutation is an insertion or deletion of nucleotides that results in a misreading of all codons downstream. Deletions or insertions in multiples of three do not cause a shift in the reading frame.

Answer C is incorrect. An insertion mutation is an addition of one or more nucleotides to the DNA.

Answer D is incorrect. A missense mutation occurs when a point mutation causes one amino acid in a protein to be replaced by a different amino acid.

Answer E is incorrect. A nonsense mutation occurs when a point mutation results in an early stop codon. This type of mutation causes a truncated protein.

Answer F is incorrect. A point mutation is the change of a single base in the DNA sequence.

Answer G is incorrect. A silent mutation occurs when a point mutation does not change the amino acid sequence of the protein. The point mutation is often in the third position of the codon.

41. **The correct answer is C.** This experimental drug is exerting its effects by acting on microtubules. Mebendazole also acts on microtubules. Other drugs that exert their effects on microtubules include paclitaxel and vincristine.

Answer A is incorrect. Cocaine is a catecholamine reuptake inhibitor. Inhibition of catecholamine reuptake proteins results in potentiation of the response to sympathetic stimulation of innervated organs and to infused catecholamine.

Answer B is incorrect. Digoxin is an Na^+-K^+-ATPase inhibitor. The Na^+-K^+-ATPase pump in cells plays a key role in creating the electrochemical gradient that is needed in order for pumps on the cell surface to work correctly. Na^+-K^+-ATPase pumps are located throughout the body. Digoxin is primarily used in the treatment of congestive heart failure.

Answer D is incorrect. Neostigmine is a reversible acetylcholinesterase inhibitor. It is primarily used in the treatment of myasthenia gravis.

Answer E is incorrect. Procainamide is a class Ia sodium channel blocker. Procainamide decreases myocardial excitability and conduction velocity and may depress myocardial contractility by increasing the electrical stimulation threshold of ventricles and the His-Purkinje system as well as through direct cardiac effects.

42. **The correct answer is B.** Dominant negative mutation is a mutation in which the mutant product interferes with the function of the normal gene product. This is different from a condition in which the mutant product is just nonfunctional (that would be haploinsufficiency). Osteogenesis imperfecta exhibits dominant negative effects.

Answer A is incorrect. Anticipation is the term used when a disease worsens or the age of onset of the disease is earlier in successive generations. Huntington's disease, like all trinucleotide repeat diseases, shows anticipation.

Answer C is incorrect. Incomplete penetrance indicates that not all individuals with a mutant genotype exhibit the mutant phenotype. Treacher Collins syndrome is an example of a disease with incomplete penetrance.

Answer D is incorrect. Mosaicism occurs when cells in the body have a different genetic makeup. Patients with Turner's syndrome can have a mosaic genotype, with some cells having 45,XO and some 46,XX.

Answer E is incorrect. Pleiotropy is a term used when one gene has more than one effect on a person's phenotype.

43. **The correct answer is C.** The cause of this patient's findings is an aneurysm of the right common iliac artery. The common iliac arteries lie posterior and medial to the ureters. Common iliac artery aneurysms are uncommon but can present with unilateral hydronephrosis if the ureters are compressed by the growing aneurysm. The patient's age and sex, his long history of hypertension and hyperlipidemia, and his constant dull pain suggest an aneurysm as the etiology.

Answer A is incorrect. The abdominal aorta is medial but not in close proximity to the ureters. An abdominal aortic aneurysm could not compress either of the ureters.

Answer B is incorrect. The clinical presentation does not suggest a ureteral or bladder calculus. Typical symptoms would include sharp, intermittent, excruciating pain in the lower back, abdomen, or testicular region. Fever, nausea, vomiting, and hematuria are usually present as well.

Answer D is incorrect. The clinical presentation does not suggest a ureteral or bladder calculus. Typical symptoms would include sharp, intermittent, excruciating pain in the lower back, abdomen, or testicular region. Fever, nausea, vomiting, and hematuria also are usually present.

Answer E is incorrect. Urinary tract infections can lead to the development of calculi, but due to the lack of fever and hematuria, it is highly unlikely that this is the etiology responsible for this presentation.

44. **The correct answer is D.** Heparin contamination is the most common cause of spuriously elevated activated partial thromboplastin time (aPTT) levels. Intravenous lines, not running fluids, are flushed with heparin to prevent coagulation and obstruction of the line (i.e., keeping the line open). When drawing blood from a heparinized line, the first 5 cc should

be discarded before collecting blood for laboratory testing.

Answer A is incorrect. Heparin would prolong, not shorten, the activated partial thromboplastin time.

Answer B is incorrect. The International Normalized Ratio (INR) is a standardized measure derived from the prothrombin time (PT), adjusted for the particular assay type and the machine used to measure the PT. INR is increased if PT is increased.

Answer C is incorrect. Prothrombin time (PT) would not decrease with heparin and warfarin treatment. If already prolonged, vitamin K treatment would lower the PT.

Answer E is incorrect. The International Normalized Ratio (INR) is a standardized measure derived from the prothrombin time (PT), adjusted for the particular assay type and the machine used to measure the PT. INR is decreased if PT is decreased.

Answer F is incorrect. Warfarin would increase the prothrombin time.

45. **The correct answer is B.** Cluster B personality disorders include antisocial, borderline, histrionic, and narcissistic, and are characterized as dramatic or wild behavior. Patients with these types of personality disorders are characterized by persistent violation of social norms, impulsivity, emotionality, grandiosity, and "acting out." There is a genetic association with mood disorders. Patients with borderline personality disorder are impulsive, unpredictable, and labile and have fluctuations in intense moods.

Answer A is incorrect. Patients with avoidant personality disorder are sensitive to rejection, socially inhibited, and timid with overwhelming feelings of inadequacy.

Answer C is incorrect. Patients with dependent personality disorder are submissive and clinging, have low self-confidence, and have an excessive need of nurturance.

Answer D is incorrect. Patients with narcissistic personality disorder are grandiose and have a sense of entitlement. They frequently demand the 'best' of everything, including physicians and health care.

Answer E is incorrect. Patients with schizoid personality disorder exhibit voluntary social withdrawal and have limited emotional expressions.

Answer F is incorrect. Patients with schizotypal personality disorder demonstrate interpersonal awkwardness, odd thought patterns, and an odd appearance.

46. **The correct answer is B.** This patient is experiencing cardiogenic shock secondary to acute mitral regurgitation, presumably due to mitral valve leaflet rupture. At higher doses, dopamine exerts α-adrenergic effects in addition to its β_1 effects; it will thus cause positive inotropy with vasoconstriction, which would be supportive in this hypotensive patient with pump failure.

Answer A is incorrect. Amrinone, a phosphodiesterase inhibitor, causes an increase in cardiac inotropy but also causes vasodilation. Thus, its use would be inappropriate in this hypotensive patient.

Answer C is incorrect. Epinephrine is a potent α and β agonist and thus acts as a cardiac inotrope and chronotrope. It is also a vasoconstrictor that will increase blood flow to skeletal muscle and visceral organs from a combination of different receptors. However, the use of epinephrine can also induce cardiac arrhythmias, and this is not a first-line agent for the treatment of cardiogenic shock.

Answer D is incorrect. Isoproterenol is a potent β_1 agonist that increases the heart's chronotropy and inotropy. However, it is also a β_2 agonist and thus has vasodilatory effects that would be contraindicated in this hypotensive patient.

Answer E is incorrect. Because phenylephrine is a pure α agonist, it will cause vasoconstriction without any effect on the heart. Because this patient has pump failure, this drug would not be as effective as dopamine.

47. The correct answer is C. *Clostridium perfringens* can infect necrotic tissues and produce toxins. Hemolysis results because the organism destroys erythrocytes. Crepitation is present as a result of degenerative enzymes producing gas in the tissues.

Answer A is incorrect. The infection caused by *Actinomyces israelii* typically presents as a chronic, slowly progressing mass that eventually evolves into a draining sinus tract.

Answer B is incorrect. *Bacillus anthracis* can cause cutaneous anthrax, which is characterized by a painless ulcer with a black scab.

Answer D is incorrect. *Clostridium tetani* causes tetanus, which presents with severe muscle spasms. It is not associated with cellulitis.

Answer E is incorrect. *Sporothrix schenckii* is a fungus typically seen after a prick with a thorn, which accounts for the nickname, rose gardener's disease.

48. The correct answer is B. The classic histologic finding in a granulosa cell tumor of the ovary is the presence of Call-Exner bodies, which are follicles filled with eosinophilic secretions. The clinical presentation also supports this diagnosis. Granulose cell tumors are estrogen-secreting tumors. This increase in estrogen stimulates the endometrium to undergo hyperplasia with subsequent sloughing off, resulting in the vaginal bleeding with which this patient presents.

Answer A is incorrect. An endometrioid tumor, as the name suggests, histologically resembles endometrium. Call-Exner bodies would not be present, nor would vaginal bleeding.

Answer C is incorrect. Krukenberg's tumors are tumors that are metastatic to the ovaries from the gastrointestinal system, most commonly the stomach. The classic histologic finding is a mucin-secreting signet-cell ring, not a Call-Exner body.

Answer D is incorrect. Call-Exner bodies would not be found in a serous cystadenocarci-noma. Instead, one would expect to see a tumor lined with epithelium resembling that of the fallopian tube. These types of tumors are very common and account for 50% of ovarian carcinomas. They do not, however, classically present with vaginal bleeding.

Answer E is incorrect. A teratoma contains tissue derived from at least two different embryonic layers. For example, thyroid tissue, neural tissue, muscle tissue, bone, and even teeth may be present. The immature teratomas are more aggressive and are always malignant, while the mature teratomas are more well differentiated and benign. One would not expect to see Call-Exner bodies or vaginal bleeding.

49. The correct answer is E. Spironolactone is a potassium-sparing diuretic that acts as an antagonist at the aldosterone receptor. The patient's bilateral chest pain and tissue growth can be attributed to spironolactone-induced gynecomastia. Spironolactone competitively inhibits testosterone and progesterone. In men, this can result in gynecomastia; in women, it can result in dysmenorrhea. Other potassium-sparing diuretics without these adverse effects include amiloride and triamterene.

Answer A is incorrect. Enalapril is an angiotensin-converting enzyme (ACE) inhibitor associated with cough, angioedema, hyperkalemia, and other adverse effects; gynecomastia is not an adverse event associated with ACE inhibitors.

Answer B is incorrect. Hydralazine is associated with tachycardia, fluid retention, and a lupuslike syndrome but not gynecomastia.

Answer C is incorrect. Carvedilol is a β-blocker that can exacerbate asthma and result in adverse effects such as sedation and sleep alterations.

Answer D is incorrect. Nitroglycerin is associated with tachycardia, hypotension, and headache but not gynecomastia.

50. The correct answer is B. A single umbilical artery is a nonspecific finding but suggests an underlying cardiovascular abnormality. Normally, two umbilical arteries are present to carry deoxygenated blood out of the fetal circulation back to the mother.

Answer A is incorrect. Having a single allantoic duct is normal.

Answer C is incorrect. Having a single umbilical vein is normal. This vessel carries oxygenated blood from the maternal circulation to the fetus.

Answer D is incorrect. Having two umbilical arteries is normal.

Answer E is incorrect. Having two umbilical veins is abnormal but is extremely rare and is not known to be associated with any condition requiring consultation by a cardiologist.

FULL-LENGTH EXAM

Test Block 7

Common Laboratory Values

* = Included in the Biochemical Profile (SMA-12)

Blood, Plasma, Serum	Reference Range	SI Reference Intervals
* Alanine aminotransferase (ALT, GPT at 30°C)	8–20 U/L	8–20 U/L
Amylase, serum	25–125 U/L	25–125 U/L
* Aspartate aminotransferase (AST, GOT at 30°C)	8–20 U/L	8–20 U/L
Bilirubin, serum (adult)		
Total // Direct	0.1–1.0 mg/dL // 0.0–0.3 mg/dL	2–17 μmol/L // 0–5 μmol/L
* Calcium, serum (Total)	8.4–10.2 mg/dL	2.1–2.8 mmol/L
* Cholesterol, serum	140–250 mg/dL	3.6–6.5 mmol/L
* Creatinine, serum (Total)	0.6–1.2 mg/dL	53–106 μmol/L
Electrolytes, serum		
Sodium	135–147 mEq/L	135–147 mmol/L
Chloride	95–105 mEq/L	95–105 mmol/L
* Potassium	3.5–5.0 mEq/L	3.5–5.0 mmol/L
Bicarbonate	22–28 mEq/L	22–28 mmol/L
Gases, arterial blood (room air)		
P_{O_2}	75–105 mmHg	10.0–14.0 kPa
P_{CO_2}	33–44 mmHg	4.4–5.9 kPa
pH	7.35–7.45	[H+] 36–44 nmol/L
* Glucose, serum	Fasting: 70–110 mg/dL	3.8–6.1 mmol/L
	2-h postprandial: < 120 mg/dL	< 6.6 mmol/L
Growth hormone - arginine stimulation	Fasting: < 5 ng/mL	< 5 μg/L
	provocative stimuli: > 7 ng/mL	> 7 μg/L
Osmolality, serum	275–295 mOsm/kg	275–295 mOsm/kg
* Phosphatase (alkaline), serum (p-NPP at 30°C)	20–70 U/L	20–70 U/L
* Phosphorus (inorganic), serum	3.0–4.5 mg/dL	1.0–1.5 mmol/L
* Proteins, serum		
Total (recumbent)	6.0–7.8 g/dL	60–78 g/L
Albumin	3.5–5.5 g/dL	35–55 g/L
Globulins	2.3–3.5 g/dL	23–35 g/L
* Urea nitrogen, serum (BUN)	7–18 mg/dL	1.2–3.0 mmol urea/L
* Uric acid, serum	3.0–8.2 mg/dL	0.18–0.48 mmol/L
Cerebrospinal Fluid		
Glucose	40–70 mg/dL	2.2–3.9 mmol/L
Hematologic		
Erythrocyte count	Male: 4.3–5.9 million/mm³	4.3–5.9 × 10¹²/L
	Female: 3.5–5.5 million/mm³	3.5–5.5 × 10¹²/L
Hematocrit	Male: 41–53%	0.41–0.53
	Female: 36–46%	0.36–0.46
Hemoglobin, blood	Male: 13.5–17.5 g/dL	2.09–2.71 mmol/L
	Female: 12.0–16.0 g/dL	1.86–2.48 mmol/L
Hemoglobin, plasma	1–4 mg/dL	0.16–0.62 μmol/L
Leukocyte count and differential		
Leukocyte count	4500–11,000/mm³	4.5–11.0 × 10⁹/L
Segmented neutrophils	54–62%	0.54–0.62
Band forms	3–5%	0.03–0.05
Eosinophils	1–3%	0.01–0.03
Basophils	0–0.75%	0–0.0075
Lymphocytes	25–33%	0.25–0.33
Monocytes	3–7%	0.03–0.07
Mean corpuscular hemoglobin	25.4–34.6 pg/cell	0.39–0.54 fmol/cell
Platelet count	150,000–400,000/mm³	150–400 × 10⁹/L
Prothrombin time	11–15 seconds	11–15 seconds
Reticulocyte count	0.5–1.5% of red cells	0.005–0.015
Sedimentation rate, erythrocyte	Male: 0–15 mm/h	0–15 mm/h
(Westergren)	Female: 0–20 mm/h	0–20 mm/h
Proteins, total	< 150 mg/24 h	< 0.15 g/24 h

ABOUT THE SENIOR EDITORS

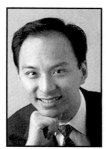
Tao Le, MD, MHS

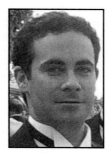
Joshua Klein, MD, PhD

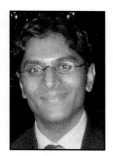
Anil Shivaram, MD

Tao Le, MD, MHS

Tao has been having fun with medical education for the past 15 years. As senior editor, he led the expansion of *First Aid* into a global educational series. In addition, he is the founder and editor-in-chief of the *USMLERx* online test bank series as well as a co-founder of the *Underground Clinical Vignettes* series. As a medical student, he was editor-in-chief of the University of California, San Francisco *Synapse,* a university newspaper with a weekly circulation of 9000. Tao earned his medical degree from the University of California, San Francisco in 1996 and completed his residency training in internal medicine at Yale University and fellowship training at Johns Hopkins University in allergy and immunology. In addition, he completed an MHS at the Johns Hopkins Bloomberg School of Public Health. At Yale, he was a regular guest lecturer on the USMLE review courses and an adviser to the Yale University School of Medicine curriculum committee. He is currently chief of allergy and immunology in the Department of Medicine at the University of Louisville.

Joshua Klein, MD, PhD

Josh is a graduate of the Medical Scientist Training Program at Yale University School of Medicine. He is originally from Roslyn, New York, and attended the University of Pennsylvania, where he studied biology and music theory. He completed his PhD dissertation in Dr. Stephen Waxman's neurology lab, where he studied activity-dependent modulation of neuronal sodium channel expression. He has authored more than ten journal articles based on his work, and has presented at numerous research conferences. His current research interests are focused on the pathogenesis and neurobiology of epilepsy. Last year, he was selected as an International Student Delegate of the Academy of Achievement. Following a year of internal medicine at Beth Israel Deaconess Medical Center, he is now a resident in neurology at Massachusetts General Hospital and Brigham and Women's Hospital. Josh has been an author and editor on multiple *First Aid* projects over the past six years. He can be contacted at joshua.p.klein@aya.yale.edu.

Anil Shivaram, MD

Anil is currently a second-year resident in ophthalmology at Boston Medical Center. He was born and raised in Chicago, Illinois, and attended college at Columbia University, where he majored in Sanskrit. After undergraduate, he went on to pursue graduate studies at Oxford University and then completed a fellowship in medical ethics at the American Medical Association. During medical school at Yale, his thesis research focused on the migration of retinal microglia in inherited retinal degenerative disorders. When he is not in pursuit of things optical, he spends time pampering his fiancée Lisa, who is finishing her final year of pediatrics residency. This is Anil's sixth year working on the *First Aid* series. He can be reached via e-mail at shivaram@aya.yale.edu.

ABOUT THE EDITORS

Paul Dieffenbach

Paul is a third-year medical student at Harvard University, where he is currently undertaking a one-year Howard Hughes Medical Institution Fellowship to study a *Drosophila* model of neurodegeneration. He earned his Bachelor of Arts degree in biochemical sciences from Harvard College in 2003 with thesis work on the protein-protein interactions of the D2 dopamine receptor. His current medical interests include emergency medicine, cardiology, and intensive care, but are subject to change at a moment's notice. During his increasingly small amounts of free time, he enjoys teaching, traveling, and the great outdoors.

Andrew H. Huang, MD

Drew is a resident in the department of surgery at the University of California-Davis. He earned his medical degree at Jefferson Medical College of Thomas Jefferson University in Philadelphia. His interests include international medical missions and the study of early New Testament Christology. During his more leisurely times, Drew enjoys reading contemporary medical memoirs, hiking, swimming, and playing his guitar.

Michael L. Rinke

Michael is a fourth-year medical student at Johns Hopkins School of Medicine interested in pediatrics and patient safety research. He completed a Bachelor of Arts degree in history from Cornell University and a post-baccalaureate premedical program at Columbia University. Michael took a year off from medical school to complete a research fellowship in patient safety and quality improvement. His interests include the New York Giants, hiking, being outdoors, and watching his dog catch a Frisbee. Michael is completely devoted to and owes everything to his parents Nomi and Ronald, his sisters Laurie and Michelle, his wonderful wife Carol, and his amazing son Coby.

Sarah Schellhorn, MD

Sarah is a resident at Beth Israel Deaconess Medical Center. She graduated in May 2006 from Weill Medical College of Cornell University. She graduated magna cum laude from Harvard University in 2000 with a Bachelor of Arts degree in biochemical sciences. In her spare time, you can find her knitting, playing poker, or rooting for her beloved Boston Red Sox—sometimes all at the same time.

Lakshmi Sonbuchner

Lakshmi is a fifth-year student in the Tri-Institutional MD/PhD program at Weill Medical College of Cornell University in New York City. Currently, she is studying transcriptional regulation in the malaria parasite *Plasmodium falciparum*. Lakshmi plans to pursue a career in teaching and medical practice. In her free time, Lakshmi takes lessons in a South Indian classical dance form called Bharatanatyam and enjoys making jewelry with semiprecious gems. She is a seasoned traveler who loves taking trips abroad with her husband whenever their schedules and finances permit.

Flora Waples-Trefil, MD

Flora is currently an intern in the University of Chicago emergency medicine program. She began working on *First Aid* and *USMLERx.com* projects while she was a second-year medical student at Weill Medical College of Cornell University. Over the past two years she has had the opportunity to be a part of several different projects for both Step 1 and Step 2 as an author, editor, and now as a senior editor. During the generous amount of free time that emergency medicine residents enjoy, Flora runs a small construction/rehab business for distressed real estate, dives, snowboards, works on the family ranch in Montana, and generally attempts to live up to the ER physician ideal of being a shiftless dilettante.

Jeffrey Weinstein, MD

Jeff is a resident at Albert Einstein Medical Center in New York City. He is a graduate of Jefferson Medical College of Thomas Jefferson University. He has many interests, including medical education, journalism, and writing.

ABOUT THE AUTHORS

Nicholas Daniel Andersen

Nicholas graduated summa cum laude from the University of Utah and currently attends Harvard Medical School. He recently completed a Howard Hughes Medical Institute Research Training Fellowship with the Department of Vascular Surgery at Beth Israel Deaconess Medical Center. For postgraduate education he will seek entry into a general surgery residency program.

Alexander Arriaga

Alex is currently a medical student at Weill Medical College of Cornell University applying for a residency position in general surgery. He completed his undergraduate education at Columbia University with a major in mathematics. His interests include surgery, digital media editing, medical animation, and medical education. He can be contacted at ala2006@med.cornell.edu.

Anna Awdankiewicz, MD

Anna grew up in Warsaw, Poland, and came to the United States at the age of 18. She completed her undergraduate education at the State University of New York at Stony Brook, where she earned a Bachelor of Science degree in biochemistry. In 2006 she graduated from Weill Medical College of Cornell University. She is currently a first-year resident at Vanderbilt Medical Center, where she pursues interests in pulmonary and critical care medicine.

Ali Behbahani, BSE

Ali is currently an MD/MBA candidate at the University of Pennsylvania in Philadelphia. He graduated summa cum laude from Duke University and received a Bachelor of Science degree in biomedical engineering and electrical engineering and a Bachelor of Arts degree in chemistry. Prior to starting medical school, Ali was an investment banker at Lehman Brothers and a venture capitalist at Morgan Stanley Venture Partners. His interests include virology, orthopedic research, and emerging medical technologies.

David T. Braun, MBA

David is currently a medical student at Temple University School of Medicine in Philadelphia. He graduated cum laude with a dual Bachelor of Arts degree in cell and molecular biology and economics from Washington and Jefferson College in Washington, Pennsylvania. As an undergraduate, David received a Howard Hughes Medical Institute grant for molecular biology research and was elected into the Phi Sigma and Phi Beta Kappa honor societies. Upon graduation, David completed a year of orthopedic research at the University of Pennsylvania and earned his Master of Business Administration degree in health care management from the Fox School of Business at Temple University. In his free time, David enjoys playing and listening to music as well as watching and competing in athletic events. His academic interests include surgical care, sports medicine, and health care economics and management.

David M. Brown, MD
Dave is a resident in the department of otolaryngology at the University of Chicago. He received his medical degree from Thomas Jefferson Medical College in Philadelphia. He completed his undergraduate education at the University of Virginia in Charlottesville followed by an amazing postgrad year in Breckenridge, Colorado. His interests include fly-fishing, skiing, and music.

Whitney K. Bryant
Whitney is currently a medical student at the Columbia University College of Physicians and Surgeons. After an 18-year stint in the Midwest, she completed her Bachelor of Arts degree in English literature at Harvard College. She received her Master of Public Health degree in the history and ethics of public health and medicine from Columbia's Mailman School of Public Health. After completing her medical degree, she intends to learn to surf.

Daniel Burdick
Dan is currently a student at Johns Hopkins University School of Medicine in Baltimore. He completed his undergraduate education at Princeton University, receiving a Bachelor's degree in economics. He worked in research at the Federal Reserve Bank of New York before completing a postbaccalaureate premedical program at Bryn Mawr College in Bryn Mawr, Pennsylvania. His interests include dementias and neurodegeneration, as well as baseball, college hockey, and choral arts. As always, he appreciates his family's continued support.

Vicki Kai Chan, MD
Vicki is currently a resident at the Jules Stein Eye Institute of the University of California–Los Angeles. She graduated from Johns Hopkins University School of Medicine in May 2006. She graduated summa cum laude from the University of Southern California, studying psychobiology and classics. She is extremely excited to return home for her ophthalmology residency. Vicki loves spending time with her friends and family, shopping, trying out new restaurants and cuisines, and playing tennis, basketball, and volleyball.

Pooja P. Chandra
Pooja grew up in New Delhi, India, and came to the United States to attend Swarthmore College, where she earned a Bachelor of Arts degree in biochemistry. She is currently a fourth-year medical student at Weill Medical College of Cornell University and will be applying to pediatric residency programs next year.

Stephen Chang, MD
Stephen is currently an intern at York Hospital in York, Pennsylvania. He graduated from Johns Hopkins University School of Medicine in May 2006 and will be starting his residency in diagnostic radiology next year at Columbia University Medical Center. Outside of medicine, his interests include reading about cars and rooting for the Redskins.

Kevin Cheung, MD
Originally from Purchase, New York, Kevin studied biochemical sciences at Harvard University, graduating magna cum laude. Following college, he attended Weill Medical College of Cornell University in New York City, where he graduated with honors in research. A member of the Alpha Omega Alpha honor society and an alumnus of the Howard Hughes Medical Institute Research Training Fellowship Program, Kevin is now starting his first year of internal medicine residency at Brigham and Women's Hospital. In his free time, he enjoys exploring Boston, catching up with friends, and playing a song or two on his Taylor guitar.

Felicia Che-Shuen Chow
Felicia is a fourth-year medical student at Johns Hopkins University School of Medicine. She recently returned from a Fogarty International Center/Ellison Medical Foundation Fellowship in Lima, Peru, where she conducted clinical research in neurological infectious diseases. She completed her undergraduate education at Columbia University in New York City, followed by two years as a middle school math and science teacher in Harlem with Teach for America.

Julia Ting Chu
Julia is currently a medical student in the Harvard-MIT Health Sciences and Technology program at Harvard Medical School. She completed her undergraduate studies at the University of California–Los Angeles with a major in biochemistry and a minor in education. She received research support from the Howard Hughes Medical Institute, the American Medical Association, and the American Society of Hematology to investigate how the early adhesive interactions between circulating hematopoietic cells and the vascular environment may establish atherosclerotic plaques. Her interests include medical education, health care for the underserved, fine arts, dancing, snowboarding, and culinary adventures. As always, she is able to pursue and enjoy her passions because of her family and friends and is very grateful for their unconditional love and support.

Christina E. Clark
Christina is currently attending medical school at Drexel University College of Medicine in Philadelphia. A native of Washington, D.C., she attended high school at Stone Ridge School of the Sacred Heart in Bethesda, Maryland, and was accepted into college before graduation. Christina completed her undergraduate education in two years at George Washington University in Washington, D.C., with a Bachelor of Science degree in biology. She is interested in increasing access to health care for underserved populations through the use of her Spanish language skills and understanding of different cultures. She has received multiple educational grants and awards and looks forward to a rewarding career in psychiatry.

Sarah K. Collins
Sarah is currently a fourth-year medical student at Weill Medical College of Cornell University. She completed her undergraduate education at Cornell, graduating with a Bachelor of Science degree in biology and society. She is planning to pursue a career in pediatrics.

Lara Devgan
Lara is an MD/MPH student at Johns Hopkins University School of Medicine, currently participating in the NIH Roadmap Predoctoral Clinical Research Training Program. She completed her undergraduate education at Yale University. Her interests include surgery and writing.

Prabhjot Singh Dhadialla
Jot is in his first year of graduate school at Rockefeller University after completing two years at Weill Medical College of Cornell University as part of the Tri-Institutional MD/PhD program. He completed undergraduate degrees in history and biology at the University of Rochester. He is a 2005 Paul and Daisy Soros Fellow, and his interests include running and rigorously protecting leisure time.

Derek J. Donegan, MD
Derek is a resident in the department of orthopedic surgery at the University of Pennsylvania. He earned his medical degree from Thomas Jefferson Medical College in Philadelphia, and completed his undergraduate education at Ithaca College in Ithaca, New York. Derek's interests include scuba diving, working out, and traveling.

John Eifler
John is a fourth-year medical student at Weill Medical College of Cornell University. He received his undergraduate education from the University of Kentucky, where he earned Bachelor of Science degrees in physics and mathematics. He pursued tumor immunology research at the surgery branch of the National Institutes of Health through the Howard Hughes Medical Institute Research Scholars program and is currently applying for residency in the field of urology.

Dawn M. Emick
Dawn is a graduate of Johns Hopkins School of Medicine and is currently a general surgical intern at Duke University. A native of Michigan, she completed her undergraduate degree at the University of Michigan in 1999. After college, she moved to New Orleans to teach high school as a Teach for America corps member. Her professional interests include health policy and medical education; when she's allowed to leave the hospital she enjoys hiking and boating with friends.

Victor Esenwa, MD
Victor graduated with a medical degree from Weill Medical College of Cornell University. He completed his undergraduate education at State University of New York at Stony Brook with a Bachelor of Science degree in biochemistry with research honors. He is currently working at New York Hospital Queens as a transitional-year intern. He will continue his residency training in the field of radiology at New York Presbyterian Hospital.

Robert Flavell
Rob is currently pursuing his PhD at the Rockefeller University under the guidance of Dr. Tom Muir. He completed his undergraduate degree at Wesleyan University, then joined the Cornell/Rockefeller/Sloan-Kettering Tri-Institutional MD/PhD program in New York. His interests include molecular mechanisms of disease and novel imaging techniques using nanotechnology.

Aaron M. Fletcher, MD
Originally from Washington, D.C., Aaron graduated from Temple University School of Medicine. He is currently a surgical intern and will be completing his residency training in otolaryngology at the University of Iowa Hospitals and Clinics. His hobbies include reading and exercising.

Kathleen Forcier
Kathleen is a student at Weill Medical College of Cornell University. She graduated from Brown University with a degree in human biology. Her career interests include pediatrics and women's health.

Jorge Galvez
Jorge is a 2006 graduate of the Yale University School of Medicine. He is currently completing a preliminary internship in the Yale primary care program, after which he will continue to the Yale anesthesiology residency program. He completed his undergraduate education at the University of Miami in Coral Gables, Florida.

Geoffrey Geiger
Geoffrey is currently a fourth-year medical student at the University of Pennsylvania School of Medicine. After completing a year of residency in the radiation oncology department under a National Institutes of Health grant, he is applying to programs in radiation oncology. He completed his undergraduate education at Bates College in 2001. His interests include radioimmunotherapy, photodynamic therapy, and medical education.

Pourya M. Ghazi, MD
Pourya is currently a senior fellow in laboratory medicine at the University of Washington in Seattle. He will be applying for residency in internal medicine and is planning for a career in endocrinology. Pourya earned his medical degree at Beheshti Medical School in Tehran, Iran. He has authored three books and contributed to five books in the *Underground Clinical Vignettes* series. Previous research activities include comparing serum parathyroid hormone levels in diabetic and nondiabetic patients on hemodialysis. Other interests include history, independent artistic cinema, and traveling.

Rani K. Hasan, MD
Rani is an intern in the department of medicine at the Hospital of the University of Pennsylvania. He earned his medical degree at Johns Hopkins University School of Medicine. A Florida native, he completed a Bachelor of Science degree in biochemistry and a Bachelor of Arts degree in economics at the University of Florida. He plans to pursue fellowship training in cardiology. Rani's interests include translational research in cardiovascular disease, health care economics, medical education, and international medical relief.

Emily Parker Hyle, MD
Emily is a resident in internal medicine at Massachusetts General Hospital. After completing her undergraduate education at Williams College with degrees in history and biology, she worked as a high school teacher before graduating from the University of Pennsylvania School of Medicine in 2006. Her interests include international health and medical education.

Daniel Jamieson, MD
Daniel received his Bachelor of Arts degree in psychology from Wesleyan University in 1999. He graduated from Weill Medical College of Cornell University in 2006. He is currently a resident in internal medicine at the University of Colorado in Denver, and plans to pursue a career in pulmonary and critical care medicine.

Bluma Lesch
Bluma is pursuing her PhD at Rockefeller University, studying the development of the nervous system. She earned her Bachelor of Science degree at Yale University before entering the Cornell/Rockefeller/Sloan-Kettering Tri-Institutional MD/PhD program. Her interests include embryology, genetics, and cellular differentiation; she occasionally kills time running and writing.

Ilya Leyngold, MD
After graduating from Johns Hopkins University School of Medicine, Ilya is currently a resident in ophthalmology at the Wilmer Eye Institute of Johns Hopkins University School of Medicine.

Mark Leyngold, MD
Mark is a first-year plastic surgery resident at the University of Nevada School of Medicine in Las Vegas. He was born in Moscow, Russia, and moved to the United States with his family when he was 13. After living in Jacksonville for seven years, Mark moved to Tallahassee to attend Florida State University, where he majored in biochemistry. He earned his medical degree from Florida State University College of Medicine. His interests include art, surgery, and medical education.

David M. Lieberman, MD
David recently completed his medical school training at Weill Medical College of Cornell University in New York City. He completed his undergraduate education at Stanford University, receiving a Bachelor's degree in human biology with a focus in neuroscience. He returned to Stanford as a resident in otolaryngology-head and neck surgery. Additional interests include international medicine, hiking, running, and movies.

Nicholas Mahoney, MD
Nick received his medical degree from the University of Pennsylvania School of Medicine and is currently an intern at Presbyterian Medical Center. He will be starting his residency at Scheie Eye Institute next year. His interests include surgical device design, optic nerve stimulators, and information and educational systems technology.

Matthew McCarthy
Matthew graduated from Yale University with a degree in molecular biophysics in 2002. He has since moved to Harvard University, where he is now a third-year medical student and a teaching fellow in the department of molecular and cellular biology.

Marcus A. McFerren, PhD, MD
Marcus received a Bachelor of Science degree in neurobiology in 1995 and a PhD in phytochemistry and natural products pharmacology from Cornell University in 2000. He was formerly a visiting assistant professor at the Swarthmore College Department of Biology, where he taught courses in botany, ecological biochemistry, and medicinal plant chemistry. He presently teaches courses in herbal supplement chemistry and pharmacology for the Weill Medical College of Cornell University Center for Complementary and Integrative Medicine.

Anuj Bharat Mehta
Anuj graduated magna cum laude from Columbia University with Bachelor of Arts degrees in biology and philosophy. He current attends Weill Medical College of Cornell University in New York City. He is scheduled to graduate medical school in May 2007, after which he will begin his residency in internal medicine. After postgraduate training, Anuj is considering a variety of subspecialties as well as pursuing a Master's degree in public health. In addition to practicing medicine, he hopes to be involved in issues related to health care reform and access to health care.

Amanda Mullins
Amanda is currently a fourth-year medical student at Drexel University College of Medicine. She completed her undergraduate education at Ohio State University, where she received a Bachelor of Arts degree in English and American literature. Her interests include dermatology and medical publication.

Anoma Nellore, MD
Anoma is a graduate of the University of Pennsylvania School of Medicine and is currently a resident in internal medicine at her alma mater. She is also a graduate of the University of Maryland–College Park with a double degree in biochemistry and government and politics.

Frank Ocasio, MD
Frank recently graduated from Weill Medical College of Cornell University. He received a Bachelor of Science degree in biology with a minor in chemistry, in addition to completing a Master's degree in biology with a focus in neuroscience at Seton Hall University in South Orange, New Jersey.

Anton Orlin
Anton is currently a fourth-year medical student at the University of Pennsylvania School of Medicine. He completed his undergraduate education at the University of Rochester. He is planning to pursue a career in ophthalmology.

Ben Eugene Paxton
Ben is a fourth-year student at Johns Hopkins University School of Medicine. He graduated summa cum laude from Brigham Young University with a Bachelor of Arts degree in philosophy. Ben is pursuing a career in interventional radiology. His interests include fishing, biking, Ultimate, and music. Ben's greatest accomplishment is that he can solve a Rubik's Cube in 72 seconds. He most enjoys spending time with his wife Juli and his daughter Elise.

Tonguc Pinar
Having completed a Howard Hughes Medical Institute fellowship studying DNA damage repair, Tonguc is currently a third-year student at Harvard Medical School. Prior to attending Harvard, he received his Bachelor of Science degree from Yale University in 2002 and completed a one-year research fellowship at the National Institutes of Health. His interests include traveling, hiking, and occasionally brewing beer.

Jason E. Portnof, DMD, MD
Jason is currently a resident in oral and maxillofacial surgery at New York Presbyterian Hospital/Cornell University in New York City. He completed his undergraduate education at Washington University in St. Louis, and received his doctorate in dental medicine from Nova Southeastern University in Ft. Lauderdale. His medical school training was completed at

Weill Medical College of Cornell University. His interests include the full scope of oral and maxillofacial surgery including orthognathic and maxillofacial reconstructive surgery, temporomandibular joint reconstructive surgery, oral and maxillofacial pathology, and dental implantology.

Arike Price, MD
Arike is a resident in the department of neurology at Albert Einstein College of Medicine in New York City. She earned her medical degree at Temple University in Philadelphia, and completed her undergraduate education at Brown University. Her interests include painting and reading. Arike would like to thank her supportive family and friends.

Pablo Recinos, MD
Pablo is a resident in the Department of Neurosurgery at Johns Hopkins University School of Medicine. He earned his medical degree at the Johns Hopkins University School of Medicine. A native Iowan, he graduated with Bachelor of Arts degrees in biochemistry, Spanish, and Portuguese from the University of Iowa and remains a passionate Hawkeye fan. His interests include soccer, traveling, and improving international health care and education.

Gabrielle Rizzuto
Gabrielle is currently an MD/PhD student in the Cornell/Rockefeller/Sloan-Kettering Tri-Institutional MD/PhD program. She completed her undergraduate education at Georgetown University. Her interests include immunology and pathology.

James S. Rosoff, MD
James is currently a surgical intern at New York Presbyterian Hospital and earned his medical degree at Weill Medical College of Cornell University. He completed his undergraduate education at Yale University, and then went on to serve as a Peace Corps volunteer in Benin, West Africa. He also worked as a science teacher in Boston for three years before starting medical school. His interests include ultimate Frisbee and jogging.

Cory Joshua Rubin, MD
Cory is currently a resident in the department of otolaryngology-head and neck surgery at University Hospitals/Case Medical Center in Cleveland. He earned his medical degree from Jefferson Medical College of Thomas Jefferson University in Philadelphia. He completed his undergraduate education at the University of Rochester in New York.

Jonathan Schoenfeld
A recipient of a Howard Hughes Medical Institute Training fellowship, Jonathan is a third-year medical student at Harvard Medical School, currently conducting research at the Dana-Farber Cancer Institute. He received his undergraduate degree from Yale University and then received a Master's degree from the University of Cambridge in the United Kingdom, where he was supported by a Gates Cambridge Scholarship.

Pritha Sen
Pritha is a third-year medical student at Harvard Medical School. She graduated magna cum laude from Harvard University with Bachelor of Arts degrees in biology and women's studies. After college, Pritha conducted research on the vector transmission of Chagas' disease through an Emerging Infectious Disease fellowship at the Centers for Disease Control and Prevention. Currently, as a recipient of a Howard Hughes Medical Institute Research fellowship, she is studying the importance of cytotoxic T lymphocytes in controlling HIV infection. In her free time, Pritha loves to read, dance, travel, and eat good food.

Mohummad Minhaj Siddiqui, MD
Mohummad is an intern at Massachusetts General Hospital and graduated from the Harvard-MIT Division of Health, Science, and Technology. He is performing his residency in urology with a concurrent academic interest in kidney tissue engineering research. When not at the hospital, he enjoys sleeping, with the occasional interest in skiing and kayaking.

Amandeep Singh
Amandeep is a fourth-year student in the Cornell/Rockefeller/Sloan-Kettering Tri-Institutional MD/PhD program. He is currently a Paul and Daisy Soros Fellow, pursuing his PhD in molecular genetics, focusing on obesity. Amandeep earned a Bachelor of Arts degree in biology from Cornell University in 2002. Outside of school he is a professional bhangra choreographer who has danced in music videos and concerts with world-renowned artists, and directs the annual Surat Sikh Conference.

Joanna Louise Spencer
Joanna is a fourth-year student in the Tri-Institutional MD/PhD program of Cornell/Rockefeller/Sloan-Kettering in New York City. She is pursuing her PhD in the Harold and Margaret Milliken Hatch Laboratory of Neuroendocrinology at Rockefeller University. She graduated from Yale University in 2003 with a Bachelor of Arts degree in music. Outside the lab and hospital, she appreciates the performing arts, the culinary arts, traveling, and good friends and family. Her parents are the most inspiring figures in her life.

Tessa A. Sundaram, PhD
Tessa earned dual degrees in biomedical engineering and computer science at Johns Hopkins University, where she also earned her Master's in biomedical engineering. She is currently finishing her MD degree at the University of Pennsylvania School of Medicine. Her research interests include dynamic modeling of the lungs and heart using medical image processing techniques. She is also involved in developing radiology teaching tools for medical students. Tessa intends to pursue a career in radiology after graduating in 2007.

Venée N. Tubman, MD
Venée is a resident in the pediatrics departments of Children's Hospital Boston and Boston Medical Center. She earned her medical degree at the University of Pennsylvania School of Medicine. She completed her undergraduate education at Harvard University, earning a Bachelor of Arts degree in chemistry. Venée's career interests include medical education, blood disorders, and advocacy for underserved populations. She enjoys baking, arts and craftwork, and travel.

April Troy
April is currently a fourth-year medical student at Johns Hopkins University School of Medicine. She completed her undergraduate education at the University of Scranton. During medical school, she has been very active in the Baltimore community with various community service projects and also serves on the school's Interaction Council, a group that helps students interested in community service. She has recently completed a Master's degree in public health from Johns Hopkins Bloomberg School of Public Health. She hopes to pursue a career in pediatrics.

Jenica Upshaw
Jenica earned a Bachelor of Arts degree in religion from Columbia University and is currently a medical student at Weill Medical College of Cornell University. She is interested in helping to solve the problems of the uninsured and underinsured in the United States and in pursuing holistic approaches to healing such as meditation, yoga, and energy medicine. She can be contacted at jeu2002@med.cornell.edu.

Konstantina M. Vanevski, MD
Konstantina is a native of the Republic of Macedonia, where she obtained her Medical Doctorate degree at the Faculty of Medicine, University of Ss. Cyril and Methodius, followed by a postgraduate internship and part of a residency in obstetrics and gynecology. She continued her training in the United States as a postdoctoral fellow in developmental endocrinology (NIH/NICHD) and neuroimmunology (NIH/NINDS), respectively, while remaining fully engaged in clinical research. Presently, she is pursuing her PhD in interdisciplinary neuroscience at the Uniformed Services University of the Health Sciences. Her greatest passions are medical education and mentoring, which are coupled with pursuit of her hobbies, including writing, reading, cooking, foreign languages and traveling, swimming, and competitive skiing. Konstantina dedicates this project in memory of her late beloved father, General Metodija N. Vanevski.

Marissa A. Wagner
Marissa is currently a third-year student at Harvard Medical School. She earned her undergraduate degree at Yale University and received her Master of Philosophy degree from the University of Cambridge. Her research interests are centered around parasitology, and she worked in malaria and schistosomiasis labs between college and medical school. She will be spending ten months of next year working on a malaria-filaria coinfection study in Mali and will likely pursue a residency in internal medicine. She enjoys running, swimming, trying to surf, and cooking.

Adam M. Weitzman
Adam is currently a fourth-year medical student at Weill Medical College of Cornell University in New York City. He will be applying for residency in obstetrics and gynecology and is planning for a career in reproductive endocrinology and infertility. Adam earned his undergraduate degree at Tufts University. His interests include getting into residency, feeding the seagull that sits on his ledge, and long walks on the beach.

Elizabeth Winter, MD
Elizabeth is an intern in the Department of Medicine at Mount Sinai Hospital. She earned her medical degree at Johns Hopkins University in Baltimore. She also completed her undergraduate degree at Johns Hopkins with a Bachelor of Arts degree in cognitive science. Past research interests have included neuropsychological deficits following stroke and procedures such as elective aneurysm clipping. She will be applying for a residency in the field of psychiatry.

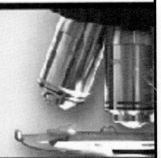